McGraw-Hill Medical Coding
An Introduction

Jean H. Jurek

MS, RHIA, CPC

Stacey Mosay

RHIA, CCS-P, CPC-H, CMRS

Daphne Neris

CPC, CCS-P

Cynthia Newby

CPC

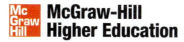

Mc Graw Hill McGraw-Hill Higher Education

Boston   Burr Ridge, IL   Dubuque, IA   New York   San Francisco   St. Louis
Bangkok   Bogotá   Caracas   Kuala Lumpur   Lisbon   London   Madrid   Mexico City
Milan   Montreal   New Delhi   Santiago   Seoul   Singapore   Sydney   Taipei   Toronto

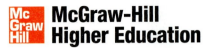
**McGraw-Hill
Higher Education**

McGRAW-HILL MEDICAL CODING: AN INTRODUCTION

Published by McGraw-Hill, a business unit of The McGraw-Hill Companies, Inc., 1221 Avenue of the Americas, New York, NY, 10020. Copyright © 2009 by The McGraw-Hill Companies, Inc. All rights reserved. No part of this publication may be reproduced or distributed in any form or by any means, or stored in a database or retrieval system, without the prior written consent of The McGraw-Hill Companies, Inc., including, but not limited to, in any network or other electronic storage or transmission, or broadcast for distance learning.

Some ancillaries, including electronic and print components, may not be available to customers outside the United States.

This book is printed on acid-free paper.

1 2 3 4 5 6 7 8 9 0 DBQ/DBQ 0 9 8

ISBN   978-0-07-340185-0
MHID   0-07-340185-4

Vice President/Editor in Chief: *Elizabeth Haefele*
Vice President/Director of Marketing: *John E. Biernat*
Senior sponsoring editor: *Debbie Fitzgerald*
Managing developmental editor: *Patricia Hesse*
Executive marketing manager: *Roxan Kinsey*
Lead media producer: *Damian Moshak*
Media producer: *Marc Mattson*
Director, Editing/Design/Production: *Jess Ann Kosic*
Project manager: *Marlena Pechan*
Senior production supervisor: *Janean A. Utley*
Designer: *Marianna Kinigakis*
Senior photo research coordinator: *Carrie K. Burger*
Media project manager: *Mark A. S. Dierker*
Typeface: *10.5/13 Palatino*
Compositor: *Aptara*
Printer: *Quebecor World Dubuque*
Cover image courtesy of: the Medical Management Institute, a Contexo Media Company
Credits: *The credits section for this book begins on page 509 and is considered an extension of the copyright page.*

Library of Congress Cataloging-in-Publication Data

McGraw-Hill medical coding : an introduction / Jean H. Jurek ... [et al.].
      p. ; cm.
   Includes index.
   ISBN-13: 978-0-07-340185-0 (alk. paper)
   ISBN-10: 0-07-340185-4 (alk. paper)
   1. Nosology—Code numbers. 2. Clinical medicine—Code numbers. I. Jurek, Jean H.
II. Title: Medical coding.
   [DNLM: 1. Forms and Records Control—methods—Case Reports. 2. Medical Records—Case Reports. W 80 M4784 2009]
RB115.M34 2009
651.5'04261—dc22

2007043931

www.mhhe.com

Brief Contents

Contents

Welcome to *McGraw-Hill Medical Coding: An Introduction.* This text/workbook introduces you to the foundational concepts, knowledge, and skills you will need for a successful career in medical coding.

Your Career in Medical Coding

Medical coding is one of the fastest-growing allied health occupations. This employment growth is the result of the increased medical needs of an aging population, advances in technology, and the growing number of health care providers—both hospitals and physicians—who require trained coders on their staffs. Medical coders play important roles in gathering and analyzing data for improved health care. They also help ensure the financial well-being of health care organizations in every delivery setting. Because coding is the basis for billing for services in health care, medical coders must be familiar with the rules and guidelines of each health care plan to build the basis for maximum appropriate reimbursement for services provided.

Medical coding is a challenging, interesting career, where you are compensated according to your level of skills and how effectively you put them to use. Those with the right combination of skills and abilities may have the opportunity to advance to management positions, such as coding supervision, or to higher-paid specialty coding positions, such as anesthesiology or radiology coding. Education, coupled with national certification, brings more employment options and advancement opportunities. Individuals who have a firm understanding of the medical coding process will find themselves well prepared to enter this ever-changing field.

Overview of This Program

Whether your course of study is medical coding, medical assisting, medical insurance and billing, or health information technology/management, this text/workbook gives you a strong foundation in medical coding basics. The program focuses on four key aspects of the medical coding process:

1. Knowledge of HIPAA-mandated medical code sets, which are the ICD-9-CM diagnosis code set, the CPT procedure code set, and the HCPCS supply code set.
2. Skill in applying the HIPAA-compliant guidelines for the correct use of these medical code sets, such as the *Official Guidelines for Coding and Reporting* that define correct diagnosis coding.
3. Understanding of correct procedures for code assignment, which are explained in carefully sequenced presentations of coding principles and in flow charts that reinforce proper steps to follow.
4. Ability to access available Internet and other resources to keep current in the field.

To the Student

The instructional parts of the text/workbook follow a logical sequence. The first part, *Medical Coding and the Health Care Environment,* is an introduction to the program. The second and third parts, *Introduction to ICD-9-CM* and *Introduction to CPT,* cover diagnosis and procedure coding, respectively. The fourth part, *Coding Case Studies,* presents clinical case studies to reinforce skills in assigning both diagnosis and procedure codes in typical medical settings.

The chapter coverage is as follows:

- Chapter 1 introduces the field of medical coding. It covers the types of work settings in which coders are employed and the documentation that is the basis for coding, HIPAA regulations, the general coding process, and career advancement.
- Chapter 2 overviews the ICD-9-CM code set structure, conventions for code selection, and general coding resources.
- Chapters 3, 4, and 5 are structured according to the *ICD-9-CM Official Guidelines for Coding and Reporting,* which explain general diagnosis

coding rules and then the specific guidance for the inpatient and the outpatient settings.

- Chapter 6 overviews the CPT code set structure, conventions for code selection, and general coding resources.

- Chapters 7, 8, and 9 each cover major sections of the CPT code set, including evaluation and management (E/M) codes as well as anesthesia, surgery, radiology, pathology/laboratory, and medicine codes.

- Chapter 10 covers the supply codes contained in the HCPCS code set.

- Chapter 11 presents 70 assignments that require application of both diagnosis and procedure coding skills to clinical case studies taken from various medical settings.

What Every Instructor Needs to Know

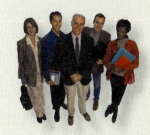

Welcome to the new McGraw-Hill Medical Coding introductory text!

The medical coding profession that you are training students to enter is evolving. Different jobs and employer settings are available to qualified graduates of your programs. The McGraw-Hill Medical Coding (MMC) series addresses an equally varied range of student abilities and aspirations. This text/workbook, *McGraw-Hill Medical Coding: An Introduction*, provides strong academic preparation. Moving forward from this foundation, students will gain experience in the practical application of coding principles and preparation for certification in the second and third books in the series, *McGraw-Hill Medical Coding: Moving Ahead* and *McGraw-Hill Medical Coding: Becoming an Expert Coder* that will be published.

THE STORY BEHIND THE NEW SERIES. . . .

What kind of instructional program would meet this variety of needs? To answer this question, McGraw-Hill pulled together key coding instructors in a Coding Symposium to talk over plans, ideas, and objectives. Over a weekend-long meeting, major changes were made to the initial plans to respond to what these experts said: Provide a balanced, progressive program with self-contained chapters organized into three books. The first book will present the basics, the second book will move students ahead to an in-depth understanding of the most prevalent/important coding scenarios, and the third book will be designed so that students can build a portfolio demonstrating their expertise in diagnostic and procedural professional and facility coding. This group has served as a sounding board throughout the writing and reviewing, ensuring implementation of these key features:

- **Balanced coverage of coding topics** Students must prepare for work in various health care environments: hospital-based, outpatient clinics, physician practices, and others. MMC provides a thorough understanding of both inpatient and outpatient coding.

- **Focused coverage of coding topics** Certain diseases and medical procedures are predominant in health care. Based on the Medical Group Management Association (MGMA) and Medicare analyses of the most common, MMC focuses on the need-to-know topics that students will continually encounter in their work, and presents the highlights of additional topics at the familiarization level.

- **Authoritative coverage of coding topics** The authors of MMC are seasoned instructors of coding and are also employed in the medical coding profession. This hands-on experience in both areas benefits students as difficult topics and clearly explained with examples from common clinical situations.

- **Structure of ICD-9-CM chapters based on the *Official Guidelines for Coding and Reporting*** Students gain greatest understanding of correct ICD-9-CM coding by learning and applying these HIPAA-mandated coding rules for diagnoses.

- **Graphic tools support coding rules** Flow charts support and reinforce the learning of key coding principles by showing the decision-making process and yes/no branching for assigning codes.

- **Customizable content and lesson plans** Instructors who wish to cover diagnosis coding or procedural coding in separate courses can easily customize the chapters for their curriculum.

- **Online Coding Tool** *McGraw-Hill Medical Coding: An Introduction* includes access to CodeItRightOnline™, an online coding tool from Medical Management Institute, a Contexo Media Company, that is available for use with Chapter 11.

- **Effective instructional design supports effective teaching** The instructional design of *McGraw-Hill Medical Coding: An Introduction* supports effective teaching each with balanced chapters that include learning outcomes, key terms, critical thinking questions, applications, summaries, and other well-established pedagogical features, as well as hundreds of coding exercises.

- **Online Learning Center** www.mhhe.com/JurekIntroMedCoding includes Power Point® Slides, links to professional organizations, and coding updates, including the ICD-9-CM *Official Guidelines for Coding and Reporting*. Also provided for student review are games, flashcards, and additional questions.

TEACHING SUPPLEMENTS

For the Instructor

Instructor's Manual (0-07-725184-9) includes:

- Course overview
- Information on accessing and using Medical Management Institute's online coding tool, CodeItRightOnline™
- Chapter-by-chapter lesson plans
- Checkpoint and end-of-chapter solutions
- Correlation tables: AHIMA CCA, CCS, CCS-P; AAPC CPC; SCANS; AAMA Role Delineation Study Areas of Competence (2003); and AMT Registered Medical Assistant Certification Exam Topics.

Instructor Productivity Center CD-ROM (packaged with the Instructor's Manual) includes:

- Instructor's PowerPoint® presentation of Chapters 1 through 10.
- Electronic testing program featuring McGraw-Hill's EZ Test. This flexible and easy-to-use program allows instructors to create tests from book specific items. It accommodates a wide range of question types and

instructors may add their own questions. Multiple versions of the test can be created and any test can be exported for use with course management systems such as WebCT, Blackboard, or PageOut.

- Instructor's Manual.

Online Learning Center (OLC), www.mhhe.com/JurekIntroMedCoding

Instructor Resources include:

- Instructor's Manual in Word and PDF format
- PowerPoint® files for each chapter
- Links to professional associations
- PageOut link

For the Student

Online Learning Center (OLC), www.mhhe.com/JurekIntroMedCoding

includes additional chapter quizzes and other review activities.

Medical Insurance Coding Workbook for Physician Practices, 2007-2008 edition
(0-07-352205-8)

The *Medical Insurance Coding Workbook* is available for additional practice and instruction in coding and compliance skills for physician (professional) coding and billing. The workbook reinforces and enhances skill development by applying the coding principles introduced in *McGraw-Hill Medical Coding: An Introduction,* providing coding guideline reinforcement, examples, compliance tips, and case studies.

McGraw-Hill ICD-9-CM Code Book 2008 Edition (ISBN 0-07-723688-2)

Online Coding Tool, CodeItRightOnline™, 21-day free use.

About the Authors

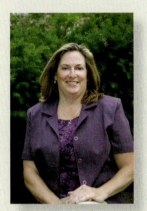

JEAN JUREK, MS, RHIA, CPC

Jean has over 25 years of experience in medical coding and the health information profession. She is an Associate Professor in the Health Information Technology Program at Erie Community College. Her primary responsibilities include teaching all medical coding courses, billing courses, on-line course development, and instruction in quality management, computer applications and health care statistics. As a consultant, she also is able to continue with "hands on" experience in medical coding and auditing. Her work consists of medical coding for a variety of health care providers, conducting medical coding audits and education for health care providers in documentation and coding issues.

Jean has served as president of the Health Information Management Association of Western New York (HIMAWNY), and received their Distinguished Member Award in 2005. Recently, Jean has served as Education Director and Finance Director for the New York Health Information Management Association (NYHIMA). Currently Jean is the NY Community Education Coordinator for the Personal Health Record (PHR) campaign sponsored by AHIMA. She is also a participating member of the American Health Information Management Association (AHIMA), the American Academy of Professional Coders (AAPC), and UNYPHIED (Upstate New York Professional Healthcare Information and Education Demonstration Project).

Her Master's Degree was awarded from the State University of New at Buffalo, Department of Social and Preventive Medicine in 2000.

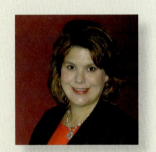

STACEY MOSAY, RHIA, CCS-P, CPC-H, CMRS

Stacey has over 15 years experience in health information management, including working as director of medical records for a multihospital health system and in coding, quality improvement, business office management, medical staff credentialing, regulatory compliance, reimbursement analysis, and physician office consulting. She served five years as the Medical Record Coder Program Coordinator for the academic Coding Certificate program in the Division of Allied Health at Trident Technical College. She is a graduate of the Medical University of South Carolina with a B.S. in Health Information Management. She served as chairman of the CCA test construction committee for AHIMA from 2006-2007. She is a registered member of the American Health Information Management Association and the American Academy of Professional Coders. She is a member of the Low Country Coders Association, the Palmetto Coder Association, AHIMA's Assembly of Education, American Medical Billing Association, Healthcare Billing and Management Association, and a participant in Low Country Coding Roundtables.

Daphne has been in the healthcare field since 1984. She currently has her own consulting business and is an approved American Academy of Professional Coders (AAPC) Instructor. Previously, she was the Compliance Auditor for the Department of Internal Medicine at Yale University's School of Medicine, and the Manager of Clinical and Reimbursement Services at the School of Medicine. Her first years in healthcare were as the Clinic Manager for a large surgical group in Connecticut. She is one of the founders of the Connecticut Chapter of AAPC and is a past President. She has been an AAPC member since 1995, and a CPC since 1996. Daphne has spoken nationally at the AAPC National Conferences in Minnesota and Washington DC, and previously at the National Physician's Coding Summit in Las Vegas. She is a member of the Connecticut Medical Group Management Association (CMGMA) and the Connecticut Women in Healthcare Management Association (CWHCM), serving on their Career Development Committee. Daphne also has a Bachelor of Science degree from the University of New Haven and majored in Financial Accounting.

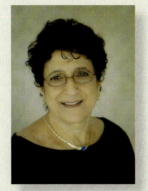

DAPHNE NERIS, CPC, CCS-P

Cynthia has developed and written text programs for McGraw-Hill for over seventeen years. Her publishing career began with McGraw-Hill in New York, where she was employed for 15 years, first as a copyeditor trainee, last as Executive Editor, Business & Marketing/Office Technology Group, Gregg Division. Before founding Chestnut Hill Enterprises in 1990, Cynthia was vice president for product marketing at Dialogue Systems, Inc., in New York. She is certified as a professional coder by the American Academy of Professional Coders, and is a graduate of Hood College.

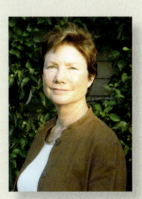

CYNTHIA NEWBY, CPC

Walkthrough

WHAT EVERY STUDENT NEEDS TO KNOW

Many tools to help you learn have been integrated into your text.

CHAPTER FEATURES

Learning Outcomes—present a list of the most important points you should focus on in the chapter.

Key Terms—list the important vocabulary words alphabetically to build your insurance terminology. Key terms are highlighted and defined when introduced in the text.

Chapter Outline—gives you an overview of the key concepts and organization.

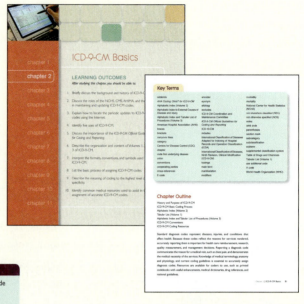

HIPAA Tips, Billing Tips, and Compliance Guidelines—connect you to the real world of coding. These tips on HIPAA rules, billing points, and ensuring compliance with correct coding practices are located in the margins near the related chapter topics.

HIPAA TIP
Mandated Code Set

ICD-9-CM is the mandated code set for medical diagnoses and hospital inpatient services.

BILLING TIP
Inpatient and Outpatient Procedures

Use Volume 3 of ICD-9-CM for *inpatient* procedures, and use CPT (covered in Chapters 6 through 10 of your program) for *outpatient* procedures.

COMPLIANCE GUIDELINE
Use Current Codes

Compliant coding under HIPAA requires codes to be current as of the date of service. Do not report codes that are no longer in the code set.

Coding Tips, Cautions, and Alerts—these pointers on correct coding procedures and processes (color-coded green for "go," yellow for "proceed with care," and red for "stop") are also located in the margins near the related coding concepts.

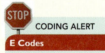 **CODING ALERT**
E Codes

E codes are never reported alone or first.

 CODING TIP
Follow the *Official Guidelines*

Always base assignment of ICD-9-CM codes on the *Official Guidelines*.

⚠ **CODING CAUTION**

When Four Digits Are Correct

When a five-digit code is not available, a four-digit code is correct. For example, if a patient has a malignant neoplasm of the stomach (category 151), a fourth digit is required to reflect the exact location of the neoplasm in the stomach, such as 151.4 for a malignant neoplasm of the body of the stomach.

> *I feel the level and depth of information is appropriate for the beginning and intermediate student.*
>
> *The author has offered many examples and covers the guidelines in a student friendly and efficient manner.*
>
> **Denise Wallen, CPC, Academy of Professional Careers**

Figures, Flow Charts, and Websites—illustrate the key concepts in the chapter visually.

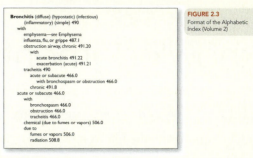

Bronchitis (diffuse) (hypostatic) (infectious) (inflammatory) (simple) 490
    with
        emphysema—see Emphysema
        influenza, flu, or grippe 487.1
        obstruction airway, chronic 491.20
            with
                acute bronchitis 491.22
                exacerbation (acute) 491.21
        tracheitis 490
            acute or subacute 466.0
                with bronchospasm or obstruction 466.0
            chronic 491.8
    acute or subacute 466.0
        with
            bronchospasm 466.0
            obstruction 466.0
            tracheitis 466.0
        chemical (due to fumes or vapors) 506.0
        due to
            fumes or vapors 506.0
            radiation 508.8

FIGURE 2.3
Format of the Alphabetic Index (Volume 2)

Checkpoints—challenge you to stop and think through the questions that are posed at major points in the chapter.

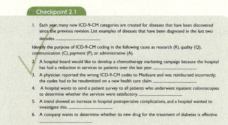

Checkpoint 2.1

1. Each year, many new ICD-9-CM categories are created for diseases that have been discovered since the previous revision. List examples of diseases that have been diagnosed in the last two decades. _____

Identify the purpose of ICD-9-CM coding in the following cases as research (R), quality (Q), communication (C), payment (P), or administrative (A).

2. A hospital board would like to develop a chemotherapy marketing campaign because the hospital has had a reduction in services to patients over the last year. _____
3. A physician reported the wrong ICD-9-CM codes to Medicare and was reimbursed incorrectly; the codes had to be resubmitted on a new health care claim. _____
4. A hospital wants to send a patient survey to all patients who underwent inpatient colonoscopies to determine whether the services were satisfactory. _____
5. A trend showed an increase in hospital postoperative complications, and a hospital wanted to investigate this. _____
6. A company wants to determine whether its new drug for the treatment of diabetes is effective. _____

CHAPTER REVIEW

Summary—provides a helpful review of the chapter's key concepts.

Review Questions—reinforce the important facts and points made in the chapter. Question formats include matching, true-false, completion, and short answer.

Applying Your Knowledge—utilizes cases that ask you to apply the coding skill gained by studying the chapter for correct answers.

Internet Resources and Activities—describe relevant websites and direct you to use the Internet to research and report your findings. The goal of the activities is to extend your knowledge of the selected topics and to learn to use the Internet as a research tool.

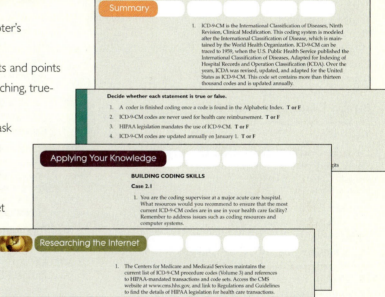

Summary

1. ICD-9-CM is the International Classification of Diseases, Ninth Revision, Clinical Modification. This coding system is modeled after the International Classification of Disease, which is maintained by the World Health Organization. ICD-9-CM can be traced to 1959, when the U.S. Public Health Service published the International Classification of Diseases, Adapted for Indexing of Hospital Records and Operation Classification (ICDA). Over the years, ICDA was revised, updated, and adapted for the United States as ICD-9-CM. This code set contains more than thirteen thousand codes and is updated annually.

Decide whether each statement is true or false.

1. A coder is finished coding once a code is found in the Alphabetic Index. **T or F**
2. ICD-9-CM codes are never used for health care reimbursement. **T or F**
3. HIPAA legislation mandates the use of ICD-9-CM. **T or F**
4. ICD-9-CM codes are updated annually on January 1. **T or F**

Applying Your Knowledge

BUILDING CODING SKILLS

Case 2.1

1. You are the coding supervisor at a major acute care hospital. What resources would you recommend to ensure that the most current ICD-9-CM codes are in use in your health care facility? Remember to address issues such as coding resources and computer systems.

Researching the Internet

1. The Centers for Medicare and Medicaid Services maintains the current list of ICD-9-CM procedure codes (Volume 3) and references to HIPAA-mandated transactions and code sets. Access the CMS website at www.cms.hhs.gov, and link to Regulations and Guidelines to find the details of HIPAA legislation for health care transactions.

CHAPTER 11's CODING CASE STUDIES

The coding case studies in Chapter 11 place you in the coder's role in various medical settings and ask for the selection of correct code sets followed by the assignment of accurate, compliant codes for both the patients' diagnoses and procedures.

REIMBURSEMENT REVIEWS AND PATHOPHYSIOLOGY REFRESHERS

Reimbursement reviews introduce key billing and payment topics at appropriate points; pathophysiology refreshers also review key disease processes and how they related to assignment of ICD-9-CM codes.

ABBREVIATIONS and GLOSSARY

The most important coding abbreviations, acronyms, and definitions are found at the back of the text for easy reference.

ONLINE LEARNING CENTER (OLC)

www.mhhe.com/JurekIntroMedCoding

The OLC offers additional learning and teaching tools.

> *The organization of the sections, symbols, graphs, questions, and the detailed information will give the student a better understanding of the introductory material on CPT coding.*
>
> **Irma Rodriquez, Med, RHIA, CCS, South Texas College**

Acknowledgments

For insightful reviews and helpful suggestions, we would like to acknowledge the following:

Teresa Barbour, CPC
Pittsburgh Technical Institute
Oakdale, PA

Dorine Bennett, MBA, RHIA, RAHIMA
Dakota State University
Madison, SD

Darlene Boschert, BS, CPC, CPC-H
Career Institute of Florida
St. Petersburg, FL

Christine M. Cole, CCA
Williston State College
Williston, ND

Janelle Ciaussen, CPC
Mt. Hood Community College
Gresham, OR

Michelle Crissman, JD, MS, BS
Colorado Technical University
Sioux Falls, SD

Barbara Desch, LVN, CPC, AHI
San Joaquin Valley College, Inc.
Visalia, CA

Linda H. Donahue, RHIT, CCS, CCS-P, CPC
Health Information Technology Instructor,
Delgado Community College
New Orleans, LA

Yolande Gardner, MA
Lawson State Community College
Bessemer, AL

Mack Henderson, PhD, CCS-P, CPC
Durham Technical Community College
Durham, NC

Judy Hurtt, MEd
East Central Community College
Decatur, MS

Pat King, MA, RHIA
Baker College of Cass City
Cass City, MI

Jennifer Lame', MPH, BS, RHIT
Southwest Wisconsin Technical College
Fennimore, WI

Martha Luebke, BA
High-Tech Institute
Las Vegas, NV

Marjorie H. McNeill, PhD, RHIA, CCS
Division of Health Information Management,
School of Allied Health Sciences,
Florida A&M University
Tallahassee, FL

Sandra Moaney Wright, MEd, CMA
Atlanta Medical Academy
College Park, GA

Irma Rodriguez, MEd, RHIA, CCS
South Texas College
McAllen, TX

Maggie M. Scott, MPH, BA, RHIT
Victor Valley College
Victorville, CA

Carol G Skelton, CPC
Augusta State University
Augusta, GA

Lynn G. Slack, BS, CMA
Kaplan Career Institute – ICM Campus
Pittsburgh, PA

Diane Swift, RHIT
State Fair Community College
Sedalia, MO

Linda Templeton, CCS-P, CPC, CPC-H
Stautzenberger College
Maumee, OH

Denise Wallen, CPC
Academy of Professional Careers
Nampa, ID

Lynette Williamson, MBA, RHIA, CCS, CPC
Camden County College
Camden, NJ

Carole A. Zeglin, MS, BS, RMA,
Director Medical Assisting Program
Westmoreland County Community College
Youngwood, PA

SYMPOSIUM ATTENDEES

Rita Anderson
San Joaquin Valley College
Rancho Cucamonga, CA

Patricia Bucho
Long Beach Community College
Long Beach, CA

Lisa Campbell
South Suburban College
South Holland, IL

Susan Dengler
Prince George's Community College
Largo, MD

Barbara Desch
San Joaquin Valley College
Largo, CA

Angela Kuhn
Harrison Career Institute
Voorhees, NJ

Sharon McCaughrin
Ross Learning, Inc
Southfield, MI

Lynn Slack
Kaplan Career Institute – ICM Campus
Pittsburg, PA

Denise Wallen
Academy of Professional Careers
Nampa, ID

PART ONE

Medical Coding and the Health Care Environment

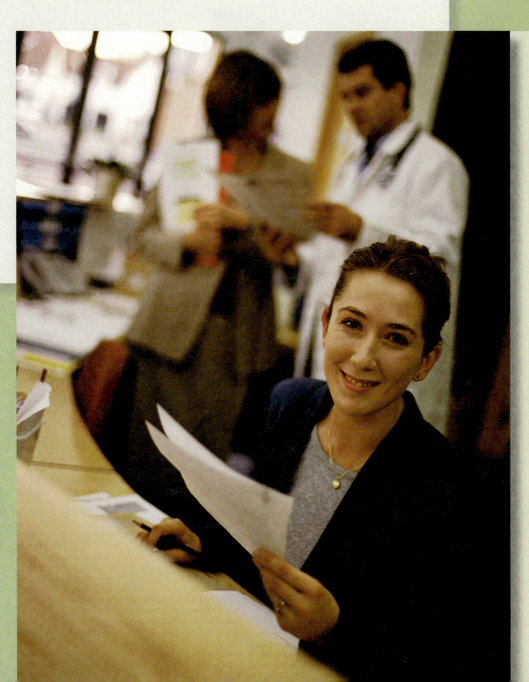

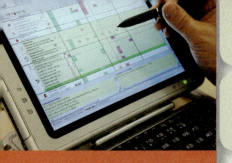

Your Career as a Medical Coder

LEARNING OUTCOMES

After studying this chapter, you should be able to:

1. Describe the purposes of medical coding.

2. Define medical necessity, and discuss the way that medical coding links diagnoses and procedures to establish it.

3. Discuss the types of health care organizations that employ medical coders, comparing facility (inpatient and outpatient) and physician practice coding environments.

4. Describe the importance of the documentation in medical records to the medical coding process.

5. Understand the requirements for and procedures to guard the confidentiality of patients' protected health information under HIPAA.

6. Briefly describe the purpose of the HIPAA Privacy Rule, the HIPAA Security Rule, the HIPAA Electronic Health Care Transactions and Code Sets standards, and National Identifiers.

7. List the basic steps in the medical coding process.

8. Describe the laws that regulate accurate and compliant medical coding.

9. Identify the skills, attributes, and ethical behaviors that successful medical coders exemplify.

10. Define the opportunities for professional certification as a medical coder.

Key Terms

abuse
ambulatory
authorization
Centers for Medicare and Medicaid Services (CMS)
certification
code set
compliance
compliance plan
computer-assisted coding (CAC)
de-identified health information
diagnosis code
documentation
electronic medical records (EMR)
encounter
ethics
facility

fraud
health care claim
health information management (HIM)
Health Insurance Portability and Accountability Act (HIPAA) of 1996
health plan
HIPAA Electronic Health Care Transactions and Code Sets (TCS)
HIPAA Privacy Rule
HIPAA Security Rule
hybrid record
informed consent
inpatient (IP)
The Joint Commission
medical coder
medical coding
medical insurance

medical necessity
medical standards of care
minimum necessary standard
Office for Civil Rights (OCR)
Office of the Inspector General (OIG)
outpatient (OP)
payer
procedure code
professional
protected health information (PHI)
provider
release of information (ROI)
revenue cycle
treatment, payment, and health care operations (TPO)

Chapter Outline

The Importance of Medical Coding
A Medical Coder's Working Environment
The Medical Record
HIPAA
Medical Coding: Accurate and Compliant
Professionalism as a Medical Coder

Spending on health care in the United States is rising, for two major reasons. The first factor is the cost of advances in medical technology that improve health care. The second factor is that the American population is aging and requires more health care services. More than half the money spent on health care goes to managing chronic diseases, such as diabetes, hypertension, chronic obstructive pulmonary disease (COPD), and arthritis, which are more common in older people.

The rising medical costs affect federal and state government budgets and employers that pay for medical insurance for employees. Rising costs also increase the financial pressure on hospitals and physicians. To continue to serve their patients' needs, these health care providers must carefully manage their business functions. Because knowledgeable medical coders help ensure the maximum appropriate payment for medical services, they are in demand. Successful completion of this program is your first step on the path to a rewarding career as a medical coder.

The Importance of Medical Coding

When health care providers examine or treat patients, they use clinical terms to document the patients' medical diagnoses and procedures in medical records. To be able to analyze and track how these conditions are treated and to bill for the medical services, medical codes must be assigned to the narrative clinical text. Code numbers are efficient, translating long descriptions so that they can be universally understood and exchanged regardless of the different medical terms physicians might use.

Determining the correct codes for these diagnoses and procedures is the role of a **medical coder.** Coders are health information practitioners who are skilled in classifying medical data from patient records. Various job titles are *health information coders, medical record coders, coder/ abstractors*, and *medical coding specialists*. Medical coders use standardized codes and medical coding software programs to assign codes that accurately report the medical services provided and facilitate the payment for the billed services.

Can a code, like a picture, be worth a thousand words? It is clear from the following example that numbers can be very effective in portraying complex meanings. Consider this code combination:

> **EXAMPLE** **Diagnosis code 650:** Normal delivery: delivery requiring minimal or no assistance, with or without episiotomy, without fetal manipulation or instrumentation of spontaneous, cephalic, vaginal, full-term, live-born infant.
>
> **Procedure code 59400 (Obstetrician):** Routine obstetric care including antepartum care, vaginal delivery, and postpartum care.
>
> **Procedure code 73.59 (Hospital):** Assisted spontaneous delivery.

The patient's primary illness or symptoms and other treated conditions are assigned **diagnosis codes** selected from the codes in the International Classification of Diseases, Ninth Revision, Clinical Modification (ICD-9-CM). Similarly, procedures that are performed are assigned **procedure codes** that stand for particular services, treatments, or tests. Most procedure codes are selected from the Current Procedural Terminology (CPT). A large group of CPT codes covers the physician's evaluation and management of a patient's condition at particular places of service, such as an office, a hospital, or a nursing home. Other codes cover specific procedures, such as surgery, pathology, and radiology. Another group of codes called HCPCS covers supplies and other services. Facilities use a separate set of codes from the ICD-9-CM to code for and bill the costs of procedures that occur in the hospital setting.

GATHERING ACCURATE DATA FOR BETTER HEALTH CARE

Scientists and medical researchers have long gathered information from medical records about patients' morbidity (impairment due to disease) and mortality (death). In place of the written descriptions of many different symptoms and conditions that used to be stored, the coded data that the **medical coding** process produces are easier to study and analyze. The clinical data that medical coders provide may be used to help plan for needed health care services, to improve patient care, to control costs, in legal actions, and for research studies. Examples are:

- *Pay-for-performance* measurements that reward physicians financially for following the best medical practices to ensure patients' health, such as prescribing a beta blocker after a patient has had a myocardial infarction (MI, or heart attack).
- Cancer (tumor) registries that collect information about cancer—the types diagnosed, their locations in the body, the extent of the cancers when diagnosed, the treatments provided, and the outcomes—to improve care.
- Alerts that advise providers about preventive immunizations such as flu shots.
- Reports of patients' mortality, of births, and of cases of abuse that must be released to state health or social services departments under state law.
- Reports of communicable diseases such as tuberculosis, hepatitis, and rabies that also must be reported to authorities to monitor public health and risks.
- A special category of communicable disease control for patients with diagnoses of human immunodeficiency virus (HIV) infection and acquired immunodeficiency syndrome (AIDS). Every state requires AIDS cases to be reported, and most states also require reporting of the HIV infection that causes the syndrome.
- Data that identify fraudulent activities.
- Data that help consumers compare costs and outcomes of treatment options.

Study the coding tips in the margin. Throughout your text, these notes in the margin guide and advise you on correct coding.

ESTABLISHING MEDICAL NECESSITY FOR PAYMENT

Medical coding also provides a bridge between the clinical data and the billing process that generates payment for medical services to physicians and facilities (Figure 1.1). The billing process is called the **revenue cycle,** because the business side of medicine is a continual process of providing clinical services, billing, collecting payments, and then using these funds to pay for the cost of operations, such as salaries and medical equipment.

The costs for most medical services that patients receive are covered, in part or in full, by medical insurance. Nearly 250 million people in the United States have some form of insurance, through either their employers or government programs. To be paid for by insurance companies (called the **payers**), treatments and procedures must be medically necessary. **Medical necessity** means that the services are reasonable and are required for the diagnosis or treatment

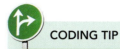
CODING TIP

Green is the color for "go," and these tips help build coding skill.

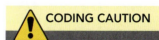
CODING CAUTION

Yellow means "proceed with caution," and these notes explain how to move ahead carefully in the particular coding situation.

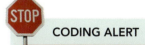
CODING ALERT

Red means "stop before moving ahead," and these alerts point out coding mistakes you can avoid.

Clinical Services Provided to Patient → Medical Codes Assigned → Health Care Claims Transmitted → Reimbursement for Clinical Services

FIGURE 1.1
Medical Coding Links Clinical Services to Reimbursement

Medical Insurance

Medical (health) **insurance** is a written policy between an individual, called the *policyholder*, and a **health plan**—an insurance company or government program that is the *payer*. The policyholder pays a specified amount of money called a *premium*. In exchange, the payer provides benefits—defined by the Health Insurance Association of America as payments for covered medical services—for a specific period of time.

The Major Types of Payers Are:

- *Private payers*: Nationwide insurance companies that dominate the national market and offer all types of health plans, such as WellPoint, UnitedHealth Group, Aetna, Kaiser Permanente, and the members of the Blue Cross and Blue Shield Association.
- *Self-funded health plans*: Health plans, set up by employers, that assume the risk of paying directly for medical services.
- *Government-sponsored health care programs*: Four major government-sponsored health care programs offer benefits for which various groups in the population are eligible:

Medicare is a 100 percent federally funded health plan that covers people who are sixty-five and over and those who are disabled or have permanent kidney failure (end-stage renal disease, or ESRD).

Medicaid, a federal program that is jointly funded by federal and state governments, covers low-income people who cannot afford medical care. Each state administers its own Medicaid program, determining the program's qualifications and benefits under broad federal guidelines.

TRICARE, a Department of Defense program, covers medical expenses for active-duty members of the uniformed services and their spouses, children, and other dependents; retired military personnel and their dependents; and family members of deceased active-duty personnel.

CHAMPVA, the Civilian Health and Medical Program of the Department of Veterans Affairs, covers veterans with permanent service-related disabilities and their dependents. It also covers surviving spouses and

---

CODING TIP

Look it up!

Successful coders research the meaning of unfamiliar medical terms to improve their coding skill.

of a condition, illness, or injury or to improve the functioning of a malformed body part. Services also may not be elective, experimental, or performed for the convenience of the patient or the patient's family.

EXAMPLES
Medically necessary:
   Diagnosis: Nasal obstruction
   Procedure: Nasal surgery
Not medically necessary:
   Diagnosis: Overly large nose
   Procedure: Cosmetic nasal surgery performed to improve a patient's appearance

The **provider** of the service must also meet the payer's professional standards. Providers include all types of licensed health care **professionals,** such as physicians, nurse-practitioners, physician's assistants, and therapists, as well as **facilities** (hospitals and their departments for therapy and radiology, for example) and suppliers such as pharmacies and medical supply companies. Providers must hold the payer's required medical credentials and follow the payer's other *conditions of participation* relating to patient care.

Study the "Medical Insurance" Reimbursement Review. At appropriate points in your text, these overviews provide you with background information on the key components of the revenue cycle and explain how they are related to medical coding.

dependent children of veterans who died from service-related disabilities.

Note that under the federal Emergency Medical Treatment and Active Labor Act (EMTALA), hospital emergency departments must provide care for all patients in need of medical services regardless of their ability to pay. More than $100 billion in unpaid health care is provided annually for uninsured and underinsured patients.

Covered services are listed on the schedule of benefits. These services may include primary care, emergency care, medical specialists' services, and surgery. Coverage of some services is mandated by state or federal law; coverage of others is optional. Some policies provide benefits only for loss resulting from illnesses or diseases, while others also cover accidents or injuries. Many health plans cover *preventive medical services*, such as annual physical examinations, pediatric and adolescent immunizations, prenatal care, and routine screening procedures such as mammograms.

The medical insurance policy also describes non-covered services (excluded)—those for which it does not pay—which may include all or some of the following:

- Most medical policies do not cover dental services, eye examinations or eyeglasses, employment-related injuries, cosmetic procedures, or experimental procedures.
- Policies may exclude specific items such as vocational rehabilitation or surgical treatment of obesity.
- Many policies do not have prescription drug benefits.
- If a new policyholder has a medical condition that was diagnosed before the policy took effect—known as a *preexisting condition*—medical services to treat it are often not covered.

Providers send a **health care claim**—a formal insurance claim in either electronic or hard copy format that reports data about the patient and the services provided—to the payer on behalf of the patient. Payers scrutinize the need for medical procedures, examining each bill to make sure it meets their medical necessity guidelines.

Checkpoint 1.1

In your opinion, is each of the following diagnoses and procedures correctly linked to show medical necessity? Why?

A. Diagnosis: deviated septum
    _____ Procedure: nasal surgery

B. Diagnosis: mole on a female patient's cheek, questionable nature
    _____ Procedure: surgical removal and biopsy

C. Diagnosis: male syndrome hair loss
    _____ Procedure: implant hair plugs on scalp

D. Diagnosis: probable broken wrist
    _____ Procedure: comprehensive full-body examination, with complete set of lab tests, chest X-ray, and ECG

A Medical Coder's Working Environment

Medical coders are part of the trillion-dollar health care industry, a fast-growing and dynamic sector of the American economy that includes pharmaceutical companies, hospitals, doctors, medical equipment makers, nursing homes, assisted-living centers, and insurance companies. According to the U.S. Department of Labor, employment in the field of medical coding is expected to grow much faster than average through 2014. Job prospects for employees who work with medical records are very good, and people with strong backgrounds in medical coding will be in particularly high demand (see Figure 1.2).

Medical coders may work in traditional health care delivery environments or in nontraditional jobs. Traditional employers include both facilities and physician practices:

- Acute care hospitals
- Various hospital departments, such as same-day surgery, radiology, and laboratory departments, and emergency rooms

U.S Department of Labor
Bureau of Labor Statistics

Occupational Outlook Handbook

Health Information Technicians

- Health Information technicians are projected to be one of the 20 fastest growing occupations.
- Job prospects for formally trained technicians should be very good. Employment of health information technicians is expected to grow much faster than the average for all occupations through 2010, due to rapid growth in the number of medical tests, treatments, and procedures which will be increasingly scrutinized by third-party payers, regulators, courts, and consumers.
- Most technicians will be employed in hospitals, but job growth will be faster in offices and clinics of physicians, nursing homes, and home health agencies.

Medical Assistants

- Employment of medical assistants is expected to grow much faster than the average for all occupations through 2010 as the health services industry expands due to technological advances in medicine and a growing and aging population. It is one of the fastest growing occupations.
- Employment growth will be driven by the increase in the number of group practices, clinics, and other health care facilities that need a high proportion of support personnel, particularly the flexible medical assistant who can handle both administrative and clinical duties. Medical assistants work primarily in outpatient settings, where much faster than average growth is expected.
- Job prospects should be best for medical assistants with formal training or experience, particularly those with certification.

Medical Administrative Support

- Growth in the health services industry will spur faster than average employment growth for medical support staff.
- Medical administrative support employees may transcribe dictation, prepare correspondence, and assist physicians or medical scientists with reports, speeches, articles, and conference proceedings. They also record simple medical histories, arrange for patients to be hospitalized, and order supplies. Most medical administrative support staff need to be familiar with insurance rules, billing practices, and hospital or laboratory procedures.

FIGURE 1.2
USDOL Employment Projections

- Skilled nursing facilities (SNF)
- Long-term acute care facilities (LTAC)
- Rehabilitation facilities
- Home health agencies (HHA)
- Hospices
- Military treatment facilities
- Special care facilities, such as end-stage renal disease (ESRD) and cancer facilities
- Durable medical equipment suppliers (DME) and ambulance service providers
- Physician practices (solo, single specialty, multispecialty)
- Ambulatory surgery centers (ASCs)
- Clinics

FACILITY-BASED EMPLOYMENT

Facilities were the first employers of medical coders, and currently two out of five coders work in hospital settings. Because facilities are very large institutions with many employees and complex functions, they are organized into departments:

- Administrative departments perform general business support functions, such as human resources (the hiring of personnel), public relations, purchasing, and legal services.
- Financial departments perform accounting functions—including registration (collecting patient information relating to payment at admissions), patient financial services such as explaining anticipated bills, and payment plans, billing, and collections.
- Clinical departments provide medical, surgical, rehabilitation, and psychiatric services for patients. Clinical tasks also include ancillary services, such as departments for nursing; radiology; laboratory; physical, occupational, speech, and respiratory therapy; social services; and case management functions.
- Operational departments help run the facility and include the **health information management (HIM)** department—sometimes called the *medical records department*—which is responsible for collecting, organizing, maintaining, storing, and disseminating the medical records of patients both internally and externally. Several areas make up the HIM department: coding, tumor registry, transcription, and release of information (staff members who handle proper release of patients' data).

Inpatient Versus Outpatient Services   Facilities have two categories of services that are based on the status of the patient. **Inpatient (IP)** services are provided when the patient is admitted to the facility for care with the expectation of at least an overnight stay. **Outpatient (OP)** services, in contrast, are for patients who are not expected to stay overnight in the hospital. Hospital-based outpatient services may be done in the hospital or in an outside facility the hospital owns and runs. Hospital outpatient care is also called **ambulatory** service, because the patient is not bedridden.

The major hospital-based outpatient services are:

- Emergency department visits during which the patient is assessed and treated or admitted as an inpatient if required
- Diagnostic testing
- Ambulatory surgery unit visits, such as for a colonoscopy
- Observation encounters in which patients with symptoms such as shortness of breath and chest pain are assessed and either admitted or discharged from the hospital

Outpatient Care Not Provided in Facilities   Driven by advances in medical technology and anesthesia monitoring, many procedures that used to be done during a hospital stay are now provided on an outpatient basis. Examples include same-day surgical procedures and screening examinations such as colonoscopies. Outpatient services are cheaper and take less time than services in a traditional hospital operating room, so there has been explosive growth of the demand for these ambulatory procedures. Hospitals compete for outpatient business with physicians who set up outpatient clinics and ambulatory surgery centers (ASCs). Care provided in these places of service is outpatient care, but not *facility-based outpatient care.* Likewise, care in the doctor's office is outpatient care. A physician who sends a patient to a hospital on an ambulatory basis for a laboratory test is not transferring care to the hospital; the hospital provides the technical service the physician orders, and the physician continues to be responsible for the patient's care.

PHYSICIAN PRACTICE EMPLOYMENT

Many millions of visits to physicians each year are for ambulatory services. Physician practices range from solo practices to large groups of thousands of doctors. Some practices are made up of physicians of one specialty, such as family medicine, cardiology, pediatrics, and urology; others are multispecialty organizations. Seventy-five percent of physicians provide care in small practices of from one to three physicians. Specialties that require a lot of technology, such as radiology, tend to have large single-specialty medical groups.

Typically, *front office* staff members handle duties such as reception (registration) and scheduling. *Back office* staff duties are related to coding, billing, insurance, and collections. In small offices, the same person may handle both coding and billing of insurance payers and patients. In large groups, coders may handle just coding tasks and may be assigned a coding specialty, such as Medicare coding.

NONTRADITIONAL EMPLOYERS

Medical coders are also employed in many different nontraditional settings. These include working for health plans to review coded data that are sent for payment; working as a consultant to physician practices, hospitals, law firms, or other health care settings; working in educational and research institutions, public health and government agencies, and correctional facilities; and jobs with health information system computer vendors. Some coders also work for traditional employers but are home-based. Called *remote coders,* they are either employed by or have contracts with the hospital or physician practice. Coding service companies also employ qualified coders who travel to assignments in other locations.

Checkpoint 1.2

In which type of environment would you prefer to be employed? Why?

The Medical Record

The work that medical coders do is based on the medical records (charts) that providers create in physician practices and facilities. These records contain facts, findings, and observations about patients' health history that are shared among health care professionals and nonclinicians to provide continuity of care. The records help in making accurate diagnoses of patients' conditions and in tracing the course of treatment.

> **EXAMPLE** A primary care physician (PCP) creates a patient's medical record that contains the results of all tests ordered during a comprehensive physical examination. To follow up on a problem, the PCP refers the patient to a cardiologist, also sending the pertinent data for that specialist's review. By studying the medical record, the cardiologist treating the referred patient learns the outcome of previous tests and avoids repeating them unnecessarily. Instead, the cardiologist orders a needed test to be done on an outpatient basis at the hospital's radiology department, which also documents its results for interpretation by the cardiologist.

The process of creating medical records is called **documentation.** It involves organizing a patient's health record in chronological order using a systematic, logical, and consistent method. A patient's health history, examinations, tests, and results of treatments are all documented. Providers need complete and comprehensive documentation to show that they have followed the **medical standards of care** that apply in their state. Health care providers are liable (that is, legally responsible) for providing this level of care to their patients. The term *medical professional liability* describes this responsibility of licensed health care professionals.

Patient medical records are legal documents. Good medical records are part of the provider's defense against accusations that patients were not treated correctly. They clearly state who performed what service and describe why, where, when, and how it was done. Providers document the rationale behind their treatment decisions. This rationale is the basis for medical necessity—the

CODING ALERT

Medical Liability Insurance

Medical liability cases can result in lawsuits. Physicians and facilities purchase professional liability insurance to cover such legal expenses. Although they are covered under these policies, other medical professionals often purchase their own liability insurance. Medical coders are advised to have professional liability insurance called error and omission (E&O) insurance, which protects against financial loss due to intentional or unintentional failure to perform work correctly (but not against fraud and abuse cases).

CODING TIP

Documentation, Coding, and Billing: A Vital Connection

The connection between documentation and coding is essential. A service that is not documented cannot be coded—and cannot be billed.

Overview

Pathophysiology combines the study of *pathology*—the origins, causes, and course of disease—with *physiology*, the study of how living things function. Pathophysiology is the study of how diseases arise and how they affect the normal functioning of the body.

Origins and Causes of Diseases and Disorders

Diseases and disorders occur in one of two ways. They may be part of a person's genetic makeup, or they may be acquired.

Some individuals have complex genetic makeups that predispose them to a particular disease, but they may never actually get the disease. For example, Type II diabetes may tend to occur in a family, but some family members do not develop it. Other people have a genetic tendency for a particular disease but may be able to avoid it through careful lifestyle management. While people with the inherited gene for breast cancer have a greater likelihood of getting breast cancer, it is not absolutely certain that they will.

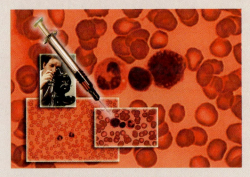

Red blood cells under a microscope.

Acquired diseases or disorders are caused by coming into contact with a *pathogen* (a disease-causing agent) or an *allergen,* or they may result from a number of factors or situations. The state of a person's immune system can determine resistance to disease. Bacteria, fungi, and viruses are some of the pathogens that cause disease. Accidents and traumas cause injuries and possible psychological disorders. Environmental causes of disease can include exposure to hazardous substances, overexposure to the ultraviolet rays of the sun, and poor diet and lack of exercise. Factors such as age, gender, genetic makeup, lifestyle, access to health care, and environment are called *predisposing* factors.

SOAP and the Understanding of Disease

When medical professionals examine patients, they often use the SOAP method of observation and treatment. Sometime the signs and symptoms of disease are reported by a patient as the chief complaint. In such cases, the physician diagnoses the disease using a standard examination process. Other times, a screening clinically logical link between a patient's condition and a treatment or procedure.

Study the Pathophysiology Refresher. At appropriate points in your text, these overviews provide you with background information on key diseases and explain how their clinical descriptions are related to medical coding.

DOCUMENTING ENCOUNTERS

An **encounter** (also called a *visit*) is a direct personal contact between a patient and a provider in any place of service (medical office, clinic, hospital, or other location) for the diagnosis and treatment of an illness or injury. At a minimum, each encounter should be documented with the following information:

- Patient's name
- Encounter date and reason
- Appropriate history and physical examination
- Review of all tests and drugs that were ordered
- Diagnosis
- Plan of care, or notes on procedures or treatments that were given

service, such as a mammogram or a blood pressure test, uncovers signs of a disease for which there is no external evidence, such as a breast tumor or hypertension. *SOAP* stands for *subjective, objective, assessment, plan:*

S: The *subjective* information is what the patient relates as the problems or complaints.

O: The *objective* information is what the physician finds during the examination of the patient. It may include the results of laboratory tests or other procedures.

A: The *assessment,* also called the "conclusion" is the physician's diagnosis.

P: The *plan,* also called "advice" or "recommendations," is the course of treatment for the patient, such as surgery, medications, other tests, further patient monitoring, follow-up, and instructions to the patient.

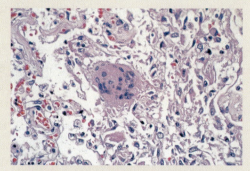

SARS cells are responsible for severe acute respiratory syndrome.

The Vocabulary of Pathophysiology

Many terms used with diseases and disorders are general terms that cover a number of diseases with certain common characteristics. For example, *cancer* is a term for any disease that involves malignant growths. A specific cancer, such as leukemia, may also include a number of different variations of the disorder. In addition, individual diseases are characterized by certain terms that indicate the type, severity, or some other aspect of the disease. Many diseases are either *acute* (brief and severe) or *chronic* (of long duration). Some symptoms may be *integral* (part of the disease process) or *nonintegral* (not directly connected with the disease). A tumor may be *benign* (located in one area and not spreading) or *malignant* (spreading in an uncontrolled manner). *Necrotic* or *necrotizing* indicates that tissue is dying; for example, *acute necrotizing pancreatitis* is a severe attack of pancreatitis with the dying of some tissue. *Suppurative* indicates the discharge of pus. *Exfoliative* indicates scaling or flaking. *Infantile* indicates very young; *senile* indicates very old. Treatments may be *invasive* (requiring incision or puncture) or *noninvasive* (not requiring incision or puncture). These and other characteristics are used to classify diseases.

- Instructions or recommendations that were given to the patient
- Signature of the physician or other licensed health care professional who saw the patient

In physician practices, the medical record for a patient usually contains these data:

- Biographical and personal information, including the patient's full name, date of birth, gender, race/ethnicity, residence address, marital status, identification numbers, home and work telephone numbers, and employer information as applicable
- Copies of all communications with the patient, including letters, telephone calls, faxes, and e-mail messages; the patient's responses; and a note of the time, date, topic, and physician's response to each communication
- Copies of prescriptions and instructions given to the patient, including refills
- Original documents that the patient has signed, such as an advance directive regarding end-of-life care
- Medical allergies and reactions, or their absence

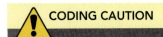
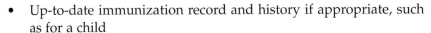

- Up-to-date immunization record and history if appropriate, such as for a child
- Previous and current diagnoses, test results, health risks, and progress, including hospitalizations
- Copies of referral or consultation letters
- Records of any missed or canceled appointments
- Requests for information about the patient (from a health plan or an attorney, for example) and release data

For each hospital encounter, additional information is recorded:

- Type of encounter
- Date of encounter, including admission and discharge dates for inpatient admissions
- Physicians involved with the patient's care
- Patient's diagnoses and procedures
- Medications prescribed
- Disposition of the patient (that is, the arrangements for the next steps in the patient's care, such as transfer to a skilled nursing facility or to home)

Hospitals need complete patient information to support high-quality medical care, and the goal is typically a unit record that brings together all documented treatment information, both inpatient and outpatient, for a patient in a single facility. The flow of information into and out of the patient record is typically funneled through a master person index (MPI)—a master list of patients—that has a unique medical record number (MRN) for each patient. This same number is used whenever the patient has an encounter with the facility.

Evaluation and Management Services Documentation

When providers diagnose a patient's condition and decide on a course of treatment to treat, or manage, it, the service is called *evaluation and management (E/M)*. There are many types of E/M encounters, such as an encounter about a patient's current complaint, a visit to decide whether surgery is needed, and a hospital postoperative visit.

Evaluation and management services often include a complete interview (history) and physical (an examination) for a new patient or for a new problem presented by a person who is already a patient. A complete history and physical (H&P) is documented with four types of information: (1) the chief complaint, (2) the history and physical examination, (3) the diagnosis/assessment, and (4) the treatment plan (see Figure 1.3).

The physician documents the patient's reason for the visit, called the chief complaint (CC), often using the patient's own words to describe the symptom, problem, condition, diagnosis, or other factor. For clarity, the physician may restate the reason as a "presenting problem," using clinical terminology. The physician also documents the patient's relevant medical history. The extent of the history is based on what the physician considers appropriate. It may include the history of the present illness (HPI), past medical history (PMH), and family and social history. There is usually also a review of systems (ROS) in which the doctor asks questions about the function of each body system considered appropriate to the problem.

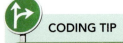

Ribielli, James E.
5/19/20--

CHIEF COMPLAINT: This 79-year-old male presents with sudden and extreme weakness. He got up from a seated position and became light-headed.

PAST MEDICAL HISTORY: History of congestive heart failure. On multiple medications, including Cardizem, Enalapril 5 mg qd, and Lasix 40 mg qd.

PHYSICAL EXAMINATION: No postural change in blood pressure. BP, 114/61 with a pulse of 49, sitting; BP, 111/56 with a pulse 50, standing. Patient denies being light-headed at this time.

HEENT: Unremarkable.

NECK: Supple without jugular or venous distension.

LUNGS: Clear to auscultation and percussion.

HEART: S1 and S2 normal; no systolic or diastolic murmurs; no S3, S4. No dysrhythmia.

ABDOMEN: Soft without organomegaly, mass, or bruit.

EXTREMITIES: Unremarkable. Pulses strong and equal.

LABORATORY DATA: Hemoglobin, 12.3. White count, 10.800. Normal electrolytes. ECG shows sinus bradycardia.

DIAGNOSIS: Weakness on the basis of sinus bradycardia, probably Cardizem induced.

TREATMENT: Patient told to change positions slowly when moving from sitting to standing, and from lying to standing.

John R. Ramirez, MD

FIGURE 1.3

Example of History and Physical Examination Documentation

The physician also performs a physical examination and documents the diagnosis—the interpretation of the information that has been gathered—or the suspected problem if more tests or procedures are needed for a diagnosis, and describes the treatment plan, or plan of care.

Physician Orders   Physician orders are another important type of documentation. Orders in the physician practice include documentation of requested laboratory, pathology, and radiology tests; consultations or referrals to other physicians; and prescriptions. In the hospital inpatient setting, orders from the physician who admits the patient (the *admitting physician*) and from the physician who is primarily responsible for taking care of the patient during the stay (the *attending physician*) include all instructions for the patient's treatment.

Procedural Services Documentation Other common types of documentation are for specific procedures done in a physician office,

---

Patient Name: Torres, Felecia
Hospital No.: 567A
Room No.: 590
Date of Surgery: 10/20/20--
Admitting Physician: Gloria Bevilacque, MD
Surgeon: Francis Lee, MD

PREOPERATIVE DIAGNOSIS: Intermittent atrial flutter/fibrillation with severe ventricular bradycardia.

POSTOPERATIVE DIAGNOSIS: Intermittent atrial flutter/fibrillation with severe ventricular bradycardia.

PROCEDURE: Implantation of permanent transvenous cardiac pacemaker.

ANESTHESIA: Local, 1% Xylocaine.

FINDINGS (including the condition of all organs examined): The patient was admitted with episodes of atrial flutter/fibrillation with very slow ventricular response in the low 40s. The patient was entirely uncooperative and combative during the course of operation. It took five people to hold him on the cath table. Also, his heart rate was between 140 and 180. He had very small veins in the region of the deltopectoral groove. All these problems led to great difficulty putting this pacemaker in. However, the electrode was finally positioned in the apex of the right ventricle, and I assumed that this threshold was satisfactory; but we could not be entirely sure of this because of his very fast ventricular rate of 140 to 160. It appeared that the threshold was an MA of 0.8, voltage 0.5, with resistance of 610 ohms. R-wave sensitivity was 7.3.

PROCEDURE IN DETAIL: With the patient in the supine position, the right pectoral region was prepped and draped in the usual fashion. As mentioned above the patient was entirely combative and uncooperative so that five people had to hold him down. After satisfactory local anesthesia and regional anesthesia were induced, a transverse incision was made and the deltopectoral groove was dissected. One vein appeared to be slightly larger than the rest of the very small venules in this area; and it was cannulated with a cardiac electrode, which with some difficulty was gotten into the apex of the right ventricle under fluoroscopic control. As mentioned above, the patient's threshold appeared to be satisfactory, though this was not entirely certain. Electrode was ligated in place with heavy silk, after which it was attached to the Medtronic pacemaker model 5985. The unit was implanted into the subcutaneous pocket. It should be noted that the patient had practically no subcutaneous fat, so that only a very, very thin layer of subcutaneous tissue and skin overlies the pacemaker. The wound was closed in two layers. Dressings were applied, and the patient was taken back to his room.

Francis Lee, MD

FL:BJ
D: 10/20/20--
T: 10/21/20--

FIGURE 1.4

Example of Operative Report

ambulatory surgery center, hospital surgical suite, or elsewhere:

- Procedure or operative reports for simple or complex surgery
- Laboratory reports for laboratory tests
- Radiology reports on the results of X-rays, CT scans, MRIs, and similar services
- Forms for a specific purpose, such as immunization records, pre-employment physicals, and disability reports

An example of an operative report is shown in Figure 1.4.

Other Chart Notes   Many other types of chart notes appear in patients' medical records. Progress notes, as shown in Figure 1.5, document a patient's progress and response to a treatment plan. They explain whether the plan should be continued or changed. Progress notes include:

- Comparisons of objective data with the patient's statements
- Goals and progress toward the goals
- The patient's current condition and prognosis
- Type of treatment still needed and for how long

Discharge summaries, as shown in Figure 1.6, are prepared during a patient's final visit for a particular treatment plan or hospitalization. Discharge summaries include:

- The final diagnosis
- Comparisons of objective data with the patient's statements

CODING TIP

Informed Consent

If the plan of care involves significant risk, as does surgery, state laws require the physician to have the patient's **informed consent** in advance. The physician discusses the assessment, risks, and recommendations with the patient and documents this conversation in the patient's record. Usually, the patient signs either a chart entry or a consent form to indicate agreement.

Delgado, Jennifer
8/14/20--

SUBJECTIVE: The patient has had epilepsy since she was 10. She takes her medication as prescribed; denies side effects. She reports no convulsions or new symptoms. She is a full-time student at Riverside Community College.

OBJECTIVE: Phenobarbital 90 mg twice a day as prescribed since 1994. The motor and sensory examination results are normal.

ASSESSMENT: Well-controlled epilepsy.

PLAN: Patient advised to continue medication regimen. Schedule for follow-up in 6 months.

Jared R. Wandaowsky, MD

FIGURE 1.5
Example of a Progress Report

Patient Name: Donaldson, Gerald
Hospital No. : 4903982
Admitted: 06/08/20--
Discharged: 06/14/20--

DIAGNOSIS:
    1. Atrophic gastritis.
    2. Irritable bowel syndrome.

OPERATION: Esophagogastroduodenoscopy 6/11/--

This 78-year-old white male was admitted for evaluation of abdominal pain, nausea, and vomiting and reports of coffee-ground emesis. Several weeks ago he was evaluated at the Rangely Hospital for similar symptoms and was told he had several ulcers in his distal esophagus and that he might require surgery. He was subsequently started on medications. He did fairly well after the initiation of medication; but over the three days prior to admission, had increasing left upper quadrant discomfort along with nausea, vomiting, and hematemesis. He also gives history of 35-pound weight loss over the last 18 months. In October 20-- he underwent evaluation at Rangely Hospital and was found to have erosive gastritis with duodenitis as well as reflux esophagitis. He also had some left upper quadrant pain at that time which was attributed to some postherpes zoster neuritis. The patient has previously had cholecystectomy and appendectomy.

Physical exam on admission showed multiple well-healed abdominal scars. No masses were palpable. There was some mild discomfort in the left upper quadrant on palpation and bowel sounds were normal.

LABORATORY DATA ON ADMISSION: Hemoglobin 13.8. WBC 8000. Urinalysis showed 3+ protein with 1 to 3 RBCs/HPF. SMAC was normal except for slight elevation of BUN at 38.

HOSPITAL COURSE: The patient underwent EGD by Dr. Arun Ramanathan on June 11 with findings of some mild erythema in the prepyloric area, but otherwise was unremarkable. CT scan of the abdomen was normal. Serum Gastrin was slightly elevated at 256 and gastric analysis was done with showed basal of 0.3 mEq/hr which was quite low, maximal acid output 7.1 which is also low and peak acid output of 10 mEQ/hr. The Zantac had been discontinued about 24 hours prior to gastric analysis. Lactose tolerance test was done and this showed normal curve. Barium enema was done which was grossly normal.

My impression is that the patient has elements of atrophic gastritis. He was started on Reglan while in the hospital and has shown marked improvement with regard to his nausea and abdominal discomfort. I suspect that he has some element of irritable bowel syndrome, and we are instituting high-fiber diet and continuing Regland and Zantac. He has been instructed to continue bland diet and to add additional foods one at a time. He is to return to my office in three weeks for follow up.

DISCHARGE MEDICATIONS: 1. Zantac 150 mg p.o. b.i.d.
                            2. Reglan 10 mg p.o. a.c. an h.s.
                            3. Restoril 30 mg h.s. p.r.n. sleep.
                            4. Darvocet-N 100 1 q.4h. p.r.n. pain.

Davida Hammett, MD

DH:BJ

D: 6/14/--
T: 6/14/--

FIGURE 1.6
Example of a Discharge Summary

- Whether goals were achieved
- Reason for and date of discharge
- The patient's current condition, status, and final prognosis
- Instructions given to the patient, noting any special needs such as restrictions in activities and medications

PAPER, ELECTRONIC, AND HYBRID MEDICAL RECORDS

Medical records are created and stored on paper, electronically, or in some combination called a **hybrid record.** Because of the advantages, health care leaders in business and government are pressing for laws to require all providers to switch to **electronic medical records (EMR).** An electronic medical record is a collection of health information that provides immediate electronic access by authorized users. In electronic medical records, documentation may be created in a variety of ways, but all words and images are ultimately viewable on a computer screen.

In the course of a lifetime, a patient may receive care from many different providers in physician offices, hospitals, emergency rooms, and home health settings. EMRs offer improved communications across the continuum of care from the primary care physician to the hospital and to other locations of patient care. These advantages are summarized in Table 1.1.

For example, one hospital's EMR system is set up so both the hospital staff and physicians who visit patients at the hospital can use it. In the hospital, an EMR contains nursing and ancillary department documentation, laboratory and radiology results, reports from the health information management (HIM) department, and electronic dates/signatures. A physician who comes to the hospital opens an

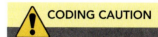 **CODING CAUTION**

EMRs?
The federal government, in Executive Order 13335, set the goal of using electronic records for all patients by 2014. However, due to cost, technical support, and privacy and security concerns, adoption of electronic records will be gradual. For the near term, most hospitals and physician practices will have hybrid systems.

Table 1.1 Advantages of Electronic Medical Records

Immediate access to health information: The EMR is simultaneously accessible to all qualified users. Compared to sorting through papers in a paper folder, an EMR database can save time when vital patient information is needed. Once information is updated in a patient record, it is available to all who need access, whether across the hall or across town.

Computerized physician order management: Physicians can enter orders for prescriptions, tests, and other services at any time, along with the patient's diagnosis.

Clinical decision support: An EMR system can provide access to the latest medical research on approved medical websites to help in medical decision making.

Automated alerts and reminders: The system can provide medical alerts and reminders for staff to ensure that patients are scheduled for regular screenings and other preventive practices. Alerts can also be created to identify patient safety issues, such as possible drug interactions.

Electronic communication and connectivity: An EMR system can provide a means of secure and easily accessible communication between physicians and staff and, in some offices, between physicians and patients.

Patient support: Some EMR programs allow patients to access their medical records and request appointments. These programs also offer patient education on health topics and instructions on preparing for common medical tests, such as cholesterol tests.

Administration and reporting: The EMR may include administrative tools, including reporting systems that enable facilities and medical practices to comply with federal and state reporting requirements.

Error reduction: An EMR can decrease medical errors that result from illegible chart notes, since notes are entered electronically on a computer or a handheld device. Nevertheless, the accuracy of the information in the EMR is only as good as the accuracy of the person entering the data; it is still possible to click the wrong button or enter the wrong letter.

Checkpoint 1.3

Nicholas J. Kramer, MD
2200 Carriage Lane
Currituck, CT 07886

Consultation Report
on John W. Wu
(Birth date 12/06/1942)

Dear Dr. Kramer:

At your request, I saw Mr. Wu today. This is a sixty-five-year-old male who stopped smoking cigarettes twenty years ago but continues to be a heavy pipe smoker. He has had several episodes of hemoptysis; a small amount of blood was produced along with some white phlegm. He denies any upper respiratory tract infection or symptoms on those occasions. He does not present with chronic cough, chest pain, or shortness of breath. I reviewed the chest X-ray done by you, which exhibits no acute process. His examination was normal.

A bronchoscopy was performed, which produced some evidence of laryngitis, tracheitis, and bronchitis, but no tumor was noted. Bronchial washings were negative.

I find that his bleeding is caused by chronic inflammation of his hypopharynx and bronchial tree, which is related to pipe smoking. There is no present evidence of malignancy.

Thank you for requesting this consultation.

Sincerely,

Mary Lakeland Georges, MD

This letter is in the patient medical record of John W. Wu.

What is the purpose of the letter?

How does it demonstrate the use of a patient medical record for continuity of care?

electronic "storage box" that contains documentation for him or her to read, correct, and sign. The documentation may have questions from coders in the HIM department for the doctor to resolve.

HIPAA

Because they work so intensively with patients' medical information in documentation, medical coders must understand the laws that govern the use of medical records. The most important legislation is called the **Health Insurance Portability and Accountability Act (HIPAA) of 1996.** This law is designed to:

- Protect people's private health information
- Ensure health insurance coverage for workers and their families when they change or lose their jobs
- Uncover fraud and abuse

Patients' medical records are legal documents that belong to the provider who created them. But the provider cannot withhold the *information* in the records from patients unless providing it would

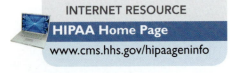

INTERNET RESOURCE
HIPAA Home Page
www.cms.hhs.gov/hipaageninfo

be detrimental to the person's health. This information belongs to the patient. Patients control the amount and type of information that is released, except for the use of the data to treat them or to conduct normal business transactions. Under HIPAA, only patients or their legally appointed representatives have the authority to authorize the release of information to anyone not directly involved in their care.

FOUR KEY HIPAA PROVISIONS

Medical coders need to protect the information in patients' records. At times, they need to know what information can be released about patients' conditions and treatments. What information can be legally shared among providers and payers? What information must the patient specifically authorize to be released? The answers to these questions are based on four parts of HIPAA:

1. *HIPAA Privacy Rule:* The privacy requirements cover patients' health information.
2. *HIPAA Security Rule:* The security requirements state the administrative, technical, and physical safeguards that are required to protect patients' health information.
3. *HIPAA Electronic Transaction and Code Sets Standards:* These standards require every provider who does business electronically to use the same health care transactions and code sets,
4. *HIPAA National Identifiers:* These standards require the use of national identifiers for employers (the Employer Identification Number or EIN, which is assigned by the Internal Revenue Service) and for providers (the National Provider Identifier or NPI assigned by the federal government).

Health care organizations that are required by law to obey the HIPAA regulations are called *covered entities*. A covered entity is an organization that electronically transmits any information that is protected under HIPAA. Three types of covered entities must follow the regulations:

1. *Health plans*: The individual or group health plan that provides or pays for medical care.
2. *Health care clearinghouses*: Companies that help providers handle such electronic transactions as submitting claims and that manage electronic medical record systems.
3. *Health care providers*: People or organizations that furnish, bill, or are paid for health care in the normal course of business. Other organizations that work for the covered entities, called *business associates,* must also agree to follow the HIPAA rules.

Study the HIPAA tip in the margin. Throughout your text, HIPAA tips help you understand HIPAA and its provisions.

HIPAA PRIVACY RULE

The HIPAA Standards for Privacy of Individually Identifiable Health Information rule is known as the **HIPAA Privacy Rule.** The HIPAA Privacy Rule is also often referred to by its number in the *Federal*

HIPAA TIP

Staying Current with HIPAA

HIPAA laws go through a lengthy review process before being released as final rules. Future changes are expected. Stay current with the changes that affect medical coders' areas of responsibility.

When a state law and the federal HIPAA provision both cover a particular situation, the law that is the strictest—the one with the toughest provisions—is followed.

Register, which is 45 CFR Parts 160 and 164. It was the first comprehensive federal protection for the privacy of health information. Its national standards protect individuals' medical records and other personal health information. Before the HIPAA Privacy Rule became law, the personal information stored in hospitals, physician practices, and health plans was governed by a patchwork of federal and state laws. Some state laws were strict, but others were not.

The Privacy Rule says that a covered entity must:

- Have a set of privacy practices that are appropriate for its health care services
- Notify patients about their privacy rights and how their information can be used or disclosed; have patients review and sign a form stating that they have received and reviewed the notice
- Train employees so that they understand the privacy practices
- Appoint a privacy official responsible for seeing that the privacy practices are adopted and followed
- Safeguard patients' records

Protected Health Information   The HIPAA privacy rule covers the use and disclosure of patients' **protected health information (PHI).** PHI is defined as individually identifiable health information that is transmitted or maintained by electronic media, such as over the Internet, by computer modem, or on magnetic tape or compact disks. This information includes a person's:

- Name
- Address (including street address, city, county, ZIP code)
- Relatives' and employers' names
- Birth date
- Telephone numbers
- Fax number
- E-mail address
- Social Security number
- Medical record number (MRN)
- Health plan beneficiary number
- Account number
- Certificate or license number
- Serial number of vehicle or other device
- Web site address
- Fingerprints or voiceprints
- Photographic images

Disclosure for Treatment, Payment, and Health Care Operations
Patients' PHI under HIPAA can be used and disclosed by providers for treatment, payment, and health care operations. Use of PHI means sharing or analysis within the entity that holds the information. Disclosure of PHI means the release, transfer, provision of access to, or divulging of PHI outside the entity holding the information.

Both use and disclosure of PHI are necessary and permitted for patients' **treatment, payment, and health care operations (TPO).** *Treatment* means providing and coordinating the patient's medical care; *payment* refers to the exchange of information with health plans; and *health care operations* are the general business management functions.

When using or disclosing protected health information, a covered entity must try to limit the information to the minimum amount of PHI necessary for the intended purpose. The **minimum necessary standard** means taking reasonable safeguards to protect PHI from incidental disclosure.

EXAMPLES

These examples comply with HIPAA:

- A medical coder does not disclose a patient's history of cancer on a workers' compensation claim for a sprained ankle. Only the information the recipient needs to know is given.

- A physician's assistant faxes appropriate patient cardiology test results before scheduled surgery at the hospital.

- A physician sends an e-mail message to another physician requesting a consultation on a patient's case.

- A patient's family member picks up medical supplies and a prescription.

Designated Record Set A covered entity must disclose individuals' PHI to them (or to their personal representatives) when they request access to, or an accounting of disclosures of, their PHI. Patients' rights apply only to a designated record set (DRS) that does not include all items. For example, in a physician office, the designated record set means the medical and billing records the provider maintains. It does not include appointment and surgery schedules, requests for lab tests, and birth and death records. It also does not include mental health information, psychotherapy notes, and genetic information.

Within this designated record set, patients have the right to:

- Access, copy, and inspect their PHI

- Request amendments to their health information

- Obtain accounting of most disclosures of their health information

- Receive communications from providers via other means, such as in Braille or in foreign languages

- Complain about alleged violations of the regulations and the provider's own information policies

Authorizations For use or disclosure other than for TPO, the covered entity must have the patient sign an **authorization** to release the information (see Figure 1.7). Processing a request for information involves careful checking and following the **release of information (ROI)** procedures.

Information about substance (alcohol and drug) abuse, sexually transmitted diseases (STDs) or human immunodeficiency virus (HIV), and behavioral/mental health services may not be released without a specific authorization from the patient. The authorization document must be in plain language and must include the following:

- A description of the information to be used or disclosed

- The name or other specific identification of the person(s) authorized to use or disclose the information

HIPAA TIP

Health Care Providers and the Minimum Necessary Standard

The minimum necessary standard does not apply to any type of disclosure—oral, written, phone, fax, e-mail, or other—among health care providers for treatment purposes.

HIPAA TIP

Protecting PHI

Take care not to discuss patients' cases with anyone not directly involved with their care, including family and friends. Avoid talking about cases, too, in areas where other patients might hear. Close charts on desks when they are not being worked on. Position computer screens so that only the person working with a file can view it.

INTERNET RESOURCE

Questions and Answers on Privacy of Health Information (HIPAA)

http://answers.hhs.gov

HIPAA TIP

PHI and Release of Information Document

A patient release of information document is not needed when PHI is shared for TPO under HIPAA. However, state law may require authorization to release data, and under HIPAA the strictest rule is enforced, so many practices and facilities ask patients to sign releases.

Patient Name: _____

Health Record Number: _____

Date of Birth: _____

1. I authorize the use or disclosure of the above named individual's health information as described below.

2. The following individual(s) or organization(s) are authorized to make the disclosure: _____

What specific information can be released

3. The type of information to be used or disclosed is as follows (check the appropriate boxes and include other information where indicated):
☐ problem list
☐ medication list
☐ list of allergies
☐ immunization records
☐ most recent history
☐ most recent discharge summary
☐ lab results (please describe the dates or types of lab tests you would like disclosed): _____
☐ x-ray and imaging reports (please describe the dates or types of x-rays or images you would like disclosed): _____
☐ consultation reports from (please supply doctors' names): _____
☐ entire record
☐ other (please describe): _____

4. I understand that the information in my health record may include information relating to sexually transmitted disease, acquired immunodeficiency syndrome (AIDS), or human immunodeficiency virus (HIV). It may also include information about behavioral or mental health services, and treatment for alcohol and drug abuse.

5. The information identified above may be used by or disclosed to the following individuals or organization(s):

Name: _____

Address: _____

Name: _____

Address: _____

To whom

For what purpose

6. This information for which I'm authorizing disclosure will be used for the following purpose:
☐ my personal records
☐ sharing with other health care providers as needed/other (please describe): _____

7. I understand that I have a right to revoke this authorization at any time. I understand that if I revoke this authorization, I must do so in writing and present my written revocation to the health information management department. I understand that the revocation will not apply to information that has already been released in response to this authorization. I understand that the revocation will not apply to my insurance company when the law provides my insurer with the right to contest a claim under my policy.

8. This authorization will expire (insert date or event): _____

If I fail to specify an expiration date or event, this authorization will expire six months from the date on which it was signed.

9. I understand that once the above information is disclosed, it may be redisclosed by the recipient and the information may not be protected by federal privacy laws or regulations.

10. I understand authorizing the use or disclosure of the information identified above is voluntary. I need not sign this form to ensure health care treatment.

Signature of patient or legal representative: _____ Date: _____

If signed by legal representative, relationship to patient

Signature of witness: _____ Date: _____

Distribution of copies: Original to provider; copy to patient; copy to accompany use or disclosure

Note: This sample form was developed by the American Health Information Management Association for discussion purposes. It should not be used without review by the issuing organization's legal counsel to ensure compliance with other federal and state laws and regulations.

FIGURE 1.7
Example of an Authorization to Use or Disclose Health Information

- The name of the person(s) or group of people to whom the covered entity may make the use or disclosure
- A description of each purpose of the requested use or disclosure
- An expiration date
- The signature of the individual (or authorized representative) and the date

In addition, the rule states that a valid authorization must include:

- A statement of the individual's right to revoke the authorization in writing
- A statement about whether the covered entity is able to base treatment, payment, enrollment, or eligibility for benefits on the authorization
- A statement that information used or disclosed after the authorization may be disclosed again by the recipient and may no longer be protected by the rule

Uses or disclosures for which the covered entity has received specific authorization from the patient do not have to follow the minimum necessary standard. Incidental use and disclosure are also allowed.

Exceptions There are a number of exceptions to the usual rules for release:

- Court orders
- Workers' compensation cases
- Statutory reports
- Research

All these types of disclosures must be logged, and the release information must be available to the patient who requests it.

De-Identified Health Information There are no restrictions on disclosing **de-identified health information** that neither identifies nor provides a reasonable basis to identify an individual. To prepare this type of document, all identifiers must be removed, such as names, medical record numbers, health plan beneficiary numbers, device identifiers (such as pacemakers), and biometric identifiers, such as fingerprints and voiceprints. Such de-identified records are also called *blinded* or *redacted* documents.

HIPAA SECURITY RULE

The **HIPAA Security Rule** requires covered entities to establish safeguards to protect PHI. The Security Rule specifies how to secure such protected health information on computer networks, the Internet, and storage disks such as CDs and flash drives. Security measures rely on *encryption*, the process of encoding information in such a way that only the person (or computer) with the key can decode it.

A number of other security measures help enforce the HIPAA Security Rule. These include:

- Access control, passwords, and log files to keep intruders out
- Backups to replace items after damage
- Security policies to handle violations that do occur

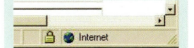

HIPAA ELECTRONIC HEALTH CARE TRANSACTIONS AND CODE SETS

The **HIPAA Electronic Health Care Transactions and Code Sets (TCS)** standards require providers and payers to exchange electronic data using a standard format and standard code sets.

Standard Transactions   The HIPAA transactions standards apply to the electronic data that are regularly sent back and forth between providers, health plans, and employers. Each standard is labeled with both a number and a name. Either the number (such as "the 837") or the name (such as the "HIPAA Claim") may be used to refer to the particular electronic document format.

Standard Code Sets   Under HIPAA, a **code set** is any group of codes used for encoding data elements, such as tables of terms, medical concepts, medical diagnosis codes, or medical procedure codes. Of great importance to medical coders are the code sets HIPAA requires for diseases, for medical procedures, and for supplies. These standards are listed in Table 1.2.

HIPAA NATIONAL IDENTIFIER STANDARDS

Likewise, HIPAA National Identifiers are assigned to employers and to providers. *Identifiers* are numbers of predetermined length and structure, such as a person's Social Security number. They are important because the unique numbers can be used in electronic transactions. These unique numbers can replace the many other numbers that are currently used.

ENFORCEMENT OF HIPAA

HIPAA privacy regulations are enforced by the **Office for Civil Rights (OCR).** When the OCR investigates a complaint, the covered entity must cooperate and provide access to its facilities, books, records, and systems, including relevant protected health information. Other rules are enforced by the **Centers for Medicare and Medicaid Services (CMS)**.

People who do not comply with HIPAA may be fined. Civil penalties for HIPAA violations are for covered entities, not for business associates, and can be up to $100 for each offense, with an annual

Table 1.2 HIPAA Standard Code Sets

Purpose	Standard	Guideline
Codes for diseases, injuries, impairments, and other health-related problems	International Classification of Diseases, Ninth Revision, Clinical Modification (ICD-9-CM), Volumes 1 and 2	*ICD-9-CM Official Guidelines for Coding and Reporting; Coding Clinic* (American Hospital Association)
Codes for procedures or other actions taken to prevent, diagnose, treat, or manage diseases, injuries, and impairments	Physicians' services: Current Procedural Terminology (CPT)	Guidelines within the code set and in the *CPT Assistant* (American Medical Association)
	Inpatient hospital services: International Classification of Diseases, Ninth Revision, Clinical Modification, Volume 3: Procedures	*ICD-9-CM Official Guidelines for Coding and Reporting; AHA Coding Clinic for ICD-9-CM* (American Hospital Association)
Codes for supplies, durable medical equipment, and other medical services	Healthcare Common Procedures Coding System (HCPCS)	Guidelines from the Centers for Medicare and Medicaid Services (CMS) and private payers

cap of $25,000 for repeated violations of the same requirement. Criminal penalties, which also apply to the covered entity but not necessarily to staff or business associates, include larger fees and/or prison sentences. Providers can also lose their contracts with payers and can be excluded from participation in all government health care programs.

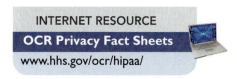

Checkpoint 1.4

Gloria Traylor, an employee of National Bank, called Marilyn Rennagel, a medical coder who works for Dr. Judy Fisk. The bank is considering hiring one of Dr. Fisk's patients, Juan Ramirez, and Ms. Traylor would like to know whether he has any known medical problems. Marilyn, in a hurry to complete the call and get back to work on this week's charts, quickly explains that she remembers that Mr. Ramirez was treated for depression some years ago, but that he has been fine since that time. She adds that she thinks he would make an excellent employee.

In your opinion, did Marilyn handle this call correctly?

What problems might result from her answers?

Medical Coding: Accurate and Compliant

Accurate and compliant medical coding follows a basic process that begins when the patient is given care in a physician office, hospital, or other setting and the provider documents the service. The medical coder works with this documentation, in full or in summary form, to follow the coding steps, which are summarized in Figure 1.8.

1. Assess the documentation for completeness and clarity.
2. Determine the appropriate provider, patient type, place, and payer for the service.
3. Abstract the diagnoses that were identified and procedures that were performed.
4. Assign accurate, complete diagnosis and procedure codes.
5. Verify that the assigned codes are compliant.
6. Release the assigned codes for billing.

STEP 1 ASSESS THE DOCUMENTATION FOR COMPLETENESS AND CLARITY

The medical coder first assesses the available documentation. Is the documentation complete, containing all the expected elements for the type of medical situation? Is the record legible, if written? Are diagnoses clearly stated, with sufficient detail about related conditions that affect the main condition?

If the answer to any of these points is *no*, the coder may query the physician for clarification. In most situations, the medical coder follows the practice or facility query procedure to secure the needed information.

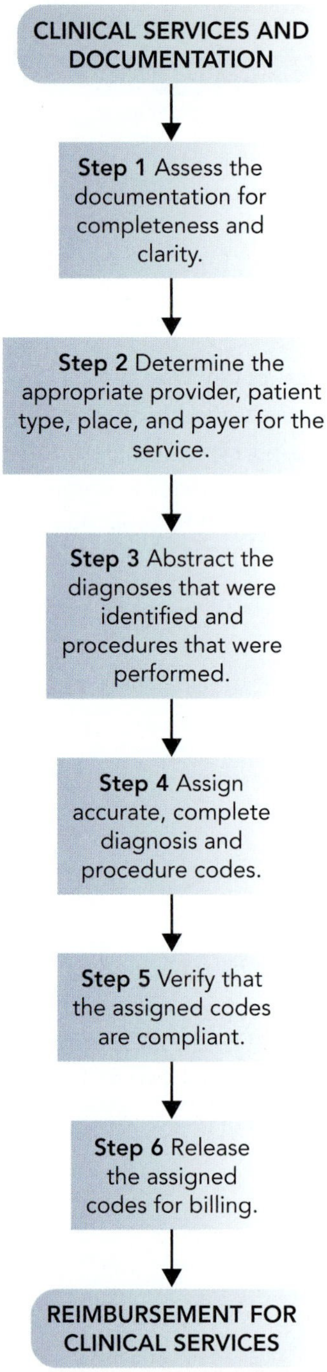

Step 1 Assess the documentation for completeness and clarity.

Step 2 Determine the appropriate provider, patient type, place, and payer for the service.

Step 3 Abstract the diagnoses that were identified and procedures that were performed.

Step 4 Assign accurate, complete diagnosis and procedure codes.

Step 5 Verify that the assigned codes are compliant.

Step 6 Release the assigned codes for billing.

REIMBURSEMENT FOR
CLINICAL SERVICES

FIGURE 1.8

Basic Code Assignment
Flow Chart

STEP 2 DETERMINE THE APPROPRIATE PROVIDER, PATIENT TYPE, PLACE, AND PAYER FOR THE SERVICE

The second step that the medical coder undertakes is to determine the appropriate provider, patient type, place, and payer for the service:

- *Provider*: The provider is the billing entity: either a physician or other professional practitioner (*professional billing*) or a facility such as a hospital (*facility billing*).
- *Patient type*: The patient type is determined by status as an outpatient (ambulatory) or inpatient.
- *Place of service*: The place of service may be an office, a facility, or another health care setting.
- *Payer*: The payer may be a private or self-funded payer, a government payer (Medicare, Medicaid, TRICARE, or CHAMPVA), or *self-pay*, the term used when the patient is responsible for the bills.

The answers that are determined direct the coder to the appropriate HIPAA code sets for researching the medical codes.

STEP 3 ABSTRACT THE DIAGNOSES AND PROCEDURES

In the third step in the medical coding process, the medical coder abstracts the diagnoses that were identified and procedures that were performed. Also included are other conditions the patient may have that affect treatment. Similarly, the procedures that the provider performed are identified. These may be medical, such as evaluation/management, diagnostic, or therapeutic, or surgical in nature.

As an example, consider this clinical chart note:

SUBJECTIVE: Patient complains of frequency of urination, urgency, and burning sensation for about 3–5 days. She denies hematuria. She has slight suprapubic discomfort. She has been treated for bladder infection in the past. Her last menstrual period was 4 days ago.

OBJECTIVE: She has very vague tenderness over the suprapubic area. Flanks are clear.

LAB: WBC 11,200. Urinalysis shows yellow, cloudy urine; specific gravity 1.015; 3–5 RBCs; 80–100 WBCs; and many bacteria.

ASSESSMENT: Urinary tract infection.

PLAN: Septra DS 1 b.i.d. × 10 days. Repeat urinalysis after that.

In this case, the patient's diagnosis can be isolated as urinary tract infection (UTI), and the procedure performed by the physician is an evaluation and management of her condition as well as a urinalysis and blood work. The doctor has prescribed medication as a result of the evaluation and orders a follow-up test postmedication.

STEP 4 ASSIGN ACCURATE AND COMPLETE DIAGNOSIS AND PROCEDURE CODES

In the fourth step in the medical coding process, the coder researches the HIPAA code sets and selects the correct medical codes to assign.

The diagnosis and the procedures that are documented in the patient's medical record should be logically connected (linked) to demonstrate the medical necessity of the charges. Codes cannot be based on what a coder assumed took place, only on what the documentation supports.

The codes assigned by coders must be accurate in terms of HIPAA. For example, HIPAA requires the use of codes that are current as of the date of service. Since codes are updated and changed every year (and sometimes more often), medical coders research the codes that are in use at that point. Medical coders also must assign codes based on the rules found in the published guidelines for the HIPAA code sets. As shown in Table 1.2 on page 26 both the diagnosis and procedure codes have particular guidelines to be observed.

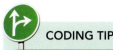

CODING TIP

Analyze; Don't Memorize!

How do coders increase their productivity? The many thousands of codes can't be memorized, but knowing the rules for assigning codes well enough to apply them efficiently is key.

STEP 5 VERIFY THAT THE ASSIGNED CODES ARE COMPLIANT

Compliance means actions that satisfy requirements. In the area of coding, compliance involves following the guidelines for correct code assignment and then following all other regulations to verify the code choice.

Regulations   Regulations are issued by the federal and state governments, as well as by other organizations that guard the interest of consumers receiving health care. The main federal government agency responsible for health care regulation is the Centers for Medicare and Medicaid Services, known as CMS (formerly the Health Care Financing Administration, or HCFA). An agency of the Department of Health and Human Services (HHS), CMS administers the Medicare and Medicaid programs to more than 90 million Americans. Every provider that receives payment from CMS, whether professional or facility, must comply with the *conditions of participation* that are issued by CMS. Individual states help CMS conduct surveys to certify Medicare and Medicaid providers and also regulate health care by licensing physicians and other clinical professionals to provide care.

A number of other nongovernmental organizations also regulate providers and health plans. Examples are:

- *The Joint Commission*: Formerly named the Joint Commission on Accreditation of Healthcare Organizations (JCAHO), **The Joint Commission** evaluates and accredits nearly fifteen thousand health care organizations and programs in the United States. For accreditation, an organization must undergo an on-site survey by a Joint Commission survey team at least every three years. (Laboratories must be surveyed every two years.) Joint Commission standards address the organization's level of performance in key functional areas, such as patient rights, patient treatment, and infection control. The Joint Commission also awards Disease-Specific Care Certification to health plans, disease management service companies, hospitals, and other care delivery settings that provide disease management and chronic care services for asthma, diabetes, congestive heart failure, coronary artery disease, chronic obstructive pulmonary disease, chronic kidney disease, skin and wound management, and primary stroke care.

INTERNET RESOURCE

CMS Home Page

www.cms.hhs.gov

INTERNET RESOURCE

The Joint Commission

www.jointcommission.org

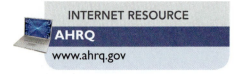
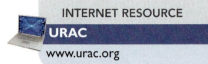
- *Agency for Healthcare Research and Quality (AHRQ):* AHRQ, a division of the federal Department of Health and Human Services, measures the various quality aspects of health care. It has established a scale of measurements called *quality indicators* that assess the results of patients' health care encounters, such as surgical complications.

- *URAC:* URAC, an independent nonprofit organization, promotes health care quality through its accreditation and certification programs. URAC offers a wide range of quality benchmarking programs and ensures that all stakeholders are represented in establishing meaningful quality measures for the entire health care industry.

Payer Policies   Through the policies they issue, payers also regulate the medical services that are covered as well as the coding and billing process used to submit health care claims. For example, some payers do not pay for certain procedure codes that are reported together for the same patient on the same day. Some policies do not cover preexisting conditions—those the patient had before signing an insurance contract—so if such a condition is the cause of the medical service, it is not paid by the insurance company.

Study the billing tip in the margin. Throughout your text, these marginal notes guide and advise you on coding-related billing points.

Fraud and Abuse   Another aspect of coding compliance is the topic of fraud and abuse. Although almost everyone involved in the delivery of health care is trustworthy and is devoted to patients' welfare, some are not. Health care fraud and abuse laws help control cheating in the health care system. Is this really necessary? The evidence says that it is. Cases filed under federal fraud laws resulted in court judgments or settlements of nearly $3.2 billion in 2006.

Fraud and Abuse Defined   **Fraud** is an act of deception used to take advantage of another person. For example, misrepresenting professional credentials and forging another person's signature on a check are fraudulent. Pretending to be a physician and treating patients without a valid medical license is also fraudulent. Fraudulent acts are intentional; the individual expects an illegal or unauthorized benefit to result.

Claims fraud occurs when health care providers or others falsely report charges to payers. A provider may bill for services that were not performed, overcharge for services, or fail to provide complete services under a contract. A patient may exaggerate an injury to get a settlement from an insurance company.

In federal law, **abuse** means an action that misuses money that the government has allocated, such as Medicare funds. Abuse is illegal because taxpayers' dollars are misspent. An example of abuse is an ambulance service that billed Medicare for transporting a patient to the hospital when the patient did not need ambulance service. This abuse—billing for services that were not medically necessary—resulted in improper payment to the ambulance company. Abuse is not necessarily intentional. It may be the result of ignorance of a billing rule or of inaccurate coding.

Fraud and Abuse Laws The major laws that address fraud and abuse are:

- The Health Care Fraud and Abuse Control Program, created under HIPAA and enforced by the HHS **Office of the Inspector General (OIG),** has the task of detecting health care fraud and abuse and enforcing all laws relating to them. The OIG works with the U.S. Department of Justice (DOJ), which includes the Federal Bureau of Investigation (FBI), under the direction of the U.S. Attorney General to prosecute those suspected of medical fraud and abuse.

- The federal False Claims Act (FCA), a related law, prohibits submitting a fraudulent claim or making a false statement or representation in connection with a claim. It also encourages reporting suspected fraud and abuse against the government by protecting and rewarding people involved in *qui tam*, or whistle-blower, cases. People who blow the whistle are current or former employees of insurance companies or of medical facilities, program beneficiaries, and independent contractors.

- The Deficit Reduction Act (DRA) of 2005 gives states financial incentives for setting up their own false claims acts to prevent false claims under the Medicaid program. This act also requires training hospital staff and outside vendors to make sure they investigate and report fraud.

INTERNET RESOURCE
OIG Home Page
http://oig.hhs.gov

OIG Enforcement The Office of the Inspector General (OIG) enforces rules relating to fraud and abuse. The intent to commit fraud does not have to be proved by the accuser for the provider to be found guilty. Actions that might be viewed as errors or occasional slips might also be seen as establishing a pattern of violations, which constitute the knowledge meant by "providers knew or should have known."

OIG has the authority to investigate suspected fraud cases and to *audit* the records of providers and payers. In an audit (which is a methodical examination), investigators review selected medical records to see whether the documentation supports the coding. The accounting records are often reviewed as well. When problems are found, the investigation proceeds and may result in charges of fraud or abuse against the provider.

Investigators look for patterns like these:

- Intentionally coding services that were not performed or documented

   EXAMPLE A lab bills Medicare for two tests when only one was done.

   EXAMPLE A physician asks a coder to report a physical examination that was just a telephone conversation.

- Coding services at a higher level than was carried out

   EXAMPLE After a visit for a flu shot, the provider bills the encounter as a comprehensive physical examination plus a vaccination.

- Performing and billing for procedures that are not related to the patient's condition and therefore are not medically necessary

EXAMPLE After reading an article about Lyme disease, a patient is worried about having worked in her garden over the summer, and she requests a Lyme disease diagnostic test. Although no symptoms or signs have been reported, the physician orders and bills for the *Borrelia burgdorferi* (Lyme disease) confirmatory immunoblot test.

Compliance Plans Because of the risk of fraud and abuse liability, facilities must be sure that rules and regulations are followed by all staff members. A wise slogan is that "the best defense is a good offense." For this reason, medical facilities have compliance plans to uncover and correct compliance problems to avoid risking liability.

A **compliance plan** is a written document that describes a process for finding, correcting, and preventing illegal activities. It is prepared by a *compliance officer* and committee that sets up the steps needed to (1) monitor compliance with government regulations, especially in the area of coding and billing, (2) have policies and procedures that are consistent, (3) provide for ongoing staff training and communication, and (4) respond to and correct errors. Having a compliance plan demonstrates to outside investigators like the OIG that honest, ongoing attempts have been made to find and fix weak areas.

Compliance plans cover more that coding and billing. They also cover other areas of government regulation, such as Equal Employment Opportunity (EEO) regulations (for example, hiring and promotion policies) and Occupational Safety and Health Administration (OSHA) regulations (for example, fire safety and handling of hazardous materials such as blood-borne pathogens).

Two parts of compliance plans are especially important to coders.

Physician Training Part of the compliance plan is a commitment to keep physicians trained in pertinent coding and regulatory matters. A medical coder may be assigned the task of briefing physicians on changed codes or medical necessity regulations. The following guidelines are helpful in conducting physician training classes:

- Keep the presentation as brief and straightforward as possible.
- In a multispecialty practice, issues should be discussed by specialty; all physicians do not need to know changed rules on dermatology, for example.
- Use actual examples, and stick to the facts when presenting material.
- Explain the benefits of coding compliance to the physicians, and listen to their feedback to improve job performance.
- Set up a way to address additional changes during the year, such as a newsletter or compliance meetings.

Staff Training The other key part of the compliance plan is a commitment to train staff members who are involved with coding and billing. Ongoing training also requires having the current annual updates, reading health plan bulletins and periodicals, and researching changed regulations. Compliance officers often conduct refresher classes in proper coding and billing techniques.

Study the compliance guideline in the margin. Throughout this program, compliance guidelines advise you on compliant coding.

COMPLIANCE GUIDELINE

Model Compliance Plans

OIG has developed a series of compliance program guidelines (CPGs) for hospitals; clinical laboratories; home health agencies; third-party billing companies; the durable medical equipment, prosthetics, orthotics, and supply industry; hospices; Medicare health plans; nursing facilities; physicians; ambulance suppliers; and pharmaceutical manufacturers. CPGs are intended to encourage the development and use of internal controls to monitor adherence to applicable statutes, regulations, and program requirements.

INTERNET RESOURCE

Model Compliance Programs

http://oig.hhs.gov/fraud/complianceguidance.html

COMPLIANCE GUIDELINE

Have It in Writing!

Do not code or bill services that are not supported by documentation, even if instructed to so do by a physician. Instead, report this kind of situation, ideally to a compliance officer, if the situation warrants doing so.

STEP 6 RELEASE THE ASSIGNED CODES FOR BILLING

The final step in the medical coding process is to release the verified codes for billing functions. Billers then develop the health care claims, transmit them to payers, and receive payments. Payments received are posted in the financial record, and patients are billed as appropriate for the amounts that insurance did not cover.

Checkpoint 1.5

Mary Kelley, a patient of the Good Health Clinic, asked Kathleen Culpepper, the employee who handles medical coding and billing, to help her out of a tough financial spot. Her medical insurance authorized her to receive four radiation treatments for her condition, one every thirty-five days. Because she was out of town, she did not schedule her appointment for the last treatment until today, which is one week beyond the approved period. The insurance company will not reimburse Mary for this procedure. She asks Kathleen to change the date on the record to last Wednesday so that it will be covered, explaining that no one will be hurt by this change and, anyway, she pays the insurance company plenty.

What type of action is Mary asking Kathleen to do?

How should Kathleen handle Mary's request?

Professionalism as a Medical Coder

Along with the importance of medical coding to physician practices and hospitals come the professional responsibilities of medical coders. Preparing for, securing, and advancing in medical coding positions require skills, attributes, ethical behavior, and achievements that demonstrate competence in the field.

SKILLS, ATTRIBUTES, AND ETHICS: THE COMPONENTS OF SUCCESS

Medical coders need three types of skills for success in their work (see Figure 1.9 on page 34):

1. Coding skill
2. Communications skill
3. Computer skill

Coding Skill Coding skill is developed through study followed by application, practice, and experience through employment. This skill is built on a strong foundation of medical terminology, anatomy, and physiology. Medical coders are knowledgeable about *pathophysiology*—identifying the clinical signs, symptoms, disease processes, and treatments of patients' conditions—and know how to relate these descriptions to diagnosis and procedure codes. They learn through training and experience to translate the clinical terms used in documentation into terms that relate directly to medical codes.

Communications Skill Communications skill—both written and verbal—is as important as knowing about specific code sets and regulations. Using a pleasant tone, a friendly attitude, and a helpful manner when gathering information increases patient satisfaction.

FIGURE 1.9
A Medical Coder's Skills

CODING SKILL
Anatomy &
physiology
Medical Terminology
Pathophysiology

HIPAA code sets
Official guidelines

COMPUTER SKILL
Microsoft Word
Electronic Health
Record (EHR)
Encoder
Grouper
Internet
Billing-related

COMMUNICATIONS
SKILL
Querying provider
Educating provider
Continuing
Education
Teamwork

Having interpersonal skills enhances the coding process by establishing professional, courteous relationships with people of different backgrounds and communication styles, both fellow workers and other people. Effective communicators have the skill of empathy; their actions convey that they understand the feelings of others.

Equally important are effective communications with physicians and other professional medical staff members. The correct terminology, used in the correct context, demonstrates knowledge of the clinical topic. Written requests for information should be brief and clear and should follow the query process and procedures. Conversations must be brief and to the point, showing that the speaker values the provider's time. People are more likely to listen when the speaker is smiling and has an interested expression, so speakers should be aware of their facial expressions and should maintain moderate eye contact.

Computer Skill Medical coders use information technology (IT)—computer hardware and software information systems—in almost all the health care environments in which they work. Computers not only improve business functions, like billing and collecting payments, but also aid the coding process in many ways.

Types of Computer Programs Because computers are used daily by most medical coders, the basic skills of file management with Microsoft Windows and document management using a word processor such as Microsoft Word are generally considered essential. Also essential is skill in Internet research. Using the Web effectively—and gaining the ability to judge the quality of information received—are valuable skills.

Building on this foundation, depending on the work setting, medical coders may receive training in the use of these major types of computer programs that relate to coding and billing work:

- *Billing-related (charge capture) programs* such as practice management programs (PMPs) that are used for billing in physician practices and charge description master (CDM) programs in facilities that hold a database of all medical services provided with their billing codes.
- *Electronic medical record (EMR) programs* that allow providers to create digital files of patients' care.
- *Encoder products—online coding tools—*that store digital versions of the HIPAA code sets, guidelines, and payer requirements.

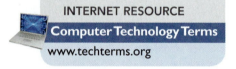

INTERNET RESOURCE
Computer Technology Terms
www.techterms.org

NOTE

You will learn more about online coding tools in Chapter 11 of your program.

- *Grouper* programs that are licensed by many facilities to analyze coded data and then produce reimbursement-related information. For example, a grouper can collect the diagnosis codes for all of a hospitalized patient's conditions and calculate the expected Medicare payment for that stay.
- *Computer-assisted coding (CAC)* products in that they can be used to electronically examine documentation and suggest codes for the medical coder to validate.

These various programs may be supplied in one of two ways in practices and facilities:

1. *Turnkey systems* are hardware and software owned by the practice or facility on which various programs are set up. These systems may be loaded on individual desktop personal computers or on a multiuser network.

2. An *application service provider (ASP)* approach, in which a vendor has software and data stored on its computers that are accessed by users over the Internet. Billed on a monthly subscription basis, ASP installations—which are also called *host-based*-- have many advantages. Data are often updated, as are HIPAA code sets with annual or more frequent code updates.

A Note of Caution: What Information Technology Cannot Do

Although computers increase efficiency and reduce errors, they are not more accurate than the individual who is entering the data. If people make mistakes while entering data, the information the computer produces will be incorrect. Computers are very precise and also very unforgiving. While the human brain knows that flu is short for influenza, the computer regards them as two distinct conditions. If a computer user accidentally enters a name as ORourke instead of O'Rourke, a human might know what is meant; the computer does not. It would probably respond with a message such as "No such patient exists in the database."

Attributes   A number of personal attributes are also very important for success as a medical coder. Most have to do with the quality of professionalism, which is key to getting and keeping employment. These factors include:

- *Appearance*: A neat, clean, professional appearance increases other people's confidence in your skills and abilities. When you are well-groomed, with clean hair, nails, and clothing, patients and other staff members see your demeanor as businesslike.
- *Attendance*: Being on time for work demonstrates that you are reliable and dependable.
- *Initiative*: Being able to start a course of action and stay on task is an important quality to demonstrate.
- *Courtesy*: Treating patients and fellow workers with dignity and respect helps build solid professional relationships at work.
- *Attention to detail:* Most aspects of the job involve paying close attention to detail, so this characteristic is essential for success.
- *Flexibility:* Working in an environment in which codes, regulations, and technology constantly change requires the ability to adapt to new procedures and to handle varying kinds of problems and interactions during a busy day.

- *Ability to work as a team member:* Patient service is a team effort. To do their part, medical coders must be cooperative and must focus on the best interests of the patients and the practice or facility.

Medical Ethics   Medical **ethics** are standards of behavior requiring truthfulness, honesty, and integrity. Ethics guide the behavior of physicians, who have the training, the primary responsibility, and the legal right to diagnose and treat human illness and injury. All individuals working in health-related professions share responsibility for observing the ethical code.

Each professional organization has a code of ethics that is to be followed by its members. In general, this code states that information about patients and other employees and confidential business matters should not be discussed with anyone not directly concerned with them. Behavior should be consistent with the values of the profession. For example, it is unethical for an employee to take money or gifts from a company in exchange for giving the company business. Study Figures 1.10 and 1.11, which are codes of ethics relating to medical coders.

AHIMA Code of Ethics 2004

Ethical Principles: The following ethical principles are based on the core values of the American Health Information Management Association and apply to all health information management professionals.

HIM professionals:

  I. Advocate, uphold, and defend the individual's right to privacy and the doctrine of confidentiality in the use and disclosure of information.
 II. Put service and the health and welfare of persons before self-interest and conduct themselves in the practice of the profession so as to bring honor to themselves, their peers, and to the health information management profession.
III. Preserve, protect, and secure personal health information in any form or medium and hold in the highest regard the contents of the records and other information of a confidential nature, taking into account the applicable statues and regulations.
IV. Refuse to participate in or conceal unethical practices or procedures.
 V. Advance health information management knowledge and practice through continuing education, research, publications, and presentations.
VI. Recruit and mentor students, peers, and colleagues to develop and strengthen professional work force.
VII. Represent the profession accurately to the public.
VIII. Perform honorably health information management association responsibilities, either appointed or elected, and preserve the confidentiality of any privileged information made known in any official capacity.
IX. State truthfully and accurately their credentials, professional education, and experiences.
 X. Facilitate interdisciplinary collaboration in situations supporting health information practice.
XI. Respect the inherent dignity and worth of every person.

FIGURE 1.10

AHIMA Code of Ethics

Copyright © 2005 American Health Information Management Association. Reprinted with permission.

FIGURE 1.11

Code of Ethical Standards, American Academy of Professional Coders
Copyright © 2007 American Academy of Professional Coders. Reprinted with permission.

SECURING AND ADVANCING ON THE JOB

Formal Education Completion of a medical coding or health information technology program at a postsecondary institution provides an excellent background for a coding position. Another possibility is to earn an associate degree or a certificate in a related curriculum area such as health care business services and learn on the job.

Job Experience Securing the first position can be challenging. Many jobs in hospitals and physician practices require both actual coding experience and coding certification. Simulated or actual experience starts with internships and/or externships. One type of internship is a capstone course in the curriculum in which students in class code de-identified patient charts, starting with simple cases and moving to more complex assignments; in another type, students are placed in doctors' offices and hospital coding departments for hands-on experience. Employers evaluate student work. Externships place students as unpaid assistants and provides mentoring, giving prospective employers a way to evaluate coding students.

Membership in Professional Organizations Moving ahead in a coding career is often aided by membership in and credentials from professional organizations. Student memberships are often available at a reduced cost. Recent graduates benefit from becoming full members, joining the local chapter of one of the national professional associations and volunteering to help with the chapter's activities. Some chapters of professional organizations may offer mentoring programs, in which a recently certified coder is employed in entry-level job under the tutelage of an established coding manager to "learn the ropes."

Certification as a Medical Coder Becoming a credentialed coder is also an important step because it shows prospective employers that the applicant has demonstrated a superior level of skill in medical coding. **Certification** is achieved by passing a written proficiency test given by a nationally recognized professional organization. Many job descriptions list certification as one of the hiring criteria for coding positions. Certification has a positive effect on the salaries of coders, as shown by the comparisons in Figure 1.12. Figure 1.12 shows that, in the AHIMA 2006 Salary Survey, average coder salaries rose with credentials (*AHIMA Advantage*, October 2006, p. 6). Further, the AAPC 2006 Salary Survey stated that certification is recognized throughout the country as adding value to the job description, with coders who are certified earning 21 percent more than those who are not (*AAPC Coding Edge*, September 26, 2006, p. 28).

AHIMA Two major organizations offer credentialing tests in the professional area of medical coding. AHIMA is the premier association of health information management (HIM) professionals. AHIMA's fifty thousand members are dedicated to the effective management of personal health information needed to deliver quality health care to the public. Founded in 1928 to improve the quality of medical records,

American Health Information Management Association (AHIMA)

233 North Michigan Avenue, Suite 2150

Chicago, Illinois 60601-5800

800-335-5535.

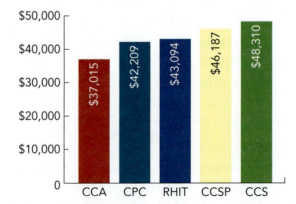

FIGURE 1.12

Effect of Certification on Salaries of Medical Coders
Source: AHIMA 2006 Salary Survey, Copyright © 2006 American Health Information Management Association. Reprinted with permission.

AHIMA is committed to advancing the HIM profession in an increasingly electronic and global environment through leadership in advocacy, education, certification, and lifelong learning.

AHIMA offers three coding certifications: the Certified Coding Associate (CCA), intended as a starting point for entering a new career as a coder; the Certified Coding Specialist (CCS); and the Certified Coding Specialist-Physician-based (CCS-P).

AAPC   The American Academy of Professional Coders' (AAPC) mission incorporates the establishment and maintenance of professional, ethical, and educational standards for all parties concerned with procedural coding. By becoming a member of the AAPC, a coder not only obtains a greater understanding of the coding field through education and networking, but also receives much deserved recognition as a coding professional. The AAPC has more than fifty-five thousand members.

The AAPC grants the Certified Professional Coder (CPC) and the Certified Professional Coder-Hospital (Outpatient) (CPC-H) certifications. It also offers the CPC-P, a payer certification; the CPC-A, an associate level for those who do not yet have medical coding work experience; and the following advanced specialty coding certifications:

- Evaluation and Management Specialist (EMS)
- General Surgery Specialist (GSS)
- Obstetrics and Gynecology Specialist (OGS)
- Orthopedics Specialist (OS)
- Emergency Medicine Specialist (EDS)
- Cardiology Specialist (CS)

Health Information Management (HIM) Education and Certification

Students who are interested in the professional area of health information management (also known as medical records) may complete an associate degree from an AHIMA-accredited college program and pass a credentialing test to be certified as a Registered Health Information Technician, or RHIT. An RHIT examines medical records for accuracy, reports patient data for reimbursement, and helps with information for medical research and statistical data.

Also offered is the Registered Health Information Administrator (RHIA), requiring a baccalaureate (four-year) degree and national certification. RHIAs are skilled in the collection, interpretation, and analysis of patient data. Additionally, they receive the training necessary to manage these functions. RHIAs interact with all levels of an organization—clinical, financial, and administrative—that use patient data in decision making and everyday operations. Both the RHIA and the RHIT national certification examinations have a coding component aimed at demonstrating the knowledge needed to supervise or manage the coding function.

Two other advanced certifications are available from AHIMA. With the National Cancer Registrars Association (NCRA), AHIMA has certification in the cancer registry profession through the Certified Tumor Registrar (CTR) examination. To show proficiency in HIPAA, AHIMA has a CHPS (Certified in Healthcare Privacy and Security) certification.

INTERNET RESOURCE
AHIMA
www.ahima.org

CODING TIP

According to AHIMA, more than 90 percent of health care executives understand the importance of continuing education for credential maintenance, and most also agree that employing credentialed professionals reduces exposure to fraud and abuse charges.

American Academy of Professional Coders

2480 South 3850 West, Suite B

Salt Lake City, Utah 84120

800-626-2633

INTERNET RESOURCE
AAPC
www.aapc.com

⚠ **CODING CAUTION**

Specialization as a Coder
The provider (facility or professional), the type and place of service (inpatient or outpatient), and the payer (insurance carrier) all affect the medical coding of patients' diagnoses and procedures. For this reason, after receiving their basic training, medical coders often specialize in either physician practice coding or facility coding. Likewise, facility coders may specialize in either outpatient or inpatient coding.

Table 1.3 Selected Job Titles and Descriptions

Job Title	Description
Entry-level coder	Coding basics/CCA or CPC-A
Coding specialist	On-the-job training/CCS, CCS-P, or CPC/CPC-H
Coding manager	Supervisory position: Bachelor of Science degree; RHIT or RHIA Certification and 5+ years of experience
Coding consultant/auditor	Consulting position: 4-year degree with management experience and business experience

CONTINUING YOUR EDUCATION THROUGHOUT YOUR CAREER

Most professional organizations require credentialed members to keep up to date by taking annual training courses to refresh or extend their knowledge. Continuing education sessions are assigned course credits by the credentialing organizations, and satisfactory completion of a test on the material is often required for credit.

Under their compliance plans, employers often approve attendance at coding seminars that apply to the practice or facility's medical setting and ask the person who attends to update other staff members.

Further baccalaureate and graduate study can enable advancement to managerial positions in physician practices and health information management departments. As shown in Table 1.3, there are many opportunities for coding and health information management personnel at all levels.

A LOOK TO THE FUTURE

Many experts think that technology will continue to change the work of medical coders. Coders' skills will remain in demand, but in a different form. It is likely that initial code assignment will increasingly be done using computer-assisted coding, but the final coding will be validated by coders who act as editors, using their critical thinking and communication skills to ensure accurate coding that reflects documentation, whether in printed or electronic form. In any event, the demand for and rewards of a medical coding career appear to have a very strong future.

CODING TIP

Moving Ahead in Your Career

Professional certification, additional study, and work experience contribute to advancement to positions such as medical coding manager. Coders may also advance through specialization in a field, such as radiology coding.

Checkpoint 1.6

Consider medical ethics, and answer the questions that follow these cases.

1. Dorita McCallister, who works for the Clark Clinic, ordered medical office supplies from her cousin, Gregory Hand. When the supplies arrived, Gregory came to the office to check on them and to take Dorita out to lunch.

Is Dorita's purchase of supplies from her cousin ethical? Why?

2. George McGrew is a medical coder in the practice of Dr. Sylvia Grets. Over the last few weeks, Dr. Grets has consistently written down codes that stand for lengthy procedures, but George knows that these visits were all very short.

Is it ethical for George to code these visits as the physician has indicated?

Summary

1. Medical coding creates coded data based on the documentation of patients' medical diagnoses and services. The data are used both to continually improve the delivery of health care and to provide a bridge between the clinical data and the billing process that generates payment for medical services to physicians and facilities.

2. Medical necessity means that the services provided to a patient are reasonable and are required for the diagnosis or treatment of the patient's condition, illness, or injury or to improve the functioning of a malformed body member. For bills to be paid by insurance companies, the medical codes must clearly show the link between the patient's diagnosis and the treatments and procedures provided.

3. Medical coders may be employed by facilities such as hospitals in the inpatient coding setting or by hospital ambulatory departments or physician practices for outpatient coding. Nontraditional employment includes positions at insurance companies and consulting, teaching, and auditing positions.

4. Patients' medical records, which contain the complete, chronological, and comprehensive documentation of their health history and status, are used by providers to communicate and coordinate health care and as the basis for medical coding. Documentation of an examination includes the chief complaint (CC), the history, the examination, the diagnosis/assessment, and the treatment plan. The process leading to the patient's informed consent for procedures is also documented. A progress report documents a patient's response to a treatment plan and provides justification for continued treatment. At the end of a treatment plan, a discharge summary documents the patient's final status and prognosis. The importance of the documentation in medical records in the medical coding process cannot be overstated: If a diagnosis or procedure is not documented, it cannot be coded, and therefore it cannot be billed.

5. Under HIPAA, covered entities are required to safeguard protected health information (PHI), defined as individually identifiable health information that is transmitted or maintained by electronic media, including data such as a patient's name, Social Security number, address, and phone number. For use or disclosure for treatment, payment, or health care operations (TPO), no release is required from the patient. To release PHI for other than TPO, a covered entity must have an authorization signed by the patient. The authorization document must be in plain language and have a description of the information to be used, who can disclose it and for what purpose, who will receive it, an expiration date, and the patient's signature.

6. The HIPAA Privacy Rule regulates the use and disclosure of patients' protected health information (PHI). The HIPAA Security Rule requires covered entities to establish administrative, physical, and technical safeguards to protect the confidentiality, integrity, and availability of health information. The HIPAA Electronic Health Care Transactions and Code Sets

establish standards for the exchange of financial and administrative data among covered entities. The standards require covered entities to use common electronic transaction methods and medical code sets. The HIPAA National Identifier standards require the use of the EIN for employers and the National Provider Identifier (NPI) for providers.

7. The basic steps in the medical coding process are to (a) assess the documentation for completeness and clarity, (b) determine the appropriate provider, patient type, place, and payer for the service, (c) abstract the diagnoses that were made and procedures that were performed, (d) assign accurate, complete diagnosis and procedure codes, (e) verify that the assigned codes are compliant, and (f) estimate the charges for the assigned codes and release them for billing.

8. HIPAA requires accurate coding using current code sets and following published coding guidelines. Federal and state regulations, voluntary accreditation organizations, and payers' policies dictate the terms of compliant medical coding.

9. Medical coders must exhibit three kinds of skills for career success: clinical coding skill, computer skill, and communication skill. Important attributes are professional appearance, punctual attendance, initiative, courtesy, attention to detail, flexibility, and ability to work as a team member. Medical ethics are standards of behavior requiring truthfulness, honesty, and integrity.

10. Certification as a medical coder is achieved by passing a written proficiency test given by one of two nationally recognized professional organizations, AHIMA and the AAPC. AHIMA has three coding certifications: the Certified Coding Associate (CCA), the Certified Coding Specialist (CCS), and the Certified Coding Specialist-Physician-based (CCS-P). The AAPC grants the Certified Professional Coder (CPC) and the Certified Professional Coder-Hospital (Outpatient) (CPC-H) certifications. The AAPC also offers the CPC-P, a payer certification; the CPC-A, an apprentice level for those who do not yet have medical coding work experience; and advanced specialty coding certifications.

Review Questions: Chapter 1

Match the key terms with their definitions.

a. health information management (HIM) _____
b. HIPAA Privacy Rule _____
c. provider _____
d. medical necessity _____
e. code set _____
f. compliance _____
g. protected health information (PHI) _____
h. treatment, payment, and health care operations (TPO) _____

i. documentation _____

j. medical coding _____

1. HIPAA law regulating the use and disclosure of patients' protected health information—individually identifiable health information that is transmitted or maintained by electronic media

2. The systematic, logical, and consistent recording of a patient's health status—history, examinations, tests, results of treatments, and observations—in chronological order in a patient's medical record

3. A coding system used to encode elements of data

4. Actions that follow and satisfy official guidelines and requirements

5. Under HIPAA, the purposes for which patients' protected health information may be shared without authorization

6. Individually identifiable health information that is transmitted or maintained by electronic media

7. Person or entity that supplies medical or health services and bills for or is paid for the services in the normal course of business; may be a professional member of the health care team, such as a physician, or a facility, such as a hospital or skilled nursing home

8. The process of analyzing the documentation of patients' diagnoses and procedures and assigning accurate, compliant codes based on HIPAA-mandated code sets

9. Payment criterion of payers that requires medical treatments to be appropriate and provided in accordance with generally accepted standards of medical practice

10. Department in a facility that manages patients' medical records to ensure quality of data

Decide whether each statement is true or false.

1. The terms *outpatient* and *ambulatory* have the same meaning. **T or F**

2. Fraud is not intentional. **T or F**

3. The chief complaint is usually documented using clinical terminology. **T or F**

4. An inpatient is usually released from a facility within fifteen to eighteen hours. **T or F**

5. When federal and state privacy laws disagree, the federal rule is always followed. **T or F**

6. Medical coders work only for hospitals. **T or F**

7. Protected health information includes the various numbers assigned to patients, such as their medical record numbers. **T or F**

8. The minimum necessary standard does not refer to the patient's health history. **T or F**

9. Patients do not have the right to access, copy, inspect, and request amendment of their medical records. **T or F**

10. A patient's authorization is needed to disclose protected information for payment purposes. **T or F**

Select the letter that best completes the statement or answers the question.

1. The correct link between a patient's condition and the services a provider performed demonstrates
   a. the minimum necessary standard
   b. HIPAA Security Rule
   c. the medical necessity of the services for payment
   d. release of information

2. An encounter is
   a. an operation
   b. an office visit
   c. a chemotherapy infusion
   d. all of the above

3. A patient's PHI may be released without authorization to

   a. local newspapers

   b. an anesthesiologist who will anesthetize the patient during a scheduled surgery

   c. friends who visit the patient during a hospital stay

   d. a lawyer who calls for information

4. Which government group has the authority to enforce the HIPAA Privacy Rule?

   a. CIA

   b. OIG

   c. OCR

   d. Medicaid

5. When PHI is correctly requested, what is the only information the HIM department releases?

   a. de-identified information

   b. code set data

   c. minimum necessary data

   d. a copy of the entire file

6. The authorization to release information must specify

   a. the number of pages to be released

   b. the Social Security number of the patient

   c. the entity to whom the information is to be released

   d. the name of the treating physician

7. Health information that does not identify an individual is referred to as

   a. protected health information

   b. authorized health release

   c. statutory data

   d. de-identified health information

8. Coding credentials that can be earned include

   a. CCP-A, CPC, CCS, and CCS-P

   b. RHIT, RHIA, and MBA

   c. CHS, ROI, and MRN

   d. none of the above

9. Medical coders assign codes based on the requirements of the

   a. HIPAA Privacy Rule

   b. HIPAA Security Rule

   c. HIPAA Electronic Health Care Transactions and Code Sets standards

   d. Health Care Fraud and Abuse Control Program

10. Skills required for medical coding include knowledge of

    a. anatomy and physiology

    b. disease processes

    c. medical terminology

    d. all of the above

Define the following abbreviations.

1. OCR _____

2. OIG _____

3. MRN _____

4. PHI _____

5. HIPAA _____

6. TPO _____

7. EMR _____

8. HIM _____

9. CMS _____

10. ROI _____

List the six steps in the medical coding process.

1. _____

2. _____

3. _____

4. _____

5. _____

Applying Your Knowledge

BUILDING CODING SKILLS

Case 1.1

In each of these cases of release of PHI, was the HIPAA privacy rule followed?

1. A laboratory communicates a patient's medical test results to a physician by phone.

2. A physician mails a copy of a patient's medical record to a specialist who intends to treat the patient.

3. A hospital faxes a patient's health care instructions to a nursing home to which the patient is to be transferred.

4. A doctor discusses a patient's condition over the phone with an emergency room physician who is providing the patient with emergency care.

5. Bedside, a doctor orally discuss a patient's treatment regimen with a nurse who will be involved in the patient's care.

6. A physician consults with another physician by e-mail about a patient's condition.

7. A hospital shares an organ donor's medical information with another hospital that is treating the organ recipient.

8. A medical assistant answers a health plan's questions about a patient's dates of service on a submitted health claim over the phone.

Case 1.2

The following chart note contains typical documentation abbreviations and shortened forms for words.

65-yo female; hx of right breast ca seen in SurgiCenter for bx of breast mass. Frozen section reported as benign tumor. Bleeding followed the

biopsy. Reopened the breast along site of previous incision with coagulation of bleeders. Wound sutured. Pt adm. for observation of post-op bleeding. Discharged with no bleeding recurrence.
Final Dx: Benign neoplasm, left breast.

Research the meaning of each abbreviation (see the abbreviations list at the end of the text), and write the meanings.

1. yo _____

2. hx _____

3. ca _____

4. bx _____

5. Pt _____

6. adm. _____

7. op _____

8. Dx _____

USING CODING TERMS

Case 1.3

In the letter from Dr. Georges to Dr. Kramer on page 20, identify and define the patient's symptom using clinical terms.

1. _____

What procedure did Dr. Georges perform?

2. _____

Case 1.4

The following chart note is on file for a female patient:

Rayelle Smith-Jones
2/14/2008

SUBJECTIVE: The mother brought in this 1-month-old female. The patient is doing very well. They have been using the phototherapy blanket. She is thirsty, has good yellow stooling, and continues on formula. Her alertness is normal. Other pertinent ROS is noncontributory.

OBJECTIVE: Afebrile. Comfortable. Jaundice is only minimal at this time. No scleral icterus. Good activity level. Normal fontanel. TMs, nose, mouth, pharynx, neck, heart, lungs, abdomen, liver, spleen, and groins are normal. Normal cord care and circumcision. Good extremities.

ASSESSMENT: Resolving physiological jaundice on phototherapy.

PLAN: Will stop phototherapy and do a bilirubin level in a couple of days to make sure there is no rebound. The patient is to be seen in one week. Push fluids. Routine care was discussed.

MD/xx

1. Identify the patient: _____

2. What abnormal condition does the patient have? _____

3. Is the abnormal condition getting better or worse? _____

4. What test is ordered? _____

Researching the Internet

1. The Internet is a valuable source of information about many topics of interest to medical coders. For example, to explore career opportunities, study the job statistics gathered by the *Occupational Outlook Handbook* of the Bureau of Labor Statistics at http://stats.bls.gov/oco. Using the site map at that home page, choose Keyword Search of BLS Web Pages, and enter a job title of interest, such as health information technicians. In particular, review the job outlook information.

2. Visit the website at www.alliedhealthcareers.com, and, using the Search feature, research positions available in the category Health Information Management/Medical Records. List five job titles that you find in the coding area.

3. Visit AHIMA's website for information about certification at www.ahima.org/certification/, and review the criteria for applying for the CCS versus the CCA examinations. Report on the major differences in their requirements.

4. Visit the AAPC website about certification at www.aapc.com/certification/index.aspx, and report on the three apprentice-level certifications that are offered.

5. Both the Computer-based Patient Record Institute (CPRI) and the Medical Record Institute promote the development of the electronic (computer-based) medical record. Go to www.cpri.org/ and www.medrecinst.com/, and research the present status of electronic medical records in the United States. From your reading, explain how electronic records can improve patient care.

Introduction to ICD-9-CM

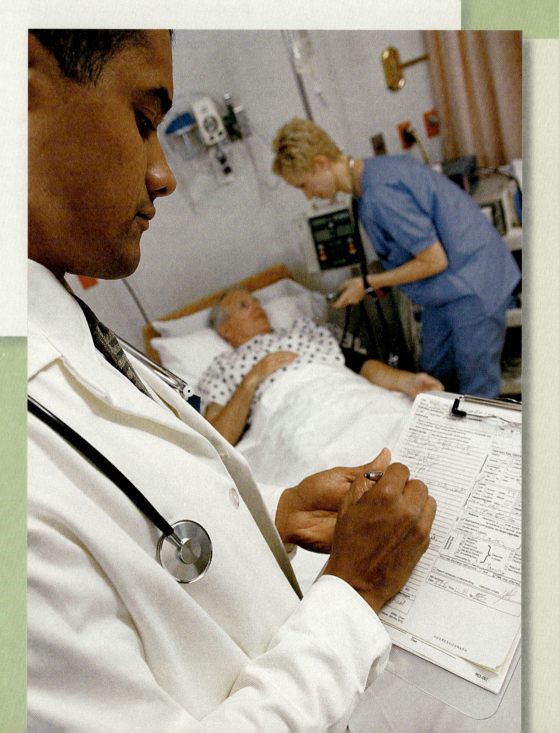

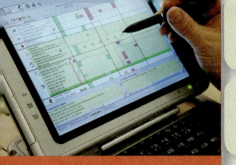

ICD-9-CM Basics

LEARNING OUTCOMES

After studying this chapter, you should be able to:

1. Briefly discuss the background and history of ICD-9-CM.

2. Discuss the roles of the NCHS, CMS, AHIMA, and the AHA in maintaining and updating ICD-9-CM codes.

3. Explain how to locate the periodic updates to ICD-9-CM codes using the Internet.

4. Identify five uses of ICD-9-CM.

5. Discuss the importance of the *ICD-9-CM Official Guidelines for Coding and Reporting.*

6. Describe the organization and content of Volumes 1, 2, and 3 of ICD-9-CM.

7. Interpret the formats, conventions, and symbols used in ICD-9-CM.

8. List the basic process of assigning ICD-9-CM codes.

9. Describe the meaning of coding to the highest level of specificity.

10. Identify common medical resources used to assist in the assignment of accurate ICD-9-CM codes.

Key Terms

addenda

AHA Coding Clinic® for ICD-9-CM

Alphabetic Index (Volume 2)

Alphabetic Index to External Causes of Disease and Injury

Alphabetic Index and Tabular List of Procedures (Volume 3)

American Hospital Association (AHA)

braces

brackets

carryover lines

category

Centers for Disease Control (CDC)

chapter

code first underlying disease

colon

conventions

cooperating parties

cross-references

E code

encoder

eponym

etiology

excludes

ICD-9-CM Coordination and Maintenance Committee

ICD-9-CM Official Guidelines for Coding and Reporting

ICD-10-CM

includes

International Classification of Diseases Adapted for Indexing of Hospital Records and Operation Classification (ICDA)

International Classification of Diseases, Ninth Revision, Clinical Modification (ICD-9-CM)

lozenge

main term

manifestation

modifiers

morbidity

mortality

National Center for Health Statistics (NCHS)

not elsewhere classified (NEC)

not otherwise specified (NOS)

notes

omit code

parentheses

section mark

subcategory

subclassification

subterm

supplemental classification system

Table of Drugs and Chemicals

Tabular List (Volume 1)

use additional code

V code

World Health Organization (WHO)

Chapter Outline

History and Purpose of ICD-9-CM

ICD-9-CM Basic Coding Process

Alphabetic Index (Volume 2)

Tabular List (Volume 1)

Alphabetic Index and Tabular List of Procedures (Volume 3)

ICD-9-CM Conventions

ICD-9-CM Coding Resources

Standard diagnosis codes represent diseases, injuries, and conditions that affect health. Because these codes reflect the reasons for services rendered, accurately reporting them is important for health care reimbursement, research, quality measurement, and management decisions. Reporting a diagnosis code communicates the reason for a medical visit, such as chest pain, and demonstrates the medical necessity of the services. Knowledge of medical terminology, anatomy and physiology, and current coding guidelines is essential to accurately assign diagnosis codes. Resources are available for coders to use, such as printed codebooks with useful enhancements, medical dictionaries, drug references, and national guidelines.

History and Purpose of ICD-9-CM

The classification system used to record all diagnoses for medical visits in the United States is the **International Classification of Diseases, Ninth Revision, Clinical Modification,** called **ICD-9-CM.** This coding system is maintained by the **National Center for Health Statistics (NCHS)** and the Center for Medicare and Medicaid Services (CMS), both of which are departments of the federal Department of Health and Human Services. The ICD-9-CM code set is organized in three volumes. Volumes 1 and 2 are used to classify diagnoses, and Volume 3 is used to classify inpatient procedures that are billed by hospitals.

ICD-9-CM BACKGROUND

HIPAA TIP

Mandated Code Set

ICD-9-CM is the mandated code set for medical diagnoses and hospital inpatient services.

The ICD-9-CM code set is modeled after the International Classification of Diseases, which is used throughout the world and maintained by the **World Health Organization (WHO).** In 1959, the U.S. Public Health Service published the **International Classification of Diseases, Adapted for Indexing of Hospital Records and Operation Classification (ICDA).** This system was revised over the years to accommodate the need to classify **morbidity,** the rate of incidences of diseases, and **mortality** (death) in the United States. In 1978, the World Health Organization published a ninth revision of ICD called ICD-9. The next year, in order to meet statistical data needs in the United States, the U.S. Public Health Service published its modified code set (the *CM* in the title means *clinically modified*). This expanded three-volume set is now known as ICD-9-CM. It includes more than thirteen thousand codes and uses more digits in those codes than does ICD-9, making it possible to specifically describe more diseases.

BILLING TIP

Inpatient and Outpatient Procedures

Use Volume 3 of ICD-9-CM for *inpatient* procedures, and use CPT (covered in Chapters 6 through 10 of your program) for *outpatient* procedures.

HIPAA considers Volumes 1 and 2 of ICD-9-CM to be the required code set for diseases, injuries, impairments, other health problems and their manifestations, and other causes of injury, disease, and impairment. Volume 3 of ICD-9-CM is the required code set for procedures or actions performed for inpatients and billed by hospitals.

ICD-9-CM TODAY

To keep current with medical trends in disease management, ICD-9-CM is updated every year. The responsibility for maintaining ICD-9-CM is divided between the National Center for Health Statistics (NCHS), a part of the **Centers for Disease Control (CDC),** which maintains Volumes 1 and 2, and CMS, which maintains Volume 3.

COMPLIANCE GUIDELINE

Use Current Codes

Compliant coding under HIPAA requires codes to be current as of the date of service. Do not report codes that are no longer in the code set.

The federal **ICD-9-CM Coordination and Maintenance Committee** considers coding modifications that have been proposed to ICD-9-CM. This committee is cochaired by representatives from CMS and NCHS. Interested parties from the public and private sectors can propose changes to ICD-9-CM. The committee's role is advisory, and the final determination of code changes is made by the administrator of CMS and the director of NCHS.

The Addenda: Updating ICD-9-CM NCHS and CMS release ICD-9-CM updates called the **addenda** that take effect on October 1 and April 1 of every year. The October 1 changes are the major updates; the April 1 changes catch up on codes that were not included in the major changes. The major new, invalid, and revised codes are posted on the

INTERNET RESOURCE

ICD-9-CM Coordination and Maintenance Committee

www.cdc.gov/nchs/about/otheract/icd9/maint/maint.htm

INTERNET RESOURCE

ICD-9-CM Code Updates

www.cms.hhs.gov/icd9providerdiagnosticcodes

CMS Internet website by the beginning of July for HIPAA-mandated use as of October 1 of the year. New codes must be used as of the date they go into effect, and invalid (deleted) codes must not be used.

Codebooks   The U.S. Government Printing Office (GPO) publishes the official ICD-9-CM code set on the Internet and in CD-ROM format every year. Various commercial publishers include the updated codes in annual coding books that are printed soon after the major updates are released. Both physician practice (Volumes 1 and 2) and hospital-based (all three volumes) codebooks are published. Many different features are available in these codebooks, ranging from straightforward code listings to enhanced manuals with many notes, illustrations, and tips helpful to coders. No matter which codebook is chosen, medical coders must have the current reference in order to select HIPAA-compliant codes.

OFFICIAL ICD-9-CM GUIDELINES

The HIPAA Final Rule, in addition to mandating the ICD-9-CM code set, also requires the use of the *ICD-9-CM Official Guidelines for Coding and Reporting* when codes are selected. These guidelines assist in standardizing the assignment of ICD-9-CM codes for all users. For example, they include the rules for selecting the principal diagnosis when a patient has more than a single condition, assist the coder in understanding the basic rules of code selection using ICD-9-CM, and explain certain coding rules for specific medical conditions. Table 2.1 outlines the *Official Guidelines.*

The *Official Guidelines* are the basis of consistent and accurate ICD-9-CM reporting. They are written by NCHS and CMS and approved by the **cooperating parties,** made up of the **American Hospital Association (AHA),** the American Health Information Management Association (AHIMA), CMS, and NCHS.

PURPOSES OF ICD-9-CM

ICD-9-CM is a statistical tool used to convert medical diagnoses and inpatient hospital procedures into numbers. The code set has five primary applications.

Reporting and Research   The statistical data are used for a variety of reasons throughout the world to provide a consistent, defined way of reporting. For example, to report that patients have the disease of chest pain, medical coders assign an ICD-9-CM code that always classifies chest pain the same way. Imagine trying to

<aside>

NOTE

The *ICD-9-CM Official Guidelines for Coding and Reporting* are provided on this program's Online Learning Center (OLC). These guidelines will be cited often as you build your coding skills.

CODING TIP

Follow the *Official Guidelines*

Always base assignment of ICD-9-CM codes on the *Official Guidelines.*

INTERNET RESOURCE

ICD-9-CM Official Guidelines

www.cdc.gov/nchs/datawh/ftpserv/ftpicd9/icdguide07.pdf

</aside>

Table 2.1 Major Sections of the *ICD-9-CM Official Guidelines for Coding and Reporting*	
Section	**Content**
I	Conventions, general coding guidelines, and chapter-specific guidelines
II	Selection of Principal Diagnosis
III	Reporting Additional Diagnoses
IV	Diagnostic Coding and Reporting Guidelines for Outpatient Services
Appendix I	Present on Admission Reporting Guidelines

gather data on diseases if the conditions were listed alphabetically; chest pain could be reported in different ways, such as "pain in the chest" and "pain: chest." Having diagnoses and procedures reported in a consistent manner is essential for a variety of uses.

ICD-9-CM codes are also very important in the study of medication effects on patients with certain diseases. For example, if a pharmaceutical company wants to research the effects of a new drug on patients with lung cancer, ICD-9-CM codes can be used to identify a patient population with that disease and to include those patients in the study. Researchers can also use ICD-9-CM to look at trends in health care among different patient groups. Federal agencies such as the CDC conduct research and report health care data using ICD-9-CM codes (see Figure 2.1). The CDC's annual report of the number of patients discharged from hospitals by disease and by age is based on ICD-9-CM codes. At the national and state levels, the code set is used to track cases of prevalent conditions such as HIV, influenza, pneumonia, and other communicable diseases.

Monitoring the Quality of Patient Care The quality of the care provided to patients can be measured in many ways, and ICD-9-CM often plays an important role. For example, all of a hospital's patients with hip replacements may be asked to complete questionnaires about their pain control after surgery. To perform this survey, researchers identify the patients who underwent hip replacements by the ICD-9-CM code listed in their medical records. Other examples include monitoring quality of care by collecting statistics on treatment for heart attacks and death rates of patients with particular diseases. Evaluating quality of care for people with certain diagnoses or procedures allows health care providers to improve services.

Communications and Transactions Because ICD-9-CM is a nationally used classification system, the code meanings are a method of consistent communication. Providers can communicate with payers about the reason for services (the diagnoses) and the services provided (the procedures) using ICD-9-CM. Payer policies often use code numbers in communications to providers. For example, a Medicare coverage policy is often explained by listing the diagnosis codes that are appropriate for a set of procedure codes.

Reimbursement Much of the focus of ICD-9-CM is insurance reimbursement. Payment for services rendered to hospital inpatients is based on their diseases and conditions. If the health care visit is not coded correctly, payment to the hospital could be incorrect. All hospital inpatients must have their visits coded in ICD-9-CM. For Medicare patients, these codes are then used to calculate a *Medicare-severity diagnosis-related group (MS-DRG)* payment. Consideration of the diagnoses and procedures and the patient's gender, disposition, and age all contribute to the MS-DRG calculation and thus to a payment.

ICD-9-CM diagnosis codes assigned to outpatients also affect payment. ICD-9-CM is used to indicate the medical necessity of (reason for) patients' health care visits to physician offices, clinics, and outpatient hospital departments. For example, a diagnosis of chest pain is the reason for a chest X-ray. The diagnosis code explains why the procedure was performed.

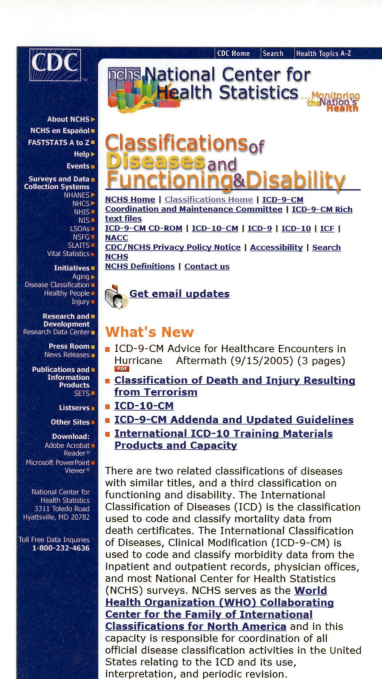

FIGURE 2.1
CDC/NCHS ICD-9-CM Home Page (The page changes as new information is included.)

Administrative Uses Because ICD-9-CM is a standardized data set used throughout the country, it is easy to use coded data to study the types of patients seen and the services provided. For example, staffing decisions can be made based on the number of patients with a certain diagnosis. Using ICD-9-CM data, a hospital director knows that the hospital performs a hundred hip replacements per month and can schedule the appropriate amount of specialized nursing care for those patients. Administrative budgeting, staffing, and marketing tasks that require the evaluation of patient types and services can be supported by review of ICD-9-CM codes reported for each patient.

ICD-10-CM

A tenth edition of the ICD code set was published by the World Health Organization (WHO) in 1990. In the United States, the new *Clinical Modification,* the **ICD-10-CM,** is being reviewed by health care professionals. ICD-10-CM is expected to be adopted as the mandatory U.S. diagnosis code set. (Other countries, such as Australia and Canada, already use their own modifications of ICD-10.) The major differences are:

- The ICD-10 contains more than two thousand categories of diseases, many more than the ICD-9. This creates more codes to permit more-specific reporting of diseases and newly recognized conditions.

- Codes are alphanumeric, containing a letter followed by up to five numbers.

- A sixth digit is added to capture clinical details. For example, all codes that relate to pregnancy, labor, and childbirth include a digit that indicates the patient's trimester.

- Codes are added to show which side of the body is affected for a disease or condition that can be involved with the right side, the left side, or bilaterally. For example, separate codes are listed for a malignant neoplasm of right upper-inner quadrant of the female breast and for a malignant neoplasm of left upper-inner quadrant of the female breast.

When ICD-10-CM is mandated for use, a crosswalk (a printed or computerized resource that connects two sets of data) will be made available. Although the code numbers look different, the basic systems are very much alike. People who are familiar with the current codes will find that their training quickly applies to the new system.

Checkpoint 2.1

1. Each year, many new ICD-9-CM categories are created for diseases that have been discovered since the previous revision. List examples of diseases that have been diagnosed in the last two decades. _____

Identify the purpose of ICD-9-CM coding in the following cases as research (R), quality (Q), communication (C), payment (P), or administrative (A).

2. A hospital board would like to develop a chemotherapy marketing campaign because the hospital has had a reduction in services to patients over the last year. _____

3. A physician reported the wrong ICD-9-CM codes to Medicare and was reimbursed incorrectly; the codes had to be resubmitted on a new health care claim. _____

4. A hospital wants to send a patient survey to all patients who underwent inpatient colonoscopies to determine whether the services were satisfactory. _____

5. A trend showed an increase in hospital postoperative complications, and a hospital wanted to investigate this. _____

6. A company wants to determine whether its new drug for the treatment of diabetes is effective. _____

ICD-9-CM Basic Coding Process

Diagnostic coding requires knowledge of the format of each ICD-9-CM volume and of the conventions and rules each uses to assist the coder in finding different types of codes, such as those describing external causes of injuries rather than codes describing the injuries themselves. A codebook is the source of the codes; the *Official Guidelines* are the source of the conventions and rules.

The three volumes of the *Official Guidelines* are:

1. *Diseases and Injuries: Tabular List:* Volume 1 is made up of seventeen chapters of disease descriptions and codes with two supplementary classifications and five appendixes.
2. *Diseases and Injuries: Alphabetic Index:* Volume 2 provides (a) an index of the disease descriptions in the Tabular List, (b) an index in table format of drugs and chemicals that cause poisoning, and (c) an index of external causes of injury, such as accidents.
3. *Procedures: Tabular List and Alphabetic Index:* Volume 3 covers inpatient procedures billed by hospitals.

Although the Tabular List and the Alphabetic Index are labeled Volume 1 and Volume 2, they are related like the parts of a book. They cover diagnostic coding, and the coding process starts with looking up words. Thus the **Alphabetic Index (Volume 2),** which contains medical terms, is used first. After a code has been located in Volume 2 based on the diagnostic statement, it is verified in **Volume 1,** known as the **Tabular List.** This two-step process must be followed in order to code correctly (Figure 2.2). This chapter follows the same order of use, with the Alphabetic Index discussed first, followed by the Tabular List. (Some publishers' versions of the ICD-9-CM place the Alphabetic Index before the Tabular List for the same reason.)

Volume 3 contains both the **Alphabetic Index and Tabular List of Procedures.** To use this volume correctly, the coder finds the procedural term in the Index and verifies the associated code in the Tabular List of Procedures.

Alphabetic Index (Volume 2)

Volume 2, the Alphabetic Index, is organized alphabetically by medical term, as its title suggests. It has three main sections:

1. Alphabetic Index to Diseases and Injuries
2. Table of Drugs and Chemicals
3. Alphabetic Index to External Causes of Disease and Injuries

The Alphabetic Index lists words that describe diseases or injuries, such as *pneumonia, bronchitis, infection,* and *fracture.* The **Table of Drugs and Chemicals** is an alphabetical listing of different drugs and chemicals such as aspirin, alcohol, gasoline, and penicillin. In coding external causes of diseases, coders start with words such as *fall, accident, burn,* and *cut* that can be found in the **Alphabetic Index to External Causes of Disease and Injuries.** Examples of entries in the three main sections of Volume 2 are listed in Table 2.2.

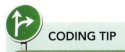

CODING TIP

Official Guidelines: **Conventions and Rules**

The first part of Section I of the *Official Guidelines* is "A. Conventions for the ICD-9-CM."

CODING TIP

Coding Process

The correct coding process is to locate a term and its code in the Alphabetic Index and to verify the code selection in the Tabular List.

Step 1.
Review complete medical documentation.

↓

Step 2.
Abstract the medical conditions and procedures that should be coded.

↓

Step 3.
Identify the main term for each condition and procedure.

↓

Step 4.
Locate the main terms in the Alphabetic Index.

↓

Step 5.
Verify the code in the Tabular List by reading all notes and applying appropriate conventions and guidelines.

FIGURE 2.2
Basic ICD-9-CM Code Assignment Process

Table 2.2 Organization of the Alphabetic Index (Volume 2)

Section Description	Sample Entries
Alphabetic Index to Diseases and Injuries (A-Z)	Angina Fracture Pneumonia
Table of Drugs and Chemicals (A-Z)	Aspirin Coumadin Petroleum
Alphabetic Index to External Causes of Disease and Injuries (A-Z)	Fire Hit Sting

MAIN TERMS AND SUBTERMS

The Alphabetic Index lists **main terms** that represent diseases, injuries, problems, complaints, drugs, and external causes of diseases or conditions. Main terms are shown in bold print. In addition to common nouns, main terms can be abbreviations (such as AAT) or **eponyms,** names or phrases based on people's names, such as Gamstorp's disease.

Usually the main term in the Alphabetic Index is a disease, not a site of disease. This point is demonstrated by studying the underlined words in these entries, which are examples of the main terms the medical coder locates in the Alphabetic Index to begin the coding process. Note that for a broken arm, for example, the term *fracture* (not *humerus*) is printed.

- Urinary tract <u>infection</u>
- Benign prostatic <u>hypertrophy</u>
- Aspiration <u>pneumonia</u>
- <u>Fractured</u> humerus
- Chronic obstructive pulmonary <u>disease</u>

Main terms are followed by indented words that provide additional specifications of a disease. Words that are indented under a main term are called **subterms.** Each subterm under a main term may have additional indented terms (*sub-subterms*). A subterm or a sub-subterm is indented three character spaces from the term above it. For example, as shown in Figure 2.3, the first subterm under the main term *bronchitis* is *with*. The second subterm under the main term *bronchitis* is *acute or subacute*. Subterms are listed alphabetically except for those *with* or *without*, which are always the first listed subterms.

EXAMPLE   To code acute chemical bronchitis, first locate the main term *bronchitis*, then the subterm *acute*, and then the sub-subterm *chemical*. This results in code 506.0.

Figure 2.3 illustrates some of the entries in ICD-9-CM relating to bronchitis, a common respiratory condition. Coders will need familiarity with the disease processes relating to respiratory illnesses, which are reviewed in the Pathophysiology Refresher on pages 60–61.

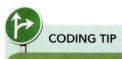

CODING TIP

Alphabetizing Words

The entries in the Alphabetic Index are organized on letter-by-letter alphabetizing, but the following are ignored: (1) single spaces between words, (2) single hyphens within words, and (3) the *s* in the possessive form of a word.

FIGURE 2.3

Format of the Alphabetic Index (Volume 2)

```
Bronchitis (diffuse) (hypostatic) (infectious)
        (inflammatory) (simple) 490
    with
        emphysema—see Emphysema
        influenza, flu, or grippe 487.1
        obstruction airway, chronic 491.20
            with
                acute bronchitis 491.22
                exacerbation (acute) 491.21
        tracheitis 490
            acute or subacute 466.0
                with bronchospasm or obstruction 466.0
            chronic 491.8
    acute or subacute 466.0
        with
            bronchospasm 466.0
            obstruction 466.0
            tracheitis 466.0
        chemical (due to fumes or vapors) 506.0
        due to
            fumes or vapors 506.0
            radiation 508.8
```

INDENTION AND CARRYOVER LINES

The use of the indented format helps coders see that the word *chemical* (in Figure 2.3) refers specifically to *acute or subacute,* which refer to the main term *bronchitis.* It is important to always observe this pattern of indention. The subterm indentions are listed in strict letter-by-letter alphabetical order below the term that is modified, with the exception of the subterm *with*, which is always listed first.

There are other types of indentions. Indentions that are six characters in length represent **carryover lines.** These lines are used when an entry will not fit on a single line. For example, the terms in parentheses after the main term *bronchitis (diffuse, hypostatic, infectious, inflammatory, simple)* are related to bronchitis, but because they all do not fit on one line, they are carried over to the next line.

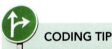

CODING TIP

Alphabetizing Numbers

In the Alphabetic Index, numeric subterms appear before alphabetic subterms. Numbers appear in numerical order even if they are spelled out in words (*first, second, third*).

Checkpoint 2.2

Using the Alphabetic Index of ICD-9-CM, answer the following questions.

1. In which section of the Volume 2 would you locate the term *carbon monoxide*? _____

2. In which section of Volume 2 would you locate the word *laceration*? _____

3. In which section of Volume 2 would you locate the word *parachuting*? _____

4. What main term is used to code *burn of the hand*? _____

5. What main term is used to code *fall from tree*? _____

6. What main term used to code *poisoning from cocaine*? _____

7. What is the first subterm under the main term *earth falling*? _____

8. What is the first subterm under the main term *pain*? _____

9. Using the Alphabetic Index only, code *urinary tract infection*. _____

10. Using the Alphabetic Index only, code *progressive atrophic paralysis*. _____

The Respiratory System

The respiratory tract consists of two major parts: the upper respiratory tract (generally regarded as including the sinuses, nose, nasopharynx, and larynx) and the lower respiratory tract (the trachea, bronchi, and lungs). Both the upper and lower tracts are the sites of infections, including major diseases that occur and are treated in the United States and around the world. In addition, allergies and environmental hazards cause many disorders of the respiratory system.

Respiratory Infections

Sinusitis is a common upper respiratory infection. It is classified as *accessory* (in addition to the nose), *nasal* (primarily in the nasal sinuses), *hyperplastic* (accompanied by swelling), *nonpurulent* (without the production of pus), *purulent* (with the production of pus), and *chronic* (recurrent over time). In addition, sinusitis is categorized by location as *ethmoidal* or *frontal*. *Tonsillitis* is classified in a number of ways (such as *acute, staphylococcal,* and *ulcerative*).

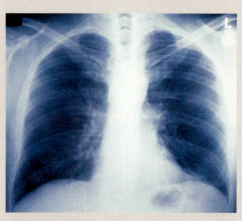

A chest X-ray.

It is often found along with *adenoiditis*, which itself can be *chronic* or *acute*. *Pharyngitis*, an inflammation of the pharynx, is classified in a number of ways. For example, it can be *influenzal, herpetic* (associated with Herpes), *streptococcal,* or *chronic,* among other classifications. Similarly, *laryngitis* is categorized in a numbers of ways, such as *acute, infective, pneumococcal,* and *spasmodic*. The general term *sore throat* usually refers to pharyngitis but can include laryngitis and other inflammations of the area around the pharynx. *Epiglottitis, rhinitis* (nasal inflammation or a runny nose), and *laryngotracheitis* are just a few examples of other upper respiratory infections. Some respiratory infections are caused by allergies and are thus classified as *allergic*.

The lower respiratory tract is also the site of acute respiratory infections. *Bronchitis* is classified as *acute, simple, infectious, inflammatory,* or *hypostatic* (caused by hypostasis, lowered blood flow). It is also categorized based on whether it is *viral, purulent,* or *with tracheitis,* as well as in a number of other ways. *Pleurisy* is an inflammation of the serous membranes of the lungs and is

Tabular List (Volume 1)

As shown in Table 2.3, the Tabular List has three divisions:

1. The chapters containing the diagnosis codes
2. The supplementary classification containing codes for nondisease factors and for external causes of injury and poisoning
3. Appendixes

CHAPTERS

The first major section of the Tabular List includes the seventeen chapters of disease and injuries. These chapters represent different categories of disease and body systems such as respiratory diseases and circulatory diseases. The codes are listed in numerical order and range from 001.0 through 999.9.

The chapters of diagnosis codes are used to verify codes first looked up in the Alphabetic Index. For example, to verify the code 486, the coder looks in Chapter 8, Diseases of the Respiratory System, of Volume 2.

classified in a number of ways, including *acute*, *chronic*, *residual* (remaining in an organ following another condition), and *unresolved* (ongoing and not cured). *Empyema* is a purulent infection in the pleural space. It is classified as *interlobar* (between the lobes of the lungs) or *encapsulated* (localized), among other ways. In addition, it may appear with or without a fistula.

COPD, Pneumonia, and Influenza

As mentioned above, the lower respiratory tract is the site of a number of infections. It is also the site of serious respiratory disorders. The category *Chronic Obstructive Pulmonary Disease and Allied Conditions* includes chronic bronchitis, asthma, emphysema, and other chronic airway obstructions. Some of these conditions may result from allergies or chemical exposure. *Asthma* is classified as *bronchial* (with bronchial obstructions), *catarrh* (with inflammation of mucous membranes), or *spasmodic* (occurring intermittently). It is also categorized in a variety of other ways, such as by cause (*allergic* or *exercise-induced*), by accompanying conditions (*with hay fever*), or by age (*childhood*). *Emphysema* is also classified in a number of ways, such as *atrophic* (accompanied by *wasting*), *chronic*, and *postural* (intensified when standing), and it can be categorized as accompanying other conditions (such as *with bronchitis*).

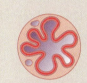

Normal bronchiole

Asthmatic bronchiole, showing constriction

A normal airway compared with one obstructed by asthma.

Pneumonia is classified in many ways (*acute*, *hemorrhagic*, or *septic*, for example). It is divided into two main types: *viral* and *bacterial*. Viral pneumonias are usually categorized by the specific virus (such as *pneumonia due to SARS-associated coronavirus*), just as bacterial pneumonias are categorized by the specific bacteria (as *Streptococcus, unspecified* or *Streptococcus, Group A*). Pneumonia can also be due to other specified organisms or to other infectious disease such as *whooping cough*, or it may be caused by aspiration.

Other Respiratory Conditions

There are many other respiratory conditions, some of which are mechanical, such as a *deviated septum* or the *mechanical complication of a tracheostomy*. Pneumothorax is the accumulation of air or gas in the pleural cavity, sometimes leading to a lung collapse. A pneumothorax may be *acute* or *chronic*. It is also categorized by timing or cause (*congenital* if at birth, *postoperative*, or *due to an accidental puncture*).

SUPPLEMENTARY CLASSIFICATIONS

To report or classify events or circumstances, a **supplemental classification system** must be used. The supplementary codes are ICD-9-CM codes, but they do not reflect diagnoses or injuries.

V Codes V codes, codes that start with the letter *V*, are the Supplementary Classification of Factors Influencing Health Status and Contact with Health Services. They are found immediately after code 999.9 in the first section of the Tabular List. This classification reports circumstances other than disease or injury such as the following:

- A person who is not currently sick encounters health care services.

  EXAMPLES A well-child visit; a visit for a routine chest X-ray.

- A person with a resolving disease or injury or a long-term chronic condition encounters the health care system for specific aftercare or service for that disease.

  EXAMPLE V58.11: Encounter for chemotherapy.

Table 2.3 Organization of the Tabular List (Volume 1)

Chapter	Category	Code Range
Classification of Diseases and Injuries		
1	Infectious and Parasitic Diseases	001–139
2	Neoplasms	140–239
3	Endocrine, Nutritional, and Metabolic Diseases, and Immunity Disorders	240–279
4	Diseases of the Blood and Blood-Forming Organs	280–289
5	Mental Disorders	290–319
6	Diseases of the Central Nervous System and Sense Organs	320–389
7	Diseases of the Circulatory System	390–459
8	Diseases of the Respiratory System	460–519
9	Diseases of the Digestive System	520–579
10	Diseases of the Genitourinary System	580–629
11	Complications of Pregnancy, Childbirth, and the Puerperium	630–677
12	Diseases of the Skin and Subcutaneous Tissue	680–709
13	Diseases of the Musculoskeletal System and Connective Tissue	710–739
14	Congenital Anomalies	740–759
15	Certain Conditions Originating in the Perinatal Period	760–779
16	Symptoms, Signs, and Ill-Defined Conditions	780–799
17	Injury and Poisoning	800–999
Supplementary Classifications		
V Codes	Supplementary Classification of Factors Influencing Health Status and Contact with Health Services	V01–V86
E Codes	Supplementary Classification of External Causes of Injury and Poisoning	E800–E999
Appendixes		
A	Morphology of Neoplasms	
B	Glossary of Mental Disorders (deleted in 2004)	
C	Classification of Drugs by American Hospital Formulary Services List Number and Their ICD-9-CM Equivalents	
D	Classification of Industrial Accidents According to Agency	
E	List of Three-Digit Categories	

- When a patient is being evaluated preoperatively, a code from category V72.8 is listed first, followed by a code for the condition that is the reason for the surgery.

  EXAMPLES V72.81: Preoperative cardiovascular examination. 414.01: Arteriosclerotic heart disease of native coronary artery.

- A circumstance or problem influences a patient's health status, but is not itself a current illness or injury. For example, codes V10–V19 cover history. If a person with a family history of colon cancer presents with rectal bleeding, the problem is listed first, and the V code is assigned as an additional code.

EXAMPLES 569.3: Hemorrhage of rectum and anus.
V16.0: Family history of malignant neoplasm.

- In the case of a newborn, the V code indicates the birth status.

EXAMPLE V30.01: Single liveborn born in hospital via cesarean delivery.

V codes classify the reasons for health care services or provide supplemental information about a person's health.

A V code can be used either as a primary code for an encounter or as an additional code. It is researched the same way as other codes, using the Alphabetic Index to point to the term's code and the Supplementary Classification in the Tabular List to verify it.

The terms that indicate the need for V codes, however, are not the same as other medical terms. They usually have to do with a reason for an encounter other than a disease or its complications. When found in diagnostic statements, the words listed in Table 2.4 often point to V codes.

E Codes Following the V code section are the **E codes,** the Supplemental Classification of External Causes of Injury and Poisoning. These codes classify the causes of injury, poisoning, and adverse events and are used to gather statistics relating to these occurrences. They are unique in that they are never listed alone or first; rather, the condition is reported first, followed by the E code to reflect the circumstance. For example, if a patient presented to the office for a sprained finger (diagnosis) after falling from a chair at home (E codes), three codes would

BILLING TIP

Use V Codes to Show Medical Necessity

V codes such as family history or a patient's previous condition help demonstrate why a service was medically necessary.

CODING ALERT

E Codes

E codes are never reported alone or first.

BILLING TIP

Use E Codes to Show Who Is Responsible for Payment

E codes for trauma and accidents help payers determine which insurance applies. They are especially useful on workers' compensation claims.

Table 2.4 Terminology Associated with V Codes

Term	Example
Contact	V01.1: Contact with tuberculosis
Contraception	V25.1: Insertion of intrauterine contraceptive device
Counseling	V61.11: Counseling for victim of spousal and partner abuse
Examination	V70: General medical examination
Fitting of	V52: Fitting and adjustment of prosthetic device and implant
Follow-up	V67.0: Follow-up examination following surgery
Health, healthy	V20: Health supervision of infant or child
History (of)	V10.05: Personal history of malignant neoplasm, large intestine
Replacement	V42.0: Kidney replaced by transplant
Screening/test	V73.2: Special screening examination for measles
Status	V44: Artificial opening status
Supervision (of)	V23: Supervision of high-risk pregnancy
Therapy	V57.3: Speech therapy
Vaccination, inoculation	V06: Need for prophylactic vaccination and inoculation against combinations of disease

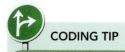

CODING TIP

Locate the Appendixes

Take the time to find the appendixes in the codebook you are using; each publisher determines the extent to which these appendixes are included.

be used to report the visit: a code for sprained finger (Chapter 17 in the Tabular List), a code for falling from a chair (Ecode), and a code to show that the fall happened at home (E code). Without the E codes, the circumstances and places of injury would not be known.

APPENDIXES

The last section of the Tabular List includes the appendixes. They are used for specific coding purposes and by specific types of facilities. For example, Appendix A, Morphology of Neoplasms, lists the morphology codes that are used to report cancers in specialized cancer facilities. The following appendixes are part of Volume 1 and are typically located in the back of the codebook, depending on the publisher:

Appendix	Topic
A	Morphology of Neoplasms
B	Glossary of Mental Disorders (officially removed October 1, 2004)
C	Classification of Drugs by American Hospital Formulary Service List Number and ICD-9-CM Equivalents
D	Classification of Industrial Accidents
E	List of Three-Digit Categories

Checkpoint 2.3

In what section of the Tabular List would each of the following codes be found, and on what page numbers in your codebook? For example, code V45.1 is found in the Tabular List of V codes.

1. 486 _____

2. E816.1 _____

3. 28:12 _____

4. M9044/3 _____

5. V 02.51 _____

TABULAR LIST FORMAT

ICD-9-CM diagnosis codes range from three digits (numbers) to five digits in length. The first three digits identify the broad category of the disease, and the additional digits are used to more specifically identify the details of the disease. The format of the Tabular List reflects this method of identifying diagnoses:

Chapter	Range of codes
Section	Range of codes within a chapter
Category	Three-digit code
Subcategory	Four-digit code
Subclassification	Five-digit code

Chapters and Sections   Each of the seventeen **chapters** in the Tabular List contains a series of three-digit codes that represent a body system or group of diseases. Chapters are divided into sections. A section contains a group of numbers related to a more specific disease group. For example, Chapter 1 covers infectious and parasitic diseases (001–139). The first section in the chapter is titled Intestinal Infectious Diseases (001–009), and the second section is titled Tuberculosis (010–018). The sections in ICD-9-CM are not specifically labeled, but they are important in understanding the format of the tabular list. Figure 2.4 shows a chapter and the first section in that chapter.

FIGURE 2.4
Example of Tabular List Entries

1. INFECTIOUS AND PARASITIC DISEASES (001–139)
Note: Categories for "late effects" of infectious and
      parasitic diseases are to be found at 137–139.
Includes: Diseases generally recognized as communicable or transmissible as
      well as a few diseases of unknown but possible infectious origin.
Excludes:
acute respiratory infections (406–466)
carrier or suspected carrier of infectious organism (V02.0–V02.9)
certain localized infections
influenza (487.0–487.8)

INTESTINAL INFECTIOUS DISEASES (001–009)
   Excludes:
   helminthiases (120.0–129)

001 CHOLERA

   001.0 DUE TO VIBRIO CHOLERAE

   001.1 DUE TO VIBRIO CHOLERAE EL TOR

   001.9 CHOLERA, UNSPECIFIED

002 TYPHOID AND PARATYPHOID FEVERS

   002.0 TYPHOID FEVER
       Typhoid (fever) (infection) [any site]

   002.1 PARATYPHOID FEVER A

   002.2 PARATYPHOID FEVER B

   002.3 PARATYPHOID FEVER C

   002.9 PARATYPHOID FEVER, UNSPECIFIED

003 OTHER SALMONELLA INFECTIONS
   Includes: Infection or food poisoning by
       Salmonella [any serotype]

   003.0 SALMONELLA GASTROENTERITIS
       Salmonellosis

   003.1 SALMONELLA SEPTICEMIA

   003.2 LOCALIZED SALMONELLA
       INFECTIONS

      003.20 LOCALIZED SALMONELLA INFECTION,
         UNSPECIFIED

      003.21 SALMONELLA MENINGITIS

      003.22 SALMONELLA PNEUMONIA

      003.23 SALMONELLA ARTHRITIS

      003.24 SALMONELLA OSTEOMYELITIS

      003.29 OTHER

The Endocrine System

The endocrine system consists of a group of glands that secrete hormones. The oversecretion or undersecretion of these hormones is responsible for many disorders of the body. Endocrine disorders are closely related to the functions of the body's metabolism.

Metabolic Disorders

Diabetes is a major contributor to rising health care costs in the United States. Approximately 7 percent of the population has diabetes, and the rate of growth of cases of diabetes is increasing rapidly. In addition, adult-onset diabetes is now appearing at much younger ages. Much of this is attributed to lifestyle factors—less exercise and greater intake of calories starting at an early age.

There are two basic types of *diabetes mellitus*: *Type I* (*juvenile type*)

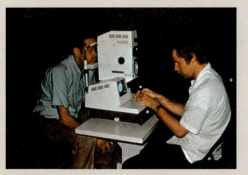

A yearly diabetic eye exam is essential to maintain eye health.

and *Type II.* Diabetes may be described in documentation as *brittle* (unpredictable, with large fluctuations in blood sugar), *congenital* (present at birth), *familial* (present in close relations), *uncontrolled, severe, slight,* or *without complication.* Diabetes is either controlled (with blood glucose measured often and kept within reasonable limits) or uncontrolled (with great variations in the

blood glucose readings). Reflecting this, there are four subclassifications (0 = Type II or unspecified; 1 = Type I not stated as uncontrolled; 2 = Type II or unspecified type uncontrolled; 3 = Type I uncontrolled). *Gestational diabetes* is Type II diabetes that appears only during pregnancy.

Diabetes is also related to many complications, such as *neuropathy* (nerve disease), *retinitis* (inflammation of the retina), *peripheral vascular disease with ulcers,* and *coma with ketoacidosis.* Diabetic wound care is necessitating the opening of new wound care centers as the incidence of Type II diabetes increases. Diabetes is also classified as *without mention of complication.* Diabetes often affects kidney and heart functioning, so some of the classifications have to do with kidney conditions or blood vessel disease. *Hypoglycemia* (abnormally low glucose level in the blood) may occur if too much insulin is taken to control diabetes, or it may be *spontaneous.* It is also classified in a number of different ways, such as *infantile* or *reactive.*

Obesity is calculated according to growth charts supplied by the *Centers for Disease Control and Prevention* (www.cdc.gov). There are pediatric growth charts (ages two to twenty) and adult growth charts (over age twenty) that calculate

Categories, Subcategories, and Subclassifications Three terms are used to identify the types of specific codes: category, subcategory, and subclassification. **Category** codes are three digits in length; **subcategory** codes have four digits; and **subclassification** codes are five digits long. To interpret each code, the medical coder reads the description at the category level, subcategory level, and subclassification level. Notes at the chapter or section levels apply to the entire chapter or section.

> **EXAMPLE** To find the correct code for transient arthropathy of the upper arm, which is 716.42, first read the information with 716.4 in the Tabular List. Note that a fifth digit is required. Next, read the fifth-digit subclassification at the beginning of the category to choose the correct digit.

An important coding rule is that *a disease must be classified to its highest level of specificity.* This means that all digits assignable for a specific disease must be used. For example, code 250.00–diabetes

the *BMI (body mass index)*. Obesity and *morbid obesity* are based on the weights listed in those charts. Obesity is classified in a number of ways, including *familial* and *nutritional*. Other metabolic disorders include disorders of *carbohydrate metabolism* and *lipid metabolism*. Lack of absorption of various minerals, such as calcium, can also cause disorders.

Other Glandular Disorders

A *goiter* is an enlargement of the thyroid gland. Goiters have many different causes and are classified in a variety of ways. For example, there are *juvenile goiters, goiters due to iodine deficiency,* and *internal goiters. Hypothyroidism* (deficiency of thyroid secretions) may have a number of causes. *Hyperthyroidism* (overabundance of thyroid secretions) is also categorized in a variety of ways, such as *preadult* and *recurrent. Grave's disease* is one form of hyperthyroidism. *Thyrotoxicosis,* excessive concentrations of thyroid secretions in the body, can be fatal.

A diabetic patient receives instruction on glucose monitoring.

The pituitary gland plays an important role in normalizing growth. *Acromegaly* (abnormal head, hand, and foot enlargement), *dwarfism* (abnormally diminished growth), and *gigantism* (abnormally large stature) are all pituitary disorders.

The secretions of the testes and ovaries—the male and female sex glands—control menstrual cycles in the female and sexual functioning in both sexes. *Premature menopause* before age forty may result from surgical removal of the ovaries or from unknown causes. *Hormone replacement therapy* is used to treat this condition as well as the symptoms of menopause occurring at a normal age. *Erectile dysfunction* may also be treated with hormones and other medications. There are other conditions, such as *polycystic ovaries,* that are controlled by the sex glands.

Cushing's syndrome results from hypersecretion of the adrenal glands. *Addison's disease* is the result of hyposecretion of the adrenal glands. *Aldosteronism* (oversecretion of aldosterone from the adrenal glands) can cause hypertension and fluid retention.

mellitus—requires the use of five digits. Using only the first three digits—category code 250—reports only that the patient has diabetes, rather than a specific type or degree of control. Correct diagnosis coding using ICD-9-CM requires adding both a fourth digit (subcategory) to explain the presence of diabetic complications (such as 250.7 to report peripheral circulatory disorders) and a fifth digit (subclassification) to provide detail regarding the type and control of diabetes.

Fifth-digit subcategory codes are found throughout the Tabular List. For example, as shown for category 250 in Figure 2.5, the fifth digits may be shown in a table at the category level (right below the category entry). Figure 2.5 illustrates the entries in ICD-9-CM relating to diabetes mellitus, a common disease of the endocrine system. Coders will need familiarity with these disease processes, which are reviewed in the Pathophysiology Refresher at the top.

Another typical format for presenting required fifth digits is shown in Figure 2.6, where five-digit codes are indented under a subcategory

FIGURE 2.5

Fifth Digits for Reporting Diabetes Mellitus

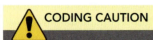

CODING CAUTION

When Four Digits Are Correct

When a five-digit code is not available, a four-digit code is correct. For example, if a patient has a malignant neoplasm of the stomach (category 151), a fourth digit is required to reflect the exact location of the neoplasm in the stomach, such as 151.4 for a malignant neoplasm of the body of the stomach.

250 DIABETES MELLITUS

Excludes
gestational diabetes (648.8)
hyperglycemia NOS (790..6)
neonatal diabetes mellitus (775.1)
nonclinical diabetes (790.29)

The following fifth-digit subclassification is for use with category 250:

0 TYPE II OR UNSPECIFIED TYPE, NOT STATED AS UNCONTROLLED
Fifth-digit 0 is for use for type II patients, even if the patient requires insulin.
Use additional code, if applicable, for associated long-term (current) insulin use (V58.67)

1 TYPE I [JUVENILE TYPE], NOT STATED AS UNCONTROLLED

2 TYPE II OR UNSPECIFIED TYPE, UNCONTROLLED
Fifth-digit 2 is for use for type II patients, even if the patient requires Insulin.
Use additional code, if applicable, for associated long-term (current) insulin use (V58.67)

3 TYPE I [JUVENILE TYPE], UNCONTROLLED

FIGURE 2.6

Five-Digit Codes for Reporting Obstructive Chronic Bronchitis

CODING ALERT

E Code Format

E codes are the exception to the format rule that all diagnosis codes contain three digits before the decimal point. E codes have four digits before the decimal point.

CODING TIP

Select the Most Specific Code

Always code to the highest level of specificity—the most number of digits available.

491.2 OBSTRUCTIVE CHRONIC BRONCHITIS

Bronchitis:
  Emphysematous
  Obstructive (chronic) (diffuse)
Bronchitis with:
  Chronic airway obstruction
  Emphysema

Exclude
asthmatic bronchitis (acute) NOS (493.9)
chronic obstructive asthma (493.2)

491.20 WITHOUT EXACERBATION

Emphysema with chronic bronchitis

491.21 WITH (ACUTE) EXACERBATION

Acute exacerbation of chronic obstructive pulmonary disease [COPD]
Decompensated chronic obstructive pulmonary dsease [COPD}
Decompensated chronic obstructive pulmonary disease [COPD] with exacerbation

Excludes
chronic osbstructive asthma with acute exacerbation (493.22)

491.22 WITH ACUTE BRONCHITIS

code, as shown for code 491.2 . In other instances, the fifth digits are listed and described at the section level, as is done under the codes for complications mainly related to pregnancy (640–648). In all these instances, the fifth digit has to be assigned for the ICD-9-CM code to report the disease completely. Fifth-digit notations are also found in the Tabular List to External Causes of Injury. For example, code E905 requires a fifth digit to reflect the type of animal or plant that caused poisoning or a toxic reaction.

Checkpoint 2.4

Using Volume 1, write the narrative description for the following codes.

1. 486 _____
2. 585.2 _____
3. 153.3 _____
4. 250.71 _____
5. E812.0 _____
6. V21.32 _____
7. 493.90 _____
8. 718.65 _____
9. 808.41 _____
10. 276.51 _____

Alphabetic Index and Tabular List of Procedures (Volume 3)

Volume 3 of ICD-9-CM classifies procedures performed in the hospital inpatient setting, and the codes are used only by the facility. They are not used to classify procedures performed by physicians in any setting. Volume 3 contains both an Alphabetic Index to Procedures and a Tabular List of Procedures.

ALPHABETIC INDEX TO PROCEDURES

The Alphabetic Index to Procedures is formatted alphabetically by type of procedure, eponym, or operation. Some of the main terms in this volume are *reduction, removal, incision, appendectomy,* and *Keller* (eponym). The format of subterms and carryover lines applies in this volume as well. The subterms *as, by,* and *with* are unique to the Alphabetic Index to Procedures; they immediately follow the main terms to which they refer. The remaining subterms are listed in alphabetical order. For example, the main term *repair* and subterm *knee* are used to find the code for repair of the knee. 81.47. If the repair was of the collateral ligament of the knee, code 81.46 would be assigned.

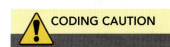

CODING CAUTION

Use the Alphabetic Index *and* the Tabular List

All codes found in the Alphabetic Index must be verified in the Tabular List before the final codes are assigned.

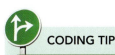

CODING TIP

Coding Volume 3 Procedures

Always look at all the subterms to obtain the most specific code representing the procedure performed.

TABULAR LIST OF PROCEDURES

Once a code has been located in the Alphabetic Index to Procedures of Volume 3, the code is verified in the Tabular List of Procedures. The format of the Volume 3 Tabular List is similar to the format of the Volume 1 Tabular List to Diseases and Injuries. Volume 3 procedure codes contain three or four digits, with two characters placed to the left of the decimal point. Coding to the highest level of specificity is required, meaning that the code must include the most digits available.

EXAMPLES 21.1: Incision of the nose.
21.22: Biopsy of the nose.

The two codes in the example are two completely different procedures. Figure 2.7 shows an example from Chapter 7, Operations on the Cardiovascular System (35–39). Code 35.11 is assigned to classify an open heart valvuloplasty of aortic valve without replacement.

FIGURE 2.7

Example from Tabular List of Procedures

35 OPERATIONS ON VALVES AND SEPTA OF HEART
Includes: Stenotomy (median) (transverse), as operative approach
           Thoracotomy, as operative approach
Code also cardiopulmonary bypass [extracorporeal circulation] [heart-lung machine] (39.61)

35.0 CLOSED HEART VALVOTOMY
Excludes:
percutaneous (balloon) valvuloplasty (35.96)

35.00 CLOSED HEART VAVLOTOMY, UNSPECIFIED VALVE
NON-SPECIFIC O.R. PROC

35.01 CLOSED HEART VALVOTOMY, AORTIC VALVE

35.02 CLOSED HEART VALVOTOMY, MITRAL VALVE

35.03 CLOSED HEART VALVOTOMY, PULMONARY VALVE

35.04 CLOSED HEART VALVOTOMY, TRICUSPID VALVE

35.1 OPEN HEART VALVULOPLASTY WITHOUT REPLACEMENT
Includes:
Open heart valvotomy
Code also cardiopulmonary bypass, if performed [extracorporeal circulation] [heart-lung machine] (39.61)

Excludes:
percutaneous (balloon) valvuloplasty (35.96)
that associated with repair of:
endocardial cushion defect (35.54, 35.63, 35.73)
valvular defect associated with atrial and ventricular septal defects (35.54, 35.63, 35.73)

35.10 OPEN HEART VALVULOPLASTY WITHOUT REPLACEMENT, UNSPECIFIED VALVE
NON-SPECIFIC O.R. PROC

35.11 OPEN HEART VALVULOPLASTY OF AORTIC VALVE WITHOUT REPLACEMENT

35.12 OPEN HEART VALVULOPLASTY OF MITRAL VALVE WITHOUT REPLACEMENT

35.13 OPEN HEART VALVULOPLASTY OF PULMONARY VALVE WITHOUT REPLACEMENT

35.14 OPEN HEART VALVULOPLASTY OF TRICUSPID VALVE WITHOUT REPLACEMENT

CODING TIP

What Type of ICD-9-CM Code Is It?

It is easy to determine whether an ICD-9-CM code represents a diagnosis or a procedure. A diagnosis code has three to five digits with a decimal point after the third digit. A procedure code contains three or four digits with a decimal point after the second digit. For example, 434.91 is a diagnosis code, and 45.23 is a procedure code.

ICD-9-CM Conventions

Just as the basic rules of the road help people drive safely, so do coding conventions guide the use of ICD-9-CM. **Conventions** or notations appear throughout ICD-9-CM. The cardinal rule is that codes are never selected from one volume alone; always start with the Alphabetic Index and finish by verifying the code in the Tabular List. Specific details and examples of coding conventions follow and are summarized in Tables 2.5 and 2.6.

MODIFIERS

Modifiers (also called parenthetical or nonessential modifiers) are found in the Alphabetic Index (Volume 2) and in the Alphabetic Index to Procedures in Volume 3. The modifiers are terms surrounded by parentheses. The presence or absence of these parenthetical terms in diagnostic statements has no affect on code assignment. For example, in the Alphabetic Index for the entry *diabetes*, the nonessential modifiers *brittle, congenital, familial, mellitus*, and so on are listed. If documentation states that the diagnosis of diabetes is familial diabetes or poorly controlled diabetes, the same code is researched in the Tabular List.

EXAMPLE
Diabetes, diabetic (brittle) (congenital) (familial) (mellitus) (poorly controlled) (severe) (slight) (without complication)   250.0

Other modifiers, the *subterms*, do affect code assignment because they provide clarification, such as differences or specifics about the site. Each of these modifiers (*subterms*) is presented in an individual line entry under the main term:

EXAMPLE
Ganglion   727.43
   joint   727.41
   of yaws (early) (late)   102.6
   periosteal (*see also* Periostitis)   730.3
   tendon sheath (compound) (diffuse)   727.42
   tuberculous (*see also* Tuberculosis)   015.9

CODING TIP

Follow the *Official Guidelines* for Conventions

ICD-9-CM conventions and rules are also covered in Section I, Part A of the *Official Guidelines*.

Table 2.5 Summary List of Conventions Used in ICD-9-CM Volumes 1 and 2

Convention	Convention Location (Volume)	Meaning
Abbreviations		
NEC	1, 2, 3	Not elsewhere classified or other specified, or a more specific category is not provided
NOS	2	Not otherwise specified, or unspecified
Punctuation		
Brackets [ ]	1	Enclose synonyms or explanations
Slanted brackets *[ ]*	2	Enclose manifestation codes, or codes that should be listed second
Parentheses ( )	1, 2	Enclose supplemental words or nonessential modifiers
Colon :	1	Placed after an incomplete term that needs one or more of the following modifiers to assign that code
Braces { }	1	Enclose a series of terms, each of which is modified by the statement to the right of the brace; both terms must be present to assign that code
Section marks §	1	Instruct the coder to reference a footnote
Lozenges □	1	Identify a code unique to ICD-9-CM (not the same in ICD-9)
Terms		
Includes	1	Further defines or gives examples of terms included in that code or code section
Excludes	1	Lists terms that are excluded from or are to be coded elsewhere (not included)
Note	1, 2	Defines terms or gives coding instruction
Cross-References		
See	2	Follows a main term and provides a new main term that should be referenced
See also	2	Follows a main term to see additional entries (subterms) that may apply
See category	2	Go directly to the Tabular List
Typeface		
Bold	1	Font of all codes and titles
	2	Font of all main terms
Italics	1	Font of excludes notes and identifies codes that are not to be used as primary
Instructions		
Use additional code	1	Instructs the coder to assign an additional code to give more information if known
Code first underlying disease	1	Instructs the coder to code the underlying disease first, then the other code second (the code containing the instruction)

The example on page 71 shows individual subterms (modifiers) describing the site and type of disease (manifestation). This type of modifier must be present in documentation in order for the specific code to be assigned. In this example, the modifying subterms are *joint* and *tendon sheath*, and a ganglion of the joint would result in code 727.41, whereas a

Table 2.6 Summary List of Conventions Used in ICD-9-CM Volume 3

Convention	Location: Alphabetic Index (A) or Tabular List (T)	Meaning
Abbreviations		
NEC	A, T	Not elsewhere classified, or indication that specified forms of the procedure are classified separately. Only used if more specific information is not available. OR term for which a more specific code is not available, even with additional information provided.
NOS	T	Not otherwise specified or unspecified
Punctuation		
Brackets [ ]	T	Enclose synonyms or explanations
Slanted brackets *[ ]*	A	Enclose codes representing components of a procedure that should be reported second
Parentheses ( )	A	Enclose supplemental words or nonessential modifiers whose absence or presence does not affect code assignment
	T	Enclose supplemental word or nonessential modifiers
Colons :	T	Placed after an incomplete term that needs one or more of the following modifiers
Braces { }	T	Enclose a series of terms, each of which is modified by the statement to the right of the brace; both terms must be present
Section marks §	T	Instruct the coder to reference a footnote
Lozenges □	T	Identify a code unique to ICD-9-CM (not the same in ICD-9)
Terms		
Includes	T	Further defines or gives examples of terms included in that code or code section
Excludes	T	Lists terms that are excluded from or are to be coded elsewhere (not included)
Note	A, T	Defines terms or gives coding instruction
Cross-References		
See	A	Follows a main term and provides a new main term that should be referenced
See also	A	Follows a main term to see additional entries (subterms) that may apply
See category	A	Go directly to the Tabular List
Typeface		
Bold	T	Font of all codes and titles
	A	Font of all main terms
Italics	T	Font of excludes notes and identifies codes that are not to be used as primary
Instructions		
Code also	T	An instruction to code each component of a procedure when completed at the same time
Omit code	A	Instruction in the Alphabetic Index to not use the incision code when an incision is performed only for completing an additional surgery

ganglion of a tendon sheath would result in code 727.42. This example also shows the nonessential modifiers *compound* and *diffuse* following the subterm *tendon sheath*.

ABBREVIATIONS

Abbreviations are used in all three volumes of ICD-9-CM.

Not Elsewhere Classified (NEC) NEC, **not elsewhere classified**, means that ICD-9-CM does not have a code for the documented condition. The abbreviation appears in the Alphabetic Index, and the code must be verified in the Tabular List. Often the Tabular List uses a grouping of such conditions. When NEC is used, additional information will not alter the code assignment; often there is a precise statement but no correlated code.

EXAMPLE
Household circumstance affecting care V60.9
    specified type NEC   V60.8

In this example from the Alphabetic Index, NEC is used to classify a specified type of household circumstance affecting care (V60.8). When verified in the Tabular List (Volume 1), code V60.8 means "other specified housing or economic circumstances." This application of NEC refers to the facts that a more specific category is not provided and that additional information will not alter code assignment. Many household circumstances could affect care, so ICD-9-CM does not separately classify each and every one of them. The entries in the Tabular List for codes V60.8 and V60.9 are as follows.

EXAMPLES
V60.8 OTHER SPECIFIED HOUSING OR ECONOMIC CIRCUMSTANCES
V60.9 UNSPECIFIED HOUSING OR ECONOMIC CIRCUMSTANCE

Not Otherwise Specified (NOS) NOS, **not otherwise specified**, is used in the Tabular List to indicate a code that should be used when the documentation does not supply a more specific condition for code assignment. In other words, typically the coder does not have information to code a specific disease and would need such information to assign a different code.

EXAMPLE
414.9 CHRONIC ISCHEMIC HEART DISEASE, UNSPECIFIED
Ischemic heart disease NOS

This code ends in a 9. Often, codes that end in 9 classify conditions that are unspecified or not otherwise specified.

EXAMPLES
- 728.9: Unspecified disorder of muscle, ligament, and fascia.
- V75.9: Screening examination for unspecified infectious diseases.
- E987.9: Falling from a high place, undetermined whether accidentally or purposely inflicted, unspecified means.

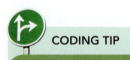

CODING TIP

NEC versus NOS

Essentially, NEC indicates a classification failure of the ICD-9-CM, and NOS indicates a documentation failure.

Code the following using Volumes 1 and 2, and identify the conventions that apply: NEC, NOS, nonessential modifier, or subterm modifier.

		Codes	Conventions
1.	Contraception management	_____	_____
2.	Flash pneumonia	_____	_____
3.	Food poisoning	_____	_____
4.	Conjunctivitis	_____	_____
5.	Closed fracture, phalanx of foot	_____	_____

NOTES

Notes are used to define terms and give coding instruction. For example, in the Alphabetic Index the main term *fracture* is followed by a note that defines an open fracture and related terms as compared to a closed fracture and related terms. Similarly, a note follows the main term *diabetes* that instructs the coder to use a fifth digit. In the Alphabetic Index to Procedures in Volume 3, a note at the main term *transplant* instructs the coder on how to report a donor source.

EXAMPLE
Infarct, infarction

. . .

myocardium, myocardial (acute or with a stated duration
of 8 weeks or less) (with hypertension)   410.9

> Note—Use the following fifth-digit subclassification with category 410:
> 0 episode unspecified
> 1 initial episode
> 2 subsequent episode without recurrence

CROSS-REFERENCES

In the ICD-9-CM, the terms *see, see also,* and *see category* indicate **cross-references,** meaning that the coder must look elsewhere to code a particular condition.

See   The cross-reference *see* refers the coder to another main term under which all the information about a specific disease or injury will be found.

EXAMPLES
Parkinson's Disease, syndrome or tremor—*see Parkinsonism*
Myringitis with otitis media—*see Otitis Media*
Plastic Repair—*see Repair, by site*
Deformity, leg, congenital, reduction—*see Deformity, reduction, lower limb*

Notice that the comma separates a main term from a subterm when the cross-reference refers to a more specific disease. In the example of deformity above, the coder would follow the cross-reference to the main term *Deformity*, then the subterm *reduction*, and finally the sub-subterm *lower limb*.

CODING TIP

Following Cross-References

When the cross-reference *see* appears, look at the new main term and all subterms listed.

See Also The cross-reference term *see also* directs the coder to check another main term that may have additional information if the first main term the coder looks up does not provide a correct match for the diagnostic statement.

EXAMPLES
Paresthesia—*see also Disturbance, sensation*
Dilation, heart (acute) (chronic)—*see also Hypertrophy, cardiac*
Neuroma—*see also Neoplasm, connective tissue, benign*
Neuropathy, neuropathic—*see also Disorder, Nerve*

In the first example, to code paresthesia of smell, the cross-reference *Disturbance, sensation* tells the coder to go to the main term *Disturbance.* By following this cross-reference, the specific code for disturbance of smell can be located (781.1).

See (or See Also) Category The cross-reference *see category* directs the coder to go immediately to the Tabular List, specifically to a category or range of codes. In such a case, the Tabular List contains specific information regarding the use of the codes, and the coder can determine the exact code assignment from the notes.

EXAMPLES
Septicemia, with ectopic pregnancy—*see also Categories 633.0–633.9*
Fever, brain, late effect,—*see category 326*

Checkpoint 2.7

Answer the following questions using all three volumes of ICD-9-CM.

1. What does the note at the main term *asthma* instruct the coder to do?

   _____

2. What is the cross-reference used to code embolic cerebrovascular disease?

   _____

3. What does the note refer to at the main term *fracture*?

   _____

4. Which cross-reference should the coder follow when coding *depressive psychosis*?

   _____

5. What does the note specify at code 777.9?

   _____

6. What does the note at category 299 instruct the coder to do?

   _____

7. Which cross-reference is used in coding the procedure incision with removal of foreign body?

   _____

8. What does the note located at the main term *endarterectomy* instruct the coder to do?

   _____

9. Which cross-reference is used when coding a late effect of an intracranial abscess?

   _____

10. What does the note at category 532 instruct the coder to do?

   _____

PUNCTUATION

ICD-9-CM uses various punctuation marks that direct the coder to follow certain rules, provide additional meaning, or explain terms.

Brackets   Brackets [ ] are used to enclose synonyms, alternative wordings, and explanatory phrases in the Tabular List of Diseases and Injuries.

> **EXAMPLE**
> **483.0 MYCOPLASMA PNEUMONIAE**
> Eaton's agent
> Pleuropneumonia-like organism [PPLO]

Slanted Brackets   Some conditions may require two codes, one for the **etiology,** the cause or origin of the condition, and a second for the **manifestation,** a disease resulting from the underlying disease or disorder. For example, diabetes (underlying cause) can manifest to diabetic peripheral angiopathy. When slanted brackets *[ ]* appear, both codes must be reported; the etiology code should be listed first and the manifestation code in slanted brackets reported second.

> **EXAMPLE**
> Phlebitis
> . . .
> gouty 274.89 *[451.9]*

The Alphabetic Index entry above indicates that the diagnostic statement "gouty phlebitis" requires two codes, one for the etiology (gout) and one for the manifestation (phlebitis). The use of slanted brackets around the code means that it cannot be used as the primary code; it is listed after the etiology code.

> **EXAMPLE**
> **Anthrax**   022.9
> with pneumonia   022.1 *[484.5]*

In this example from the Alphabetic Index, both codes 022.1 and 484.5 would be reported. When these codes are verified in the Tabular List, code 022.1 represents anthrax (etiology) with the manifestation of pneumonia.

Slanted brackets in the Alphabetic Index to Procedures in Volume 3 require the coder to code both procedures (if performed). For example, the main term *ileocystoplasty* lists two codes, 57.87 and *[45.51],* so both should be reported.

Parentheses   Parentheses ( ) are used in both the Alphabetic Index and the Tabular List to enclose terms that are supplementary, that may or may not be present in the disease statement, and that do not affect code assignment. They are always used to enclose these nonessential terms.

Colon   The **colon** : is used in the Tabular List after an incomplete term that needs one or more of the terms or modifiers that follow it.

> **EXAMPLE**
> **462 ACUTE PHARYNGITIS**
> Acute sore throat NOS
> Pharyngitis (acute)**:**
> NOS
> Gangrenous

CODING TIP

Verify All Codes

Verify all codes, even those presented in brackets or slanted brackets.

Infective
Phlegmonous
Pneumococcal
Staphylococcal
Suppurative
Ulcerative
Sore throat (viral) NOS
Viral pharyngitis

In this example, other diseases such as gangrenous pharyngitis, ulcerative pharyngitis, and infective pharyngitis as well as acute pharyngitis are coded as 462. Both the term to the left of the colon and the term to the right of the colon must be present in order to assign that code.

Braces   Braces { } are occasionally used in the Tabular List to enclose a series of terms that, when combined with the statement to the right of the brace, results in that specific code assignment.

EXAMPLE
INTERNAL INJURY OF THORAX, ABDOMEN, AND PELVIS (860–869)
Includes:

{
blast injuries
blunt trauma
bruise
concussion injuries (except cerebral) of internal organs
crushing
hematoma
laceration
puncture
tear
traumatic rupture
}

The example above, which depicts the Internal Injury of Thorax, Abdomen, and Pelvis (860–869) section, means that that internal injury of the abdomen includes a tear of an internal organ, a blast injury of an internal organ, a crushing of an internal organ, or other listed type of injury.

SYMBOLS

Special symbols instruct the coder that there is a special circumstance regarding that code.

Lozenge   The **lozenge** □ indicates that a code—296.3 in the example that follows—is unique to ICD-9-CM. In other words, the ICD-9-CM code does not appear in ICD-9. The lozenge symbol is located in the ICD-9-CM Tabular List only and can be ignored by coders.

EXAMPLE
□ 296.3 MAJOR DEPRESSIVE DISORDER, RECURRENT EPISODE

Section Mark   A **section mark** symbol § precedes a code to indicate that there is a footnote with special instructions. This symbol is found in all three volumes of ICD-9-CM.

EXAMPLE
§ 675 INFECTIONS OF THE BREAST AND NIPPLE ASSOCIATED WITH CHILDBIRTH

---

§ Requires fifth digit. Valid digits are in [brackets] under each code. See beginning of section 640–649 for codes and definitions.

Includes: The listed conditions during pregnancy, childbirth, or the puerperium

§ 675.0 INFECTIONS OF NIPPLE
[0–4] Abscess of nipple

For example, code 675.0 instructs the coder to look at the footnote at the bottom of the page. The footnote then instructs the coder to see the beginning of the applicable section for definitions of the fifth digits. A section mark can also be found at procedure code 78.7 in the Tabular List of Procedures (Volume 3).

Typeface   Boldface and italic type are special typeface settings that provide coding instructions.

Bold   **Boldface** print is used to identify main terms and titles in the Alphabetic Indexes. Bold type in the Tabular List depicts each code and code title.

Italics   In the Tabular List of Diseases and Injuries, *italics* indicate that the code should not be reported alone or listed first. In other words, the code in italics typically represents a manifestation of disease, and the underlying cause should be reported first, before the code in italics.

EXAMPLE

484.8 *PNEUMONIA IN OTHER INFECTIOUS DISEASES CLASSIFIED ELSEWHERE*
Code first underlying disease, as:
Q fever (083.0)
Typhoid fever (002.0)

In the example, code 484.8 *Pneumonia in other infectious disease classified elsewhere* is in italics. This disease is a manifestation of an underlying disease.

> **NOTE**
>
> Sequencing of multiple codes is covered in Chapter 4 of your program.

Checkpoint 2.8

Apply the punctuation, symbols, and typeface conventions to answer the following questions.

1. Would the diagnosis of sprue be classified to code 579.1? _____

2. Which two codes should be reported when coding lupus nephritis? _____

3. What does the section mark at category 651 refer to? _____

4. What symbol is located at code 312, and what is the meaning of this symbol? _____

5. Code waxy kidney. _____

6. Would the diagnosis of acute coronary embolism without myocardial infarction be classified to code 411.81? _____

7. Explain the significance of the italics for code 774.5. _____

8. Code Ebstein's disease, Type 2, in control. _____

9. What is the significance of the terms in parenthesis located at the main term *bronchitis*?

_____

10. Code glaucoma in anterior dislocation of the lens. _____

INSTRUCTIONAL NOTATIONS

ICD-9-CM also includes terms that are instructional in nature. These notations tell the coder to do something, or let the coder know what types of diseases are included or excluded. These notations are found in the Tabular List and the Tabular List of Procedures.

Includes   The notation **includes** refers to a code title to give an example or define the contents of the code or code series. Therefore, an includes note at the section level, such as for the section of Tuberculosis codes, instructs the coder that infection by *Mycobacterium* tuberculosis (human or bovine) is included for any code ranging from 010 to 018.

EXAMPLE
TUBERCULOSIS (010–018)
Includes: Infection by Mycobacterium tuberculosis (human) (bovine)

An includes note at the category level gives definitions or examples for that category.

EXAMPLE
433 OCCLUSION AND STENOSIS OF PRECEREBRAL ARTERIES
Includes: Embolism, of basilar, carotid, and vertebral arteries
Narrowing, of basilar, carotid, and vertebral arteries
Obstruction, of basilar, carotid, and vertebral arteries
Thrombosis, of basilar, carotid, and vertebral arteries

In this example, category 433 includes the conditions of embolism of basilar, carotid, and vertebral arteries.

EXAMPLE
830 DISLOCATION OF JAW
Includes: Jaw (cartilage) (meniscus)
Mandible
Maxilla (inferior)
Temporomandibular (joint)

Looking at the includes note at category 830 helps the coder review the jaw anatomy cited in the documentation.

Excludes   An **excludes** note in the Tabular List of Disease and Injuries and the Tabular List of Procedures instructs the coder about words and conditions that should be coded elsewhere. In other words, these conditions are not included in the code.

EXAMPLE
455 HEMORRHOIDS
Includes: Hemorrhoids (anus) (rectum)
Piles
Varicose veins, anus or rectum
Excludes:
that complicating pregnancy, childbirth, or the puerperium (671.8)

In this example, the excludes note is at the category level. This means that if documentation states that a hemorrhoid complicates pregnancy, childbirth, or the puerperium, that condition should not be coded (or is excluded) from category 455.

EXAMPLE

464.1 ACUTE TRACHEITIS

Tracheitis (acute):
>   NOS
>   Catarrhal
>   Viral
>   *Excludes:*
>   *chronic tracheitis (491.8)*

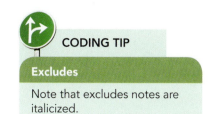

CODING TIP

Excludes

Note that excludes notes are italicized.

The excludes note here is at the subcategory level and states that chronic tracheitis is excluded from code 464.1, acute tracheitis.

Use Additional Code

The instruction **use additional code** tells the coder to also code further information if it is documented. For example, in the Alphabetic Index to Procedures, this instruction means to use an additional code for a procedure if in fact that procedure was carried out.

EXAMPLE

599.0 URINARY TRACT INFECTION, SITE NOT SPECIFIED

Use additional code to identify organism, such as Escherichia coli [E. coli] (041.4)

This notation instructs the coder that the organism causing a urinary tract infection should be coded if it is identified in the documentation. The following example shows the notation instructing the coder to identify a drug (E code) if the disease was drug induced.

EXAMPLE

333.90 UNSPECIFIED EXTRAPYRAMIDAL DISEASE AND ABNORMAL MOVEMENT DISORDER

Medication-induced movement disorders NOS
Use additional E code to identify drug, if drug-induced

Code First Underlying Disease

The instruction **code first underlying disease** is located only in the Tabular List with codes that are not intended to be selected as a primary disease because they are manifestations of other underlying diseases. Sometimes, these codes are in italics. The underlying disease should be coded first, followed by the code with the notation *code first underlying disease*.

EXAMPLE

517 LUNG INVOLVEMENT IN CONDITIONS CLASSIFIED ELSEWHERE

Excludes:
rheumatoid lung (714.81)
517.1 RHEUMATIC PNEUMONIA
Code first underlying disease (390)

Code 517.1 should be coded second, and the underlying cause of the rheumatic pneumonia—code 390, rheumatic fever—should be coded and sequenced first. Notice the italics in the next example:

EXAMPLE

337.1 PERIPHERAL AUTONOMIC NEUROPATHY IN DISORDERS CLASSIFIED ELSEWHERE

Code first underlying disease, as:
Amyloidosis (277.30–277.39)
Diabetes (250.6)

The code 337.1 is in italics and contains the instructional notation to code first the underlying disease of peripheral autonomic neuropathy. Therefore, the underlying cause of the neuropathy should be reported first, followed by the neuropathy code 337.1. The underlying cause could be amyloidosis or diabetes.

Omit Code   The instructional notation **omit code** is found only in the Alphabetic Index to Procedures in Volume 3. It is seen next to a term listing an incision, such as *laparotomy*. This means that when an incision was made for the purpose of performing further surgery, the code for the incision should be omitted, or not coded.

EXAMPLE

Arthrotomy 80.10
As operative approach—omit code

In the above example, the main term in the Alphabetic Index to Procedures is arthrotomy. The notation, under the subterm "as operative approach" tells the coder that if the arthrotomy was completed as the operative approach and additional surgery was performed, the code for arthrotomy should not be assigned.

Checkpoint 2.9

Using all three volumes of ICD-9-CM, answer the following questions.

1. What site is excluded from malignant neoplasm of the intrahepatic bile ducts, code 155.1?

   _____

2. Is emphysema due to fumes or vapors excluded from subcategory 498.2? _____

3. Which sites are included when a code from category 27 is assigned from the Tabular List of Procedures? _____

4. Would assigning code 34.59 be appropriate for biopsy of the pleura? _____ Why?

   _____

5. Do the codes in section 410–414 include ischemic heart disease with mention of hypertension? _____

Code the following using Volumes 1 and 2 of ICD-9-CM.

6. Acute cystitis due to *Escherichia coli (E coli)* _____

7. Tuberculosis of bone with necrosis of the knee _____

8. Type II controlled diabetic gangrene _____

9. Coronary artery bypass of one coronary artery while on cardiopulmonary bypass (heart-lung machine) _____

10. Streptococcal septicemia with SIRS _____

TABLES

Three tables in ICD-9-CM are used to provide an organized structure for the coding of certain diseases and drugs. The format of each table is based on the need to classify different types of disease, sites of diseases, or circumstances of disease. These tables are the:

1. Hypertension Table
2. Neoplasm Table
3. Table of Drugs and Chemicals

Hypertension Table The hypertension table is located at the main term *hypertension* in the Alphabetic Index. It contains a complete listing of conditions associated with hypertension (subterms) and requires classification of the hypertensive conditions as malignant, benign, or unspecified.

> **EXAMPLE** Benign cardiorenal hypertension is classified as code 404.10. The main term is *hypertension*; the subterm is *cardiorenal*, and the second column lists *benign*.

Neoplasm Table Neoplasm codes can be located two different ways in the Alphabetic Index. The first way is by morphology, meaning the histologic type such as carcinoma, sarcoma, adenoma, and histiocytoma. The second listing is found in the Neoplasm Table. The table is organized alphabetically by body or anatomical site. The first column lists the anatomical location , and the next six columns relate to the behavior of the neoplasm, described as a malignant tumor, a benign tumor, a tumor of uncertain behavior, or a tumor of unspecified nature.

There are three types of malignant tumors. Each is progressive, rapid-growing, life-threatening, and made of cancerous cells:

1. *Primary*: The neoplasm that is the encounter's main diagnosis is found at the site of origin.
2. *Secondary*: The neoplasm that is the encounter's main diagnosis metastasized (spread) to an additional body site from the original location.
3. *Carcinoma in situ*: The neoplasm is restricted to one site (a noninvasive type); this may also be referred to as *preinvasive cancer*.

A benign tumor is slow-growing, usually not life-threatening, and is made of normal or near-normal cells. A tumor of uncertain behavior was not classifiable when the cells were examined, and one of unspecified nature is one for which there is no documentation of the nature of the neoplasm.

The following entries are shown in the Neoplasm Table for a neoplasm of the colon:

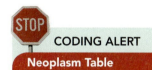

CODING ALERT

Neoplasm Table

Never go directly to the Neoplasm Table. The specific morphology is referenced first.

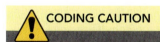

CODING CAUTION

Neoplasms

Go to the main term Neoplasm only when directed to do so based on the morphology of the neoplasm.

	MALIGNANT					
	Primary	Secondary	Cancer in situ	BENIGN	UNCERTAIN BEHAVIOR	UNSPECIFIED
Colon	154.0	197.5	230.4	211.4	235.2	239.0

Coders will need familiarity with these diseases, which are reviewed in the Pathophysiology Refresher on cancer shown on the following pages.

Table of Drugs and Chemicals The Table of Drugs and Chemicals is used to classify *poisoning* (intentionaly taken or administered toxic drug overdose) or *adverse effects* (conditions inadvertently caused

Cancer

Cancer is a general term for any of a number of diseases with malignant growths. *Tumors* or *neoplasms* are growths. Cancerous tumors are also known as *carcinomas*. *Benign* growths are generally located within a limited area and do not spread. *Malignant* growths sometimes spread within the organ or part in which they originate. If they spread to other organs or parts, they are said to *metastasize*.

Neoplasms are grouped according to whether they are *primary* (located in a specific originating site, except for lymphatic tissue), *primary of lymphatic tissue, secondary* (originating from another site), *unspecified* (as to location), *benign, carcinoma in situ* (meaning a localized cluster of malignant cells), or of *uncertain behavior*. In addition, neoplasms are categorized by where they occur, such as *abdominopelvic, brain,* and *breast*. Subcategories within the sites indicate more specific locations (for example, brain cancer is subcategorized as *basal ganglia, cerebrum, cerebellum, midbrain,* and so on).

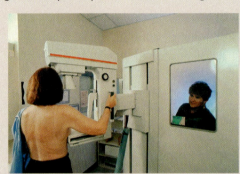

A mammogram.

Neoplasms are also *staged* (graded) by the TNM system. *T* stands for tumor; *N* stands for spread to the lymph nodes; and *M* stands for metastasis (spreading to other sites). The TNM system rates tumors from 1 to 4 depending on the severity of the malignancy.

Cancer is the second leading cause of death in the United States, following heart disease, the number one killer. The most deadly form of cancer is lung cancer.

Common Cancers

Cancer can occur anywhere in the body. For women, breast, cervical, and ovarian cancers occur frequently. *Breast cancer* is classified by *glandular tissue* or *soft tissue,* and it is categorized by location (such as the quadrant or the nipple). *Cervical cancer* is categorized by location (*endocervix* or *external os,* for example). *Ovarian cancer* may be categorized according to the parts involved, such as *fallopian tube* or *parametrium*.

For men, *prostate cancer* may be aggressive and require treatment, or it may be slow-growing and just need watching. *Testicular cancer* is more common in men who have had an undescended testicle or abnormal testicular development.

Lung cancer is widespread, especially among smokers. It is categorized by location (for example, *middle lobe* or *main bronchus*). *Colon cancer* is also categorized by loca-

by the correct use of a drug). The table is organized alphabetically by drug or chemical name. Columns across the table provide codes to identify that a poisoning occurred. The columns located after the poisoning code are the external cause codes (E codes). The E code identifies the circumstances of the poisoning or adverse effect for the specific drug or chemical.

Checkpoint 2.10

Using the tables in the Alphabetic Index (Volume 1) of ICD-9-CM, answer the following questions.

1. What are the three types of hypertension noted in the hypertension table? _____

2. What is the code for benign hypertension with chronic kidney disease? _____

3. Which type of term is used as a subterm in the neoplasm table: site, etiology, or manifestation?
   _____

4. What is the code for benign neoplasm of the lung? _____

5. What is the poisoning code for aspirin? _____

tion (for example, *sigmoid* or *ascending*). Some glandular cancers can be fairly contained and easily treated; for example, *thyroid cancer* usually requires removal and limited treatment, followed by hormone replacement. However, others, such as *pancreatic cancer,* are difficult to treat and are usually fatal.

Skin cancer is categorized by location, such as *hand* or *thigh.* Moles on the skin are either benign or malignant (the latter are usually dark and irregular). Skin cancer is on the rise as a result of increasing exposure to ultraviolet rays from the sun.

Leukemia is a general term for blood or bone marrow cancer. Leukemias are classified either *without mention of remission* or *with remission*. They are either *acute* (having an overgrowth of immature blood cells) or *chronic* (having an overgrowth of mature blood cells). There is also an early stage of leukemia called *myelodysplastic syndrome (MDS)* in which bone marrow does not produce enough blood cells.

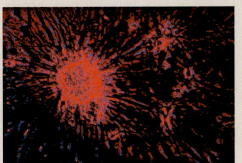
A cancer cell.

is the best way to prevent it. Some known carcinogens are tobacco smoke, asbestos, ultraviolet rays of the sun, and certain chemicals. The next best thing to total avoidance is early detection. Some symptoms clearly indicate possible cancer: rectal bleeding; dark, irregular skin moles; breast lumps; and persistent coughing of unknown cause. Other symptoms are more subtle, but can be detected by cancer screenings, now common procedures. Mammograms (breast cancer screening) are recommended at certain intervals for women depending on age and family history. PSA tests (prostate cancer screening) are routine for males at certain ages and with certain histories. A colonoscopy provides a clear picture of any suspicious polyps. Chest X-rays can detect lung cancer, and MRIs and CAT scans can see tumors in various locations.

Cancer treatment has advanced greatly in the past decade. Radical surgeries are still sometimes necessary, but radiation and chemotherapy have replaced some surgical procedures. New targeted therapies, such as hormone receptor treatments, show promise for limiting tumor growth in certain cases.

Cancer Prevention and Treatment

Cancer is not always preventable; however, avoidance of *carcinogens* (things that are known to cause cancer)

ICD-9-CM Coding Resources

To assign ICD-9-CM codes correctly, the coder must use the current code set and follow the *Official Guidelines*. Knowledge of medical terminology and reference to other medical resources are also required.

AHA CODING CLINIC® FOR ICD-9-CM

AHA Coding Clinic® for ICD-9-CM is published by the American Hospital Association (AHA). The AHA Central Office handles all ICD-9-CM coding-related issues and works with NCHS and CMS to maintain integrity of the coding system. *AHA Coding Clinic* provides advice on coding certain diseases and includes:

- Official coding advice and guidelines
- Correct code assignments for new diseases and technologies
- Articles offering practical information to improve data quality
- A communication process to disperse code changes or corrections to health care providers

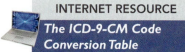

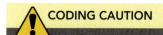

- An "Ask the Editor" section that includes practical examples
- Information on question submission

Coding Clinic is published quarterly or as needed and can be purchased from the AHA. The coding advice is approved by CMS for Medicare reimbursement and is also accepted by many other payers.

NCHS WEBSITE

A list of all ICD-9-CM diagnosis code changes can be found at the NCHS website. Also available is an ICD-9-CM conversion table that shows new and replaced codes used to classify the same conditions. This conversion table includes code changes made between 1986 and the current year. Coders use this resource to update old codes reported in earlier years. For example, dehydration was coded differently before 2005 than it is today (it is currently code 276.51).

MEDICAL REFERENCES

A basic understanding of medical terms, the disease process, and current medical procedures is required in medical coding, but no one can possibly remember all the medical terms and anatomy, physiology, disease, and procedural information. It is important for coders to have references available to help when a documented health issue needs further investigation. For example, if a medical record includes terms a coder has never seen before, a medical dictionary would be helpful. If a physician documents a blockage of a specific artery, the coder may need to consult an anatomy book to locate that artery in the vascular system.

Documented medications can be investigated in a drug manual to determine the category of drug. Internet research is helpful in understanding new technology in the treatment of disease. Researching and understanding a new medical technique can help a coder assign the correct ICD-9-CM procedure code. Pathophysiology books discuss the disease process and treatment, including the signs and symptoms of disease. Table 2.7 is a basic listing of medical references used by coders.

COMPUTER-AIDED CODING

Today many larger health care facilities use computer programs to assign ICD-9-CM codes. Such computer-aided coding software is called an **encoder.** Encoder software can be based on the logic behind selecting codes or on a computerized version of the actual ICD-9-CM code set.

Logic-based encoders contain a system of questions and answers that help the coder assign the correct ICD-9-CM code. Book-based encoders provide computerized versions of the actual ICD-9-CM codebook, allowing the coder to access the Tabular List and Alphabetic Index on-screen. Built into these software encoding systems are alerts, edits, and references. For example, if the coder enters an invalid ICD-9-CM code, the software alerts the coder to make a correction. If the coder selects a code for a male when the patient is female, the encoder system alerts the coder about that error. Other types of edits alert the coder that two codes that should not be reported together were assigned, or that a fifth digit is required.

Table 2.7 Recommended Medical Coding Resources

Coding Resource	Information
ICD-9-CM Official Guidelines for Coding and Reporting	Contains the most current rules for ICD-9-CM coding
AHA Coding Clinic® for ICD-9-CM	Provides official advice on coding issues
Centers for Medicare and Medicaid website at www.cms.gov	Lists most current ICD-9-CM procedure codes (Volume 3)
National Center for Health Care Statistics website at www.cdc.gov/nchs	Lists most current ICD-9-CM diagnosis codes (Volumes 1 and 2)
Medical dictionary	Defines medical terms
Anatomy and physiology book	Identifies location of body organs and explains different body systems
Pathophysiology book	Explains the disease process
Drug reference	Lists different medications and their actions, indications, and side effects
Abbreviation book	Lists abbreviations and their meanings
Internet medical sites	Resource for new technology and endless health care information
Medical terminology book	Defines medical terms

References to *Coding Clinic* can also be linked to codes in the Tabular List, allowing the coder to access specific guidelines immediately.

The use of encoders does not replace the need for knowledge of the ICD-9-CM coding guidelines. These computer-aided systems provide a tool for coders that can be useful to improve consistency, efficiency, and accuracy by putting alerts, edits, and references at the coder's fingertips. A list of diagnosis codes and their description in a billing software package or file is not the same as using an encoder. The list in billing software primarily includes the diagnoses most commonly used in a physician practice. It does not contain specific coding edits, alerts, or references.

> **NOTE**
>
> CPT codes for procedures are covered in Chapters 6 through 10 of your program.

Checkpoint 2.11

Which coding resource would be used to find the medical information below?

1. The meaning of *CHF* _____
2. Coding advice regarding a patient who has uncontrolled diabetes _____
3. The medical indications for the drug Zantac _____
4. The ICD-9-CM procedure code changes effective October 1, 2007 _____
5. The signs and symptoms of gastric ulcer _____
6. In which part of the body the talus is located _____
7. The code for sleep apnea effective October 1, 2005 _____
8. The latest technology for heart transplants _____
9. The rules for sequencing diagnosis codes _____
10. Medical term for gallbladder removal _____

1. ICD-9-CM is the International Classification of Diseases, Ninth Revision, Clinical Modification. This coding system is modeled after the International Classification of Disease, which is maintained by the World Health Organization. ICD-9-CM can be traced to 1959, when the U.S. Public Health Service published the International Classification of Diseases, Adapted for Indexing of Hospital Records and Operation Classification (ICDA). Over the years, ICDA was revised, updated, and adapted for the United States as ICD-9-CM. This code set contains more than thirteen thousand codes and is updated annually.

2. The responsibility for maintaining ICD-9-CM is divided between the National Center for Health Statistics (NCHS; part of the Centers for Disease Control, CDC) for Volumes 1 and 2, and CMS for Volume 3. The ICD-9-CM Coordination and Maintenance Committee considers proposed coding modifications to ICD-9-CM. In order to maintain the coding system, the cooperating parties, which represent NCHS, CMS, AHIMA, and AHA, meet regularly. Interested parties from either the public or private sector can propose a change in ICD-9-CM. Changes are published annually on October 1 and April 1.

3. The best way to keep up-to-date on ICD-9-CM code changes is to use the Internet. The website for ICD-9-CM updates from the National Center for Health Care Statistics (www.cms.gov/nchs/icd9.htm) contains the latest information on ICD-9-CM codes. This website also includes a crosswalk from old codes to new codes along with the addenda and updated guidelines.

4. ICD-9-CM is the medical coding system used throughout the United States for reporting medical conditions and procedures. The three-volume code set is used to transform medical words into code numbers for data reporting. The codes are used by a variety of health care providers, payers, and agencies for data reporting. The actual coded data are used for health care payment, health care communication, measurement of health care quality, research and education, and administrative decision making.

5. For all health care providers to use ICD-9-CM accurately and consistently, national guidelines for its use must be followed. ICD-9-CM guidelines are published in the *ICD-9-CM Official Guidelines for Coding and Reporting,* and HIPAA legislation mandates their use. The guidelines address basic coding steps, conventions, sequencing, and chapter-specific guidelines. National guidelines provide coders with consistent, comprehensive instructions on the use of ICD-9-CM.

6. The structure and content of ICD-9-CM differs depending on which volume is being used. For example, the Alphabetic Index to Diseases and Injuries (Volume 2) is formatted in three main sections: the Alphabetic Index to Diseases and Injuries, the Table of Drugs and Chemicals, and the Alphabetic Index to External Causes of Disease and Injuries. The Tabular List of Diseases and Injuries (Volume 1) contains three main sections as well: the Tabular List of Diseases and Injuries, the Supplemental Classifications, and the Appendixes.

Volume 3 of ICD-9-CM is structured differently. This volume includes both the Alphabetic Index to Procedures and the Tabular List of Procedures. The format of each volume helps direct the coder. In the Alphabetic Index, main terms are used to identify the patient's condition. Subterms provide further specification to a condition, such as location, type of condition, or cause of disease. The indented format of the Alphabetic Index helps the coder assign the most specific code available. Verification of the code in the Tabular List requires use of the indented format as well. In the Tabular List, the format of chapters, sections, categories, subcategories and subclassifications assist the coder in assigning the most specific code available.

7. Conventions, or rules of coding, are specific to the use of ICD-9-CM. For example, punctuation such as parentheses, brackets, and colons instruct the coder. Other conventions such as notes, includes, and excludes instruct the coder regarding certain conditions and how those conditions should be coded. Cross-references and terms such as *code also* or *code first underlying disease* also provided instructions. It is imperative to understand and apply these conventions in order to assign codes accurately.

8. The basic coding process begins with review of complete medical documentation and abstraction of conditions. Each condition is coded by identifying the main term representing it. The main term is one word in the diagnostic statement that the coder uses to find the code. For example, the diagnosis of urinary tract infection would require the coder to look up the main term *infection*. Indented subterms are used to provide specificity in coding a condition. Once a code has been located in the Alphabetic Index, that code is verified in the Tabular List. All conventions and instructions must be followed for accuracy in coding.

9. The requirement to code to the highest level of specificity means that the most digits available for a particular code must be assigned. The use of the fifth digit subclassification is prominent throughout the codebook. The fourth and fifth digits assigned to a particular category may have an indented format, or instructions to use a fourth or fifth digit may be located in notes. Remember to always code to the highest level of specificity.

10. Having the resources to assign ICD-9-CM codes accurately is essential. Access to national coding guidelines, published coding advice, medical dictionaries, and medical Internet sites and use of encoders are some of the resources coders use to keep current with medical practice, understand medical documentation, and assign accurate codes.

Review Questions: Chapter 2

Match the key terms with their definitions.

a. WHO _____

b. cooperating parties _____

c. *ICD-9-CM Official Guidelines for Coding and Reporting* _____

d. Alphabetic Index to External Causes of Disease and Injury _____

e. slanted brackets _____

f. section _____

g. includes note _____

h. subclassification _____

i. colon _____

j. omit code _____

1. Coding convention that encloses codes that should be reported second; these codes represent manifestation of a disease

2. Organization responsible for maintaining ICD-9 and ICD-10

3. Instruction in Alphabetic Index to Procedures

4. An ICD-9-CM code with five digits

5. Publication that contains rules on ICD-9-CM coding and sequencing

6. A range of codes within a chapter

7. A coding convention that combines a term on the left with a term on the right

8. A coding convention that instructs the coder that these conditions are not excluded

9. The group of organizations that includes representative from the NCHS, CMS, AHIMA, and AHA

10. A portion of Volume of ICD-9-CM

Decide whether each statement is true or false.

1. A coder is finished coding once a code is found in the Alphabetic Index. **T or F**

2. ICD-9-CM codes are never used for health care reimbursement. **T or F**

3. HIPAA legislation mandates the use of ICD-9-CM. **T or F**

4. ICD-9-CM codes are updated annually on January 1. **T or F**

5. An E code can never be used as a principal diagnosis. **T or F**

6. The first step in assigning an ICD-9-CM code is reviewing complete documentation. **T or F**

7. When coding to the highest level of specificity, the coder must assign a code using the most digits available. **T or F**

8. The comma is a convention used in ICD-9-CM to list nonessential modifiers. **T or F**

9. An encoder can replace a knowledgeable coder. **T or F**

10. The Tabular List of V codes is located in Volume 3 of ICD-9-CM. **T or F**

Select the letter that best completes the statement or answers the question.

1. Which codes would be used to classify uncontrolled type II diabetic neuropathy?
   a. 250.60, 357.2
   b. 250.62, 583.81
   c. 250.60, 583.81
   d. 250.62, 357.2

2. Which convention instructs the coder to read a footnote?
   a. lozenge
   b. section mark

  c. colon

  d. brace

3. Which of the following would not be found in the ICD-9-CM Tabular List of Disease and Injuries (Volume 2)?

  a. 486

  b. 434.91

  c. 45.23

  d. V10.05

4. Which codes represent open fracture of the distal tibia due to fall from a ladder at home?

  a. 823.90, E881.0, E849.9

  b. 824.9, E888.9, E849.9

  c. 824.8, E888.9, E849.0

  d. 824.9, E881.0, E849.0

5. Which codes represent acute pyelonephritis due to pseudomonas in a patient with a history of urinary tract infections?

  a. 590.10, V13.02, 041.7

  b. 590.00, V18.69, 041.7

  c. 590.10, V18.69, 041.7

  d. 590.10, V13.02

6. Code 098.0 describes

  a. gonorrhea not otherwise specified

  b. acute gonococcal infection of the lower genitourinary tract

  c. gonococcal urethritis

  d. all of the above

7. Which code or codes represent acute and chronic cholecystitis with choledocholithiasis?

  a. 575.12, 574.80

  b. 574.40

  c. 574.30, 574.40

  d. 574.5, 575.12

8. Which codes represent hypertension with stage V chronic kidney disease?

  a. 403.01, 585.5

  b. 403.91, 585.5

  c. 403.90, 585.5

  d. 403.9, 585.5

9. Which E code would be assigned when coding a suicide attempt by morphine?

  a. E850.2

  b. E935.2

  c. E950.0

  d. E962.0

10. Which codes represent pyrophosphate crystal induced arthritis of the knee?

  a. 275.49, 712.25

  b. 712.25, 275.49

  c. 275.49, 712.26

  d. 274.0, 712.26

1. List the three main sections of the ICD-9-CM Alphabetic Index. _____
_____

2. List the three main sections of the ICD-9-CM Tabular List. _____
_____

3. Describe the difference between an ICD-9-CM diagnosis code and an ICD-9-CM procedure code.
_____

4. Identify whether the fifth digit subclassification classifies the site of disease, the cause of disease (etiology), or the type of disease.
   a. 250.63 _____
   b. 053.14 _____
   c. 038.43 _____
   d. 552.21 _____
   e. 945.33 _____

5. What are the steps in the coding process? _____

6. Code the following.
   a. Cerebral *concussion* with loss of consciousness for forty-five minutes _____
   b. Family *history* of colonic polyps _____
   c. *Myelopthisis* due to malignant neoplasm of the central portion of the female breast _____
   _____
   d. *Abnormal* electrocardiogram _____
   e. Alcohol *intoxication* with alcoholism, continuous use of alcohol _____

Applying Your Knowledge

BUILDING CODING SKILLS

Case 2.1

1. You are the coding supervisor at a major acute care hospital. What resources would you recommend to ensure that the most current ICD-9-CM codes are in use in your health care facility? Remember to address issues such as coding resources and computer systems.

2. Why is it important to follow the *ICD-9-CM Official Guidelines for Coding and Reporting*?

3. Which of the following codes are not coded to the highest level of specificity?
   a. 250.1
   b. 410.3
   c. E812
   d. V58.1

Case 2.2

The following chart note is on file for a female patient.

Rayelle Smith-Jones
2/14/2008

SUBJECTIVE: The mother brought in this 3-week-old female. The patient is doing very well. They have been using the phototherapy blanket. She is thirsty, has good yellow stooling, and continues on formula. Her alertness is normal. Other pertinent ROS is noncontributory.

OBJECTIVE: Afebrile. Comfortable. Jaundice is only minimal at this time. No scleral icterus. Good activity level. Normal fontanel. TMs, nose, mouth, pharynx, neck, heart, lungs, abdomen, liver, spleen, and groins are normal. Normal cord care. Good extremities.

ASSESSMENT: Resolving physiological jaundice on phototherapy.

PLAN: Will stop phototherapy and do a bilirubin level a couple of days to make sure there is no rebound. The patient is to be seen one week. Push fluids. Routine care was discussed.

MD/xx

---

1. After review of the documentation, which diagnosis should be coded?

2. What main term would you use to begin the coding process?

3. Is this patient a newborn (twenty-eight days old or less)?

4. What ICD-9-CM code is assigned for this visit?

Case 2.3

The following chart note is on file for a male patient.

Joseph Baldwin
2/15/2008

SUBJECTIVE: Joseph is a 56-year-old male who presents to the office with nausea, vomiting, and diarrhea over the past two days. He has no fever and no history of gastrointestinal problems, and he has had a hard time keeping food down. Other pertinent ROS is noncontributory.

OBJECTIVE: Afebrile, appears weak and ill. Oral mucosa is dry; ENT is normal; neck, heart, lungs, liver, spleen, and groins are normal. Abdomen is nontender with no masses. Bowel sounds are normal. Good extremities.

ASSESSMENT: Viral gastroenteritis with mild dehydration.

PLAN: Patient should rest, drink plenty of fluids. If symptoms do not subside or worsen within 48 hours, return to the office. Watch for signs of worsening dehydration. Care was discussed.

MD/xx

---

1. What diagnoses should be reported for this visit?

2. What main term should be used to begin the coding process?

3. What are the diagnosis codes for this visit?

Case 2.4

The following chart note is on file for a female patient.

Sandy Wright
4/15/2008

SUBJECTIVE: Patient complains of a mole on her back and a red, swollen lump on her thigh. The mole on the back has not changed in size and is not painful. However, the lump on the thigh is red, swollen, and painful.

OBJECTIVE: Back: the mole is 1 cm uniform, brown in color with irregular borders.

THIGH: There is an indurate area measuring 3 cm in diameter in the proximal medial right thigh. In the center there is a small pustule and a wider area of erythema surrounding this, consistent with cellulitis. There are no red streaks present.

ASSESSMENT: Abscess with cellulitis; nevus of the back.

PLAN: The abscess was cleansed with Betadine and anesthetized with 1% Xylocaine. An incision and drainage was done with #11 blade. A pocket was created and packed with Iodoform gauze. The patient was given Ancef 1 gm IM. She was given a prescription for Keflex 500 mg and Tylenol #3 for pain. Sandy will be referred to a dermatologist for evaluation of the possible basal cell carcinoma of the back.

1. Which diagnoses should be reported for the lump on the thigh?

2. Which diagnosis should be reported for the mole on the back?

3. Assign the codes for this patient.

4. Where is the instructional notation to use an additional code found?

5. Can the additional code be assigned? Why?

Case 2.5

The following chart note is on file for a female patient.

Joann Adamson
4/10/2008

SUBJECTIVE: Patient complains of sore throat, dysphagia, fever, and chills this morning. Patient has had two documented Strep throat cases this year.

OBJECTIVE: Temperature is 100.2 degrees. Ears are clear. Throat is deeply injected with 4+ cryptic hypertrophic tonsils with exudate. Neck had marked tender cervical lymphadenopathy and submandibular adenopathy.

   LAB: Quick Strep is positive for Strep.

ASSESSMENT: Acute suppurative *Streptococcal* tonsillitis and pharyngitis.

PLAN: She was given 1.2 C-R Bicillin IM. She was observed for 20 minutes. She is to rest for the next 24 hours and use Tylenol PRN.

1. What are the signs and symptoms?

2. Which conditions would be coded?

3. What main terms would the coder use to begin the coding process?

4. Which terms are supplementary terms (in parentheses) when assigning the code for tonsillitis?

5. Assign the code or codes for this outpatient visit.

6. When verifying the code or codes, which convention is used to show that the code assigned in correct for *Streptococcal* pharyngitis and tonsillitis?

Case 2.6

The following chart note is on file for a male patient.

Derek Appleton
4/12/2008

SUBJECTIVE: This 61-year-old male has a problem with nosebleeds. No history of nose trauma. Hemorrhage comes on spontaneously about every two weeks. They start at rest and occasionally with exertion. He has no other bleeding problems. He has been on antihypertensive medications in the past.

OBJECTIVE: Blood pressure, 174/70; pulse 80. He has some dried blood in the right nostril. There is no active bleeding at this time, but there is a small clot over the anterior midseptum, which may be the bleeding site.

ASSESSMENT: 1. Benign hypertension
2. Recurrent epistaxis

PLAN: Patient was given Procardia sublingually with blood pressure dropping to 140/70. Vaseline jelly was applied to the right nostril anteriorly. Follow-up for blood pressure check in two weeks.

1. List the diagnoses that would be reported for this visit.

2. What main terms would be used to code the diagnoses?

3. Which column should the coder use in coding hypertension?

4. Which diagnosis codes would be reported for this visit?

Case 2.7

The following chart note is on file for a female patient.

Catherine Gregory
4/18/2008

SUBJECTIVE: This 25-year-old female complains of nausea and epigastric discomfort, which she describes as constant burning, for several weeks. She states that she gets nauseated when she is around food. No vomiting, melena, or hematemesis. She admits that she is taking aspirin 81 mg, QID for headaches, and on weekends she has four to eight drinks. She has not consumed any chocolate, tea, pop, or coffee.

OBJECTIVE: Abdomen is soft, flat, and nontender with normal bowel sounds; no masses or organomegaly.

ASSESSMENT: 1. Acute gastritis, due to therapeutic use of aspirin
2. Headaches

PLAN: She is to stop using aspirin and is to use Extra-Strength Tylenol for headaches. She was given a sample of Prilosec 20 mg QD for one month. Patient should return for follow-up in four weeks.

1. Abstract the diagnoses from this office visit.

2. Identify the main terms that would used to code the diagnoses.

3. Which column from the Table of Drugs and Chemicals is used in this case to show the adverse effect of aspirin?

4. Where is the note regarding the use of a fifth digit when coding gastritis located?

5. Verify and assign the correct diagnosis codes.

Case 2.8

The following chart note is on file for a male patient.

Ross Henderson
5/15/2008

SUBJECTIVE: Ross is an 81-year-old male who is diabetic. He in on Humulin insulin 30 NPH and 15 regular. He developed a diabetic ulcer on the ventral aspect of his left foot several months ago, and he has been treating the ulcer. Today he feels that there is too much callous formation around the ulcer.

OBJECTIVE: There is definite callous formation around the ulcer; the ulcer is smaller today than it was two weeks ago. Debridement of the skin was done, and the ulcer was dressed with Neosporin.

ASSESSMENT: 1. Diabetic ulcer of left foot
2. Type II diabetes mellitus, treated with long-term use of insulin

PLAN: Patient will keep soaking his foot and applying new dressings daily. Patient is to return in two weeks for follow-up.

1. Which diagnosis reflects the use of insulin over a long period of time?

2. Abstract the diagnoses from this office visit.

3. Abstract the procedure from the office visit.

4. Identify the main terms used to code all diagnoses and procedures.

5. Which convention instructs the coder regarding sequencing of the diagnosis codes?

6. Which convention instructs the coder to assign an additional code?

7. Assign the diagnosis and procedure codes for this visit.

Case 2.9

The following chart note is on file for a female patient.

Anna Starship
5/17/2008

HISTORY: Patient complains of severe pain in the right lateral abdomen, around to the back. No fever, chills. She had a kidney stone that required lithotripsy.

EXAM: There is tenderness over the right costovertebral angle and flank area.

DIAGNOSTICS: IVP shows a small calcified fleck in the right ureter. Urinalysis reveals 2+ blood cells. White blood cell count is 11,900.

DIAGNOSIS: Right ureteral stone; acute pyelonephritis.

PLAN: She is given codeine #3 for pain. Push fluids. She is to strain all urine and save any stones. Septra DS for five days.

1. Abstract the diagnoses from this office visit.

2. Identify the main terms used to code these diagnoses.

3. Which coding reference would be used to define *IVP*?

4. Which cross-reference is used when coding the stone?

5. Assign the correct ICD-9-CM diagnosis codes.

Case 2.10

The following chart note is on file for a male patient.

Jeremy Hoffman
5/20/2008

SUBJECTIVE: Patient complains of right inguinal cramping and sharp, constant pain that was brought on by lifting heavy objects at work today. Patient is status post vasectomy.

OBJECTIVE: Abdomen is soft and nontender with positive bowel sounds. There is fullness in the right groin area. Palpation of the inguinal canal reveals a bulge that is made worse with coughing. The hernia is reducible, and there is no question of incarceration or strangulation.

ASSESSMENT: Right direct inguinal hernia.

PLAN: Testicular self-exam was discussed. He is being referred to a surgeon for probable herniorrhaphy.

1. Abstract the diagnosis from this visit.

2. Locate the main term that would be used to code the diagnosis. Which convention is used to instruct the coder?

3. What is the first subterm located under the main term used to code this diagnosis?

4. Assign the diagnosis code for this patient.

Case 2.11

The following chart note is on file for a female patient.

Denise Golden
5/25/2008

HISTORY OF PRESENT ILLNESS: Denise fell off her bike and injured her right wrist and right knee.

PHYSICAL EXAM: The right wrist is swollen with obvious deformity. There is normal sensation of fingers with normal motion of the fingers. She has pain with movement of the wrist. Right knee patella is tender to palpation. There is joint effusion of the knee. Sensation and motor distal to the injury is normal.

X-RAY: X-ray of the right wrist reveals a Colles fracture with displacement of 30% from the normal position. Right knee X-ray shows a fracture of the patella with no displacement of the fragments.

IMPRESSION: 1. Colles fracture, right wrist
2. Communited patellar fracture, right knee

TREATMENT: Leg immobilizer was placed. Patient was given one crutch and instructed in crutch walking. She should bear as little weight as possible on the right knee. Posterior splint with Ace wrap was placed on the forearm. She is given Tylenol #3 for pain. Appointment will be made with Orthopedics for tomorrow for possible surgery.

1. What injuries did Denise sustain?

2. How did these injuries occur?

3. What is a Colles fracture? Which coding resource could be used to locate the definition of a Colles fracture?

4. Which main terms would the coder look up in the Alphabetic Index to Diseases and Injuries and the Alphabetic Index to External Causes?

5. Which convention instructs the coder regarding the definition of open versus closed fracture? What type of fractures did this patient sustain (open or closed)?

6. Assign the fracture codes for this visit.

7. Assign the E code or codes for this visit.

Researching the Internet

1. The Centers for Medicare and Medicaid Services maintains the current list of ICD-9-CM procedure codes (Volume 3) and references to HIPAA-mandated transactions and code sets. Access the CMS website at www.cms.hhs.gov, and link to Regulations and Guidelines to find the details of HIPAA legislation for health care transactions.

2. The National Center for Health Care Statistics (NCHS) oversees the changes and modifications to ICD-9-CM, Volumes 1 and 2. The Coordination and Maintenance Committee provides a mechanism for change in codes. Locate the meeting minutes of the Coordination and Maintenance Committee at www.cdc.gov/nchs (search for Top Ten Links to include ICD-9 information) to see how this committee addresses applications for code changes and modifications.

3. ICD-9-CM codes are used for statistical reporting by federal health agencies such as the Centers for Disease Control (CDC). Access the CDC website at www.cdc.gov, and find one study or survey that included ICD-9-CM codes. How are the codes used to provide information?

4. Knowledge of new technology is essential for keeping up with medical practice and treatment for ICD-9-CM coding. Find a medical website that provides information on the latest technology used to treat heart disease. List the name and URL of the website, and describe the new technology.

5. Understanding the disease process can make ICD-9-CM coding easier. One website that lists a variety of diseases and conditions is Web MD. Access the Web MD at http://boards.webmd.com, and find information about the causes, signs and symptoms, treatment, and prevention of asthma. For example, ICD-9-CM codes classify the different types of asthma, so knowledge of this information allows the coder to understand coding issues about this disease.

6. With ICD-9-CM codes changing every year under the National Center for Health Statistics, it is important to be able to access new codes and keep track of codes you reported in the past. Locate code 276.51 using the ICD-9-CM coding conversion table at the National Center for Health Statistics website at www.cdc.gov/nchs/datawh/ftpserv/ftpicd9/ftpicd9.htm#guidelines. What disease does this code represent, and what code was used to report this disease before 2005? Why is it important to have access to this information?

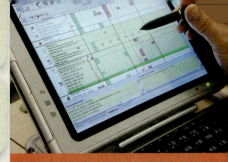

ICD-9-CM *Official Guidelines (Section I):* General Rules

LEARNING OUTCOMES

After studying this chapter, you should be able to:

1. Understand the content and source of ICD-9-CM "General Coding Guidelines."

2. Describe how the correct coding process uses both the Alphabetic Index and the Tabular List to assign codes.

3. Apply the coding guidelines on the level of detail.

4. Explain the coding of conditions that are an integral part of the disease process.

5. Explain the coding of conditions that are not an integral part of the disease process.

6. Differentiate coding guidelines for multiple codes and combination codes.

7. Understand the guidelines for coding acute and chronic conditions.

8. Explain the rules governing the coding of the late effects of previous diseases and conditions.

9. Understand the coding implications of diagnostic terms stated as *impending* or *threatened.*

10. Briefly discuss the content of the chapter-specific coding guidelines.

Key Terms

acute

causal condition

chapter-specific guidelines

chronic

code first notes

combination code

impending

integral

late effect

mandatory multiple coding

Neoplasm Table

residual condition

sign

specificity

symptom

threatened

Chapter Outline

"General Coding Guidelines": Inpatient and Outpatient

Use of Both the Alphabetic Index and the Tabular List

Level of Detail in Coding

Coding Decisions for Signs, Symptoms, and Integral Conditions

Multiple Coding for a Single Condition

Acute and Chronic Conditions

Combination Codes

Late Effects

Impending or Threatened Condition

Chapter-Specific Coding Guidelines

This chapter covers the basic coding guidelines found in Sections IB and IC of the *ICD-9-CM Official Guidelines for Coding and Reporting*. The major benefit of the national standard for reporting is data consistency. HIPAA legislation requires the use of ICD-9-CM for reporting diagnoses in all patient care settings and also stipulates following the *Official Guidelines*.

Understanding these guidelines is essential in assigning accurate ICD-9-CM codes. The basic guidelines clarify the use of both the Alphabetic Index and Tabular List and the need to code to the highest level of specificity. Guidelines also address the coding of conditions that may or may not be integral to a disease process. The coder learns when to assign multiple codes for a single condition and combination codes to reflect multiple conditions. The rules on coding both acute and chronic conditions are covered, as are the definition of a late effect and the way to code conditions that are impending or threatened. The chapter-specific coding guidelines, which are briefly summarized here, provide point-by-point rules for the various common coding situations.

"General Coding Guidelines": Inpatient and Outpatient

The Centers for Medicare and Medicaid Services (CMS) and the National Center for Health Statistics (NCHS), two departments in the federal Department of Health and Human Services (DHHS), provide guidelines for coding and reporting using ICD-9-CM (see Figure 3.1). These guidelines have been approved by the four organizations that make up the cooperating parties for ICD-9-CM: the American Hospital Association (AHA), the American Health Information Management Association (AHIMA), CMS, and NCHS. The guidelines are included on the official government version of ICD-9-CM, and they also appear in *Coding Clinic® for ICD-9-CM* published by the AHA.

The coding guidelines apply to all settings and all providers of health care. For example, a physician, a hospital, and a nursing home utilize these guidelines for all diagnosis reporting. The guidelines apply whether coding in the outpatient or the inpatient setting.

Use of Both the Alphabetic Index and the Tabular List

Points 1 and 2 of the "General Coding Guidelines," as shown in Figure 3.1, explain the basic correct coding process. The coder must use both the Alphabetic Index and the Tabular List when locating and assigning codes and must not rely solely on only one volume, as errors will occur in code assignment if only one volume is used. For example, by using the Alphabetic Index only to code the condition of abdominal pain, the code 789.0 would be assigned. This code is incorrect; the Tabular List indicates that a fifth digit is required to identify the specific location of pain. Code 789.00 correctly reports the diagnosis of abdominal pain. It is also important for the coder to read and follow any notes that appear in either volume.

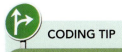

CODING TIP

Correct Coding Process

The Alphabetic Index drives code assignment; verification of codes is completed using the Tabular List.

Level of Detail in Coding

Points 3, 4, and 5 of the "General Coding Guidelines" (see Figure 3.1) explain how to assign the most specific code. The primary rule states that both diagnosis and procedure codes are to include the highest number of digits available for the highest level of **specificity.**

ICD-9-CM DIAGNOSIS CODES

ICD-9-CM diagnosis codes are composed of either three, four, or five digits, with three digits always before the decimal point. Codes with three digits are categories, and a category may be subdivided by a fourth digit and possibly a fifth digit. Typically the fourth and fifth digits provide additional specificity regarding the type of disease, the cause of disease, or the site of disease.

In other words, a three-digit code is to be used only if it is not further subdivided. If a particular category includes fourth-digit subcategories and fifth-digit subclassifications, they must be assigned. A code is incorrect or invalid if it has not been coded to the full number of digits available. Example of coding to the highest level of specificity follow.

1. Use of both Alphabetic Index and Tabular List

Use both the Alphabetic Index and the Tabular List when locating and assigning a code. Reliance on only the Alphabetic Index or the Tabular List leads to errors in code assignments and less specificity in code selection.

2. Locate each term in the Alphabetic Index

Locate each term in the Alphabetic Index and verify the code selected in the Tabular List. Read and be guided by instructional notations that appear in both the Alphabetic Index and the Tabular List.

3. Level of detail in coding

Diagnosis and procedure codes are to be used at their highest number of digits available. ICD-9-CM diagnosis codes are composed of codes with either 3, 4, or 5 digits. Codes with three digits are included in ICD-9-CM as the heading of a category of codes that may be further subdivided by the use of fourth and/or fifth digits, which provide greater detail.

A three-digit code is to be used only if it is not further subdivided. Where fourth-digit subcategories and/or fifth-digit subclassifications are provided, they must be assigned. A code is invalid if it has not been coded to the full number of digits required for that code. For example, Acute myocardial infarction, code 410, has fourth digits that describe the location of the infarction (e.g., 410.2, Of inferolateral wall), and fifth digits that identify the episode of care. It would be incorrect to report a code in category 410 without a fourth and fifth digit.

ICD-9-CM Volume 3 procedure codes are composed of codes with either 3 or 4 digits. Codes with two digits are included in ICD-9-CM as the heading of a category of codes that may be further subdivided by the use of third and/or fourth digits, which provide greater detail.

4. Code or codes from 001.0 through V84.8

The appropriate code or codes from 001.0 through V84.8 must be used to identify diagnoses, symptoms, conditions, problems, complaints, or other reason(s) for the encounter/visit.

5. Selection of codes 001.0 through 999.9

The selection of codes 001.0 through 999.9 will frequently be used to describe the reason for the admission/encounter. These codes are from the section of ICD-9-CM for the classification of diseases and injuries (e.g., infectious and parasitic diseases; neoplasms; symptoms, signs, and ill-defined conditions, etc.).

6. Signs and symptoms

Codes that describe symptoms and signs, as opposed to diagnoses, are acceptable for reporting purposes when a related definitive diagnosis has not been established (confirmed) by the provider. Chapter 16 of ICD-9-CM, Symptoms, Signs, and Ill-Defined Conditions (codes 780.0–799.9) contain many, but not all codes for symptoms.

7. Conditions that are an integral part of a disease process

Signs and symptoms that are associated routinely with a disease process should not be assigned as additional codes, unless otherwise instructed by the classification.

8. Conditions that are not an integral part of a disease process

Additional signs and symptoms that may not be associated routinely with a disease process should be coded when present.

9. Multiple coding for a single condition

In addition to the etiology/manifestation convention that requires two codes to fully describe a single condition that affects multiple body systems, there are other single conditions that also require more than one code. "Use additional code" notes are found in the tabular at codes that are not part of an etiology/manifestation pair where a secondary code is useful to fully describe a condition. The sequencing rule is the same as the etiology/manifestation pair—"use additional code" indicates that a secondary code should be added.

For example, for infections that are not included in chapter 1, a secondary code from category 041, Bacterial infection in conditions classified elsewhere and of unspecified site, may be required to identify the bacterial organism causing the infection. A "use additional code" note will normally be found at the infectious disease code, indicating a need for the organism code to be added as a secondary code.

"Code first" notes are also under certain codes that are not specifically manifestation codes but may be due to an underlying cause. When a "code first" note is present and an underlying condition is present the underlying condition should be sequenced first.

"Code, if applicable, any causal condition first" notes indicate that this code may be assigned as a principal diagnosis when the causal condition is unknown or not applicable. If a causal condition is known, then the code for that condition should be sequenced as the principal or first-listed diagnosis. Multiple codes may be needed for late effects, complication codes and obstetric codes to more fully describe a condition. See the specific guidelines for these conditions for further instruction.

10. Acute and chronic conditions

If the same condition is described as both acute (subacute) and chronic, and separate subentries exist in the Alphabetic Index at the same indentation level, code both and sequence the acute (subacute) code first.

11. Combination code

A combination code is a single code used to classify:
- Two diagnoses, or
- A diagnosis with an associated secondary process (manifestation)
- A diagnosis with an associated complication

Combination codes are identified by referring to subterm entries in the Alphabetic Index and by reading the inclusion and exclusion notes in the Tabular List.

Assign only the combination code when that code fully identifies the diagnostic conditions involved or when the Alphabetic Index so directs. Multiple coding should not be used when the classification provides a combination code that clearly identifies all of the elements documented in the diagnosis. When the combination code lacks necessary specificity in describing the manifestation or complication, an additional code should be used as a secondary code.

12. Late effects

A late effect is the residual effect (condition produced) after the acute phase of an illness or injury has terminated. There is no time limit on when a late effect code can be used. The residual may be apparent early, such as in cerebrovascular accident cases, or it may occur months or years later, such as that due to a previous injury. Coding of late effects generally requires two codes sequenced in the following order: The condition or nature of the late effect is sequenced first. The late effect code is sequenced second.

An exception to the above guidelines are those instances where the code for late effect is followed by a manifestation code identified in the Tabular List and title, or the late effect code has been expanded (at the fourth and fifth-digit levels) to include the manifestation(s). The code for the acute phase of an illness or injury that led to the late effect is never used with a code for the late effect.

13. Impending or threatened condition

Code any condition described at the time of discharge as "impending" or "threatened" as follows:

If it did occur, code as confirmed diagnosis.

If it did not occur, reference the Alphabetic Index to determine if the condition has a subentry term for "impending" or "threatened" and also reference main term entries for "Impending" and for "Threatened." If the subterms are listed, assign the given code.

If the subterms are not listed, code the existing underlying condition(s) and not the condition described as impending or threatened.

FIGURE 3.1

Section IB, "General Coding Guidelines," October 1, 2007

466 ACUTE BRONCHITIS AND BRONCHIOLITIS

Includes: That with:
Bronchospasm
Obstruction

466.0 ACUTE BRONCHITIS

Bronchitis, acute or subacute:
Fibrinous
Membranous
Pneumococcal
Purulent
Septic
Viral
With trachetitis
Tracheobronchitis, acute

Excludes:
acute bronchitis with chronic obstructive pulmonary
disease (491.22)

466.1 ACUTE BRONCHIOLITIS

Bronchiolitis (acute)
Capillary pneumonia

466.11 ACUTE BRONCHIOLITIS DUE TO RESPIRATORY SYNCYTIAL VIRUS (RSV)

466.19 ACUTE BRONCHIOLITIS DUE TO OTHER INFECTIOUS ORGANISMS

Use additional code to identify organism

This example represents category 466, acute bronchitis and bronchiolitis. It is incorrect to assign code 466 alone. A fourth digit is required to identify the type of disease, either acute bronchitis (466.0) or acute bronchiolitis (466.11 or 466.19), and the fifth digit for category 466.1 classifies more detail about the cause of acute bronchiolitis.

142 MALIGNANT NEOPLASM OF MAJOR SALIVARY GLANDS

Includes: Salivary ducts
Excludes:
malignant neoplasm of minor salivary glands:
NOS (145.9)
buccal mucosa (145.0)
soft palate (145.3)
tongue (141.0–141.9)
tonsil, palatine (146.0)

142.0 PAROTID GLAND

142.1 SUBMANDIBULAR GLAND

Submaxillary gland

142.2 SUBLINGUAL GLAND

142.8 OTHER MAJOR SALIVARY GLANDS

Malignant neoplasm of contiguous or overlapping sites of salivary glands and ducts whose point of origin cannot be determined

142.9 SALIVARY GLAND, UNSPECIFIED

Salivary gland (major) NOS

Category 142 classifies malignant neoplasms of major salivary glands. A fourth digit must be added to identify the specific site or type of salivary gland, such as code 142.0 to identify a malignant neoplasm of the parotid gland.

Using the Tabular List of the ICD-9-CM, determine whether the following codes classify the cause of the disease (Cause), the site of the disease (Site), or the type of disease (Type).

1. What does the fifth digit classify for code 715.3? _____

2. What does the fourth digit classify for category code 047? _____

3. What does the fourth digit classify for category code 588? _____

4. What does the fifth digit classify for subcategory code 535.5? _____

5. What does the fifth digit classify for subcategory code 038.4? _____

ICD-9-CM PROCEDURE CODES

ICD-9-CM Volume 3 procedure codes have either three or four digits. The two-digit category codes serve as the heading, and the category is further subdivided into three-digit and sometimes four-digit codes that provide greater detail. For example, procedure category code 22 identifies operations on nasal sinuses.

EXAMPLE

22 OPERATIONS ON NASAL SINUSES
   22.0 ASPIRATION AND LAVAGE OF NASAL SINUS
      22.00 ASPIRATION AND LAVAGE OF NASAL SINUS NOS
      22.01 PUNCTURE OF NASAL SINUS FOR ASPIRATION OR LAVAGE
      22.02 ASPIRATION OR LAVAGE OF NASAL SINUS THROUGH NASAL OSTIUM
   22.1 DIAGNOSTIC PROCEDURES ON NASAL SINUS
      22.11 CLOSED [ENDOSCOPIC] [NEEDLE] BIOPSY OF NASAL SINUS
      22.12 OPEN BIOPSY OF NASAL SINUS
      22.19 OTHER DIAGNOSTIC PROCEDURES ON NASAL SINUSES
      Endoscopy without biopsy

   Excludes:
   transillumination of sinus (89.35)
   x-ray of sinus (87.15–87.16)

This category is broken down to both three and four digits to provide greater detail. For example, code 22.1, aspiration and lavage of nasal sinuses, a specific type of procedure on the nasal sinuses, is broken down into more detail about the technique used to aspirate the nasal sinuses, such as 22.01, puncture of nasal sinus for aspiration or lavage.

Coding Decisions for Signs, Symptoms, and Integral Conditions

Coders are required to make decisions about whether to include aspects of the patient's diagnosis that are not clear-cut. Points 6, 7, and 8 of the "General Coding Guidelines" (Figure 3.1) explain how to proceed.

SIGNS AND SYMPTOMS

A diagnosis is not always readily established for a patient's condition. Often a series of workups, tests, and examinations during follow-up visits are required before the physician determines a diagnosis. During this process, signs and symptoms, rather than an uncertain diagnosis, are reported for reimbursement of service fees.

A **sign** is an objective indication that can be evaluated by the physician, such as weight loss. A **symptom** is a subjective statement by the patient that cannot be confirmed during an examination, such as pain. Figure 3.2 shows a flow chart to guide the basic process for coding signs and symptoms.

EXAMPLE
DIAGNOSTIC STATEMENT: Middle-aged male presents with abdominal pain and weight loss. He had to return home from vacation due to acute illness. He has not been eating well because of vague upper-abdominal pain. He denies nausea, vomiting. He denies changes in bowel habit or blood in stool. Physical examination revealed no abdominal tenderness.
PRIMARY DIAGNOSIS: 789.06, abdominal pain, epigastric region
COEXISTING CONDITION: 783.2, abnormal loss of weight

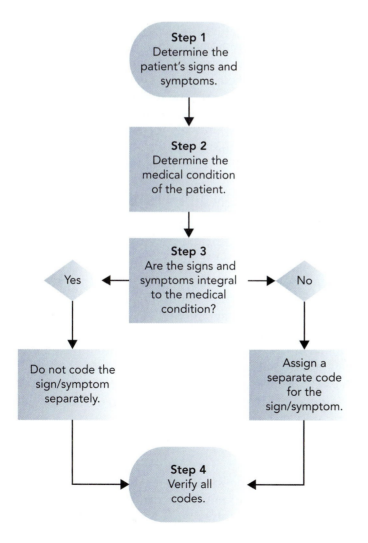

FIGURE 3.2
Signs and Symptoms Code Assignment Flow Chart

Point 6 of the "General Coding Guidelines" states:

> Codes that describe symptoms and signs, as opposed to diagnoses, are acceptable for reporting purposes when a related definitive diagnosis has not been established (confirmed) by the provider. Chapter 16 of ICD-9-CM, "Symptoms, Signs, and Ill-Defined Conditions" (codes 780.0–799.9), contains many, but not all codes for symptoms.

Some examples of signs are fever, tachycardia, and seizure. Symptoms such as abdominal pain, headache, and chest pain are also reported in Chapter 16 of ICD-9-CM. More specific guidelines are based on whether a sign or symptom is integral to a disease process.

CONDITIONS THAT ARE AN INTEGRAL PART OF A DISEASE PROCESS

Point 7 of the "General Coding Guidelines" (Figure 3.1) covers conditions that are an integral part of a disease process. For example, pneumonia presents with certain signs and symptoms that are considered **integral.** This means that the signs and symptoms are always seen in patients with the disease. The coding rule states that codes for signs and symptoms that are routinely associated with a disease process should not be assigned.

Consider the typical signs and symptoms of pneumonia. Objective and measurable signs of pneumonia include the patient's temperature (fever). Symptoms (subjective and not easily measured) include difficulty breathing (dyspnea). A patient with pneumonia might have the signs of fever and cough and the symptom of difficulty breathing. This guideline explains that the coder would code only pneumonia, since the signs and symptoms are integral to pneumonia and not separately reportable.

To decide how to handle a case, the coder asks whether the sign or symptom would be routinely present in all cases of the disease. If so, it would not be coded. In correct coding language, we would say that cough, fever, and dyspnea are integral to pneumonia, so only pneumonia would be reported.

CONDITIONS THAT ARE NOT AN INTEGRAL PART OF A DISEASE PROCESS

In contrast to the guideline covering integral conditions, point 8 of the "General Coding Guidelines" states that "additional signs and symptoms that may not be associated routinely with a disease process should be coded when present." For example, a patient may have cirrhosis of the liver and the symptom of ascites. Since ascites is not routinely associated with cirrhosis, it would be reported in addition to the code for cirrhosis. Another example of a symptom that is not integral to the disease process is a coma. A coma is not routinely associated with a stroke. If a patient suffering from a stroke goes into a coma, the coma code would be reported in addition to the code for stroke.

DETERMINING SIGNS, SYMPTOMS, AND INTEGRAL CONDITIONS

How can a coder determine whether a sign or symptom is integral to the disease process? This knowledge can be obtained through the study of disease and pathophysiology. Online coding resources can also be used to research a disease process. Another option is to refer to the AHA *Coding Clinic* guidelines, which often discuss signs and symptoms of specific diseases and conditions.

EXAMPLE Hematuria (blood in the urine) is integral to a renal or ureteral calculus. In other words, if a patient has a renal calculus, hematuria (599.7) would be expected. Hydronephosis (fluid collection in the kidney), however, is not integral to a renal calculus (592.0), so this condition (591) should be reported separately. Some symptoms are coded in their specific ICD-9-CM chapter by body system. Hydronephrosis is one such symptom.

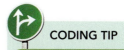

CODING TIP

Know—or Research— the Disease Process

Use your coding resources to determine whether a sign or symptom is integral to a disease or condition.

Checkpoint 3.2

Using ICD-9-CM Volumes 1 and 2, code the following.

1. Antral gastritis, with hemorrhage and abdominal pain _____
2. Closed fracture of the wrist with wrist pain _____
3. Acute pancreatitis with abdominal ascites _____
4. Acute asthma exacerbation with hypoxia _____
5. Urinary tract infection with dysuria _____

Multiple Coding for a Single Condition

In addition to the etiology and manifestation convention that requires two codes to fully describe a single condition that affects multiple body systems, other single conditions also require more than one code. Point 9 of the "General Coding Guidelines" (Figure 3.1), referred to as **mandatory multiple coding,** indicates when two codes may be required to report a condition.

CODE FIRST NOTE

The **code first notes** are used when there is an underlying condition. When a code first note and an underlying condition are both present, the underlying condition code should be sequenced first.

EXAMPLE
785.4 GANGRENE
    Gangrene:
        NOS
        Spreading cutaneous
    Gangrenous cellulitis
    Phagedena
    Code first any associated underlying condition:
        Diabetes (250.7)
        Raynaud's syndrome (443.0)

CODING TIP

Code First Note

Code first notes indicate mandatory coding of both conditions.

The Genitourinary System

The genitourinary system consists of the urinary tract and the male and female reproductive systems. The urinary tract organs are the kidney, bladder, ureters, and urethra. The male and female reproductive systems are both susceptible to sexually transmitted diseases (STDs) as well as to problems related to fertility and sexual functioning.

Urinary Tract Disorders

Nephritis is a general term for any inflammation of the kidneys. It is classified in a number of ways, such as *albuminuric* (with the presence of albumin in the urine), *infantile, degenerative,* and *granulomatous* (with inflamed granulated tissue). It is also categorized in a number of ways, such as by what accompanies it (as *with edema* or *with membranous lesions*) or by its cause (as *due to diabetes mellitus*). *Glomerulonephritis* (inflammation of the glomeruli of the kidneys) and *pyelonephritis* (inflammation of the renal pelvis of the kidney) are also classified as

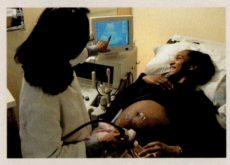
An ultrasound.

acute or *chronic* and are categorized in various other ways. *Kidney* or *renal failure* is classified as *acute* or *chronic* and is also categorized in other ways, such as *with hypertensive disease* or *following an ectopic pregnancy.*

Calculi (stones; the singular is *calculus*), cysts, and fistulas are common occurrences in various parts of the urinary tract. Renal calculi are classified as *impacted* (causing a blockage), *recurrent,* or *congenital.* Bladder calculi are classified as *impacted, encysted* (enclosed in a cyst), or *urinary.* A calculus can also be classified as *calculus of lower urinary tract, unspecified. Cystitis* is a general term for inflam-

mation of the urinary bladder. It is classified in a number of ways, such as *recurrent, exudative* (with oozing), *hemorrhagic,* and *ulcerative.* It is also categorized in a variety of ways, such as *with fibrosis* or *chronic. Ureteritis* and *urethritis* are inflammations of the ureters and urethra, respectively. *Urinalysis* is one of the most common diagnostic tests used for the genitourinary system as well as for most of the body's other systems.

Female Reproductive Disorders

The female reproductive cycle is disrupted by pregnancy or complications that affect the menstrual cycle. In addition, each part of the female reproductive is susceptible to various diseases and disorders. Once menstruation ceases and menopause begins, other symptoms and disorders can occur. *Complications of pregnancy, childbirth, and the puerperium* (the six weeks following childbirth) can occur at the very earliest stages.

An *abortion* may be *spontaneous* (as in a *missed abortion* or *miscarriage*), or it may be *legal.* Abortions are classified as *complete* or *incomplete* (with some material remaining in the uterus). There are many categories of abortion, such as *early, self-induced, with complications,* and *with damage to a pelvic organ.* Complications of abortion are also categorized by type (for example, *hemorrhage* or *sepsis.*

If the pregnancy progresses, an ultrasound is usually given within the first three months to see whether the fetus is progressing normally and the pregnancy itself is viable. Some complications of pregnancy are mechanical, such as *placenta previa* (placenta abnormally implanted in the lower part of the uterus), which is classified in various

The code first note appears at code 785.4, gangrene. When assigning the code for gangrene, the coder should first code any underlying condition that is documented, such as diabetes or Raynaud's syndrome. In coding Raynaud's syndrome with gangrene, the coder reports both codes 443.0 and 785.4.

USE ADDITIONAL CODE NOTE

The *use additional code* notes found in the Tabular List identify codes that are not part of etiology and manifestation pairs. In these cases, a secondary code is used to fully describe the condition. For example,

ways (*partial, complete,* and *lateral,* for example). Other complications involve infections, such as *toxoplasmosis,* which can cause damage to the fetus. Other complications, such as *pre-eclampsia, hemorrhage, hypertension,* and *edema,* may result from other diseases (as renal disease). Complications of pregnancy are also classified according to when the complication arises (*antepartum,* before delivery, or *postpartum,* after delivery).

Endometriosis (the presence of uterine lining in other pelvic organs) is usually categorized by location (*endometriosis of ovary*). Inflammations may appear in various parts of the female reproductive system (for example, *cervicitis, inflammatory disease of the breast,* and *vaginitis*). Lumps in the breast may become cancerous. Cysts may form in various parts, such as the ovaries. *Dysmenorrhea* (painful menstruation) is classified in several ways, such as *primary* and

exfoliative (with scaling). *Menopausal* and *postmenopausal disorders* may involve bleeding and/or a group of uncomfortable symptoms, sometimes treated with hormones. *Infertility* may be a female or a male reproductive problem.

Male Reproductive Disorders

Male infertility may be due to *azoospermia* (absence of sperm) or *oligospermia* (low sperm count). A PSA (*prostate-specific antigen*) test is routine in male physical examinations. It can show the presence of prostate cancer or simply of a prostate irritation (*prostatitis*). *Benign prostatic hypertrophy (BPH)* is prostate enlargement that restricts urination. A *hydrocele,* accumulation of fluid around the testes, is classified in a variety of ways, such as *infantile* and *calcified* (hardened). Inflammations, such as *orchitis* and *epididymitis,* occur throughout the male reproductive system. *Impotence* can be *sexual* or *psychogenic* (psychological in origin). It may also result from medication or other disorders. *Erectile dysfunction* is treated with medication. Other penile disorders are *priapism* (painful erection) and *Peyronie's disease* (severe curvature of the erect penis).

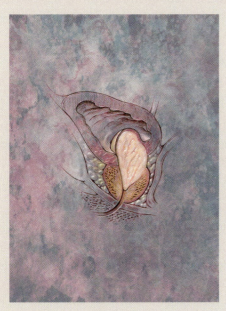

An inflamed prostate.

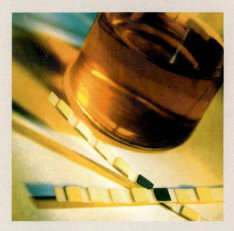

A urinalysis.

for infections not included in Chapter 1 of the ICD-9-CM Tabular List, a secondary code is required to identify the bacterial organism causing the infection, if the organism is documented.

EXAMPLE
OTHER DISEASES OF URINARY SYSTEM (590–599)
590 INFECTIONS OF KIDNEY
Use additional code to identify organism, such as Escherichia coli
[E. coli] (041.4)
590.0 CHRONIC PYELONEPHRITIS
Chronic pyelitis

Chronic pyonephrosis
Code, if applicable, any causal condition first
590.00 WITHOUT LESION OF RENAL MEDULLARY NECROSIS
590.01 WITH LESION OF RENAL MEDULLARY NECROSIS
590.1 ACUTE PYELONEPHRITIS
Acute pyelitis
Acute pyonephrosis
590.10 WITHOUT LESION OF RENAL MEDULLARY NECROSIS
590.11 WITH LESION OF RENAL MEDULLARY NECROSIS

The example shows a *use additional code note* requiring the coder to also report the organism causing the infection of the kidney. To code the specific organism causing the infection, the main term *infection* is located in the Alphabetic Index. Reporting the condition of pyelonephritis due to *Streptococcus* B requires reporting two codes: 590.80 (pyelonephritis) and 041.02 (streptococcal B infection).

Coders will need familiarity with the disease processes relating to genitourinary illnesses as illustrated in the example. These diseases are reviewed in the Pathophysiology Refresher on pages 108–109.

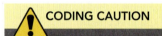
CODING CAUTION

Code Only What Is Documented

If the infectious organism causing an infection is not documented, the code for the infection should be reported alone.

CODE, IF APPLICABLE, ANY CAUSAL CONDITION FIRST NOTE

Code, if applicable, any causal condition first notes indicate that the codes may be assigned as principal diagnoses when the **causal condition**— the medical illness that has brought on the documented disease—is unknown or not applicable. If a causal condition is known, the code for that condition should be sequenced as the principal or first-listed diagnosis. In the example above, the notation is located at the subcategory level code 590.0. Therefore, if the chronic pyelonephritis was due to renal calculus, the code for renal calculus (592.0) would be sequenced first, followed by the code for the chronic pyelonephritis (590.00). Another notation in the Tabular List instructs the coder to use two codes if documentation is supportive. If a patient had chronic *E. coli* pyelonephritis due to renal calculus, the coder would assign three codes: renal calculus (592.0), chronic pyelonephritis (590.00), and *E. coli* infection (041.4).

Checkpoint 3.3

Using ICD-9-CM Volumes 1 and 2, code the following conditions.

1. Acute cystitis due to proteus mirabilis infection _____
2. Diverticulitis of the sigmoid with peritonitis _____
3. Benign prostatic hypertrophy with urinary obstruction and urinary frequency _____
4. Vaginal wall prolapse with stress urinary incontinence _____
5. Systemic Inflamatory Response Syndrome (SIRS) with septic shock due to *E. coli* septicemia

_____

Acute and Chronic Conditions

Point 10 of the "General Coding Guidelines" explains:

> If the same condition is described as both acute (subacute) and chronic, and separate subentries exist in the Alphabetic Index at the same indentation level, code both and sequence the acute (subacute) code first.

This guideline instructs the coder to look carefully at the indentation level to determine whether two codes should be assigned when the condition is both acute (subacute) and chronic. An **acute** illness or condition is one that has severe symptoms and a short duration, whereas a **chronic** illness or condition has a long duration. *Acute* can also refer to a sudden exacerbation of a chronic condition.

EXAMPLE
Pancreatitis   577.0
    acute (edematous) (hemorrhagic) (recurrent)   577.0
    annular   577.0
    apoplectic   577.0
    calcereous   577.0
    chronic (infectious)   577.1
        recurrent   577.1

When coding acute and chronic pancreatitis, as in the example above, both subterms, *acute* and *chronic*, are located at the same indentation level. Therefore, both codes 577.0 and 577.1 would be assigned if the patient had both conditions. The acute condition code should be listed first, followed by the code for the chronic condition.

Acute and *chronic* can also be sub-subterms.

EXAMPLE
Cholelithiasis (impacted) (multiple)   574.2

Note—Use the following fifth-digit subclassification with category 574:
        0 without mention of obstruction
        1 with obstruction

---

    with
            cholecystitis   574.1
                acute   574.0
                chronic   574.1

The Alphabetic Index shows that cholelithiasis (the main term) with cholecystitis (the subterm) has the sub-subterms *acute* and *chronic* at the same indentation level. Therefore, the condition of acute and chronic cholecystitis with cholelithiasis is assigned two codes—574.00 and 574.10—sequencing the acute code (574.00) first. The basic coding process for acute and chronic conditions is shown in Figure 3.3.

Combination Codes

As explained in point 11 of the "General Coding Guidelines" (Figure 3.1), a **combination code** is one code that classifies:

- Two diagnoses
- A diagnosis with an associated manifestation
- A diagnosis with an associated complication

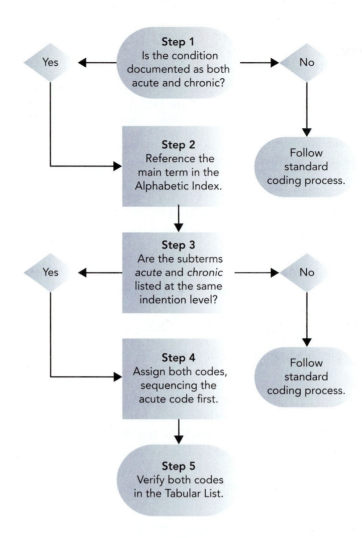

FIGURE 3.3

Acute and Chronic Conditions Code Assignment Flow Chart

Step 1
Is the condition documented as both acute and chronic?

Yes

No

Step 2
Reference the main term in the Alphabetic Index.

Follow standard coding process.

Step 3
Are the subterms *acute* and *chronic* listed at the same indention level?

Yes

No

Step 4
Assign both codes, sequencing the acute code first.

Follow standard coding process.

Step 5
Verify both codes in the Tabular List.

Combination codes are identified by referring to subterm entries in the Alphabetic Index and by reading the inclusion and exclusion notes in the Tabular List. Often the subterm *with* will result in the classification of two diagnoses in one code. For example, if a patient has the diagnoses of diverticulitis *with* bleeding, code 562.13 classifies the two conditions together. This example illustrates the disease processes associated with the digestive system, a major area about which medical coders must be familiar. The Pathophysiology Refresher on pages 114–115 provides information on key conditions and processes in this body system.

When a combination code reflects both a disease and its manifestation, the subterm *due to* often appears. For example, for pneumonia *due to* adenovirus, code 480.0 identifies the disease pneumonia with the causal organism adenovirus. Although this example uses the phrase *due to*, neither *due to* nor the equally common *with* is required to assign a combination code.

An example of a combination code that classifies a diagnosis and an associated complication is a postoperative hemorrhage, where code 998.11 indicates that the hemorrhage is a post-op complication.

When documentation supports a relationship between two conditions, multiple codes should not be used if a combination code clearly identifies all the elements. If the combination code lacks the necessary specificity in describing the manifestation or complication, an additional code should be reported.

Code the following conditions using ICD-9-CM Volumes 1 and 2.

1. Acute and chronic cystitis _____

2. Acute and chronic cholecystitis _____

3. Acute appendicitis with perforation _____

4. Postoperative hematoma _____

5. Chronic bronchitis due to tobacco smoking _____

Late Effects

A **late effect** is the residual condition produced after the acute phase of an illness or injury has terminated. Based on point 12 of the "General Coding Guidelines" (Figure 3.1), there is no time limit on when a late effect code can be used; a late effect may be apparent early, or it may occur some months or years later. For example, a patient may have a **residual condition,** such as paralysis (residual), soon after a stroke (cause of the residual condition, no longer present). On the other hand, a patient may not develop a residual condition from an accident, such as a nonunion of a fracture, until much later. Terms often used to describe late effects include *old, previous, due to previous, malunion,* and *nonunion.*

As shown in Figure 3.4, a late effect generally requires two codes, with the code for the condition or nature of the late effect (code the

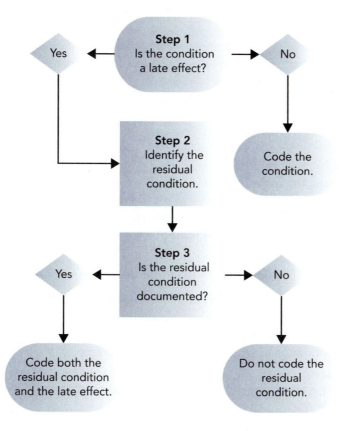

FIGURE 3.4
Late Effects Code Assignment Flow Chart

The Digestive System

The digestive system involves the intake and digestion of nutrients in the upper gastrointestinal tract through absorption and elimination processes in the lower gastrointestinal tract. Diseases of the mouth affect the ability to take in life-sustaining nutrients. Diseases of the accessory digestive organs (salivary glands, liver, gallbladder, and pancreas) affect the ability to digest nutrients. The stomach and intestines are crucial in furthering the digestion and elimination processes.

Diseases of the Mouth, Esophagus, Stomach, and Duodenum

Glossitis is an inflammation of the tongue, and *cheilitis* is an inflammation of the lips. *Esophagitis* is a general term for any inflammation of the esophagus. It is classified in several ways, such as *postoperative* or *regurgitant* (caused by acid reflux). *Gastroesophageal reflux disease (GERD)* is one type of esophagitis.

Ulcers appear in many parts of the digestive system. Ulcers of the esophagus may be *fungal* (caused by a fungus) or *peptic* (caused by digestive secretions).

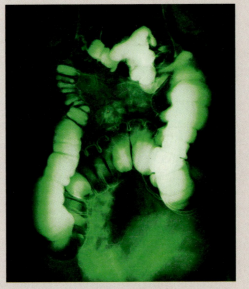

An X-ray of the lower gastrointestinal tract.

Gastric or *stomach ulcers* are classified as *eroded, peptic,* or *round* and with or without *obstruction.* Ulcers can become complicated when something such as *bleeding* or *perforation* occurs. *Duodenal ulcers* have similar classifications.

Gastritis is a general term for an inflammation of the stomach (stomach upset, acute stomach inflammation). It is categorized in many ways, such as *irritant, allergic,* or *alcoholic. Gastroenteritis* (the general term for inflammation of both the stomach and the intestines) also has many classifications, such as *acute* and *infectious.* Surgeries and procedures to treat obesity, such as *gastric bypass* and *gastric banding,* can lead to *postgastric surgery syndrome,* postoperative *diarrhea,* or *vomiting.*

Diseases of the Intestines

Enteritis is a general term for any inflammation of the intestines. It is classified in a number of ways, such as *diarrheal, presumed noninfectious,* and *infantile;* by cause (*allergic* or *bacterial*); or by type (*E. coli*). Inflammations of particular areas of the intestines, such as *colitis,* are also classified in a number of ways, such as *acute, ulcerative,* and *noninfectious.* The intestines are also the site

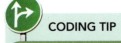

CODING TIP

Possible Use of an E Code

An E code may be needed to reflect the circumstances of a late effect of an injury.

condition/residual) listed first, followed by the code for the late effect (code using the main term *late*).

There are three exceptions to the general guidelines. First are instances in which the code for the late effect is followed by a manifestation code identified in the Tabular List.

EXAMPLE

myelitis (*see also* Late, effect(s) (of), encephalitis)—*see* category 326

To code a late effect of myelitis, the Alphabetic Index instructs the coder to see category 326. The instructions at category 326 in the Tabular List direct the coder to use an additional code (reported second) to identify the condition, as shown in the following example.

EXAMPLE

326   LATE EFFECTS OF INTRACRANIAL ABSCESS OR PYOGENIC INFECTION

of obstructions. Some of them are caused by an *intussusception* (the slipping of one part into another) or a *volvulus* (a twisting of the intestine). There may also be an *impaction* (a wedging together of waste matter). An intestinal obstruction can also appear with or without a hernia. *Hernias* can appear throughout the body but are most common in the abdominal region. They are classified as *acquired* or *recurrent*.

Many other intestinal disorders can occur. They are further categorized by location and/or characteristics, such as *colon with gangrene* or *gastrointestinal with obstruction*. *Diverticulitis* is *with* or *without* *hemorrhage*. *Constipation* may be *unspecified, drug-induced,* or *other*. *Irritable bowel syndrome* may include an irritable colon or a spastic colon. *Fistulas* (abnormal passages or ducts) can appear throughout the body. An *anal fistula* may be accompanied by an *abscess*. *Peritonitis* (inflammation of the serous membrane lining the abdominal cavity) is classified in a number of ways, such as *acute, idiopathic* (of unknown cause), and *localized*. It is further categorized by cause (*due to bile*), by location (*pelvic*), or by other characteristics. *Polyps* may appear throughout the intestines and in the rectum and anus. They are usually categorized by

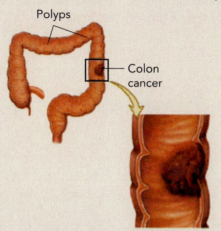

Polyps

Colon cancer

Polyps and Colon Cancer

Colon polyps may become malignant.

location (*colon*). If they become malignant, they are classified under neoplasms.

Diseases of the Accessory Organs

The liver, pancreas, appendix, and gallbladder are all sites of digestive disorders. Some of these organs are also part of other body systems (for example, the pancreas plays a crucial role in endocrine disorders, such as diabetes). *Cirrhosis* of the liver is often categorized by cause (such as *alcoholic cirrhosis*). *Hepatitis* is a general term for an inflammation of the liver. There are many subcategories of hepatitis. *Viral hepatitis* itself is classified in many ways depending on its origin (*type B*) and other characteristics or causes (such as *with hepatic coma*). Nonviral hepatitis may be *alcoholic* or *chronic*. There are other liver diseases, such as *chronic liver disease* and *liver abscess*.

Pancreatitis can be *acute, chronic,* or *malignant*, as well as a number of other classifications. *Appendicitis* can also be classified in a number of ways, such as *acute* and *chronic*. The gallbladder and the bile ducts are often the sites of calculus or stones in a condition known as *cholelithiasis* (gallstones) or *choledocholithiasis* (bile duct stones). This condition is usually classified as *with* or *without obstruction*.

Note: This category is to be used to indicate conditions whose primary classification is to 320–325 [excluding 320.7, 321.0–321.8, 323.0–323.4, 323.6–323.7] as the cause of late effects, themselves classifiable elsewhere. The "late effects" may include conditions specified as such, or as sequelae, which may occur at any time after the resolution of the causal condition,
Use additional code to identify condition, as:
Hydrocephalus (331.4)
Paralysis (342.0–342.9, 344.0–344.9)

Second are situations in which the late effect code has been expanded (at the fourth- and fifth-digit levels) to include the manifestations or residuals. In this case, to code the late effect of a cerebrovascular accident, subterms include listings of the different manifestations such as hemiplegia (342.90).

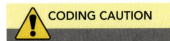

CODING CAUTION

Coding Late Effects

Do not use the code for the acute phase of an illness or injury that led to the late effect with a code for the late effect of that illness or injury.

EXAMPLE

Late effect(s) (of)

cerebrovascular disease (conditions classifiable to 430–437 438.9)

with

alterations of sensations	438.6
aphasia	438.11
apraxia	438.81
ataxia	438.84
cognitive deficits	438.0
disturbances of vision	438.7
dysphagia	438.82
dysphasia	438.12

The third exception is when the manifestation (residual) was not documented, such as late effect of skull fracture due to a car accident. Code only late effect, fracture, skull, code 905.0 and the E code E-929.0; the residual condition is not coded.

Checkpoint 3.5

Code the following late effects using ICD-9-CM Volumes 1 and 2, and underline the residual condition.

1. Painful scar due to old burn injury, left leg _____

2. Leg paralysis due to previous poliomyelitis _____

3. Neurogenic dysphagia due to old cerebrovascular accident _____

4. Hydrocephalus due to previous encephalitis _____

5. Malunion of the tibia due to old fracture _____

Impending or Threatened Condition

As explained in point 13 of the "General Coding Guidelines" (Figure 3.1), if a condition documented at the time of discharge as **impending** or **threatened** did occur, it should be coded as a confirmed diagnosis.

If the condition did not occur, first reference the Alphabetic Index to determine whether the condition has a subterm for *impending* or *threatened*. Also reference the main terms *impending* and *threatened* to determine whether there is a specific code for the condition. If so, assign the code after verifying it in the Tabular List.

EXAMPLE

Impending

cerebrovascular accident or attack	435.9
coronary syndrome	411.1
delirium tremens	291.0
myocardial infarction	411.1

An impending cerebrovascular accident would be reported using code 435.9.

If, on the other hand, the subterm *impending* or *threatened* is not listed, code the existing underlying condition, *not* the condition described as impending or threatened.

EXAMPLE

Gangrene, gangrenous(anemia)(artery)(cellulitis)(dermatitis)(dry) (infective)(moist)(pemphigus)(septic)(skin)(stasis)(ulcer)

.
.
.

    hernia—see Hernia, by site, with gangrene
    hospital noma   528.1
    intestine, intestinal (acute) (hemorrhagic) (massive)   557.0
        with
            hernia—see Hernia, by site, with gangrene
            mesenteric embolism or infarction   557.0
        laryngitis   464.00

This example illustrates how to code impending gangrene due to decubitus ulcer of the lower back. There is no subterm for *impending* gangrene in the Alphabetic Index. Therefore, the code for gangrene would not be assigned, and the decubitus ulcer would be coded as documented (707.03).

Checkpoint 3.6

Code the following conditions using Volumes 1 and 2 of ICD-9-CM.

1. Threatened abortion _____

2. Impending delirium tremens _____

3. Impending gangrene of the heel due to decubitus ulcer _____

4. Impending respiratory failure due to COPD exacerbation _____

5. Impending myocardial infarction _____

Chapter-Specific Coding Guidelines

NOTE

Detailed coverage of the chapter-specific coding guidelines is provided in the second book *McGraw-Hill Medical Coding: Moving Ahead.*

In addition to the "General Coding Guidelines," there are guidelines for specific diagnoses and/or conditions in the Tabular List of the ICD-9-CM code set. Unless otherwise indicated, these guidelines apply to all health care settings. The **chapter-specific guidelines** comprise Section IC of the *ICD-9-CM Official Guidelines for Coding and Reporting.* They provide detailed instructions for coding conditions and situations that are specific to certain ICD-9-CM chapters.

INFECTIOUS AND PARASITIC DISEASES—CODES 001–139

Codes in Chapter 1 of the ICD-9-CM Tabular List classify communicable infectious and parasitic diseases. Most categories describe conditions and the types of organisms that cause them.

NEOPLASMS—CODES 140–239

Neoplasms are coded from Chapter 2 of the ICD-9-CM. Also called tumors, neoplasms are growths that arise from normal tissue. This category does not include a diagnosis statement with the word *mass,* which is a separate main term.

Neoplasm Table   The Alphabetic Index contains the **Neoplasm Table** that points to codes for neoplasms. The first column of the table lists the anatomical location, and the next six columns relate to the behavior of the neoplasm. In the Tabular List, neoplasms are listed under categories 140 through 239 in Chapter 2.

M Codes   In the regular Alphabetic Index entries, the pointers for neoplasms also show morphology codes, known as M codes. An M code is made up of the letter *M* followed by four digits, a slash, and a final digit. M codes (listed in Appendix A of ICD-9-CM) are used by pathologists and cancer registry departments of hospitals to report on and study the prevalence of various types of neoplasms. They are not used in physician practice (outpatient) coding. However, pathologists' reports help in selecting the correct code for a neoplasm. In the M code, the digit after the slash indicates the behavior of the neoplasm:

/0	Benign
/1	Uncertain whether benign or malignant/borderline malignant
/2	Carcinoma in situ: intraepithelial, noninfiltrating, or noninvasive
/3	Malignant, primary site
/6	Malignant, metastatic site, secondary site

The M codes are related to the Neoplasm Table and the Tabular List as follows:

M Code	Neoplasm Table	Tabular List
/0	Benign neoplasm	210–229
/1	Neoplasm of unspecified nature	239
	Neoplasm of uncertain behavior	235–238
/2	Carcinoma in situ	230–234
/3	Malignant neoplasm, stated or presumed to be primary	140–195 200–208
/6	Malignant neoplasm, stated or presumed to be secondary	196–198

For example, a pathologist's report might indicate the presence of an endometrioid adenofibroma. If it is benign, the M code is M8381/0, the equivalent of diagnosis code 220. If it is borderline malignant, the M code is M8381/1, and the diagnosis code is 236.2. If it is malignant, the M code is M8381/3, and the diagnosis code is 183.0.

For a metastasized neoplasm, if the secondary site is the main reason for treatment, the primary site is listed as a coexisting condition if it is still being treated. If the primary site is not documented, the code 199.1, malignant neoplasm without specification of site, other, is used. After the neoplasm is removed or is in remission and not being treated, a V code for the personal history of malignant neoplasm is used.

ENDOCRINE, NUTRITIONAL, AND METABOLIC DISEASES AND IMMUNITY DISORDERS—CODES 240–279

Codes in Chapter 3 of ICD-9-CM classify a variety of conditions. The most common disease in Chapter 3 is diabetes mellitus, which is a progressive disease of either type I or type II. Ninety percent of cases are type II.

DISEASES OF THE BLOOD AND BLOOD-FORMING ORGANS—CODES 280–289

Codes in this brief ICD-9-CM chapter classify diseases of the blood and blood-forming organs, such as anemia and coagulation defects.

MENTAL DISORDERS—CODES 290–319

Codes in Chapter 5 of ICD-9-CM classify the various types of mental disorders, including conditions of drug and alcohol dependency, Alzheimer's disease, schizophrenic disorders, and mood disturbances. Most psychiatrists use the terminology found in the *Diagnostic and Statistical Manual of Mental Disorders (DSM)* of the American Psychiatric Association for diagnoses, but the coding follows ICD-9-CM. This specialty coding area is described in the Pathophysiology Refresher on pages 120–121.

DISEASES OF THE NERVOUS SYSTEM AND SENSE ORGANS—CODES 320–389

Codes in Chapter 6 of ICD-9-CM classify diseases of the central nervous system, the peripheral nervous system, the eye, and the ear.

DISEASES OF THE CIRCULATORY SYSTEM—CODES 390–459

Because the circulatory system involves so many interrelated components, the disease process can create complex interrelated conditions. Many types of cardiovascular system disease, such as acute myocardial infarction (heart attack), require hospitalization of patients. The notes and *code also* instructions in Chapter 7 of the Tabular List must be carefully observed to code circulatory diseases accurately.

Ischemic heart disease conditions—those caused by reduced blood flow to the heart—are coded under categories 410 through 414. Myocardial infarctions that are acute or have a documented duration of eight weeks or less are located in category 410. Chronic myocardial infarctions, or those that last longer than eight weeks, are coded to subcategory 414.8. An old or healed myocardial infarction without current symptoms is coded 412.

Other chronic ischemic heart diseases are coded under category 414. Coronary atherosclerosis, 414.0, requires a fifth digit for the type of artery involved and includes arteriosclerotic heart disease (ASHD), atherosclerotic heart disease, and other coronary conditions. A diagnosis of angina pectoris—an episode of chest pain from a temporary insufficiency of oxygen to the heart—is coded 413.9 unless it occurs only at night (413.0) or is diagnosed as Prinzmetal (angiospastic) angina (413.1).

Arteriosclerotic cardiovascular disease (ASCVD)—hardening of the arteries affecting the complete cardiovascular system—is coded 429.2. A second code for the arteriosclerosis, 440.9, is also needed for this diagnosis. Likewise, 440.9 is never the primary code when ASCVD is a diagnosis.

Hypertension is a diagnosis related to high (elevated) blood pressure. Almost all cases have unknown causes. This is called essential hypertension and is the primary diagnosis. In the few cases where the

Mental Disorders

Mental disorders account for a large portion of health care costs in the United States. Alzheimer's disease is the third most costly disease nationwide, after heart disease and cancer. Mental disorders are divided into three categories: organic psychotic conditions; neurotic, personality, and other nonpsychotic mental disorders; and mental retardation.

Organic Psychotic Conditions

Dementia is a general term for any mental disorder caused by organic damage to the brain. In certain mental disorders, changes in the brain can be seen on a brain scan. *Alzheimer's disease* is classified both as a disorder of the nervous system with cerebral degeneration (characterized by plaques on the brain) and as a mental disorder (*dementia with behavioral disturbances* or *without behavioral disturbances*). Other dementias may be *alcohol-induced* or *drug-induced*. They may also occur due to other conditions, such as delirium associated with epilepsy.

Other organic psychoses include *schizophrenia* (a severe mental disorder with delusions, disordered thinking, and a complex of other symptoms) and *episodic mood disorders* (including *bipolar disorder* and *major depressive disorder*), among others. Schizophrenia is subclassified as *unspecified, subchronic, chronic, subchronic with acute exacerbation, chronic with acute exacerbation,* or *in remission.* Types of schizophrenia are also given separate classifications. Some examples are: *paranoid type, latent type, catatonic type,* and *simple type.* Many disorders can be single episodes or recurrent episodes. There are other psychotic conditions such as *paranoia* (delusions and projections of personal conflicts onto others) and *delusional disorder.*

Neurotic, Personality, and Other Nonpsychotic Mental Disorders

Nonpsychotic mental disorders, such as *anxiety,* may result from *neurosis* (a fairly mild personality disorder with obsessive thoughts, physical complaints, anxiety, and other symptoms), a *reaction* to a specific trauma or incident, or a *state* of mind (as one caused by alcohol or drugs or by another condition). *Drug abuse* is the excessive use of a drug. *Drug dependence* is the compulsive use of a drug or other substance in spite of negative reactions and consequences.

A comparison of a normal brain with the brain of a patient with Alzheimer's disease.

cause is known, the hypertension is called secondary, and its code is listed after the code for the cause.

DISEASES OF THE RESPIRATORY SYSTEM—CODES 460–519

Codes in Chapter 8 of ICD-9-CM classify respiratory illnesses such as pneumonia, chronic obstructive pulmonary disease (COPD), and asthma. Pneumonia, a common respiratory infection, may be caused by one of a number of organisms. Many codes for pneumonia include the condition and the cause in a combination code, such as 480.2, pneumonia due to parainfluenza virus.

DISEASES OF THE DIGESTIVE SYSTEM—CODES 520–579

Codes in Chapter 9 of ICD-9-CM classify diseases of the digestive system. Codes are listed according to anatomical location, beginning with the oral cavity and continuing through the intestines.

Drug dependence is also known as *addiction*. Substance or drug abuse may be *unspecified, continuous, episodic,* or *in remission*. Both abuse and dependence are sometimes categorized by the specific substance involved (such as cocaine, alcohol, amphetamines, and so on).

Other nonpsychotic disorders include eating disorders (*anorexia nervosa* and *bulimia nervosa*) and various sleep disorders of nonorganic origin. In addition, there are a number of physical symptoms (skin rashes, vomiting, diarrhea, and so on) that are classified as *physiological malfunctions arising from mental factors*.

Some childhood disorders are also nonpsychotic. *Attention deficit disorder without mention of hyperactivity* or *with hyperactivity* usually begins in early childhood but may also be present in adults. *Specific delays in development*, such as *alexia* (inability to understand written language) and *developmental dyslexia* (serious impairment of reading skills), are developmental disorders. There are other emotional disorders of childhood and adolescence, such as *oppositional defiant disorder* (extreme defiance of

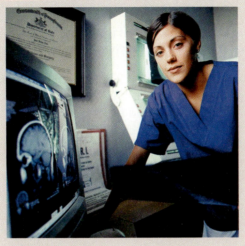
A doctor examining a brain scan.

authority). In addition, *shyness* or *sensitivity* (both when unusually intense) or adjustment disorders are also common in children and adolescents.

Some nonpsychotic disorders result from a traumatic event or series of events. *Posttraumatic stress disorder* is one such disorder. Some nonpsychotic mental disorders are due to brain damage. *Postconcussion syndrome* is an example of a disorder caused by brain damage.

Some conduct disorders, including disorders of impulse control, are usually categorized by the major symptom displayed, such as *pathological gambling, kleptomania,* or *pyromania.* There is also a group of *sexual and gender identity disorders*, such as *pedophilia* and *exhibitionism*, that are nonpsychotic disorders.

Mental Retardation

Mental retardation may be caused by various birth defects. Mental retardation is categorized as *unspecified,* or it is graded according to an IQ number as mild, moderate, severe, or profound.

DISEASES OF THE GENITOURINARY SYSTEM—CODES 580–629

Codes in Chapter 10 of ICD-9-CM classify diseases of the male and female genitourinary (GU) systems, such as infections of the genital tract, renal disease, conditions of the prostate, and problems with the cervix, vulva, and breast.

COMPLICATIONS OF PREGNANCY, CHILDBIRTH, AND THE PUERPERIUM—CODES 630–677

Codes in Chapter 11 of ICD-9-CM classify conditions that are involved with pregnancy, childbirth, and the puerperium (the six-week period following delivery). Many categories require a fifth digit that is based on when the complications occur (referred to as the episode of care): either before birth (antepartum), during birth, or after birth (postpartum).

DISEASES OF THE SKIN AND SUBCUTANEOUS TISSUE—CODES 680–709

Codes in ICD-9-CM Chapter 12 classify skin infections, inflammations, and other diseases. An entire chapter or section may be subject to excludes or includes notes, based on the notes' location. For example, the first section in this chapter (680–686) begins with a note excluding certain skin infections that are classified in Chapter 1.

DISEASES OF THE MUSCULOSKELETAL SYSTEM AND CONNECTIVE TISSUE—CODES 710–739

Codes in Chapter 13 of ICD-9-CM classify conditions of the bones and joints—arthropathies (joint disorders), dorsopathies (back disorders), rheumatism, and other diseases.

CONGENITAL ANOMALIES—CODES 740–759

Codes in the brief ICD-9-CM Chapter 14 classify anomalies, malformations, and diseases that exist at birth. Unlike acquired disorders, congenital conditions are either hereditary or due to influencing factors during gestation.

CERTAIN CONDITIONS ORIGINATING IN THE PERINATAL PERIOD—CODES 760–779

Codes in Chapter 15 of ICD-9-CM classify conditions of the fetus or the newborn infant, the neonate, up to twenty-eight days after birth. These codes are assigned only to conditions of the infant, not those of the mother.

SYMPTOMS, SIGNS, AND ILL-DEFINED CONDITIONS—CODES 780–799

Codes in this sixteenth chapter of ICD-9-CM classify patients' signs, symptoms, and ill-defined conditions for which definitive diagnoses cannot be made. In outpatient coding, these codes are always used instead of coding rule-out, probable, or suspected conditions.

INJURY AND POISONING—CODES 800–999

Codes in Chapter 17 of ICD-9-CM classify injuries and wounds (fractures, dislocations, sprains, strains, internal injuries, and traumatic injuries), poisoning, and the late effects of injuries and poisoning. Often, E codes are also used to identify the causes of injuries or poisoning.

Fractures   Fractures are coded using categories 800 through 829. A fourth digit indicates whether the fracture is closed or open. When a fracture is closed, the broken bone does not pierce the skin. An open fracture breaks through the skin. If the fracture is not indicated as open or closed, it is coded as closed. A fifth digit is often used for the specific anatomical site.

Burns   Burns appear in categories 940 through 949, where they are classified according to the cause, such as flames or radiation. They are grouped by severity and by how much body surface is involved.

CLASSIFICATION OF FACTORS INFLUENCING HEALTH STATUS AND CONTACT WITH HEALTH SERVICE—SUPPLEMENTAL—V01–V86

This section of the chapter-specific guidelines covers the use of V codes in specific situations.

SUPPLEMENTAL CLASSIFICATION OF EXTERNAL CAUSES OF INJURY AND POISONING—E CODES—E800–E999

This section covers the correct reporting of E codes.

Checkpoint 3.7

Code the following conditions using ICD-9-CM Volumes 1 and 2.

1. Septicemia due to *Escherichia coli* _____
2. Dermatofibroma of the leg _____
3. Non-Hodgkin's lymphoma of intrapelvic lymph nodes _____
4. Endothelial sarcoma of the arm _____
5. The morphology code for malignant melanoma of the breast _____
6. Grave's disease _____
7. Anemia due to acute blood loss _____
8. Chronic alcoholism, in remission _____
9. Paranoid schizophrenia, chronic _____
10. Myopathy in Addison's disease _____
11. Arteriosclerotic carciovascular disease (ASCVD) _____
12. Acute inferior wall myocardial infarction, initial episode of care _____
13. Bilateral carotid artery stenosis _____
14. Benign hypertensive cardiovascular disease _____
15. Acute exacerbation of asthma with COPD _____
16. Diverticulosis with diverticulitis _____
17. Acute salpingitis with oophoritis _____
18. Severe hyperemesis gravidarum, antepartum _____
19. Pustular acne _____
20. Incomplete cleft palate on the right _____
21. Newborn respiratory distress syndrome _____
22. Urge and stress urinary incontinence _____
23. Overdose of Librium in a suicide attempt at home _____
24. Compound fracture of the phalanx, right hand _____
25. Second degree burn of the left ankle, occurred at a bonfire at camp _____

1. Section IB, "General Coding Guidelines," of the *Official Guidelines for Coding and Reporting* (effective November 15, 2006) covers basic coding guidelines that all coders must follow in order to accurately assign ICD-9-CM codes. Mistakes in coding can occur if these basic rules are not followed. The rules apply to both the inpatient and outpatient settings and should be used by all health care providers, including hospitals, physicians, nursing homes, and home health care agencies.

2. Both the Alphabetic Index and the Tabular List should be used for all ICD-9-CM coding. Skipping a step in the coding process can result in coding errors.

3. Always code to the highest level of specificity. This means that if a fourth digit is available for a category (three-digit code), the fourth digit must be assigned, and if a fifth digit is also available, it too must be assigned. ICD-9-CM uses an indented format and conventions to direct the coder to the fourth-and fifth-digit levels. Each additional subcategory (fourth digit) and subclassification (fifth digit) provides a higher level of detail for a particular condition.

4. Conditions that are an integral part of a disease process should not be coded separately. Signs and symptoms that are not integral to the disease process should be reported separately.

5. Multiple codes are often required to report a single condition. Conventions such as code first, use additional code, and code also notations help the coder understand when an additional code is required. Documentation in the medical record must support the use of the additional code.

6. The *Official Guidelines* address the use of combination codes. In a combination code, one code reflects more than one condition. Combination codes can reflect two diseases, a combination of a disease and its underlying cause, or a complication of care.

7. When coding both acute and chronic conditions, the coder must remember to determine whether the subterms *acute* (subacute) and *chronic* are located at the same indentation level. When they are located at the same indentation level, both codes are assigned, and the acute condition code is sequenced first.

8. For late effect coding, the acute condition is no longer present, but a residual condition remains. When coding late effects, the residual condition (manifestation) is coded first, followed by a code for the cause of the late effect. The main term *late* is used to locate the code for the cause of the late effect. Terms in the diagnostic statement such as *old* and *previous* alert the coder that the patient has a late effect and that late effect coding rules apply. There are exceptions to the requirement of reporting late effects with two codes.

9. Impending and threatened conditions should first be coded by looking up the main terms *impending* or *threatened* or by searching for these terms as subterms. If a specific code is not available for an impending or threatened condition, the code for the actual condition should be reported. Typically, documentation of

threatened or impending implies that the patient does not actually have the condition but is at risk for developing it.

10. Section IC of the *ICD-9-CM Official Guidelines for Coding and Reporting*, "Chapter-Specific Coding Guidelines," contains guidelines for specific diagnoses and/or conditions in the classification. Unless otherwise indicated, these guidelines apply to all health care settings.

Review Questions: Chapter 3

Match the key terms with their definitions.

a. specificity _____
b. integral _____
c. combination code _____
d. chapter-specific guidelines _____
e. causal condition _____
f. code first _____
g. impending condition _____
h. mandatory multiple coding _____
i. late effect _____
j. acute condition _____

1. The fact that a symptom is a component part of a disease process

2. Two codes required to fully classify a condition

3. A medical condition that develops suddenly and resolves quickly

4. A condition that has not developed yet, but may develop

5. A set of rules specific to a chapter in ICD-9-CM

6. One code that reflects two conditions

7. An instructional notation about which code should be listed before another

8. The medical cause of a condition or illness

9. A circumstance in which a residual condition is present

10. The use of additional ICD-9-CM digits to provide more detail

Decide whether each statement is true or false.

1. The *ICD-9-CM Official Guidelines for Coding and Reporting* apply only to the inpatient setting. **T or F**

2. A patient presents to the physician office with epigastric pain. The physician documents the diagnosis as gastroesophageal reflux. In this case, the epigastric pain should not be coded, as this symptom is integral to the disease. **T or F**

3. The statement "scar from previous burn" would be coded as a late effect. **T or F**

4. All impending conditions should be coded as if they exist. **T or F**

5. The coder must verify all codes in the Tabular List. **T or F**

6. The main tern *late* is used to code the cause of the late effect. **T or F**

7. When coding the presence of a disease that is both acute and chronic, the code for the chronic condition is sequenced first. **T or F**

8. The sign of a coma is integral to a cerebrovascular accident. **T or F**

9. The neoplasm table is organized alphabetically by location of the neoplasm. **T or F**

10. An open fracture involves a break through the skin. **T or F**

Select the letter that best completes the statement or answers the question.

1. Which codes would be reported for a patient with a seizure disorder from previous viral encephalitis?
   a. 345.9, 139.0
   b. 345.90, 139.0
   c. 345.9, 139.8
   d. 345.90, 049.9

2. Which code or codes would be reported for a patient with impending cerebrovascular accident with dysphagia?
   a. 435.9, 787.20
   b. 435.9, 784.5
   c. 434.91, 787.20
   d. 435.9

3. Which instruction at code 370.44 directs the coder to assign a mandatory code for the underlying cause of keratoconjunctivitis?
   a. code first the underlying disease
   b. excludes
   c. use additional code to identify the underlying disease
   d. None of the above

4. Which code is not coded to its highest level of specificity?
   a. 466.0
   b. E804
   c. 789.2
   d. 535.50

5. Which codes report an open fracture of the distal tibia and fibula due to collision on the highway when the injured person was the driver?
   a. 823.82, E812.0
   b. 823.92., E813.0
   c. 823.90, 823.91, E813.0
   d. 823.92, E812.0

6. Mary presented with abdominal pain, hematemesis, and dehydration due to an acute gastric ulcer with hemorrhage. Which code or codes are reported?
   a. 531.30, 276.51
   b. 531.20, 276.51
   c. 531.00, 276.51
   d. 531.00

7. Joseph presented with fever, tachycardia, chest pain, and headache. Identify any complaint(s) that are symptoms.
   a. fever
   b. fever and tachycardia
   c. chest pain, headache, and tachycardia
   d. chest pain and headache

8. Which code is reported for primary malignant neoplasm of the breast, outer quadrant?
   a. 174.9
   b. 174.8
   c. 174.5
   d. 198.81

9. Which code or codes are reported for type I diabetes, uncontrolled, with diabetic ketoacidosis?
   a. 250.11
   b. 250.11, 250.01
   c. 250.13
   d. 250.13, 250.03

10. A patient presented with acute and chronic prostatitis due to pseudomonas and also has dysuria. Which codes are reported? (*Hint:* Consider sequencing guidelines.)
    a. 601.0, 041.7, 788.1
    b. 601.0, 601.1, 788.1
    c. 601.0, 601.1, 788.1, 041.7
    d. 601.1, 601.0, 788.1, 041.7

Provide the codes for the following diagnoses.

1. Malunion of the femur due to previous fracture six months ago. The patient had fallen out of a tree. _____

2. Fever, cough, and dyspnea due to rickettsia pneumonia. _____

3. Hemiplegia and aphasia due to old cerebrovascular accident. _____
   _____

4. Stress urinary incontinence, female. _____

5. Infertility from panhypopituitarism origin. _____

6. Methicillin resistant *Staphylococcus* aureas cellulitis of the leg. _____
   _____

7. Perforated sigmoid diverticulitis with hemorrhage and bacterial peritonitis. _____

8. Bleeding esophageal varices in cirrhosis of the liver. _____

9. Acute and chronic appendicitis. _____

10. Chest pain due to acute inferior wall myocardial infarction (initial episode of care) with respiratory failure. _____

Applying Your Knowledge

BUILDING CODING SKILLS

Answer the questions using the case scenarios provided.

Case 3.1

The following chart note is on file for a female patient.

> Mary Wisely
> 4/21/08
>
> **HISTORY OF PRESENT ILLNESS:** This is a 62-year-old female with a history of antithrombin-3 deficiency in the past who was followed in the Medicine Clinic and Hematology Clinic for bilateral swelling of the legs for three to four days prior to admission with increased swelling and tenderness more on the right side than on the left side in both calves. On routine follow-up visit in the clinic, she was seen for a diagnosis of deep venous thrombosis. She was taking Coumadin [an anticoagulant] at home, 3 mg a day for the past two years.

1. What are Mary's signs and symptoms?

2. What main term would you look up to code the long-term use of Coumadin?

3. What is the cause of Mary's symptoms?

4. Assign the correct ICD-9-CM codes for this outpatient visit.

Case 3.2

The following chart note is on file for a female patient.

> Borden, Lois
> May 15, 2008
>
> **HISTORY OF PRESENT ILLNESS:** The patient is a 66-year-old female with a past medical history of hypertension and type I diabetes mellitus. The patient also has a history of coronary artery disease of the native vessels. She was admitted to the hospital for chest pain associated with nausea, vomiting, and diaphoresis. The patient was given nitroglycerin in Emergency Services, which relieved the chest pain.
>
> Medications included 10 mg b.i.d., Nitropatch, and insulin NGH 35 units q. a.m.
>
> **SOCIAL HISTORY:** Smokes one pack per day, no drinking, and no IV drug abuse.
>
> **FAMILY HISTORY:** Positive for coronary artery disease in her father.
>
> **DIAGNOSIS:** Chest pain due to native vessel coronary artery disease, hypertension, diabetes and tobacco dependence.

1. What signs and symptoms did the patient have on admission?

2. What was the cause of the these symptoms?

3. What other diseases does this patient have?

4. How does the family history contribute to the patient' illness?

5. Does the patient have any social habits that might contribute to disease?

6. Code all the diagnoses for this case.

Case 3.3

The following chart note is on file for a female patient.

> Denise Gordon
> May 20, 2008
>
> **SUBJECTIVE:** Abdominal pain for four days. Admits to fairly heavy drinking over the past week or so. Emesis originally, but that has stopped, and patient is now able to keep down some fluids. Denies diarrhea. Patient has a past history of hepatitis secondary to alcoholism. She also has seizures due to previous bacterial meningitis. She does need a refill of her antiseizure medication.
>
> **OBJECTIVE:** Pleasant female in no distress. Appears well-hydrated. Lungs are clear. No neurological deficits. Heart sounds are normal. Abdomen is benign.
>
> **LAB:** White count 11,100. Hemoglobin 15.2. Electrolytes are normal. Liver functions tests elevated showing AST of 32; Bilirubin, 0.5; alkaline phospatase, 97; amylase, 24.
>
> **ASSESSMENT:** Alcoholic gastritis, alcoholism, seizure disorder due to previous bacterial meningitis.
>
> **PLAN:** Patient was given Toradol 60 mg IM with some relief. She will take antacids at home, avoid alcohol, and begin a bland diet. She will continue to take her antiseizure medication daily.

1. What are the patient's signs and symptoms?

2. Has the underlying cause of the signs or symptoms been determined? If yes, what is the underlying cause?

3. Are the symptoms integral to the underlying cause?

4. Which conditions should be reported for this visit?

5. Assign ICD-9-CM diagnosis codes for this visit.

Case 3.4

Mary presents to the hospital ER with hematuria, flank pain, and fever. She has known chronic pyelonephritis. IVP is positive for kidney stones and hydronephrosis. Urine culture is positive for pseudomonas. The patient will be admitted for further treatment. The ER documents the following diagnoses: acute pyelonephritis due to pseudomonas, hydronephrosis, chronic pyelonephritis, and renal calculus with obstruction.

1. What are the patient's signs and symptoms?

2. Which conditions should be coded?

3. Assign ICD-9-CM codes for this ER visit.

4. Which of the following coding rules apply to this case scenario
    a. use additional code
    b. acute and chronic conditions sequencing
    c. symptoms that are integral to the disease
    d. All of the above

Case 3.5

Lolita is an 84-year-old women with a lengthy medical history. She now complains of pain 8/10 in her left ankle, with swelling, and erythema. She has a fever of 101.8, and she is unable to bear weight on the left. This is complicated by her other medical conditions of status post left knee replacement, osteoarthritis of the lumbar spine, and right-sided hemiplegia from an old cerebrovascular accident.

LAB: Joint fluid aspiration was positive for *Streptococcus,* Group B.

PLAN: Admit the patient for further workup; treat with antibiotics.

DX: The physician documented the following diagnoses:
Septic arthritis of the ankle, due to *Streptococcus* Group B
Osteoarthritis of the lumbar spine
Status post left total knee replacement
Hemiplegia from previous CVA

1. Assign the correct ICD-9-CM codes.

Case 3.6

Joseph has pain, redness, and swelling with an ulcer of his lower right shin. He has severe arteriosclerosis of the femoral artery causing the ulcer of his right shin. He now presents with worsening symptoms after completion of antibiotics three weeks ago. He is concerned about keeping his leg given his infection with ulcer. The plan is to admit Joseph to the hospital for IV antibiotics. The physician documents the following diagnosis: arteriosclerotic ulcer of the shin with impending gangrene.

1. What are the signs and symptoms of Joseph's illness?

2. What diagnosis should be coded?

3. Assign the correct ICD-9-CM codes for this visit.

Case 3.7

John presents to his dermatologist for an excision of a painful scar from a previous burn to his palm. His hand was burned when he accidentally spilled hot coffee at work.

1. Does this visit reflect a condition that is a late effect? If yes, what is the residual condition? What is the cause of the residual condition (or late effect)?

2. What main term would be used to assign the code for the previous burn?

3. What main term would be used to assign the E code?

4. Assign the correct ICD-9-CM diagnosis codes for this visit.

Case 3.8

Marie presented to the ER after sustaining a head injury in a car collision. Marie was the driver of the vehicle. She had a loss of consciousness at the scene for five minutes. She also sustained an abrasion of the lower leg. The ER physician documented the following diagnoses: concussion and leg abrasion.

1. Assign the correct ICD-9-CM diagnosis codes for this visit.

2. Which code or codes are combination codes?

Case 3.9

Leo Rumboldt
4/10/08

SUBJECTIVE: This 56-year-old with emphysema has shortness of breath and increasing weakness. For the last 1.5 months, he has had paroxysmal nocturnal dyspnea up to 3x/night but denies problems of orthopnea. He is not smoking. He states that he uses an albuterol inhaler for asthma, and its use seems to relieve the symptoms. He has also had a cough with some white sputum. No fevers or chills. No lower extremity edema.

OBJECTIVE: Thin, gaunt gentleman appearing older than his stated age. BP is 150/62. Pulse is 95. Respirations are 30; barrel chested.

> **Heart:** Regular rhythm.
>
> **Lungs:** Fair to good air movement with diffuse expiratory wheezing and prolongation of the expiratory phase.
>
> **Extremities:** Without edema.
>
> **LAB:** PA and lateral chest films reveal flattened diaphragm, increased AP diameter, and boxcar lung shapes consistent with severe emphysema.
>
> **TREATMENT:** Pulmonary function testing before and after albuterol treatments reveals severe obstructive changes with no improvement following treatment.

ASSESSMENT: Shortness of breath secondary to COPD exacerbation with asthma.

PLAN: Refer to Pulmonary Medicine.

1. What are the patient's signs and symptoms?

2. What does the abbreviation *COPD* mean?

3. Assign the correct ICD-9-CM codes for this outpatient visit.

4. Which of the following coding conventions are demonstrated in this scenario?

   a. mandatory multiple coding

   b. combination codes

   c. symptoms integral to the underlying condition

   d. both B and C

Case 3.10

Ned Long
4/26/08

SUBJECTIVE: Ned comes in for a 15-month-old examination (routine). His mother has no complaints. He is feeding himself and putting two words together when talking. He is actually in motor and growth development at the 22-month level. Most recent hemoglobin was 12.3. He is above the 95th percentile for height; at the 95th percentile for weight.

OBJECTIVE: Head is normal. Ears are clear. Pupils are equal, round, and reactive. Throat is clear. Nose is clear. Neck has good range of motion without nodes. Lungs are clear. Heart has regular rate and rhythm. Abdomen is soft without masses. Testicles are descended. Back is straight. He is walking well. He has good muscle tone. See development form in chart.

ASSESSMENT: Normal well-baby examination.

PLAN: Continue present diet and advance as tolerated. Measles, mumps, and rubella immunization given; see immunization chart. Recheck in three months, sooner if needed.

1. Does this visit represent a well-baby examination?

2. What is another term for *immunization*?

3. Assign the diagnosis codes for this visit.

Case 3.11

Rhonda Elders
4/15/08

SUBJECTIVE: Renee is a 26-year-old female who presents with swelling, redness, and tenderness in the left lower extremity, present for the past 24 hours, becoming more swollen. She has some pain with walking. It is worse after being on her feet throughout the day, but she denies any direct trauma to this area.

OBJECTIVE: Left lower extremity: She has localized erythema, induration, tenderness, swelling, and obliteration of the femoral vein.

ASSESSMENT: Superficial thrombophlebitis of the femoral vein with deep vein thrombosis.

PLAN: Coumadin, ibuprofen 600 mg BID with food, and warm compresses to the affected area for 30–60 minutes TUD. Back in two weeks or sooner if symptoms worsen.

1. What are the patient's signs and symptoms?

2. Assign the ICD-9-CM codes for this visit.

3. Which of the following ICD-9-CM conventions applies here?
   a. discretionary multiple coding
   b. mandatory multiple coding
   c. combination codes
   d. impending or threatened conditions

Read each of the following cases and assign codes using all three volumes of the ICD-9-CM.

Case 3.12

Joseph presents to the hospital for a coronary artery bypass graft to treat his native vessel coronary artery disease. On the second hospital day, Joseph underwent a coronary artery bypass using aortocoronary graft of the left anterior descending (LAD) artery. The patient required the use of the heart-lung machine during the procedure.

Case 3.13

Mary was diagnosed with primary carcinoma of the sigmoid colon. She underwent sigmoid colon resection with side to side anastamosis (large to large intestine).

Case 3.14

Mark presented to the hospital due to chronic cough and hemoptysis. He underwent bronchoscopy with biopsy of the lung which confirmed the presence of asbestosis.

Case 3.15

Justine underwent total abdominal hysterectomy with bilateral salpingo-oophorectomy to treat her submucous uterine fibroids.

Case 3.16

Inpatient hospitalization was required for Jane due to non-ruptured cerebral artery aneurysm. She underwent repair of the aneurysm using endovascular coiling.

Case 3.17

Maureen presented to the hospital for scheduled cesarean section. Maureen had a previous cesarean delivery (delivery complicated by previous cesarean section) two years ago for the delivery of her first child. She underwent low transverse cesarean section delivery of a healthy, full-term baby boy.

Case 3.18

John presented with abdominal pain. Work-up was positive for incarcerated inguinal hernia on the left. He underwent repair of his direct inguinal hernia using mesh (graft).

Case 3.19

Michael presented with new onset of pain and swelling of the left leg. Lower extremity Doppler was positive for deep vein thrombosis with thrombophlebitis of the femoral vein. Michael underwent percutaneous transluminal angioplasty of the femoral vein with stent insertion.

Case 3.20

Larry presented with urinary frequency and obstruction due to benign prostatic hypertrophy. He underwent transurethral resection of the prostate.

Case 3.21

Margaret was admitted for elective joint replacement due to localized osteoarthritis of the hip. She underwent total hip replacement with bearing surface of ceramic-on-ceramic.

USING CODING TERMS

Case 3.22

The following information is sent by a health plan to the coding department:

> Hyaluronan is FDA-approved for the treatment of osteoarthritis of the knee. There is no specific ICD-9-CM code that designates the knee only. Noridian Administrative Services (NAS) will therefore use the ICD-9-CM codes for the lower leg to indicate the knee. Effective 45 days following publication of this notice, ICD-9-CM diagnosis coding acceptable for Hyaluronan knee injections will be as follows:
>
> | Code | Description |
> | --- | --- |
> | 715.16 | Osteoarthritis, localized, primary, lower leg |
> | 715.26 | Osteoarthritis, localized, secondary, lower leg |
> | 715.36 | Osteoarthritis, localized, not specified whether primary or secondary, lower leg |
> | 715.96 | Osteoarthritis, unspecified whether generalized or localized, lower leg |

Based on these instructions, what ICD-9-CM code should be used for a patient who has a documented diagnosis of secondary osteoarthritis of the left knee?

Case 3.23

These questions are based on the coding principles covered in this chapter and on the disease processes defined in the chapter's pathophysiology refreshers. Assign all ICD-9-CM codes to the following:

1. Alzheimer's dementia with behavioral disturbance

2. Chronic paranoid schizophrenia with acute exacerbation

3. Chest pain due to anxiety attack

4. Cocaine dependence with drug withdrawal; patient uses cocaine continuously

5. Headache due to post-concussion syndrome

6. Severe mental retardation

7. Hematuria due to renal calculus versus bladder lesion

8. Acute and Chronic cystitis

9. Incomplete spontaneous abortion

10. Acute on chronic renal failure

11. Abdominal pain due to possible erosive gastritis

12. Fecal impaction

13. Acute duodenal ulcer with perforation and hemorrhage due to Helicobacter pylori (H. pylori)

14. Jaundice, Cirrhosis of the liver suspected

15. Crohn's ileitis

1. Locate five medical conditions at the Web MD website at www.webmd.com. Identify the medical condition and the symptoms that are integral to it. For example, symptoms of asthma include difficulty breathing, wheezing, coughing, and shortness of breath.

2. Knowledge of new technology is essential for keeping up with medical practice and treatment for ICD-9-CM coding. Find a medical website that provides information on the latest technology used to treat heart disease. List the address of the website, and describe the new technology.

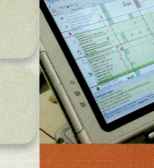

ICD-9-CM *Official Guidelines (Sections II and III)*: Selection of Principal Diagnosis/Additional Diagnoses for Inpatient Settings

LEARNING OUTCOMES

After studying this chapter, you should be able to:

1. Describe the patient care flow and associated documentation in the inpatient setting.

2. Discuss the importance of the UHDDS and its relationship to diagnostic coding.

3. Define the term *principal diagnosis* as it relates to the inpatient setting.

4. Describe the specific sequencing rule that is followed when multiple diagnoses are documented.

5. Apply diagnostic coding sequencing rules to these coding situations: (a) two or more principal diagnoses, (b) treatment plan not carried out, (c) complications, and (d) uncertain diagnoses.

6. Understand the use of E codes in reporting complications in the inpatient setting.

7. Describe the guideline for selecting the principal diagnosis following admission from an observation unit and outpatient surgery.

8. Discuss the criteria for reporting additional diagnoses.

9. Discuss the assignment of present on admission (POA) indicators.

10. Based on diagnostic statements, correctly assign diagnosis codes for the inpatient setting.

Key Terms

837I

abnormal finding

admitting physician

attending physician

comorbidity/complication (CC)

comparative or contrasting condition

definitive diagnosis

diagnosis-related group (DRG)

discharge summary

disposition

face sheet

ill-defined condition

Inpatient Prospective Payment System (IPPS)

Major Comorbidity and Complication (MCC)

medical observation

Medicare-Severity DRG (MS-DRG)

nonoutpatient

nonscheduled admission

observation unit

POA exempt from reporting

postoperative observation

present on admission (POA)

principal diagnosis

query

scheduled admission

secondary diagnosis

sequenced

treatment plan

UB-04 (CMS-1450)

uncertain diagnosis

Uniform Hospital Discharge Data Set (UHDDS)

Chapter Outline

The Uniform Hospital Discharge Data Set (UHDDS)—Guidance

Documentation in the Inpatient Setting

Section II: Selection of the Principal Diagnosis in the Inpatient Setting

Section III: Reporting Additional Diagnoses

Present on Admission (POA) Guidelines

Inpatient care is an enormous health cost, amounting to nearly $800 billion for 39 million hospital stays, according to recent data. Many patients, particularly elderly or very ill patients, do not have only one diagnosis or condition. According to the Centers for Medicare and Medicaid Services (CMS), almost a quarter of Medicare beneficiaries (usually adults age 65 or over) have five or more chronic conditions. When these patients are admitted for hospital treatment, in many cases, documentation for a single visit supports classifying multiple conditions, health care factors, and circumstances. For example, an admission to the hospital to evaluate a patient with chest pain, hypertension, and diabetes requires many ICD-9-CM diagnosis codes. How do coders decide which code is listed first?

In the inpatient setting, the first listed diagnosis code is the **principal diagnosis** code for the encounter. The **Uniform Hospital Discharge Data Set (UHDDS)** guidelines state that the principal diagnosis is "that condition established after study to be chiefly responsible for occasioning the admission of the patient to the hospital for care."

This chapter covers the ways in which the circumstances of inpatient admission govern the selection of the principal diagnosis. Specific guidelines explain the unique rules for selecting the principal diagnosis in different circumstances, such as when two or more conditions meet the definition of principal diagnosis and when a symptom is listed as the principal diagnosis by the attending physician. Other guidelines address selection of the principal diagnosis when a patient is admitted from observation or from an ambulatory surgery unit. Still others determine which conditions should be reported as additional or secondary diagnoses. Coders who understand and can apply these specific guidelines when assigning ICD-9-CM codes for inpatient visits will be correct, consistent, accurate, and complete in their code assignments.

The Uniform Hospital Discharge Data Set(UHDDS)—Guidance

The Uniform Hospital Discharge Data Set (UHDDS) is a common core of data. This standardized minimum data set is applied to the inpatient setting (acute care, short-term hospitals) and to **nonoutpatient** care settings (psychiatric hospitals, home health agencies, rehabilitation facilities, nursing homes, and so on). The goal of UHDDS data collection is to obtain uniform comparable discharge data on all inpatients. A list of all data elements appears in Table 4.1.

The data elements can be categorized into:

- Patient identification
- Provider information
- Clinical information of the patient episode of care
- Financial information

Coders are most concerned about the clinical information regarding the patient episode of care. These data elements and their definitions drive the coding process in the inpatient setting. Based on applying the documentation guidelines, coders correctly select the principal diagnosis, the principal procedure, and secondary diagnoses.

> **HIPAA TIP**
>
> **UHDDS**
>
> The UHDDS definitions are incorporated into the ICD-9-CM *Official Guidelines for Coding and Reporting* mandated by HIPAA.

Documentation in the Inpatient Setting

The patient care flow and clinical documentation in the medical record provide the foundation for ICD-9-CM code assignment. To uncover all relevant diagnostic information, coders review the entire medical record from admission through discharge when coding an inpatient visit. Deciphering the content of the record can help the coder understand the documentation, which ultimately is required for accurate code assignment. The flow chart in Figure 4.1 outlines the physician-documented components of the inpatient medical record that develop as the inpatient visit progresses and then ends.

The flow begins with the medical orders written by the **admitting physician.** Admission—the formal acceptance by the hospital of a patient—can be either a **scheduled admission,** in which arrangements have been made prior to the patient's appearing, or a **nonscheduled admission,** such as via the emergency room. The patient's information is summarized on a **face sheet,** also called an inpatient admission form, or using an electronic program to record the data.

> **CODING TIP**
>
> **A Reminder: The Vital Connection—Documentation, Coding, and Billing**
>
> The connection between documentation and coding is essential. A service that is not documented cannot be coded—and cannot be billed.

Table 4.1 Uniform Hospital Discharge Data Set Definitions*

Data Element	Description
Personal Identification	A unique number identifying the patient, applicable to the individual regardless of health care source or third-party arrangement
Date of Birth	Month, day, year
Sex	Male or female
Race and Ethnicity	Race (1) American Indian/Eskimo/Aleut (2) Asian or Pacific Islander (3) Black (4) White (5) Other race (6) Unknown Ethnicity (1) Spanish/Hispanic origin (2) Not of Spanish/Hispanic origin (3) Unknown
Residence	Usual residence, full address, and ZIP code; nine-digit ZIP code if available
Hospital Identification	NPI* (A unique institutional number across data systems)
Admission Date	Month, day, and year of admission
Type of Admission	Scheduled: an arrangement with the admissions office at least 24 hours before the admission Unscheduled: all other admissions
Discharge Date	Month, day, and year of discharge
Physician Identification—Attending	National Provider Identifier (NPI)*
Physician Identification—Operating	The NPI* for the clinician who performed the principal procedure
Other Diagnoses	All conditions that coexist at the time of admission, or develop subsequently, that affect the treatment received and/or the length of stay; diagnoses that relate to an earlier episode that have no bearing on the current hospital stay are to be excluded. Code conditions that affect patient care in terms of requiring: Clinical evaluation Therapeutic treatment Diagnostic procedures Extended length of hospital stay Increased nursing care Monitoring
External Causes of Injury Code	The ICD–9-CM code for the external cause of an injury, poisoning, or adverse effect
Birth Weigh of Newborns	The specific birth weight of the newborn, preferably recorded in grams
Procedures and Dates	All significant procedures are to be reported. A significant procedure is one that: (1) Is surgical in nature (2) Carries a procedural risk (3) Carries an anesthetic risk (4) Requires specialized training Surgery includes incision, excision, amputation, introduction, destruction, suture, and manipulation. The date must be reported for each significant procedure. When more than one procedure is reported, the principal endoscopy, repair, procedure is to be designated. In determining which of several procedures is principal, the following criteria apply: The principal procedure is one that was performed for definitive treatment rather than for diagnostic or exploratory purposes, or was necessary to take care of a complication. If two procedures appear to be principal, the one most related to the principal diagnosis should be selected as the principal procedure.
Disposition of Patient	Home, nursing facility, other health care facility, left against medical advice, expired.
Expected Sources of Payment	Primary source: the primary source that is expected to be responsible for the largest percentage of the patient's current bill Other source(s): other sources, if any, that are expected to be responsible for a portion of the patient's current bill; more than one can be identified
Total Charges	All charges billed by the hospital for this hospitalization; professional charges for individual patient care by physicians are excluded

Source: http://www.cdc.gov/nchs/data/ncvhs/nchvs92.pdf.
*UPIN has been updated to NPI to reflect current practice.

Admitted patients are then housed appropriately and treated by the medical staff. The **attending physician**—the medical professional who supervises the patient's care during hospitalization—directs the medical work that needs to be done to evaluate and treat the patient's conditions.

Following treatment, the patient is released, or discharged, from the hospital. The documentation must contain a **discharge summary** (or progress note) of the patient's medical condition and **disposition** or arrangements, indicating whether the patient is returning home, moving to another facility (such as a rehabilitation facility), or has died.

The discharge summary is typically the best place to begin the coding process because this document contains a recap of the entire hospitalization (that is, hospital course), summarizing the reason for admission and the tests, medications, and services provided.

The easiest way to grasp the concept of medical record documentation flow is to look at a case scenario.

As shown in the case scenario, the various documents incorporated into the medical record are generated over the course of an inpatient

NOTE

Details about the reports listed in Figure 4.1, such as the history and physical, are covered Chapter 1 of your program.

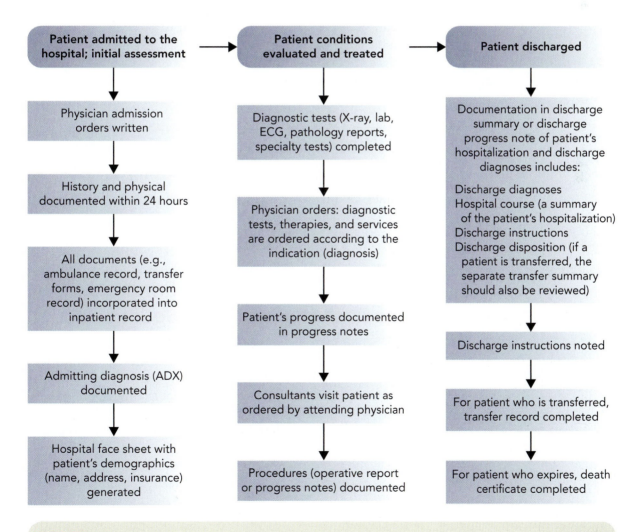

FIGURE 4.1

Inpatient Medical Record Documentation Flow

Case Scenario: Inpatient Documentation Flow

Mary Jane presents to the hospital Emergency Department (ED) because of chest pain. Diagnostic tests completed in the ED are suspicious for heart disease, so her physician, Dr. Jones, admits her to the hospital with possible unstable angina. Dr. Jones documents Mary Jane's medical history in the history and physical. Here we learn that Mary Jane has no history of coronary artery disease, but she does have type II diabetes, benign hypertension, and a family history of coronary artery disease. Dr. Jones orders a diabetic diet, Avalide 300 mg for hypertension, serial ECGs, cardiac enzymes, and nitroglycerin for chest pain. He also orders a chest X-ray and routine blood work.

During the course of the hospitalization, Mary Jane also undergoes an upper endoscopy to rule out digestive causes of her chest pain. The endoscopy report supports the presence of reflux esophagitis. After admission, Mary Jane develops hypokalemia and is treated with potassium supplements. Mary Jane's progress is documented in the physician progress notes. The physician orders, medication sheets, and test results are all placed in the medical record. After three days, Mary Jane is feeling much better, and Dr. Jones orders her discharge.

Upon discharge, Dr. Jones's discharge summary documents the hospital course and discharge diagnoses of chest pain due to esophageal reflux, type II diabetes mellitus, hypertension, hypokalemia, and family history of coronary artery disease. Mary Jane is to follow a diabetic diet, take her medications as instructed, and return to the office in one month. Prevacid is prescribed for the reflux esophagitis.

FIGURE 4.2

Inpatient Code Assignment Flow Chart

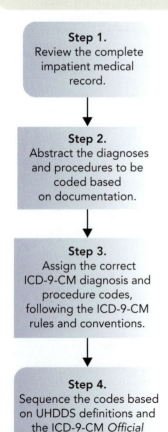

Step 1.
Review the complete impatient medical record.

Step 2.
Abstract the diagnoses and procedures to be coded based on documentation.

Step 3.
Assign the correct ICD-9-CM diagnosis and procedure codes, following the ICD-9-CM rules and conventions.

Step 4.
Sequence the codes based on UHDDS definitions and the ICD-9-CM *Official Guidelines.*

hospitalization. The physician documentation found in the history and physical, discharge summary, progress notes, orders, and operative report include the information the coder needs to assign ICD-9-CM codes. Understanding the content and flow of documentation assists the coder in selecting the principal and secondary diagnoses that should be reported in the inpatient setting.

Section II: Selection of the Principal Diagnosis in the Inpatient Setting

The UHDDS defines the principal diagnosis for the inpatient setting as "that condition established after study to be chiefly responsible for occasioning the admission of the patient to the hospital for care." For example, a patient is admitted with unstable angina, but a diagnostic cardiac catheterization with coronary angiography (a diagnostic procedure) shows that the principal diagnosis is coronary artery disease.

The basic coding rules and conventions for determining principal diagnosis in ICD-9-CM Volumes 1, 2, and 3 take precedence over the *Official Guidelines*. As shown in Figure 4.2, the process involves applying the rules and conventions before the guidelines.

The guidelines in the following sections apply to the selection of the principal diagnosis in the various presenting situations encountered by coders.

CODES FOR SYMPTOMS, SIGNS, AND ILL-DEFINED CONDITIONS

"Codes for symptoms, signs, and **ill-defined conditions** from Chapter 16 are not to be used as principal diagnosis when a related definitive diagnosis has been established." The codes in Chapter 16 of ICD-9-CM range from 780.0 to 799.0 and include such diagnoses as fever, dizziness, chest pain, and hematuria. If the related **definitive diagnosis** has been identified, the symptom code should not be **sequenced** first.

> **EXAMPLES**   A patient presents with fever and cough, and if further study and documentation support the diagnosis of pneumonia, the code for pneumonia is sequenced first. Since the basic coding guidelines show that the symptoms of fever and cough are integral to pneumonia, these symptoms are not reported separately. Code 486 is reported.
>
> A patient presents with jaundice and abdominal ascites, further investigation results in documentation of the diagnosis of cholelithiasis. Jaundice due to cholelithiasis requires one code, and the code for ascites is reported as an additional diagnosis because the symptom of ascites is not integral to the definitive condition of cholelithiasis. The reported codes are 574.20 and 789.59.

Sometimes incomplete or inconsistent documentation requires a physician **query,** a written communication from the coder asking the physician for clarification. For example, a physician may document chest pain as a principal diagnosis, but an upper endoscopy is positive for gastric ulcer. The physician should be queried about the definitive diagnosis that is causing the chest pain. In this instance, the coder may think that the ulcer is causing the chest pain and may report the symptom of chest pain as the principal diagnosis (786.50). However, the query results may support the principal diagnosis of gastric ulcer as the cause of chest pain, and the principal diagnosis would be reported as 531.90.

The American Health Information Management Association (AHIMA) has developed a *Practice Brief* that outlines the recommended process of developing a physician query.

NOTE

Note that the coding rules and conventions for the ICD-9-CM are presented in Chapter 2 of your program.

INTERNET RESOURCE

AHIMA Practice Brief on the Query Process

http://library.ahima.org/xpedio/groups/public/documents/ahima/bok1_009224.hcsp?dDocName=bok1_009224

COMPLIANCE GUIDELINE

Use of *Coding Clinic* for Queries

The publication *Coding Clinic* is a resource for when queries are appropriate; containing numerous examples of the correct way to write a query about a specific coding situation without appearing to "lead" the physician.

Checkpoint 4.1

Using Volumes 1 and 2 of ICD-9-CM, code the following, and identify the symptom and definitive diagnosis of each.

	Symptom	Diagnosis	Code(s)
1. Abdominal pain due to gastritis	_____	_____	_____
2. Hematuria due to renal calculus	_____	_____	_____
3. CVA with aphasia	_____	_____	_____
4. Sprained knee with pain	_____	_____	_____
5. Cirrhosis of the liver with ascites	_____	_____	_____

The Circulatory (or Cardiovascular) System

The circulatory system includes the heart and the body's network of blood vessels (arteries, veins, and capillaries). Diseases of the circulatory system can occur anywhere in this system or as a result of disorders of functions of the heart. Most circulatory diseases can be grouped into categories. Some of the most common categories are *ischemic disease, heart failure, hypertensive disease, conduction (or rhythm) disorders, cerebrovascular disorders,* and *diseases of blood vessels.* Other diseases, such as various inflammations, also affect parts of the circulatory system. In addition, the heart valves can be affected by untreated rheumatic fever.

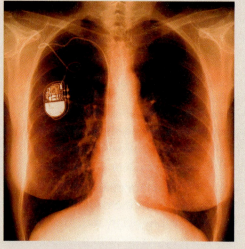

A pacemaker is used to treat conduction disorders.

Ischemic Disease

Heart disease is the leading cause of death in the United States. The term *heart disease* includes several conditions, but it most commonly refers to *coronary heart disease (CHD).* Also called coronary artery disease (CAD) and arteriosclerotic heart disease (ASHD), coronary heart disease is the buildup of plaque in the arteries (called *atherosclerosis*). This leads to ischemic heart disease, which is any disease that cuts off or lessens blood supply to the heart. *Angina* (or chest pain) is the most common symptom of ischemic heart disease. The major ischemic disease is a *heart attack* or *myocardial infarction.* An acute myocardial infarction can occur either in a specified site such as on the lateral wall of the heart or at an unspecified site. CHD can also lead to other conditions in which blood supply is lessened but a myocardial infarction does not occur. Some of these conditions are *coronary syndrome,* also known as *unstable angina,* and *angina pectoris* (pain in the chest radiating to the arms). Hardening and thickening of the arteries (atherosclerosis) is treated with medications, with a bypass graft, or with a stent.

Heart Failure

Heart failure, commonly known as *congestive heart failure* (mostly on the left side of the heart) or *chronic heart failure,* is the inability of the heart to pump enough blood to meet the needs of the body's other organs. The cause may be unspecified, or heart failure may occur as a result of a specific problem, such as systolic or diastolic malfunction. Heart failure may be *compensated* (accompanied by a physiological change in the body to compensate for the failure) or *decompensated* (not accompanied by such change).

Hypertensive Disease

The *Centers for Disease Control and Prevention* (www.cdc.gov) estimate that one of every three Americans has *hypertension*

TWO OR MORE INTERRELATED CONDITIONS, EACH POTENTIALLY MEETING THE DEFINITION FOR PRINCIPAL DIAGNOSIS

According to the *Official Guidelines*:

> When there are two or more interrelated conditions (such as diseases in the same ICD-9-CM chapter or manifestations characteristically associated with a certain disease) potentially meeting the definition of principal diagnosis, either condition may be sequenced first, unless the circumstances of the admission, the therapy provided, the Tabular List, or the Alphabetic Index indicate otherwise.

Sometimes a patient is admitted because of interrelated conditions. One condition aggravates the other. For example, congestive heart failure can be related to atrial fibrillation. If a patient presents in atrial fibrillation (427.31) and congestive heart failure (428.0) and the conditions are equally treated, both conditions should be coded, or *high blood pressure. Hypertensive disease* is hypertension or high blood pressure over a period of time. Infrequent incidents of high blood pressure with normal blood pressure most of the time (diagnosed as *isolated* or *incidental* hypertension) is not considered to be a disorder. Only when the high blood pressure is maintained consistently or requires treatment does hypertensive disease exist.

There are three types of hypertension: *essential hypertension, secondary hypertension*, and *pregnancy-related hypertension*. Secondary hypertension is caused by another condition, such as kidney disease or a congenital abnormality. It is usually resolved once the underlying condition is treated. Pregnancy-related hypertension is treated during pregnancy and usually resolves once the pregnancy is over.

Essential hypertension usually has no known treatable cause. It is further labeled *malignant* (very high and difficult to treat), *benign* (controllable with medication or lifestyle changes), or *unspecified*.

Conduction (or Rhythm Disorders)

The heart's conduction system regulates the heartbeat or pulse. *Cardiac dysrhythmias* occur in a variety of forms. Sometimes the heartbeat is too fast *(tachycardia)*, too slow *(bradycardia)*, or irregular *(atrial fibrillation)*. These rhythm irregularities may occur in a specific part of the heart, or they may be *unspecified*. There are other types of dysrh-

thymias, such as *premature beats*. Pacemakers are often inserted to regulate heart rates. Arrhythmias are often detected by ECGs.

Cerebrovascular Disorders

The arteries that supply blood to the brain can rupture and cause bleeding in the brain. Such *hemorrhages* may occur in specific areas, such as a *subarachnoid hemorrhage*, or they may be *unspecified*. They may be accompanied by hypertension. The disease may be *nontraumatic* and may occur due to occlusion of a specific artery. Occlusion of an artery to the brain is a cause of *stroke* (either a nonbleeding or a bleeding stroke).

Diseases of Blood Vessels

The blood vessels of the body (arteries, veins, and capillaries) can be the sites of various disorders. A general term for degenerative changes in the arteries is *arteriosclerosis*. The most common form of arteriosclerosis is *atherosclerosis*, which involves the accumulation of plaque in the artery. The sites are either specific (such as *atherosclerosis of renal arterioles*) or generalized to an area (*atherosclerosis of the extremities*). Certain diseases (such as *phlebitis*) can also be located in specific sites or may be generalized or unspecified. A specific blood vessel condition, such as *varicose veins* or *hemorrhoids*, is often labeled with a specific site as well as with a complicating factor.

Blood vessel

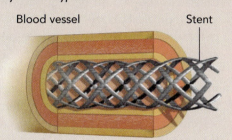 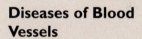

Stent

A stent.

sequencing either code first. In this case, no coding convention (such as brackets or code first guideline) directs the coder to sequence differently.

This example is based on common illnesses of the circulatory system. Coders will need familiarity with the disease processes relating to this system, which are reviewed in the Pathophysiology Refresher above.

Another example of interrelated conditions is:

EXAMPLE A patient presents with bleeding esophageal varices and active cirrhosis of the liver. The coding convention of slanted brackets requires the code for cirrhosis to be sequenced first, followed by the code for bleeding esophageal varices. So even though these are interrelated conditions that equally meet the definition of principal diagnosis, the code for cirrhosis is listed first because the ICD-9-CM Alphabetic Index and conventions indicate sequencing.

How does the coder decide which code to sequence first when either code can be reported? Typically the code that results in the highest payment from a payer for the hospitalization is listed first in the rare instance when this guideline applies.

TWO OR MORE DIAGNOSES THAT EQUALLY MEET THE DEFINITION OF PRINCIPAL DIAGNOSIS

The previous guideline addresses two conditions that are interrelated, but what should the coder do when two conditions that are not related equally meet the definition of principal diagnosis? For example, a patient presents with exacerbation of chronic obstructive pulmonary disease and atrial fibrillation. If both conditions occasioned the admission and were treated equally throughout the inpatient stay, either diagnosis code could be sequenced first.

As indicated above, when two or more diagnoses equally meet the criteria for principal diagnosis as determined by the circumstances of admission, diagnostic workup, and/or therapy, and when the Alphabetic Index, Tabular List, or other coding guidelines do not provide sequencing direction, any one of the diagnoses may be sequenced first. The circumstances of inpatient admission always govern the selection of the principal diagnosis, and this guideline applies only in the rare instance when two conditions occasion the admission to the hospital and both conditions are equally treated.

Checkpoint 4.2

Indicate whether the following scenarios meet the criteria under which the coder may sequence either code first when two conditions are either related or unrelated.

1. Mary presents to the hospital with chest pain and shortness of breath. Further study confirms both pneumonia and congestive heart failure. Mary is treated equally using medications and respiratory therapy. _____

2. Joseph presents with atrial fibrillation. After admission, he develops syncope due to a medication.

   _____

3. Pamela is admitted due to epigastric pain. Further evaluation by an upper endoscopy is positive for both gastritis and esophagitis. _____

TWO OR MORE COMPARATIVE OR CONTRASTING CONDITIONS

Occasionally, documentation supports the presence of two or more **contrasting or comparative conditions.** In such a case, the documentation indicates that the two diagnoses are comparative, using *either/or* (or similar terminology), and both conditions are coded as if the diagnoses were confirmed. The sequencing of the diagnoses is determined according to the circumstances of the admission. If no determination of which diagnosis should be principal can be made, either diagnosis may be sequenced first.

> **EXAMPLE** A patient presents with dizziness. The physician documentation supports the diagnosis of benign position vertigo versus labrynthitis.

In this case, both conditions are reported, and either can be sequenced first because both the comparative and the contrasting conditions are present. The documentation is worded in this way: The patient has both *this and that condition*, or *either this or that is causing the admission*. The documentation of contrasting and comparative diagnoses requires the coder to choose either condition as the principal diagnosis; either will be correct.

A SYMPTOM FOLLOWED BY CONTRASTING OR COMPARATIVE DIAGNOSES

At times, two or more conditions cause a symptom or set of symptoms. The *Official Guidelines* for this situation state that:

> When a symptom(s) is followed by contrasting/comparative diagnoses, the symptom code is sequenced first. All the contrasting/comparative diagnoses should be coded as additional diagnoses.

For example, the patient presents with chest pain caused by coronary artery disease and/or by gastroesophageal reflux. In this case, the symptom of chest pain is coded first, followed by the codes for coronary artery disease and gastroesophageal reflux. (All three codes are assigned.) In other words, this guideline instructs the coder to code the symptom and the diagnoses when two separate conditions may be the cause of the symptom.

If the presenting symptom is integral to both conditions, such as a patient who has abdominal pain due to gastritis or duodenitis (the symptom of abdominal pain is integral to both conditions), the case is coded according to the guidelines of comparative or contrasting conditions. The coder assigns a code for gastritis and a code for duodenitis, and either code is sequenced first.

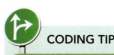

CODING TIP

Two Principal Diagnoses

In the rare instance that two conditions equally meet the definition of principal diagnosis, the coder may sequence either condition first.

Checkpoint 4.3

Code the following statements using ICD-9-CM Volumes 1 and 2. Also note which guideline applies.

	Codes(s)	Guideline
1. Chest pain due to anxiety or reflux esophagitis	_____	_____
2. Back pain due to lumbar stenosis versus lumbar osteoarthritis	_____	_____
3. Hypotension versus hypoglycemia	_____	_____
4. Pneumonia versus congestive heart failure	_____	
5. Shortness of breath due to either pneumonia or congestive heart failure	_____	_____

ORIGINAL TREATMENT PLAN NOT CARRIED OUT

Sometimes a patient is admitted to the hospital with a specified **treatment plan,** but the plan may not be carried out for one or more reasons. The ICD-9-CM coding guidelines direct the coder to sequence the principal diagnosis as the condition that after study occasioned the admission. Even though the original treatment plan is not carried out, the reason for admission is still considered the principal diagnosis.

EXAMPLES

- A patient admitted for coronary artery bypass surgery to treat coronary artery disease develops a fever prior to surgery. The surgery is cancelled, and the patient is discharged. In this case, the coronary artery disease (414.01) is sequenced as the principal diagnosis, followed by a code for the fever (780.6) and a code to indicate that the surgery was cancelled due to a contraindication (V64.1). An ICD-9-CM procedure code is not reported because the surgery was not done.

- A patient is admitted for gastrointestinal bleeding due to diverticulitis (562.13). The initial treatment plan is for the patient to undergo a sigmoid resection, but the patient decides to postpone the surgery for personal reasons. The principal diagnosis is still the condition that after study occasioned the admission to the hospital—diverticulitis with bleeding. Again, a code from V64.1 to V64.3, Surgery not done, is assigned as an additional diagnosis code; in this case, V64.2 is assigned to reflect the fact that the patient's decision was the reason the surgery was not done.

- The original treatment plan is not carried out, but other treatment is done: The patient is admitted with a intertrochanteric femur fracture after falling from a ladder at home, and surgical reduction of the fracture is required. When the patient is taken to surgery, the surgeon discovers that the patient needs metal-on-metal total hip replacement. The ICD-9-CM procedure of total hip replacement is reported and the principal diagnosis remains the fractured femur (820.21, E881.0, E849.0, 81.51, 00.75)

COMPLICATIONS OF SURGERY AND OTHER MEDICAL CARE

The *Official Guidelines* state that:

> When the admission is for treatment of a complication resulting from surgery or other medical care, the complication code is sequenced as the principal diagnosis. If the complication is classified to the 996–999 series and the code lacks the necessary specificity in describing the complication, an additional code for the specific complication should be assigned. (See the ICD-9-CM Tabular List for "use additional code" notes.)

Complications may be difficult to determine, but the coder can look for such documentation as "post-op infection," "post-op hematoma," "hip pain due to loose hip prosthesis," or "infected bypass graft." The complication code identifies the presence of a type of complication, and the additional code where directed classifies it.

For example, the code 998.12 for the diagnostic statement of postoperative hematoma not only classifies the hematoma but also indicates that the hematoma was a complication. Only one code is required because the type of complication is specific and is included in the code description. In other instances, a second code is required, such as when a patient has post-op pneumonia. The first listed code is the complication code (997.3, Complication, respiratory, post-op). The Tabular List directs the coder to use an additional code to identify the specific respiratory condition, so the additional code for pneumonia is also reported (486). The complication code is listed first if, after study, it is the reason for admission.

The main term *complication* is a good place to start in order to assign a complication code. It is sometimes also possible to find the correct complication code by looking up the type of complication with the subterm *postoperative*.

Documentation of complications may also indicate the need for an E code—that is, External Causes of Injury Code–for complete coding. (As a reminder, E codes are supplementary classifications for the causes of injury, poisoning, and adverse events, and are always sequenced after the condition code.) This data element, as shown in Table 4.1, is a required part of the UHDDS elements if applicable. E codes can be located under the main term *reaction, abnormal to or following* (a medical or surgical procedure) or *misadventure*.

EXAMPLE

Patient had a postoperative hemorrhage following tonsillectomy. Codes reported would be 998.11 and E code E878.6 for the abnormal reaction to the removal of an organ.

Checkpoint 4.4

Code the following complications, sequencing the code(s) in order. Verify all codes in the Tabular List, and read all coding notes and conventions. Do not assign E codes.

1. Post-op urinary retention _____

2. Loosening of a prosthetic hip joint replacement _____

3. Post-op seroma _____

4. Infected urinary catheter with cystitis _____

5. Mechanical complication of a pacemaker _____

UNCERTAIN DIAGNOSIS

The *Official Guideline* covering diagnoses that are not definitive states that a condition associated with an **uncertain diagnosis** should be coded as if it existed or was established if the documented diagnosis at discharge is probable, suspected, likely, questionable, possible, or still to be ruled out. The reason for coding the possible condition in the inpatient setting is based on the diagnostic workup, the arrangements for further workup or observation, and the initial therapeutic approach that corresponds most closely with the diagnosis. For example, if documentation states that the discharge diagnosis for an inpatient hospital visit is probable gastroenteritis, the coder assigns the code for gastroenteritis (558.9).

On the other hand, conditions that are ruled out should not be coded as if they exist. There is a different between conditions that are *ruled out* and conditions that are *rule out*. One letter changes the coding rule drastically.

EXAMPLES

Nausea and vomiting, gastroenteritis ruled out: only the nausea and vomiting are coded; gastroenteritis was ruled out. Code 787.01 is assigned.

Nausea and vomiting, rule out gastroenteritis: code the gastroenteritis because conditions that are possible or probable or not ruled out should be coded as if they exist. Code 558.9 is assigned.

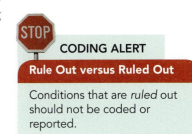

CODING ALERT

Rule Out versus Ruled Out

Conditions that are *ruled* out should not be coded or reported.

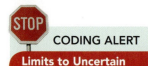
Exceptions to this rule are certain illnesses such as multiple sclerosis, AIDS, and epilepsy. If documentation states "possible multiple sclerosis," the coder should discuss the coding with the attending physician. Many physicians are not aware of the coding rule, and reporting these unconfirmed diagnoses may have social or employment ramifications for the patient. Therefore, discussion with the physician to check is essential.

ADMISSION FROM AN OBSERVATION UNIT

Sometimes a patient is admitted from an **observation unit** for either medical reasons or following surgery. The guidelines on sequencing the principal diagnosis in these circumstances must be clarified.

Admission Following Medical Observation
The principal diagnosis is the medical condition that leads to the hospital admission. Often a patient will present to the observation unit for a condition that needs monitoring, a status referred to as **medical observation**. If that condition does not improve or if it worsens, the patient may require hospital admission. In this case, the principal diagnosis for the inpatient hospital stay is the medical condition that led to the admission. For example, a patient enters observation due to acute diastolic congestive heart failure. Intravenous medications do not improve the patient's condition, and hospital admission is required. The principal diagnosis is reported as acute diastolic congestive heart failure (428.31) followed by 428.0.

Admission Following Postoperative Observation
Under different circumstances, a patient may be admitted to the observation unit for monitoring a condition or complication following outpatient surgery (a status referred to as **postoperative observation**) and then admitted to the hospital. In this case, the UHDDS definition of principal diagnosis applies: the condition established after study to be chiefly responsible for occasioning the admission to the hospital is the principal diagnosis.

> **EXAMPLE** A patient is admitted to the observation unit following severe pain from a tonsillectomy. Pain is controlled in the observation unit, but the patient develops a postoperative hemorrhage and requires admission to the hospital. The postoperative hemorrhage is the principal diagnosis because it is chiefly responsible for occasioning the admission. The diagnosis of tonsillitis and the procedure for tonsillectomy are also reported (998.11, 463, 338.18, E878.6, 28.2).

ADMISSION FROM OUTPATIENT SURGERY

The *Official Guidelines* provide three scenarios regarding sequencing of the principal diagnosis depending on the circumstances of admission.

Admission from Outpatient Surgery Due to Complication
When a patient who has surgery in the hospital's outpatient surgery department is subsequently admitted because of a complication of surgery, the complication code is sequenced first. The additional codes for the diagnosis and surgery (the ICD-9-VM Volume 3 procedure code) are also reported. An E code is also reported when the complication code falls in the 900 code range.

EXAMPLE Mary Jane undergoes inguinal hernia repair. After surgery, she is admitted due to postoperative fever. The principal diagnosis is the post-op fever (998.89), followed by the diagnosis code for inguinal hernia (550.90). The procedure code for hernia repair (53.00; ICD-9-CM Volume 3) is also reported, along with the E code to show this was a reaction to surgery (E878.8).

Admission from Outpatient Surgery with No Complication

"If no complication, or other condition, is documented as the reason for the inpatient admission, assign the reason for the outpatient surgery as the principal diagnosis." This ICD-9-CM guideline applies when there is no complication.

EXAMPLE Mark is scheduled to undergo a laparoscopic cholecystectomy as an outpatient to treat chronic cholelithiasis. In the outpatient surgery unit, Mark undergoes open cholecystectomy and is admitted to the hospital after surgery for recovery. The principal diagnosis is chronic cholelithiasis (574.20), and the cholecystectomy (51.23) is also reported for the inpatient stay.

Admission from Outpatient Surgery for an Unrelated Condition

"If the reason for the inpatient admission is another condition unrelated to the surgery, assign the unrelated condition as the principal diagnosis." This guideline addresses a different circumstance in which a patient is admitted from outpatient surgery. Sometimes, a completely different problem that requires hospital admission arises.

EXAMPLE Donna undergoes an outpatient colonoscopy to evaluate anemia. After the surgery, her diabetes is uncontrolled, and this condition requires hospital admission. The principal diagnosis for the inpatient hospital visit is uncontrolled diabetes (250.02), and the anemia is coded second (285.9). The colonoscopy is also reported for the hospital inpatient admission (45.23).

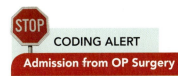

CODING ALERT

Admission from OP Surgery

The circumstances of admission are critical in assigning the principal diagnosis code.

Checkpoint 4.5

Assign ICD-9-CM codes for the following hospital inpatients using Volume 1 and Volume 2.

1. Joe is admitted to the hospital from observation after his unstable angina does not improve with medications. _____

2. Karen is admitted to the hospital due to post-op atelectasis following outpatient bronchoscopy for lung mass. _____

3. After outpatient carotid angiography for syncope, Larry's hypertension is uncontrolled, requiring admission to the hospital. _____

4. Laura is admitted to the hospital following outpatient laparoscopic hysterectomy for uterine fibroids. _____

5. Maxine undergoes cystoscopy with a biopsy for hematuria as an outpatient. She then goes to observation for pain control. In observation, Maxine develops chest pain, which requires her hospitalization. _____

Pathophysiology Refreshers

The Lymphatic, Immune, and Blood Systems

The lymphatic, immune, and blood systems are closely related to all the other systems of the body. Lymph and blood circulate throughout the body. Immunity protects the body from illnesses that affect all the body's systems.

Lymphatic Disorders

The lymph nodes and lymphatic tissue can be the sites of inflammations. *Lymphadenitis* (inflamed or swollen lymph nodes) is usually the result of an infection elsewhere in the body; however, it may also be unspecified. *Lymphangitis* (inflammation of the lymph vessels) may also result from infections elsewhere in the body. *Lymphedema* (swelling in the body due to accumulation of lymph in soft tissue) may be due to *elephantiasis* or another disorder. The lymph nodes can also become cancerous (for example, *lymphomas*).

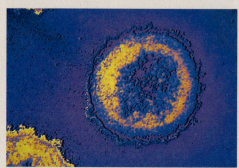

The human immunodeficiency virus (HIV) under a microscope.

Immune Disorders

The two major kinds of immune disorders are *autoimmune diseases* (diseases in which the body's immune response works against its own tissue) and *immunodefi-*

cient disorders (lack of or insufficient immunity to protect against disease). There are a number of autoimmune diseases in all the body's systems, including *rheumatoid arthritis, Type I diabetes,* and *multiple sclerosis.* In autoimmune disorders, patients' immune systems overreact to stimuli and begin attacking various organs. Another type of overreaction of the body is called an *allergic reaction.* Allergies are usually classified based on cause, such as *airborne substance* or *allergen, pollen, hay fever, food, skin contact,* or *medicinal.* Allergic reactions may also be categorized by type, such as *upper respiratory, urticaria,* or *gastrointestinal. Anaphylactic shock* is an extreme allergic reaction and is categorized by cause (such as *due to a bee sting*).

Immunodeficient disorders are either *congenital* (for example, *DiGeorge's syndrome*) or *acquired* (contracted, as from a virus). *Human immunodeficiency virus (HIV)* can be *with* or *without symptoms.* Infection by HIV is not the same as having AIDS, but it can lead to *acquired immunodeficiency syndrome (AIDS),* which is diagnosed when the virus causes a complex of AIDS-related diseases. AIDS may first appear as *AIDS-like syndrome* or *AIDS-related complex* (generally persistent fever and swollen lymph nodes). Full-blown AIDS often includes *opportunistic infections,* such as *Kaposi's sarcoma*

Section III: Reporting Additional Diagnoses

The *Official Guidelines* also indicate which conditions should be reported as **secondary diagnoses,** meaning other diagnoses. This data element of the UHDDS (see Table 4.1) defines other diagnoses as:

> all conditions that coexist at the time of admission, that develop subsequently, or that affect the treatment received and/or the length of stay. Diagnoses that relate to an earlier episode which have no bearing on the current hospital stay are to be excluded.

These definitions apply to inpatients in all inpatient and nonoutpatient settings.

GENERAL RULES FOR OTHER (ADDITIONAL) DIAGNOSES

Five key criteria are used in determining whether to report an additional diagnosis or condition. At least one criterion must be met in all cases, but many times one condition may meet one or more criteria.

CODING TIP

Reporting Order of Secondary Diagnoses

The order for reporting multiple secondary diagnoses is not mandated; however, if there is limited space for reporting, conditions should be reported in the order of their significance, with the most significant condition reported first after the principal diagnosis.

(connective tissue cancer) and *pneumocystis carinii pneumonia*. Any immune disorder, especially AIDS, causes patients to be in a state called *immunocompromised*, which means that their natural immunities are not capable of staving off infections. Such patients are at high risk for bacterial and viral infections of all kinds.

Blood Disorders

The blood can carry infections to all parts of the body. Diseases also occur in the blood itself and in the blood-forming organs. *Anemia* is a general term for a deficiency of red blood cells (also called *erythrocytes*). Anemia may occur because of hereditary, nutritional, or other factors, such as blood loss. *Thalassemia* is a term for any of group of hereditary anemias in people of Mediterranean descent. It may be classified by the particular type (as *Hb-E* or *Hb-1*). It may also be categorized as *with* or *without crisis*. *Sickle-cell anemia* (hereditary anemia in people of African descent) may also be classified by type (*Hb-S* or *Hb-C*) and may also be categorized as *with* or *without crisis*. Nutritional anemias occur either because of a deficiency of a certain nutrient (such as folate) or because of the inability of the body to absorb certain nutrients. *Pernicious* anemia occurs when there is malabsorption of vitamin B$_{12}$. *Iron-deficiency anemia* (a lack of sufficient iron in the blood) may be due to poor iron intake or may occur with sudden blood loss. Other anemias (such as *hemolytic anemia*) may result from infections or other disorders. *Aplastic anemia* (severe destruction of bone marrow) may occur with cancer or with certain medical treatments or other medical conditions.

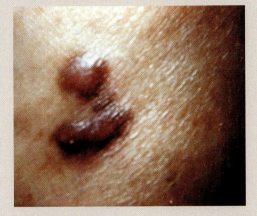
Karposi's sarcoma.

Coagulation disorders of the blood are often congenital but may also result from other disorders or conditions or even as adverse reactions to medication. *Hemophilia* is a general term for hereditary coagulation disorders. *Von Willebrand's disease* is one such disorder with slow blood coagulation. There are other disorders of red blood cells (such as *polycythemia,* an abnormally large number of red blood cells, and *thrombocytopenia*, abnormally low blood platelets). Two diseases of white blood cells are *agranulocytosis* (abnormally low number of white blood cells often caused by radiation or other medical treatments) and *eosinophilia* (abnormally high number of eosinophils, a type of *leukocyte,* white blood cell). There are disorders of both red and white blood cells, such as *leukemia* (a general term for any of several cancers of the blood).

According to the *Official Guidelines*:

> For reporting purposes the definition for "other diagnoses" is interpreted as additional conditions that affect patient care in terms of requiring:
>
> 1. clinical evaluation; or
> 2. therapeutic treatment; or
> 3. diagnostic procedures; or
> 4. extended length of hospital stay; or
> 5. increased nursing care and/or monitoring.

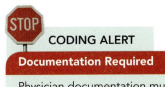

CODING ALERT

Documentation Required

Physician documentation must support the presence of additional diagnoses.

Clinical Evaluation Many conditions documented by the physician in the inpatient hospital setting may require clinical evaluation. For example, the patient may develop confusion, which requires clinical evaluation from a consultant. Confusion or the underlying cause is reported as an additional or secondary diagnosis.

Therapeutic Treatment Patients who receive medication for a particular disease are undergoing therapeutic treatment. Physical

The Medicare Inpatient Prospective Payment System and MS-DRGs

Medicare, by far the largest health plan for hospital reimbursement, pays hospitals for inpatient services based on the Medicare **Inpatient Prospective Payment System (IPPS).** This system is called *prospective* because rather than paying for each service after the fact, the rate has been set in advance. Rates are established based on Medicare's analysis of how long people are hospitalized, on average, for similar conditions. The length of stay (LOS) is a good predictor of the average use of the hospital's resource, and thus of the cost of care.

Medicare analyzes and updates a study of all the ICD-9-CM codes—both diagnosis and procedures—that are reported for care during a period of time. Medicare then groups patients into **diagnosis-related groups (DRGs).** Each DRG number is connected to a dollar amount that is payable for the patients in its category. Patients are assigned a single DRG, which is based on these elements of the UHDDS:

- Diagnoses, principal and other
- Significant procedures
- Age, sex, and discharge status

Formerly, each DRG was associated with a single payment rate. In 2008, Medicare adopted a new type of DRG called **Medicare-Severity DRGs (MS-DRGs)** to reflect the

therapy and speech therapy are also therapeutic treatment, and conditions that require such therapy should be reported.

> **EXAMPLE** An inpatient receives medication for hypertension throughout a hospitalization. Hypertension is reported as an additional diagnosis.

Diagnostic Procedures This criterion refers to conditions that require a diagnostic service, including diagnostic blood work, a radiology procedure, or another diagnostic procedure such as a colonoscopy. For example, the condition of anemia requires diagnostic testing to determine the type of anemia. Laboratory test results and physician documentation support a diagnosis of iron deficiency anemia, so the anemia should be reported as an additional diagnosis.

Many lymphatic, immune system, and blood disorders are comorbid conditions that may require diagnostic procedures during a hospitalization. Examples of these comorbidities might be rheumatoid arthritis, multiple sclerosis, AIDS, and sickle cell anemia. The Pathophysiology Refresher on pages 150-151 provides coders with an overview of the disease process for these illnesses. Remember that these conditions would be reported as additional diagnoses when the condition, after study, which occasioned the admission is due to a different condition.

Extended Length of Hospital Stay Many circumstances, such as a fever or other complications, can extend a patient's hospital stay. Typically these conditions develop after admission and may also require clinical evaluation or treatment.

> **EXAMPLE** A patient develops a severe headache the evening before his expected discharge. The discharge is cancelled, and the patient undergoes a CAT scan of the brain. Headache is reported as an additional diagnosis because this condition extended the length of stay and also required clinical evaluation.

Increased Nursing Care and/or Monitoring Many conditions required increased nursing care or monitoring. For example,

different severity of illness among patients with the same diagnosis. The system better recognizes the severity of illness and the corresponding higher cost of treating Medicare patients with more complex conditions, offset by decreasing payments for other less severely ill patients.

There are 745 DRGS, replacing the former 538. The MS-DRG system increases the importance of listing secondary conditions, because when patients have or develop them, the rate of payment hospitals receive for the hospital stay is increased.

If the secondary diagnosis represents a condition that the patient has at admission, it is called a **comorbidity.** Comorbidities are either conditions that affect a patient's recovery, such as having diabetes mellitus, or another acute illness or injury. If the secondary diagnosis represents a **complication** that affects the patient's recovery, the length of the hospital stay is increased, logically increasing payment. Complications in this context are those conditions that happen after admission that affect care.

Together, under the UHDDS, the principal diagnosis and the comorbidities/complications are known as the CCs. According to the *Journal of AHIMA* (July/august 2007, p. 18), a base MS-DRG may have three levels of severity:

1. **Major CC (MCC)**
2. CC
3. Non-CC

To achieve the correct payment level for the hospital stay, coders should code as many secondary conditions as are compliant with the rules for reporting additional diagnoses.

a patient may be legally blind, a condition that requires increased nursing care and should be reported. A patient may develop hypotension and require increased monitoring of blood pressure; hypotension should be reported as an additional diagnosis.

Based on changing rules from health plans about reimbursement, reporting secondary conditions is increasingly important for the inpatient setting. The Reimbursement Review above outlines the key points relating to the effects of secondary codes on payments.

Checkpoint 4.6

Underline the conditions that would be reported as additional diagnoses, and identify which criteria for reporting were met (1, 2, 3, 4, and/or 5). Following is an example:

Monica is admitted to the hospital for treatment of breast cancer. She is also treated with medication for her hypertension and diabetes. Criterion 2, therapeutic treatment

1. Joseph develops hypokalemia on his second hospital day. This condition requires laboratory monitoring and potassium supplements. _____

2. Kevin needs to stay in the hospital one additional day because he becomes dehydrated. _____

3. Marlene undergoes an echocardiogram because of a heart murmur heard on examination. The physician documents mitral valve prolapse as the cause of the murmur and prescribes antibiotics prior to surgery. _____

4. Paul becomes dizzy once he is able to get out of bed. The nursing staff is ordered to monitor Paul's blood pressure closely over the next twelve hours because of his dizziness. _____

5. After admission, Beth develops chest pain. The chest pain is evaluated by ECG and is treated with nitroglycerin. _____

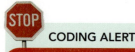
ADDITIONAL GUIDELINES FOR OTHER DIAGNOSES

According to the *Official Guidelines*, the following rules apply in designating other diagnoses when neither the Alphabetic Index nor the Tabular List provides direction.

Previous Conditions   The guidance on previous conditions is as follows:

> If the provider has included a diagnosis in the final diagnostic statement, such as the discharge summary or the face sheet, it should ordinarily be coded. Some providers include in the diagnostic statement resolved conditions or diagnoses and status-post procedures from previous admission that have no bearing on the current stay. Such conditions are not to be reported and are coded only if required by hospital policy.

> **EXAMPLE**   A physician may document the diagnosis of status post cholecystectomy on the face sheet. Review of documentation indicates that the cholecystectomy was completed five years earlier. No code is assigned for this diagnostic statement.

It is appropriate to assign history codes (V10–V19) as secondary codes if the historical condition or family history affects current care or influences treatment.

> **EXAMPLE**   The physician discharge summary lists the diagnosis of family history of coronary artery disease (CAD) for a patient with myocardial infarction. The code for family history of CAD (V17.3) is reported.

Abnormal Findings   The attending or treating physician must document clinical significance in order to code **abnormal findings** (those outside of normal ranges) such as those from laboratory, X-ray, pathology, and other diagnostic results. Without documentation of clinical significance by the treating or attending physician, these abnormal findings or conditions are not coded.

If the finding is outside the normal range and the attending provider has ordered other tests to evaluate the condition or has prescribed treatment, it is appropriate to query him or her about whether the abnormal finding should be added. Only the physician can clarify whether abnormal findings should be coded; the coder may not make the determination. If, for example, when reviewing the medical record you notice that the patient's urinalysis is positive for *E. coli* based on urine culture results alone, you should ask the physician whether these results were clinically significant. If you see that a chest X-ray supports the diagnostic impression of COPD, you need provider documentation of clinical significance before you can code the abnormal findings.

Uncertain Diagnoses   As discussed earlier, the rule governing uncertain diagnoses applies for secondary diagnoses as well. If the diagnosis documented at the time of discharge is qualified as probable, suspected, likely, questionable, possible, or still to be ruled out, code the condition as if it existed or has been established. This guideline applies only to short-term care, acute care, long-term care, and psychiatric hospitals.

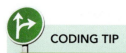

Code the following using Volumes 1 and 2, keeping in mind the ICD-9-CM *Official Guidelines* for reporting additional diagnoses.

1. Monica is admitted for acute CVA. After admission, follow-up lab work shows abnormal liver function tests, which are documented and evaluated by the attending physician. The cause of these abnormal findings is not determined. _____

2. The patient is admitted for acute renal failure. The patient had an appendectomy three years earlier. _____

3. Documentation of the discharge diagnoses states the following: Congestive heart failure, hypertension, gouty arthritis, abnormal ECG, and history of tobacco abuse. _____

4. Bonnie is admitted for treatment of breast cancer. The face sheet documentation supports the following diagnoses: carcinoma of the breast, hyponatremia, and possible allergic dermatitis. _____

5. In the outpatient setting, the patient presents to the hospital for an outpatient X-ray due to shortness of breath. Chest X-ray interpretation by the radiologist supports the diagnosis of COPD. _____

Present on Admission (POA) Guidelines

Once the diagnosis codes have been assigned and sequenced, the coder in the inpatient setting must also determine whether each principal and secondary diagnosis, as well as external cause of injury, was **present on admission (POA).** *Present on admission* means present at the time the order for inpatient admission occurs. Conditions that develop during an outpatient encounter that leads to admission—including in the emergency department, during observation, or during outpatient surgery—are considered present on admission. Whether the condition was present on admission is reported by the use of an indicator, as shown in Table 4.2. The indicator is placed next to each ICD-9-CM code reported on a hospital health care claim.

Notice that indicators U and W refer to documentation issues, or knowledge about whether the condition was present that the provider

COMPLIANCE GUIDELINE

POA Mandate

The federal requirement to report POA indicators so that Medicare does not pay hospitals for conditions the hospital caused or allowed to develop during an inpatient stay was established in the Deficit Reduction Act of 2005. The *Official Guidelines* added the reporting requirements on present on admission to Appendix I in the version effective November 15, 2006, to take effect the following year.

INTERNET RESOURCE

POA Guidelines

www.cdc.gov/nchs/datawh/ftpserv/ftpicd9/ftpicd9.htm Guidelines begin on page 92.

Table 4.2 Present on Admission (POA) Indicators

Indicator	Meaning	Definition
Y	Yes	Present at the time of inpatient admission
N	No	Not present at the time of inpatient admission
U	Unknown	Documentation is insufficient to determine whether condition is present on admission
W	Clinically undetermined	Provider is unable to clinically determine whether condition was present on admission
———	Blank	If the condition code is on the list of exempt codes, the field is left blank. (Medicare requires a "1" instead of no entry.)

was unable to clinically determine. Issues related to inconsistent, missing, conflicting, or unclear documentation must be resolved by the provider.

Leaving the POA field blank is appropriate when an ICD-9-CM diagnosis code that is listed on the **POA exempt from reporting** list is assigned. Such a code either represents conditions that are always present on admission or does not represent a current disease or injury. For example, normal delivery codes represent conditions that are always present on admission, whereas screening codes and the palliative care code do not represent current diseases. Table 4.3 summarizes the codes that are exempt from the POA indicator.

Some guidelines assist the coder in determining whether a condition or external cause (E code) is present on admission.

CONDITIONS PRESENT ON ADMISSION—INDICATOR OF Y

The Y (yes) indicator is assigned for any condition that the provider explicitly documents as being present on admission. These may be conditions that were diagnosed prior to admission (such as diabetes) or conditions that were clearly present but not diagnosed until after admission.

Conditions that are possible or probable at the time of discharge are assigned a POA of Y when the diagnosis was suspected at the time of inpatient admission. The coder also assigns a Y for chronic conditions that are present but not diagnosed until after admission. The indicator identifies whether the condition was present at admission, not whether it was diagnosed then.

> **EXAMPLE** Joe presents with chest pain from possible unstable angina. The chest X-ray reveals COPD. Evaluation and testing during hospitalization confirm that Joe has unstable angina due to coronary artery disease and COPD. Treatments are provided, and Joe is discharged. The codes reported are coronary artery disease (414.01), unstable angina (411.1), and COPD (496). The POA indicator for all the codes is Y.

Also assign the POA of Y for external causes of injury that occurred prior to admission. The patient may have fallen out of bed at home, or a patient made a suicide attempt prior to admission.

A Y indicator is also assigned for a newborn whose condition developed in utero. This includes conditions that occur during delivery (meconium aspiration, fetal distress). A newborn is not considered to be admitted until after delivery, and congenital conditions are always considered present on admission.

CONDITIONS NOT PRESENT ON ADMISSION—INDICATOR OF N

The POA indicator of N (no) refers to any condition that was not present on admission based on the provider's documentation. If the final diagnosis contains the terms *possible*, *probable*, or the like and if it was based on symptoms or clinical findings that were not present on admission, the N indicator is assigned.

Table 4.3 ICD-9-CM Diagnosis Codes Exempt from POA Indicator

137-139, Late effects of infectious and parasitic diseases
268.1, Rickets, late effect
326, Late effects of intracranial abscess or pyogenic infection
412, Old myocardial infarction
438, Late effects of cerebrovascular disease
650, Normal delivery
660.7, Failed forceps or vacuum extractor, unspecified
677, Late effect of complication of pregnancy, childbirth, and the puerperium
905-909, Late effects of injuries, poisonings, toxic effects, and other external causes

V02, Carrier or suspected carrier of infectious diseases
V03, Need for prophylactic vaccination and inoculation against bacterial diseases
V04, Need for prophylactic vaccination and inoculation against certain viral diseases
V05, Need for other prophylactic vaccination and inoculation against single diseases
V06, Need for prophylactic vaccination and inoculation against combinations of diseases
V07, Need for isolation and other prophylactic measures
V10, Personal history of malignant neoplasm
V11, Personal history of mental disorder
V12, Personal history of certain other diseases
V13, Personal history of other diseases
V14, Personal history of allergy to medicinal agents
V15, Other personal history presenting hazards to health

V16, Family history of malignant neoplasm
V17, Family history of certain chronic disabling diseases
V18, Family history of certain other specific conditions
V19, Family history of other conditions
V20, Health supervision of infant or child
V21, Constitutional states in development
V22, Normal pregnancy
V23, Supervision of high-risk pregnancy
V24, Postpartum care and examination
V25, Encounter for contraceptive management
V26, Procreative management
V27, Outcome of delivery
V28, Antenatal screening
V29, Observation and evaluation of newborns for suspected condition not found

V30-V39, Liveborn infants according to type of birth
V42, Organ or tissue replaced by transplant
V43, Organ or tissue replaced by other means
V44, Artificial opening status
V45, Other postprocedural states
V46, Other dependence on machines
V49.60-V49.77, Upper and lower limb amputation status
V49.81-V49.84, Other specified conditions influencing health status
V50, Elective surgery for purposes other than remedying health states

V51, Aftercare involving the use of plastic surgery
V52, Fitting and adjustment of prosthetic device and implant
V53, Fitting and adjustment of other device
V54, Other orthopedic aftercare
V55, Attention to artificial openings
V56, Encounter for dialysis and dialysis catheter care
V57, Care involving use of rehabilitation procedures
V58, Encounter for other and unspecified procedures and aftercare
V59, Donors
V60, Housing, household, and economic circumstances
V61, Other family circumstances
V62, Other psychosocial circumstances
V64, Persons encountering health services for specific procedures, not carried out
V65, Other persons seeking consultation
V66, Convalescence and palliative care
V67, Follow-up examination
V68, Encounters for administrative purposes
V69, Problems related to lifestyle
V70, General medical examination
V71, Observation and evaluation for suspected condition not found
V72, Special investigations and examinations
V73, Special screening examination for viral and chlamydial diseases
V74, Special screening examination for bacterial and spirochetal diseases
V75, Special screening examination for other infectious diseases
V76, Special screening for malignant neoplasms

V77, Special screening for endocrine, nutritional, metabolic, and immunity disorders
V78, Special screening for disorders of blood and blood-forming organs
V79, Special screening for mental disorders and developmental handicaps
V80, Special screening for neurological, eye, and ear diseases
V81, Special screening for cardiovascular, respiratory, and genitourinary diseases
V82, Special screening for other conditions
V83, Genetic carrier status
V84, Genetic susceptibility to disease
V85 Body Mass Index
V86 Estrogen receptor status

E800-E807, Railway accidents
E810-E819, Motor vehicle traffic accidents
E820-E825, Motor vehicle nontraffic accidents
E826-E829, Other road vehicle accidents
E830-E838, Water transport accidents
E840-E845, Air and space transport accidents
E846-E848, Vehicle accidents not elsewhere classifiable
E849.0-E849.6, Place of occurrence
E849.8-E849.9, Place of occurrence
E883.1, Accidental fall into well
E883.2, Accidental fall into storm drain or manhole
E884.0, Fall from playground equipment
E884.1, Fall from cliff
E885.0, Fall from (nonmotorized) scooter
E885.1, Fall from roller skates
E885.2, Fall from skateboard
E885.3, Fall from skis
E885.4, Fall from snowboard
E886.0, Fall on same level from collision, pushing, or shoving, by or with other person, In sports
E890.0-E89.9, Conflagration in private dwelling
E893.0, Accident caused by ignition of clothing, from controlled fire in private dwelling
E893.2, Accident caused by ignition of clothing, from controlled fire not in building or structure
E894, Ignition of highly inflammable material
E895, Accident caused by controlled fire in private dwelling
E897, Accident caused by controlled fire not in building or structure
E898.0-E898.1, Accident caused by other specified fire and flames
E917.0, Striking against or struck accidentally by objects or persons, in sports without subsequent fall
E917.1, Striking against or struck accidentally by objects or persons, caused by a crowd, by collective fear or panic without subsequent fall
E917.2, Striking against or struck accidentally by objects or persons, in running water without subsequent fall
E917.5, Striking against or struck accidentally by objects or persons, object in sports with subsequent fall
E917.6, Striking against or struck accidentally by objects or persons, caused by a crowd, by collective fear or panic with subsequent fall
E919.0-E919.1, Accidents caused by machinery
E919.3-E919.9, Accidents caused by machinery
E921.0-E921.9, Accident caused by explosion of pressure vessel
E922.0-E922.9, Accident caused by firearm and air gun missile
E924.1, Caustic and corrosive substances
E926.2, Visible and ultraviolet light sources
E927, Overexertion and strenuous movements
E928.0-E928.8, Other and unspecified environmental and accidental causes
E929.0-E929.9, Late effects of accidental injury
E959, Late effects of self-inflicted injury
E970-E978, Legal intervention
E979, Terrorism
E981.0-E981.8, Poisoning by gases in domestic use, undetermined whether accidentally or purposely inflicted
E982.0-E982.9, Poisoning by other gases, undetermined whether accidentally or purposely inflicted
E985.0-E985.7, Injury by firearms, air guns and explosives, undetermined whether accidentally or purposely inflicted
E987.0, Falling from high place, undetermined whether accidentally or purposely inflicted, residential premises
E987.2, Falling from high place, undetermined whether accidentally or purposely inflicted, natural sites
E989, Late effects of injury, undetermined whether accidentally or purposely inflicted
E990-E999, Injury resulting from operations of war

Assign N for an E code that represents an external cause of injury or poisoning that occurred during inpatient hospitalization. This might be a fall out of bed in the hospital or an adverse reaction to a medication given after admission.

EXAMPLE Maggie is admitted due to gastrointestinal bleeding and associated anemia. After a transfusion of red blood cells, she has a transfusion reaction. The code for transfusion reaction is reported with the N indicator because the reaction was not present on admission. The POA indicator for the bleeding and anemia is Y.

UNKNOWN (U) OR UNDETERMINED (W) CONDITIONS

When medical record documentation is unclear about whether a condition was present on admission, the indicator U (unknown) is assigned. This indicator is not assigned routinely, since documentation in the medical record should support a more specific indicator of Y or N. If the documentation is unclear, the physician should be queried about whether the condition was present on admission.

If the presence of the condition at admission cannot be determined clinically, the indicator W (undetermined) should be assigned.

SPECIAL CIRCUMSTANCES FOR ASSIGNING POA INDICATORS

If each code in ICD-9-CM represented one disease or condition, assignment of a POA indicator might not require an extensive explanation. But ICD-9-CM includes combination codes, acute and chronic conditions, obstetrical conditions that indicate complications of

Reimbursement Review

The Hospital Billing Process: Claims and the POA Indicator

Hospitals submit claims to health plans on behalf of patients, unless the patient is solely responsible for payment. Most hospitals, because they are regulated by HIPAA, send electronic claims, although some may bill payers using paper claims.

A large percentage of claims are sent to Medicare, and these are transmitted electronically using the HIPAA health care claim called the **837I.** This electronic data interchange (EDI) format is called *I* for *Institutional*; the corresponding physicians' claim is called 837P (*Professional*). In some situations, a paper claim form called the **UB-04** (uniform billing 2004), also known as the **CMS-1450,** is sent. The UB-04 is maintained by the National Uniform Billing Committee.

837I Health Care Claim Completion

The 837I has sections requiring data elements for the billing and the pay-to provider, the subscriber and patient, and the payer, plus claim and service level details. Most of the data elements report the same information as illustrated below for the paper claim.

UB-04 Claim Form Completion

The UB-04 claim form has eighty-one data fields, some of which require multiple entries. The information for the form locators often requires choosing from a list of codes, such as for the type of service. Medicare and private-payer-required fields may be slightly different, and other condition codes or options are often available. The completed form on page 159 shows a claim for a hospital stay of 14 days. Note the ICD-9-CM codes and the POA indicators.

1 GRACE MEMORIAL HOSPITAL	2		3a PAT. CNTL # XX871295			4 TYPE OF BILL
100 MAIN STREET			b. MED. REC. # 7650120			0111
TULSA, OK 74101			5 FED. TAX NO.	6 STATEMENT COVERS PERIOD FROM THROUGH		7
9182367007			07-1282340	033109 041409		

8 PATIENT NAME	a	9 PATIENT ADDRESS	a 201 MAGNOLIA AVE.			
b WILLIAMS, GILBERT, U.		b TULSA		c OK d 74103	e	

10 BIRTHDATE	11 SEX	12 DATE	ADMISSION 13 HR 14 TYPE 15 SRC	16 DHR	17 STAT	18 19 20 21	CONDITION CODES 22 23 24 25	26 27 28	29 ACDT STATE	30
09121920	M	033109	09 1 7	19	01	09				

31 OCCURRENCE CODE DATE	32 OCCURRENCE CODE DATE	33 OCCURRENCE CODE DATE	34 OCCURRENCE CODE DATE	35 OCCURRENCE SPAN CODE FROM THROUGH	36 OCCURRENCE SPAN CODE FROM THROUGH	37
a 18 091285						
b						

38				39 CODE VALUE CODES AMOUNT	40 CODE VALUE CODES AMOUNT	41 CODE VALUE CODES AMOUNT
			a	80 14 00		
			b			
			c			
			d			

	42 REV. CD.	43 DESCRIPTION	44 HCPCS / RATE / HIPPS CODE	45 SERV. DATE	46 SERV. UNITS	47 TOTAL CHARGES	48 NON-COVERED CHARGES	49	
1	0111	MED-SURG-GY/PVT	72000		13	9,360 00			1
2	0201	ICU/SURGICAL	170100		1	1,701 00			2
3	0230	NURSING INCREM				9,594 00			3
4	0233	NUR INCR/ICU				2,027 00			4
5	0250	PHARMACY				2,579 15			5
6	0260	IV THERAPY				1,545 20			6
7	0270	MED-SUR SUPPLIES				835 90			7
8	0300	LAB				4,942 66			8
9	0301	CHEMISTRY TESTS				125 00			9
10	0320	DX X-RAY			1	433 18			10
11	0340	NUCLEAR MEDICINE			1	784 08			11
12	0350	CT SCAN			1	421 08			12
13	0351	CT SCAN/HEAD			1	1,018 82			13
14	0352	CT SCAN/BODY			4	4,075 28			14
15	0390	BLOOD/ADMIN/STOR				1,008 00			15
16	0410	RESPIRATORY SVC			29	641 56			16
17	0450	EMERG ROOM			2	810 82			17
18	0480	CARDIOLOGY				1,289 86			18
19	0730	EKG/ECG				96 68			19
20	0761	TREATMENT RM				54 45			20
21	0921	PERI VASCUL LAB				804 65			21
22									22
23	0001	*PAGE___1___OF___1___*	CREATION DATE 042009	TOTALS ➡		44,148 37			23

50 PAYER NAME	51 HEALTH PLAN ID	52 REL INFO	53 ASG BEN.	54 PRIOR PAYMENTS	55 EST. AMOUNT DUE	56 NPI 1122999665	
A MEDICARE	00308	Y	Y			57 070089	A
B						OTHER	B
C						PRV ID	C

58 INSURED'S NAME	59 P.REL	60 INSURED'S UNIQUE ID	61 GROUP NAME	62 INSURANCE GROUP NO.	
A WILLIAMS, GILBERT, U.	18	765452817A			A
B					B
C					C

63 TREATMENT AUTHORIZATION CODES	64 DOCUMENT CONTROL NUMBER	65 EMPLOYER NAME	
A			A
B			B
C			C

66 DX	486 Y	1628 Y	1987 Y	5119 Y	7856 N	496 Y	1961 Y	4019 Y	514 Y	68
67	A	B	C	D	E	F	G	H		
	I	J	K	L	M	N	O	P	Q	

69 ADMIT DX 78600	70 PATIENT REASON DX a b c	71 PPS CODE	72 ECI a b c	73

74 PRINCIPAL PROCEDURE CODE DATE	a. OTHER PROCEDURE CODE DATE	b. OTHER PROCEDURE CODE DATE	75	76 ATTENDING NPI 1022550001	QUAL 1G 58912T
3898 033109	9904 040309			LAST FATU	FIRST LOUISE
c. OTHER PROCEDURE CODE DATE	d. OTHER PROCEDURE CODE DATE	e. OTHER PROCEDURE CODE DATE		77 OPERATING NPI 2799906111	QUAL IG 10340B
				LAST AZODI	FIRST ALI

80 REMARKS	81CC a b3 282N00000X	78 OTHER NPI	QUAL
	b	LAST	FIRST
	c	79 OTHER NPI	QUAL
	d	LAST	FIRST

UB-04 CMS-1450   APPROVED OMB NO. 0938-0997   **NUBC** National Uniform Billing Committee   THE CERTIFICATIONS ON THE REVERSE APPLY TO THIS BILL AND ARE MADE A PART HEREOF.

pregnancy, and perinatal conditions. These unique facets of ICD-9-CM require additional explanations.

POA Indicators for Combination Codes

Combination codes may represent acute exacerbations (such as a COPD exacerbation), complications (such as an ulcer with bleeding), or causal organisms (such as UTI due to *E. coli*). The guidelines instruct the coder to determine whether any part of the combination code was present on admission. If any part of the combination code was *not* present on admission, the N indicator is assigned.

> **EXAMPLE** If a patient's diabetes mellitus (250.00) becomes uncontrolled (250.02) after admission, only code 250.02 is assigned. Because the uncontrolled portion of the diabetes does not develop until after admission, code 250.02 is assigned the POA indicator N.

> **EXAMPLE** After admission, a patient with a gastric ulcer develops bleeding from the ulcer. Only the combination code for gastric ulcer with hemorrhage (531.40) is assigned. Since the hemorrhage developed after admission; the N indicator is assigned.

For some codes, acute and chronic or acute exacerbation is not reported. An example is congestive heart failure. The code 428.0 is assigned whether the heart failure is chronic or decompensated (acute exacerbation). Therefore, if the heart failure is present on admission, the indicator is Y even if the heart failure decompensates after admission.

Some combination codes include causative organisms; an example is *E. coli* septicemia (038.42). For infection codes that include the causal organism, the POA indicator of Y is assigned even if the culture results are determined after admission. Carefully determine whether the infection was present on admission. For example, if a patient presents with sepsis and the culture after admission is positive for *E. coli*, code 038.42 is assigned with the Y indicator.

Obstetrical Conditions

Whether the patient actually delivers during the current hospitalization does not affect the assignment of the POA indicator. The factor that determines the POA assignment is whether the obstetrical condition described by the code is present at the time of admission.

If the pregnancy complication or obstetrical condition is present on admission, the Y indicator is assigned. This includes such diagnoses as preterm labor and previous cesarean section. The N indicator is assigned when the condition is not present on admission, such as perineal laceration after delivery or postpartum hemorrhage. For an obstetrical combination code, if any condition represented by that code is not present on admission, the N indicator is assigned.

> **EXAMPLE** Margie presents to the hospital in labor, and the baby is full-term. Margie has gestational diabetes (648.81). After admission, Margie requires a cesarean section due to fetal distress (656.81). The pregnancy code for gestational diabetes is assigned the Y indicator, and the fetal distress code is assigned the N indicator.

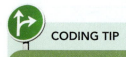

CODING TIP

Present on Admission

Review the specific POA guidelines for combination codes and obstetrical conditions.

Assign the present on admission (POA) indicators for the following scenarios.

1. A patient is admitted for a diagnostic workup of syncope. The final diagnosis is sick sinus syndrome, and the patient undergoes pacemaker insertion. _____

2. A patient presents with difficulty breathing. The diagnosis is acute asthma exacerbation. _____
   _____

3. A patient falls in the ER, sustaining a fractured hip. The patient is subsequently admitted due to hip fracture. _____

4. A patient is admitted to the hospital for knee replacement due to osteoarthritis of the knee. After surgery, the patient develops acute blood loss anemia. _____

5. A patient in active labor is admitted. During the stay, a breast abscess is noted when she starts breast feeding the baby. The provider is unable to determine whether the abscess was present on admission. _____

6. A newborn develops feeding problems after birth. _____

7. A women presents to the hospital and undergoes a normal delivery. _____

8. The patient presents with nausea and vomiting. The physician documents the discharge diagnosis as possible viral gastroenteritis. _____

9. A patient presents to the ED after a motor vehicle collision (E812.0). He requires admission due to fractured ribs and a fractured wrist. After admission and surgery, he develops a wound infection. _____

10. A homeless patient is admitted with acute renal failure. After admission, the patient develops syncope. The physician documents the diagnoses as acute renal failure and possible cardiogenic syncope. _____

Summary

1. The patient care flow and associated documentation for the inpatient setting begins with hospital admission, where the patient's face sheet with demographics as well as all medical information are compiled; continues during the evaluation and treatment of the patient, supported by appropriate notes; and is completed with the patients discharge. The documentation in the medical record must support the diagnoses and procedures reported for each patient's hospitalization. Review of the discharge summary, history and physical, progress notes, physician orders, consultations, operative reports, and diagnostic tests is essential in order to assign accurate and complete ICD-9-CM codes. The listing of the diagnoses in the patient record is the responsibility of the attending provider.

2. The Uniform Hospital Discharge Data Set (UHDDS) definitions apply to all nonoutpatient settings. The definitions in the data set are mandated by HIPAA legislation and are incorporated in the ICD-9-CM *Official Guidelines for Coding and Reporting.*

3. The definition of principal diagnosis, which is based on the UHDDS definitions, is "that condition established after study to be chiefly responsible for occasioning the admission of the patient to the hospital for care."

4. Once the diagnosis codes are assigned, their sequencing must be completed. The main rule regarding sequencing of the principal diagnosis codes is that codes for signs and symptoms should not be sequenced first when the underlying condition has been established. However, if a sign or symptom is followed by comparative or contrasting conditions, the symptom code is sequenced first.

5. (a) When each of two or more interrelated conditions potentially meets the definition of principal diagnosis, either condition can be listed first. If two or more diagnoses equally meet the definition of principal diagnosis, either condition may be sequenced first. If two principal diagnoses are contrasting or comparative in nature, either condition may be sequenced first. (b) If the original treatment plan was not carried out, the definition of principal diagnosis still applies, so the diagnosis after study is first. (c) If the reason for admission is as a complication of medical care, the complication code is sequenced first. Documentation must state that the condition is the result of a procedure or of medical care. In many instances, an additional code that specifically states the complication is assigned. (d) If a documented diagnosis at discharge is uncertain, probable, suspected, likely, questionable, possible, or still to be ruled out, the condition is coded as if it existed or was established (only for short-term care, acute care, long-term care, and psychiatric hospitals.)

6. E codes for external causes of disease and injuries are assigned as appropriate in the inpatient setting. E codes are often related to complications, such as abnormal reactions to surgery or a medical treatment.

7. For admission following medical observation, the principal diagnosis is the medical condition that leads to the hospital admission; for admission following postoperative observation, the principal diagnosis is that determined after study; and for admission after outpatient surgery, the admission circumstances determine the principal diagnosis.

8. Codes for additional diagnoses, other diagnoses, and secondary diagnoses are not sequenced first. These codes represent other conditions, comorbidities, or complications that affect the current inpatient stay. Abnormal findings from laboratory results, X-rays, pathology reports, and special diagnostic studies cannot be coded without the physician's documentation of their clinical significance. Conditions that are uncertain should also be reported.

9. Once ICD-9-CM codes have been assigned and sequenced, each code must be assigned an indicator that identifies whether the condition was present on admission (POA). The present on admission indicator represents whether the code was present. Therefore, for a combination code, the entire illness represented by that code must have been present on admission in order to assign an indicator of yes (Y). Other indicators are N (no) if the condition was not present on admission, U if the presence of the

condition on admission is unknown, and W if the presence of the condition on admission is clinically undetermined. Some codes, mostly V and E codes, are exempt from reporting the present on admission indicator, and the indicator is left blank.

10. The entire inpatient coding process requires review of complete documentation and abstraction of diagnoses and procedures from the patient record. The diagnoses are coded based on the ICD-9-CM *Official Guidelines*. Once all the conditions and procedures are coded, the codes are sequenced, listing one code as the principal diagnosis and one code as the principal procedure, and all other codes are considered additional. Then the present on admission indicators are assigned for both the principal and secondary diagnoses, including V codes and E codes in some circumstances.

Review Questions: Chapter 4

Match the key terms with their definitions.

a. UHDDS _____

b. POA _____

c. uncertain diagnosis _____

d. principal diagnosis _____

e. secondary diagnoses _____

f. comparative or contrasting conditions _____

g. abnormal findings _____

h. CC _____

i. query _____

j. IPPS _____

1. A comorbidity or complication

2. Two or more conditions documented as *either/or*

3. Condition that is probable, suspected, likely, questionable, possible, or still to be ruled out

4. Inpatient data set that includes the definitions of principal and other diagnoses

5. Test results that are outside of normal ranges

6. Condition that, after study, occasions the admission to the hospital

7. Other conditions in addition to the primary condition that are documented, coded, and reported

8. Coder's request for clarification of documentation from a physician

9. The Medicare payment system used for inpatients

10. A value assigned to each diagnosis code that represents whether the condition existed when the patient was admitted

Decide whether each statement is true or false.

1. The UHDDS definitions apply to outpatient visits only. **T or F**

2. The discharge summary is completed on patient admission to the hospital. **T or F**

3. The coder should review each lab test and X-ray in order to code the results. **T or F**

4. A patient is admitted for inguinal hernia repair. The hernia repair cannot be completed because of a new urinary tract infection. The principal diagnosis is inguinal hernia. **T or F**

5. All signs and symptoms should be coded. **T or F**

6. In the diagnostic statement "chest pain due to anxiety versus ulcer," the principal diagnosis is chest pain. **T or F**

7. An E code may be required to report complications of a medical or surgical treatment. **T or F**

8. The first thing a coder should do in assigning ICD-9-CM diagnosis and procedure codes is determine the present on admission indicator. **T or F**

9. A patient is admitted because of urinary incontinence. After admission, the patient develops chest pain. The POA indicator for the chest pain is W. **T or F**

10. The statements "postoperative hematoma" and "pain due to hip prosthesis" represent complications of surgery or medical care. **T or F**

Select the letter that best completes the statement or answers the question.

1. Which documents in the medical record should be reviewed when coding?
    a. physician progress notes
    b. physician orders
    c. discharge summary
    d. all of the above

2. The UHDDS definitions are integrated into which legislation?
    a. COBRA laws
    b. TEFRA legislation
    c. UACDS legislation
    d. HIPAA legislation

3. Under which circumstance may a sign or symptom be sequenced as the principal diagnosis?
    a. when the underlying condition is documented
    b. when the sign or symptom is followed by comparative or contrasting conditions
    c. when the underlying cause of the sign or symptom is unknown
    d. both b and c

4. Which of the following statements represents two or more diagnoses that equally meet the definition of principal diagnosis?
    a. Mary is admitted for COPD and heart failure.
    b. Joe is admitted for gallbladder removal; he also has diabetes.
    c. Max presents with hematuria due to renal calculi.
    d. Joan is admitted for thrombosis of her leg graft.

5. Which of the following statements represents an uncertain diagnosis?
    a. myocardial infarction ruled out
    b. possible myocardial infarction
    c. myocardial infarction
    d. chest pain due to myocardial infarction

6. Which of the following statements represents a complication of medical care?
    a. urinary retention
    b. possible urinary retention
    c. urinary retention due to prostate surgery
    d. urinary retention due to prostatic hypertrophy

7. Marlene presents with chest pain. After study, the attending physician determines that the chest pain is due to coronary artery disease. Marlene also has hypertension, which is treated with medication during her stay. What is the principal diagnosis?

    a. chest pain
    b. coronary artery disease
    c. hypertension
    d. either chest pain or coronary artery disease

8. Joe presents to the hospital for treatment of facial cellulitis. Joe has shortness of breath as well. The chest X-ray is positive for atelectasis, and the attending physician documents the diagnoses of facial cellulitis and bronchitis. Which of the following is coded?

    a. facial cellulitis, bronchitis, atelectasis
    b. facial cellulitis, atelectasis
    c. facial cellulitis, bronchitis
    d. bronchitis and atelectasis

9. What should the coder do when documentation supports positive test results, signs and symptoms of a disease, and treatment, but the physician does not document any corresponding diagnosis? (For example, the patient has low potassium levels on lab tests and is treated with supplemental potassium.)

    a. Code the abnormal test results.
    b. Query the physician to seek clarification.
    c. Do not code the lab results.
    d. Code the abnormal test results, and write the diagnosis on the chart.

10. Which of the following describes a condition that would have a present on admission indicator of W?

    a. After the second hospital day, the patient shows the physician that he has blood in the urine. He does not know when this started.
    b. After admission, the patient develops a drug rash.
    c. The patient presents with colon cancer and has a known history of hypertension.
    d. The code V10.03 is assigned.

1. Write the definition of *principal diagnosis*. _____

2. List the criteria that must be met in order to report a diagnosis or condition as secondary. _____
    _____

3. Explain the circumstances in which the present on admission indicator would be N. _____

4. What is the payment unit used for Medicare hospital inpatients? _____

5. If a patient is admitted from outpatient surgery due to a complication, what is the principal diagnosis? _____

6. Which terms identify the presence of comparative or contrasting conditions? _____

7. Which portion of the medical record contains documentation of the postoperative diagnosis? _____
    _____

8. Terms such as *hospital course* and *final diagnoses* are located in which report in the medical record? _____
    _____

9. When coding an inpatient medical record, the coder should review which document(s) to determine the reason a test was ordered? _____

10. What is the difference between *rule out* and *ruled out* as they pertain to inpatient coding? _____
    _____

BUILDING CODING SKILLS

Case 4.1

Anna Sandler
4/19/08

Inpatient Consultation

CHIEF COMPLAINT: Pressure and pain in the pelvic area.

SUBJECTIVE: This elderly female has had intermittent pain in the lower pelvis for several months. She was admitted to the hospital yesterday for congestive heart failure. She states that she is uncomfortable when she empties her bladder. She has occasional incontinence. She did have a GYN appointment next week for evaluation of her possible prolapsed uterus.

OBJECTIVE: Patient is alert and in no acute distress other than her breathing problems related to heart failure. She appears well hydrated. No CVA tenderness. Abdomen shows positive bowel sounds; no tenderness, no mass or distention. Pelvic exam shows a normal, atrophic vulva, normal for age. Speculum examination reveals a white atrophic vaginal mucosa. There is an apparent cystocele protruding into the vaginal vault. The uterus is not obviously prolapsed. Bimanual exam reveals no masses or tenderness.

ASSESSMENT: 1. Cystocele with questionable prolapsing uterus
2. Stress urinary incontinence

PLAN: The patient will follow up after admission for further GYN evaluation and possible surgery to include cystorrhaphy and/or uterine suspension.

---

1. What is the principal diagnosis?

2. What conditions should be reported as secondary diagnoses?

3. Assign all diagnosis codes and present on admission indicators.

Case 4.2

This four-year-old female presented to the hospital with six days of nasal congestion and cough, and she had been running intermittent low-grade fevers. Her cough has been getting worse with a decrease in energy level. Admission to the hospital was advised due to possible pneumonia. Evaluation in the hospital was positive for right lower lobe pneumonia with sputum culture positive for gram negative bacteria. The patient was also noted to be dehydrated, and IV fluids were ordered. The patient was treated with IV fluids and antibiotics and was discharged home after three hospital days.

DISCHARGE DIAGNOSES: Gram-negative bacterial pneumonia
Dehydration

---

1. What is the principal diagnosis?

2. What conditions should be reported as secondary diagnoses?

3. Assign all diagnosis codes and present on admission indicators.

Case 4.3

This patient was admitted with swelling, edema, and tenderness of her lower left leg for two weeks. This is so severe that the patient is now unable to walk, and admission was advised. Hospital course consisted of leg X-ray, and lower extremity Doppler exam. The swelling was the most troublesome to the patient. Evaluation during the hospitalization was negative, and the swelling was either due to varicose veins or vascular insufficiency.

DISCHARGE DIAGNOSIS: Pedal edema, could be secondary to varicose veins or peripheral vascular insufficiency

1. Which of the following guidelines applies to this case scenario?
   a. use of combination codes
   b. a symptom followed by comparative or contrasting conditions
   c. two comparative and contrasting conditions
   d. original treatment plan not carried out

2. What is the principal diagnosis?

3. Assign all diagnosis codes and present on admission indicators.

Case 4.4

Trent presented to the ED with weakness that had a sudden and extreme onset. Admission was advised for further workup. Trent has known congestive heart failure, coronary artery disease of his native vessels, and localized osteo-arthritis of his knees. During the hospitalization, he received medication for his heart failure and coronary artery disease. An X-ray of his knees confirmed the presence of osteoarthritis. Further evaluation of his weakness by ECG revealed sinus bradycardia. According to cardiac consultation and progress note documentation, the bradycardia was due to an adverse reaction to digoxin medication.

DISCHARGE DIAGNOSES: Bradycardia, probably digoxin induced, congestive heart failure, coronary artery disease, osteoarthritis of the knees, history of bladder cancer.

1. What was the cause of the bradycardia?
   a. an adverse reaction (medication was taken correctly)
   b. a poisoning of digoxin (medication was taken incorrectly)
   c. weakness
   d. coronary artery disease

2. Which column from the Table of Drugs and Chemicals would be used to assign the E code?

3. Would the symptom of weakness be coded? Why?

4. Assign all diagnosis codes and present on admission indicators for this patient's hospitalization.

Case 4.5

John has known chronic ulcerative colitis and now presents with abdominal pain experienced over the last several weeks. He had increasing cramps and decreasing appetite over the past week. He denies melena or blood in the stool. He also has known asthma, which is controlled with medications. John has no complaints of fever, chills, or other symptoms. Further evaluation is positive for chronic left-sided ulcerative colitis with acute exacerbation, which was treated with prednisone. John also is hyponatremic on admission, and this is attributed to his decreased appetite. On the second hospital day, John develops shortness of breath and wheezing. Physician documentation in the progress notes and orders support the presence of asthma exacerbation.

DISCHARGE DIAGNOSES: Chronic ulcerative colitis with acute exacerbation, hyponatremia, asthma exacerbation

1. Which condition is the principal diagnosis?

2. Would the symptoms of shortness of breath and abdominal pain be reported?

3. Assign the correct ICD-9-CM diagnosis codes and present on admission indicators for each code.

Case 4.6

Jamie was born in the hospital via cesarean section. He was noted to have nondescended testis and a heart murmur. Echocardiogram results were noted by the attending physician as possible pulmonary artery stenosis with ventricular septal defect. Before being transferred to Children's Hospital for further evaluation and treatment, Jamie developed newborn jaundice and was treated with phototherapy.

DISCHARGE DIAGNOSES: Single newborn, nondescended testis, possible pulmonary artery stenosis with ventricular septal defect, jaundice

1. Which conditions are considered secondary diagnoses?

2. What is the ICD-9-CM code for the principal diagnosis?

3. Assign ICD-9-CM codes and present on admission indicators for all secondary diagnoses.

Case 4.7

Marlin presented with lethargy, loss of appetite, and anuria. He was brought to the hospital by his caregiver, who states that the patient is not eating well, is drinking only small amounts, and is sleeping a lot. Condom catheter applied for urine collection yielded only 30 cc in 24 hours. Marlin also has cerebral palsy with spastic paraplegia and severe mental retardation. Urinalysis shows 10–20 WBCs/hpf, few bacteria, and few epithelial cells.

DISCHARGE DIAGNOSIS: Cystitis, possible glomerulonephritis, cerebral palsy with spastic paraplegia, severe mental retardation

1. Should the glomerulonephritis be coded? Why?

2. Assign the ICD-9-CM diagnosis codes and present on admission indicators for each code.

Case 4.8

HISTORY AND PHYSICAL   Kevin Wolters   4/29/08

CHIEF COMPLAINT: Patient is a 57-year-old white male with emphysema. He presents with complaints of increasing weakness with exertion. He also has some trouble with urinary frequency and dribbling over the past two to three years with some hesitancy and some generalized muscle aching and discomfort.

PAST MEDICAL HISTORY: Past history is significant for emphysema. He quit smoking about five months ago but continues to take occasional puff on a pipe to "loosen phlegm" in his lungs.

PHYSICAL EXAM: Thin, gaunt gentleman appearing older than his stated age; **LUNGS:** Barrel chested, flattened diaphragm, increased dullness to percussion, and poor air exchange without. **CARDIAC:** Distant heart sounds; no S3, S4, or murmur. **ABDOMEN:** benign. **RECTAL:** Digital exam reveals a 2+ symmetric, non-tender prostate, some fullness in the midline, but no nodules.

X-RAYS: PA and lateral chest films reveal flattened diaphragms, increased AP diameter, lung shapes consistent with severe emphysema.

IMPRESSION: 1. Obstructive uropathy due to prostatic hypertrophy
              2. Severe emphysema, exertional weakness, and dyspnea undoubtedly related to his lung disease

PLAN: Refer to Urology for prostatic complaints. Discussed treatment for his lungs.

---

1.   What are the signs and symptoms of this patient's urinary problems?

2.   What are the signs and symptoms of his respiratory problems?

3.   What is the principal diagnosis based only on this history and physical?

4.   Assign all codes for this visit.

Case 4.9

Arnie Stromcast   INPATIENT CHART NOTE   4/24/09

SUBJECTIVE: Arnold has left cheek numbness. He also had left arm numbness lasting about thirty minutes or so that started yesterday, and it has occurred two to three times today. There is no dizziness, headache, nausea, lightheadedness, or problem with balance or aphasia. The area involved is only the left cheek and left arm. No motor function problems. His hand had temporary paresthesia but had normal strength. He is a nonsmoker. Family history included stroke in his father; mother had multiple sclerosis.

OBJECTIVE: BP, 128/70 Temperature, 99. **HEENT:** Tympanic membranes are normal. Conjunctivae are normal; full EOMs. The area involved is only the left cheek. There is no discoloration or numbness of cheek presently. Facial expressions are normal. Pharynx appear normal. **NECK:** Cervical nodes are negative. Carotid bruits are bilaterally negative. **CHEST AND LUNGS:** Negative. Heart has normal S1 and S2. **ABDOMEN:** Normal. **EXTREMITIES AND NEUROLOGIC:** The extremities are warm. Neurologic is grossly intact. There is no particular numbness of the extremities. Reflexes are 1+ and symmetric. Romberg is normal. Gait is normal; no ataxia.

ASSESSMENT: Questionable transient ischemic attack

PLAN: CT scan and MRI. Begin aspirin.

---

1. What is the principal diagnosis?

2. Assign the principal diagnosis code.

3. What are the secondary diagnoses, if any?

4. Which inpatient coding rule applies here?

Case 4.10

Ross Elvers　　　　　INPATIENT CHART NOTE　　　　　4/26/09

SUBJECTIVE: This patient came in due to severe back pain. He is a pleasant hard-working man who has had continuous back pain since a motor vehicle accident two days ago. He was the passenger in a car that was involved in a head-on collision. He also has noticed some intermittent numbness on the left side of this face, left neck, and left arm.

HISTORY: The patient also has known stable angina due to coronary artery disease and gouty arthritis. These conditions require medications.

OBJECTIVE: Trunk range of motion is full. There is full forward extension, flexion, side bending, and rotation. He is not specifically tender at the impact site. No area of decreased sensation was detected in his face, neck, or arm on the left side.

LAB: Standing AP lateral thoracolumbar X-rays today show no change in vertebral height; there is some interval disc degeneration at the T11–T12 space shown by narrowing of the interspace. Most likely this is related to the accident.

ASSESSMENT: Traumatic fracture of the spine at T11–T12 secondary to motor vehicle accident.

PLAN: Continue pain management and consult with neurology service. Continue to treat chronic conditions with medication.

---

1. What is the principal diagnosis code?

2. What are the secondary diagnosis codes?

3. Assign the appropriate E code(s).

4. Assign the present on admission indicators for all codes.

USING CODING TERMS

Case 4.11

These questions are based on the coding principles covered in this chapter and on the disease processes defined in the chapter's pathophysiology refreshers. Assign all ICD-9-CM diagnoses codes to the following inpatient cases. Sequence the principal diagnosis first.

1. Unstable angina due to coronary artery disease of the native vessel.

2. Hypertensive cardiovascular disease with acute systolic congestive heart failure

3. Acute cerebral embolism with infarction and resulting spastic hemiplegia

4. Arteriosclerotic ulcer of the left toe and cellulitis of the foot

5. Infected vascular bypass graft of the left leg with cellulitis

6. Rheumatoid arthritis with lung involvement. Chest x-ray showed incidental finding of osteoarthritis of the spine

7. AIDS with Kaposi's sarcoma of the skin

8. Anaphylactic shock due to bee sting at home

9. Iron deficiency anemia versus acquired hemolytic anemia

10. Acquired coagulation defect. The patient was evaluated for mesenteric lymphadenitis.

Researching the Internet

1. Search the Internet for sample documents found in an inpatient medical record and study their content. See the following sites:

   Discharge summary:
   http://tulsa.ou.edu/im/Discharge%20Summary%20Guide.pdf

   Operative report:
   http://www.jointcommission.org/AccreditationPrograms/ Hospitals/Standards/FAQs/Management+of+Info/Patient+Specific +Information/Operative_Reports.htm and
   http://www.mt-resources.com/operative_report.htm

   History and physical exam:
   http://training.seer.cancer.gov/module_diagnostic/ unit01_history.html

   Laboratory tests:
   http://training.seer.cancer.gov/module_diagnostic/ unit02_lab_tests.html

   Pathology reports:
   http://training.seer.cancer.gov/module_diagnostic/ unit09_pathology.html

   Radiology reports:
   http://www.chestx-ray.com/Practice/RadiologyReport.html

2. Research Internet sites that discuss the Uniform Hospital Discharge Data Set. According to your reading, how can coders educate physicians regarding the definition of principal diagnosis and the importance of documentation? See http://www. fortherecordmag.com/archives/ftr_01222007p18.shtml and also the archives of health-information.advanceweb.com

3. Select a case from the Applying Your Knowledge questions. Research the Internet for more information about the medical condition of that patient and the health care abbreviations and terms documented. For example, for case 4.9 (transient ischemic attack, TIA), see http://www.americanheart.org/presenter. jhtml?identifier=4781.

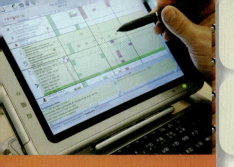

ICD-9-CM *Official Guidelines* (Section IV): Outpatient Coding and Reporting Guidelines

LEARNING OUTCOMES

After studying this chapter, you should be able to:

1. Define the outpatient settings to which Section IV of the *Official Guidelines* applies.
2. Define the term *first-listed diagnosis* as it relates to the outpatient setting.
3. Apply diagnosis code sequencing rules for a variety of outpatient encounters, such as outpatient procedures/ambulatory surgeries, observation stays, and encounters for circumstances other than disease or injury.
4. Compare and contrast coding for uncertain conditions in the outpatient and inpatient settings.
5. Understand how chronic diseases are coded in the outpatient setting.
6. Apply ICD-9-CM coding guidelines to outpatient visits when patients receive only diagnostic services, therapeutic services, or preoperative examinations.
7. Apply outpatient coding guidelines for emergency rooms visits.
8. Understand the coding and sequencing guidelines for routine outpatient prenatal visits.
9. Understand guidelines regarding reporting of additional diagnoses and E codes in the outpatient setting.
10. Based on diagnostic statements, correctly assign diagnosis codes for the outpatient setting.

Key Terms

Ambulatory Payment Classifications (APC)

ambulatory surgery

coexisting condition

contraindication

first-listed diagnosis

freestanding facility

history codes

hospital-based outpatient services

hospital-based facility

OPPS APC status indicators

outpatient procedure

Outpatient Prospective Payment System (OPPS)

Patient's Reason for Visit

therapeutic services

unscheduled outpatient visit

visit

Chapter Outline

Basic Coding Guidelines for Outpatient Settings
Selection of First-Listed Diagnosis
Reporting Secondary Diagnoses and E Codes in Outpatient Settings

The majority of health care patients' visits are to outpatient settings. In the typical year of 2003, there were more than 900 million physician office visits, nearly 100 million visits to hospital outpatient departments, and more than 113 million emergency department visits (National Ambulatory Medical Care Survey, 2005; National Hospital Ambulatory Medical Care Survey, Emergency Department Summary, 2005). These numbers compare with about 35 million inpatient hospital discharges, not counting normal newborns (National Hospital Discharge Data Survey, 2005). Correct outpatient diagnostic coding is vital for both professional and facility billing.

Assigning ICD-9-CM diagnosis codes in outpatient settings requires knowledge of specific guidelines. This chapter introduces information outpatient coders must understand, starting with the definition of an outpatient and moving to the guidelines that apply to each type of outpatient service. In many cases, these guidelines are different from inpatient guidelines. For example, the Uniform Hospital Discharge Data Set definition of *principal diagnosis* does not apply in the outpatient setting because the workup of the patient's condition typically occurs over a series of visits rather than during a single hospital stay.

These unique guidelines, though, build on the basic rules and conventions for assigning diagnosis codes using the ICD-9-CM code set, such as coding to the highest level of specificity. This chapter provides the details and guidelines for outpatient diagnostic coding.

Table 5.1 Section IV: Outpatient Coding Guidelines

These coding guidelines for outpatient diagnoses have been approved for use by hospitals/providers in coding and reporting hospital-based outpatient services and provider-based office visits.

Information about the use of certain abbreviations, punctuation, symbols, and other conventions used in the ICD-9-CM Tabular List (code numbers and titles) can be found in Section IA of these guidelines, under "Conventions Used in the Tabular List." Information about the correct sequence to use in finding a code is also described in Section I.

The terms *encounter* and *visit* are often used interchangeably in describing outpatient service contacts and, therefore, appear together in these guidelines without distinguishing one from the other.

Though the conventions and general guidelines apply to all settings, coding guidelines for outpatient and provider reporting of diagnoses will vary in a number of instances from those for inpatient diagnoses, recognizing that: The Uniform Hospital Discharge Data Set (UHDDS) definition of principal diagnosis applies only to inpatients in acute, short-term, and long-term care and psychiatric hospitals. Coding guidelines for inconclusive diagnoses (probable, suspected, rule out, etc.) were developed for inpatient reporting and do not apply to outpatients.

A. Selection of First-Listed Condition
In the outpatient setting, the term *first-listed diagnosis* is used in lieu of *principal diagnosis*.

In determining the first-listed diagnosis the coding conventions of ICD-9-CM as well as the general and disease-specific guidelines take precedence over the outpatient guidelines.

Diagnoses often are not established at the time of the initial encounter/visit. It may take two or more visits before the diagnosis is confirmed.

The most critical rule involves beginning the search for the correct code assignment through the Alphabetic Index. Never begin searching initially in the Tabular List as this will lead to coding errors.

1. Outpatient Surgery
When a patient presents for outpatient surgery, code the reason for the surgery as the first-listed diagnosis (reason for the encounter), even if the surgery is not performed due to a contraindication.

2. Observation Stay
When a patient is admitted for observation for a medical condition, assign a code for the medical condition as the first-listed diagnosis.

When a patient presents for outpatient surgery and develops complications requiring admission to observation, code the reason for the surgery as the first reported diagnosis (reason for the encounter), followed by codes for the complications as secondary diagnoses.

B. Codes from 001.0 through V84.8
The appropriate code or codes from 001.0 through V84.8 must be used to identify diagnoses, symptoms, conditions, problems, complaints, or other reason(s) for the encounter/visit.

C. Accurate Reporting of ICD-9-CM Diagnosis Codes
For accurate reporting of ICD-9-CM diagnosis codes, the documentation should describe the patient's condition, using terminology which includes specific diagnoses as well as symptoms, problems, or reasons for the encounter. There are ICD-9-CM codes to describe all of these.

D. Selection of Codes 001.0 through 999.9
The selection of codes 001.0 through 999.9 will frequently be used to describe the reason for the encounter. These codes are from the section of ICD-9-CM for the classification of diseases and injuries (e.g., infectious and parasitic diseases; neoplasms; symptoms, signs, and ill-defined conditions, etc.).

E. Codes That Describe Symptoms and Signs
Codes that describe symptoms and signs, as opposed to diagnoses, are acceptable for reporting purposes when a diagnosis has not been established (confirmed) by the provider. Chapter 16 of ICD-9-CM, Symptoms, Signs, and Ill-Defined Conditions (codes 780.0–799.9), contains many, but not all codes for symptoms.

F. Encounters for Circumstances Other Than a Disease or Injury
ICD-9-CM provides codes to deal with encounters for circumstances other than a disease or injury. The Supplementary Classification of Factors Influencing Health Status and Contact with Health Services (V01.0–V84.8) is provided to deal with occasions when circumstances other than a disease or injury are recorded as diagnoses or problems. See Section I.C.18 for information on V-codes.

G. Level of Detail in Coding
1. ICD-9-CM Codes with Three, Four, or Five Digits
ICD-9-CM is composed of codes with three, four, or five digits. Codes with three digits are included in ICD-9-CM as the heading of a category of codes that may be further subdivided by the use of fourth and/or fifth digits, which provide greater specificity.

Table 5.1 Section IV: Outpatient Coding Guidelines *(Continued)*

2. Use of full number of digits required for a code

A three-digit code is to be used only if it is not further subdivided. Where fourth-digit subcategories and/or fifth-digit subclassifications are provided, they must be assigned. A code is invalid if it has not been coded to the full number of digits required for that code. See also discussion under Section I.B.3., General Coding Guidelines, Level of Detail in Coding.

H. ICD-9-CM Code for the Diagnosis, Condition, Problem, or Other Reason for Encounter/Visit

List first the ICD-9-CM code for the diagnosis, condition, problem, or other reason for the encounter/visit shown in the medical record to be chiefly responsible for the services provided. List additional codes that describe any coexisting conditions. In some cases the first-listed diagnosis may be a symptom when a diagnosis has not been established (confirmed) by the physician.

I. Uncertain diagnosis

Do not code diagnoses documented as "probable," "suspected," "questionable," "rule out," or "working diagnosis" or other similar terms indicating uncertainty. Rather, code the conditions to the highest degree of certainty for that encounter/visit, such as symptoms, signs, abnormal test results, or other reason for the visit.

Please note: This differs from the coding practices used by short-term care, acute care, long-term care, and psychiatric hospitals.

J. Chronic Diseases

Chronic diseases treated on an ongoing basis may be coded and reported as many times as the patient receives treatment and care for the conditions.

K. Code All Documented Conditions That Coexist

Code all documented conditions that coexist at the time of the encounter/visit and that require or affect patient care, treatment, or management. Do not code conditions that were previously treated and no longer exist. However, history codes (V10–V19) may be used as secondary codes if the historical condition or family history has an impact on current care or influences treatment.

L. Patients Receiving Diagnostic Services Only

For patients receiving diagnostic services only during an encounter/visit, sequence first the diagnosis, condition, problem, or other reason for the encounter/visit shown in the medical record to be chiefly responsible for the outpatient services provided during the encounter/visit. Codes for other diagnoses (e.g., chronic conditions) may be sequenced as additional diagnoses.

For encounters for routine laboratory/radiology testing in the absence of any signs, symptoms, or associated diagnoses, assign V72.5 and V72.6. If routine testing is performed during the same encounter as a test to evaluate a sign, symptom, or diagnosis, it is appropriate to assign both the V code and the code describing the reason for the nonroutine test.

For outpatient encounters for diagnostic tests that have been interpreted by a physician when the final report is available at the time of coding, code any confirmed or definitive diagnoses documented in the interpretation. Do not code related signs and symptoms as additional diagnoses.

Please note: This differs from the coding practice in the hospital inpatient setting regarding abnormal findings on test results.

M. Patients Receiving Therapeutic Services Only

For patients receiving therapeutic services only during an encounter/visit, sequence first the diagnosis, condition, problem, or other reason for the encounter/visit shown in the medical record to be chiefly responsible for the outpatient services provided during the encounter/visit. Codes for other diagnoses (e.g., chronic conditions) may be sequenced as additional diagnoses.

The only exception to this rule is that when the primary reason for the admission/encounter is chemotherapy, radiation therapy, or rehabilitation, the appropriate V code for the service is listed first, and the diagnosis or problem for which the service is being performed is listed second.

N. Patients Receiving Preoperative Evaluations Only

For patients receiving preoperative evaluations only, sequence first a code from category V72.8, Other specified examinations, to describe the pre-op consultations. Assign a code for the condition to describe the reason for the surgery as an additional diagnosis. Code also any findings related to the pre-op evaluation.

O. Ambulatory Surgery

For ambulatory surgery, code the diagnosis for which the surgery was performed. If the postoperative diagnosis is known to be different from the preoperative diagnosis at the time the diagnosis is confirmed, select the postoperative diagnosis for coding, since it is the most definitive.

P. Routine Outpatient Prenatal Visits

For routine outpatient prenatal visits when no complications are present, codes V22.0, Supervision of normal first pregnancy, or V22.1, Supervision of other normal pregnancy, should be used as the principal diagnosis. These codes should not be used in conjunction with Chapter 11 codes.

Basic Coding Guidelines for Outpatient Settings

Table 5.1 presents the outpatient coding guidelines from Section IV of the *ICD-9-CM Official Guidelines for Coding and Reporting*. Like the inpatient guidelines, these outpatient guidelines have been developed and approved by the cooperating parties. They are approved for use by hospitals and physicians in coding and reporting diagnoses for both facility-based outpatient services and all physician services. ICD-9-CM conventions and general guidelines apply to assigning these codes, but outpatient diagnostic coding differs from inpatient coding in two ways:

1. The definition of *principal diagnosis*
2. The coding of inconclusive diagnoses

The definition of *principal diagnosis*—the diagnosis arrived at after study– in the Uniform Hospital Discharge Data Set (UHDDS) does not apply in any outpatient setting. In the outpatient setting, the study of a patient's disease is not always completed in a single visit. The patient may make many visits and have many tests and other procedures before the diagnosis is determined. Therefore, the phrase *after study*, which defines the principal diagnosis for a hospital stay, does not apply in outpatient settings.

Also, inconclusive conditions—those that are documented as possible, probable, or suspected—are not assigned codes in outpatient settings. Instead, the coder assigns codes to the condition, sign, or symptom that is known at the time of the visit. For example, if the documentation states "cough, rule out pneumonia," the outpatient coder codes the diagnosis of cough only; the inconclusive diagnosis of pneumonia is not be reported. The coding guidelines stating that codes for inconclusive diagnoses should be reported apply to inpatient reporting only.

DEFINITION OF OUTPATIENT VISIT

Since the Section IV *Official Guidelines* apply only to outpatient visits, it is important to understand that an outpatient **visit** or *encounter*—the terms are used interchangeably—is one in which the patient is not formally admitted to a facility. Such a visit occurs in an outpatient setting that is either a hospital-based or -owned facility, or a freestanding facility. **Hospital-based facility outpatient services** are the responsibility of the **hospital-based facility** and take place in emergency rooms, ambulatory surgery units, observation units, clinics (a distinct part of a facility or a separate facility used only to provide outpatient physician services), or specialized units such as physical therapy and cardiac catheterization units. A patient coming to the hospital for diagnostic testing who is not admitted is also considered a hospital outpatient.

On the other hand, a **freestanding facility** provides services to an outpatient who is not the responsibility of the hospital. Outpatient services that are not hospital based take place in such freestanding facilities as physician offices, public health clinics, and urgent care centers.

NOTE

The UHDDS rules underlying the choice of the principal diagnosis in the inpatient setting are covered in Chapter 4 of your program.

CODING ALERT

Do Not Use ICD-9-CM Volume 3 for Outpatient Coding

ICD-9-CM procedure codes (Volume 3) are used in the hospital inpatient setting only, so a reference to ICD-9-CM in this chapter is to diagnostic coding based on Volumes 1 and 2 only.

CODING ALERT

Do Not Code Inconclusive Conditions for Outpatients

Never code conditions that are documented as inconclusive in the outpatient setting.

NOTE

The 837I/UB-04 claim is introduced in Chapter 4 of your program.

This distinction is important primarily because of Medicare billing requirements; the two different settings are required to submit different types of health care claims. The facility (institutional) outpatient claim is the 837I electronic claim or its paper-based equivalent, the UB-04; nonhospital providers submit the 837P (P for professional) or its paper-based equivalent, the CMS-1500. The reason for different claim formats is that hospitals are paid for outpatient services based on different sets of fees, as explained in the Reimbursement Review on the Medicare Outpatient Prospective Payment system on pages 178–179.

The facility outpatient claim requires reporting the **Patient's Reason for Visit** for **unscheduled outpatient visits,** such as those to emergency rooms. The Patient's Reason for Visit code represents the ICD-9-CM diagnosis code for the condition the patient indicated as the reason for the visit to the provider, if applicable—in other words, the patient's chief complaint or reason for the encounter.

Checkpoint 5.1

Indicate whether the diagnostic coding for these patient services would follow the inpatient or outpatient guidelines.

1. A patient presents to the hospital emergency room for a wrist sprain and goes home. _____

2. A patient visits the physician's office for an annual physical. _____

3. A patient is transferred from the hospital to a nursing home after being in the hospital for three days. _____

4. A patient stays in the psychiatric unit at the hospital for thirty days. _____

5. A patient receives physical and occupational therapy in the outpatient clinic for two hours. _____

6. A patient has a cataract removed in the ambulatory surgery center. _____

7. A patient goes to the hospital laboratory to have blood drawn to determine cholesterol level. _____

8. A patient is admitted to the hospital and dies the same day. _____

9. A patient goes from the emergency room to the observation unit due to asthma. _____

10. A patient visits the orthopedic clinic to have a cast removed. _____

LEVEL OF DETAIL IN CODING

The ICD-9-CM *Official Guidelines* requiring the greatest detail in coding apply in the outpatient setting. The use of a fourth or fifth digit provides greater specificity regarding site, etiology, or manifestation of disease. Therefore, a three-digit code is used only when that category is not further subdivided. When a fourth-digit subcategory or a fifth-digit subclassification is provided, that code must be assigned. The coder should apply the highest number of digits available, no more and no fewer.

The Medicare Outpatient Prospective Payment System

Paralleling the Medicare Inpatient Prospective Payment System for hospital inpatient services is the Medicare **Outpatient Prospective Payment System (OPPS).** that is maintained by the Centers for Medicare and Medicaid Services (CMS). Under this system, rates are also established based on Medicare's analysis of similar outpatient medical services and procedures. The OPPS was implemented in 2000 to establish a prospective payment system for hospital-provided ambulatory procedures.

OPPS applies to covered hospital outpatient services furnished by all hospitals participating in the Medicare program. Certain services—physical, occupational, and speech therapies, orthotic and prosthetic devices, EPO for end-stage renal disease patients, durable medical equipment, ambulance, and clinical laboratory services are paid under other schedules, not OPPS.

Medicare analyzes and updates the reported costs for procedures and then groups them into **ambulatory payment classifications (APCs).** The APCs each categorize clinically similar services that require comparable resources. Each APC number is assigned a relative weight that is connected to a dollar amount that is payable. The payment rate for a new technology APC is set at the midpoint of its average cost.

Within each APC, integral items and services are packaged with the primary service and not paid

GUIDELINES FOR CODE SELECTION

The ICD-9-CM code set is used to identify the symptoms, problems, complaints, diagnoses, or other documented reasons for the outpatient visit. Reasons for outpatient visits include:

- Chest pain (symptom)
- Exposure to tuberculosis (problem)
- Palpitations (complaint)
- Diabetes mellitus (diagnosis)
- Well-child visit (other reason)

All these reasons for the encounter can be coded from ICD-9-CM, following the general process shown in Figure 5.1.

Symptoms and Signs Often, the reason for an outpatient encounter is that the patient presents with a sign or symptom. ICD-9-CM codes that describe symptoms and signs, rather than diagnoses, are acceptable for reporting purposes when the provider has not established (confirmed) a diagnosis. The code range 780.0 to 799.9 in ICD-9-CM Chapter 16, Symptoms, Signs, and Ill-Defined Conditions, contains most of the codes for symptoms; others are located in system-specific chapters. For example, the symptom of chest pain (786.50) is located in Chapter 16, whereas the symptom of hematuria (599.7) is located in Chapter 10, Genitourinary System,

Circumstances Other Than Disease or Injury (V Codes)
The Supplementary Classification of Factors Influencing Health Status and Contact with Health Services (V codes) provides codes to classify outpatient encounters for circumstances other than diseases and injuries. In such cases, the reason for the visit is not recorded as a diagnosis or a problem (sign or symptom). For example, when a patient visits the physician office for an annual vaccination or for cancer screening, the diagnosis code is a V code, not a code from the first seventeen chapters of ICD-9-CM.

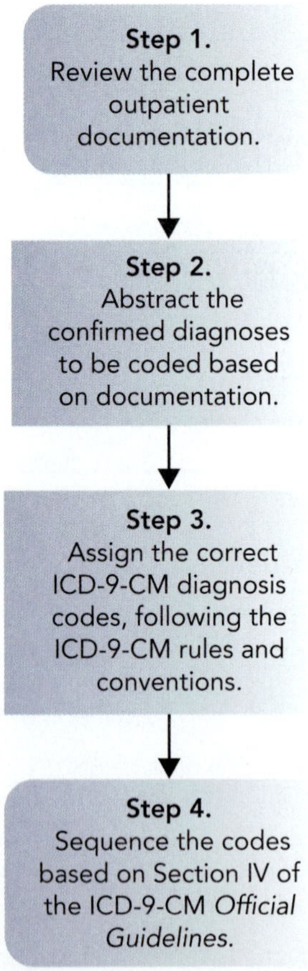

Step 1.
Review the complete outpatient documentation.

↓

Step 2.
Abstract the confirmed diagnoses to be coded based on documentation.

↓

Step 3.
Assign the correct ICD-9-CM diagnosis codes, following the ICD-9-CM rules and conventions.

↓

Step 4.
Sequence the codes based on Section IV of the ICD-9-CM *Official Guidelines.*

FIGURE 5.1
Outpatient Code Assignment Flow Chart

separately. Examples are routine supplies, anesthesia, recovery room, and most implants. A hospital may receive multiple APC payments for a single visit when multiple services have been performed during that encounter. Examples of separately paid services are

- Blood and blood products
- Surgical and diagnostic procedures
- Some observation services
- Clinic and emergency department visits
- Some drugs, biologicals, and radiopharmaceuticals

The APCs are based on the procedural coding system called CPT. CPT is the HIPAA-mandated procedure codes that are assigned by coders to each medical and surgical outpatient procedure. The CPT codes must be reported for outpatient services in place of ICD-9-CM Volume 3 codes. The ICD-9-CM Volume 1 and 2 codes, however, continue in the outpatient setting to show the medical necessity of the services provided during the encounter.

OPPS APC status indicators are used to show what procedures are paid under the system. For example, a status indicator of A means that the procedure is paid. But some procedures are typically provided *only* in the inpatient setting, and so CMS does not pay for them under the OPPS. CMS publishes a list of these procedures, to be followed for correct claim completion; these have a status indicator of C.

Checkpoint 5.2

Assign ICD-9-CM codes for the following reasons for outpatient encounters, keeping the outpatient coding guidelines in mind.

1. Shortness of breath and fever, with possible pneumonia _____
2. Screening for malignant neoplasm of the colon _____
3. Poliomyelitis vaccination _____
4. Nausea and vomiting _____
5. Well-child visit _____

Selection of First-Listed Diagnosis

In outpatient settings, diagnoses may not be established at the time of an encounter. For this reason, the definition of the principal diagnosis does not apply in the outpatient setting. In its place is the phrase **first-listed diagnosis.**

These are the outpatient coder's guidelines:

- If just one diagnosis is provided, the code for that condition is reported.
- If a definite condition is not documented, the code for the *patient's chief complaint* is reported.
- If multiple diagnoses can be assigned as the reasons for the encounter, all are coded.

In the last situation, which diagnosis should be listed first? This main sequencing guideline for all scheduled outpatient visits is that the first-listed diagnosis is the diagnosis, condition, problem, or other

CODING TIP

Outpatient First-Listed Diagnosis

The guidelines for the first-listed diagnosis differ from coding guidelines for the principal diagnosis used in short-term care, acute care, long-term care, and psychiatric hospitals.

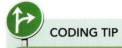

CODING TIP

Correct Coding Process

Remember that the Alphabetic Index drives the code assignment, with verification of codes completed using the Tabular List.

reason for the encounter that is shown in the medical record to be chiefly responsible for the services provided.

Note, however, that the general ICD-9-CM rules and conventions, as well as the general and disease-specific guidelines, take precedence over the outpatient guidelines. For example, conventions such as "code first underlying disease" determine the sequencing of codes for certain diagnoses, overriding an instruction in Section IV of the *Official Guidelines*.

There are specific guidelines for determining the first-listed diagnosis codes for the following outpatient cases:

- Outpatient procedures and ambulatory surgery
- Observation services
- Diagnostic services
- Therapeutic services
- Preoperative evaluations
- Routine outpatient prenatal care
- Uncertain diagnoses
- Emergency department visits

OUTPATIENT PROCEDURES AND AMBULATORY SURGERY

Typically, an **outpatient procedure** is one that is completed outside of an operating room. Examples are an outpatient colonoscopy or an outpatient cardiac catheterization. These procedures are typically performed in a specialty unit specifically designed to perform them, such a cardiac catheterization laboratory, rather than in an operating room. **Ambulatory surgery** (also called *same-day surgery)* patients typically receive services in an operating room or surgical suite. For example, cataract extraction, rotator cuff repair, and laparoscopic cholecystectomy are considered ambulatory surgeries. Note that the Reimbursement Review below shows a claim for an outpatient procedure, a commonly billed service in the OP facility setting.

COMPLIANCE GUIDELINE

POA Not Required for Outpatient Claims

By definition, POA stands for *present on admission* and so would not be reported on health care claims for outpatient services, for which a patient is not admitted.

Reimbursement Review

Outpatient Claims: Hospital (Institutional) Billing

When the patient receives outpatient care at a facility or facility-owned place of service, the facility is permitted to bill for its part of the services (the room, supplies, and so on), and the physician bills for his or her part (the surgical or other procedural work). For example, a patient visit to a same-day surgery unit for a procedure on a bunion is billed by two entities, (1) the hospital outpatient facility and (2) the physician.

The UB-04 claim on the facing page illustrates the facility bill for this outpatient procedure. Note that in place of ICD-9-CM Volume 3 codes for procedures, the CPT codes are in use, following the rules of outpatient coding. Some facilities continue to also report

an ICD-9-CM Volume 3 procedure code, although this is not required by Medicare or most private payers.

Note also that a "modifier"—an attached number that explains a special aspect of the code—is shown with the CPT code. This modifier, -RT, stands for "right" and indicates that the procedure was done on the right foot. This same CPT code and modifier would be used on the 837P (for professional) electronic claim or its paper equivalent, the CMS-1500, that is sent by the physician who did the surgery.

On claims, the ICD-9-CM diagnoses codes are critical for demonstrating the medical necessity of the services. In the example, the procedure code (CPT 28292) would be reviewed in light of the reported ICD-9-CM code (727.1) to assess the reasonableness of the claim.

¹ GRACE MEMORIAL HOSPITAL 100 MAIN STREET TULSA, OK 74101 9182367007	²		3a PAT. CNTL # 2229176 b. MED. REC. # 6003020 5 FED. TAX NO. 07-1282340	6 STATEMENT COVERS PERIOD FROM 032709 THROUGH 032709	4 TYPE OF BILL 0131

8 PATIENT NAME a b KRAUSS, WANETA	9 PATIENT ADDRESS a 216 LATIMER AVE. b TULSA	c OK d 74102	e

10 BIRTHDATE	11 SEX	12 DATE	ADMISSION 13 HR	14 TYPE	15 SRC	16 DHR	17 STAT	CONDITION CODES 18 19 20 21 22 23 24 25 26 27 28	29 ACDT STATE	30
11021957	F	032709	07	3	1	10	01			

31 OCCURRENCE CODE DATE	32 OCCURRENCE CODE DATE	33 OCCURRENCE CODE DATE	34 OCCURRENCE CODE DATE	35 OCCURRENCE SPAN CODE FROM THROUGH	36 OCCURRENCE SPAN CODE FROM THROUGH	37

38	39 CODE VALUE CODES AMOUNT	40 CODE VALUE CODES AMOUNT	41 CODE VALUE CODES AMOUNT
	a b c d		

42 REV. CD.	43 DESCRIPTION	44 HCPCS / RATE / HIPPS CODE	45 SERV. DATE	46 SERV. UNITS	47 TOTAL CHARGES	48 NON-COVERED CHARGES	49
1 0250	PHARMACY		032709	1	9 78		
2 0270	MED-SUR SUPPLIES		032709	1	32 83		
3 0360	OR SERVICES	28292RT	032709	1	410 00		
4 0370	ANESTHESIA		032709	1	40 00		
5 0710	RECOVERY ROOM		032709	1	210 00		
23 0001	PAGE 1 OF 1	CREATION DATE 033109	TOTALS ➡		702 61		

50 PAYER NAME	51 HEALTH PLAN ID	52 REL INFO	53 ASG BEN	54 PRIOR PAYMENTS	55 EST. AMOUNT DUE	56 NPI 2788000665	
A BCBS	10643	Y	Y			57 080	
B						OTHER	
C						PRV ID	

58 INSURED'S NAME	59 P.REL	60 INSURED'S UNIQUE ID	61 GROUP NAME	62 INSURANCE GROUP NO.
A KRAUSS, WANETA	18	TRS-145987	TRADITIONAL	C/107
B				
C				

63 TREATMENT AUTHORIZATION CODES	64 DOCUMENT CONTROL NUMBER	65 EMPLOYER NAME
A		TARGET, INC.
B		
C		

66 DX 7271 Y	A B C D E F G H	68
	I J K L M N O P Q	

69 ADMIT DX	70 PATIENT REASON DX a b c	71 PPS CODE	72 ECI a b c	73

74 PRINCIPAL PROCEDURE CODE DATE	a. OTHER PROCEDURE CODE DATE	b. OTHER PROCEDURE CODE DATE	75	76 ATTENDING NPI 4098120056 QUAL G2 99965X
				LAST VIVALDI FIRST JAMES
c. OTHER PROCEDURE CODE DATE	d. OTHER PROCEDURE CODE DATE	e. OTHER PROCEDURE CODE DATE		77 OPERATING NPI 4098120056 QUAL G2 99965X
				LAST VIVALDI FIRST JAMES
80 REMARKS	81CC a b3 282N00000X			78 OTHER NPI QUAL
	b			LAST FIRST
	c			79 OTHER NPI QUAL
	d			LAST FIRST

UB-04 CMS-1450 APPROVED OMB NO. 0938-0997 **NUBC** National Uniform Billing Committee THE CERTIFICATIONS ON THE REVERSE APPLY TO THIS BILL AND ARE MADE A PART HEREOF.

When a patient presents for an outpatient procedure or ambulatory surgery, the reason for the procedure or surgery is the first-listed diagnosis, unless the preoperative diagnosis and the postoperative diagnosis are different. If this happens, then the postoperative diagnosis is coded, since it is the most definitive.

> **EXAMPLE** A patient with a preoperative diagnosis of skin lesion of the cheek (709.9) undergoes an excision. After the lesion is excised and analyzed by the pathologist, documentation confirms basal cell carcinoma of the check (173.3). Only the basal cell carcinoma is reported.

If the procedure is not actually performed because of a **contraindication,** the reason for the visit code is still listed first, followed by a code to represent surgery cancelled (a code from the range V64.1–V64.3).

For instance, for a senile cataract removal, the first-listed diagnosis is senile cataract (366.10). If the surgery is cancelled, that first-listed diagnosis is still reported as the reason for surgery, and an additional code for surgery cancelled (chosen from the range V64.1–V64.3) is also reported to reflect the reason for cancellation. If the surgery is cancelled due to a contraindication (V64.1), a code for the contraindication would also be reported.

> **EXAMPLE** The patient presented to outpatient surgery for a coronary angiogram due to unstable angina. After conscious sedation, the staff noted a cardiac arrhythmia. The surgery was cancelled because of the contraindication of cardiac arrhythmia. The first-listed diagnosis is the unstable angina (411.1). Additional codes are reported for surgery not done due to contraindication (V64.1) and cardiac arrhythmia (427.9).

Figure 5.2 explains the code assignment process.

OBSERVATION STAY

Some circumstances surrounding outpatient observation care affect the first-listed diagnosis. A patient may begin care in one outpatient area and receive services in another outpatient area. For example, a patient may present to the Ambulatory Surgery department for a scheduled procedure and then require observation services.

Guidelines state that when a patient is admitted for observation due to a medical condition, a code for that medical condition should be the first-listed diagnosis. For example, a patient may be placed in the observation unit because of acute asthma exacerbation (493.92). Also, when a patient presents for an outpatient procedure or ambulatory surgery and then develops complications that require admission to observation, the reason for the surgery code is the first reported diagnosis. This reason for encounter code is followed by the codes for the complications as secondary diagnoses.

> **EXAMPLE** The patient presents to ambulatory surgery for elective laparoscopic gallbladder removal due to cholelithiasis. After surgery, he develops chest pain that requires observation services. First-listed diagnosis: cholelithiasis (574.20); secondary diagnosis: chest pain (786.50).

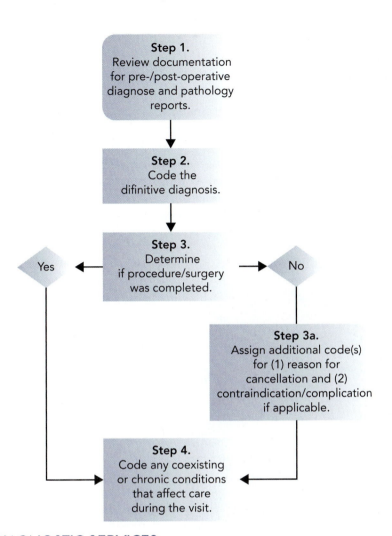

Step 1.
Review documentation
for pre-/post-operative
diagnose and pathology
reports.

Step 2.
Code the
difinitive diagnosis.

Step 3.
Determine
if procedure/surgery
was completed.

Yes

No

Step 3a.
Assign additional code(s)
for (1) reason for
cancellation and (2)
contraindication/complication
if applicable.

Step 4.
Code any coexisting
or chronic conditions
that affect care
during the visit.

DIAGNOSTIC SERVICES

Patients may present for procedures that assist the physician in making a diagnosis. Such diagnostic services include many types of laboratory/pathology tests, radiology procedures, and diagnostic surgical procedures like biopsies. Patients may or may not have signs or symptoms relating to the conditions for which they are tested. For diagnostic services, the first-listed code is the diagnosis, condition, problem, or other reason shown in the medical record to be chiefly responsible for the diagnostic services provided during the encounter. Codes for other diagnoses may be sequenced as additional codes.

As noted in the *Official Guidelines*, codes from category V72 represent special investigations and examinations (I.C, 18.d, paragraph 13). Specifically, codes V72.5 and V72.6 may be used as the first-listed diagnoses when the reason for the visit is routine testing in the absence of signs, symptoms, and associated diagnoses. If routine testing is performed at the same time as a test to evaluate a sign, symptom, or medical condition, both the V code and the code describing the reason for the nonroutine test are reported.

EXAMPLE A patient presents to the outpatient radiology center for a routine chest X-ray. Code V72.5 is reported.

EXAMPLE A patient presents for a routine chest X-ray and also undergoes an MRI of the back due to back pain. Both the code for routine exam (V72.5) and the code for back pain (724.5) are reported.

COMPLIANCE GUIDELINE

Medicare Requires a Diagnosis

When a physician orders hospital-based outpatient services for a Medicare patient, Medicare's Conditions of Participation for Hospitals require a diagnosis for the outpatient tests and procedures. If the diagnosis is not documented and signed by the ordering physician, the hospital staff contacts the physician for clarification.

The Musculoskeletal System

The musculoskeletal system includes the muscles, bones, and joints. Diseases of the musculoskeletal system can occur as a result of congenital abnormalities, injuries, or inflammation, or they may be due to or associated with another disease or condition, such as arthritis associated with diabetes. Several categories of musculoskeletal diseases are *arthritis* or *arthropathy, injuries* (most commonly, fractures, sprains, and strains), and *degenerative* disorders (for example, muscular dystrophy and osteoporosis). In addition, other musculoskeletal diseases are hereditary (such as gout), and some are conditions of unknown origin (such as a ganglion).

Arthritis or Arthropathy

Arthritis is the leading cause of disability in the United States. The terms *arthritis* and *arthropathy* refer to any inflammation of a joint. It can be *acute* (severe, sudden, and of short duration), *chronic* (occurring over a long period of time), or *subacute* (somewhere between acute and chronic; often with no symptoms). Arthritis is often *due to* or *associated with* another condition. Some examples are diabetes, gout,

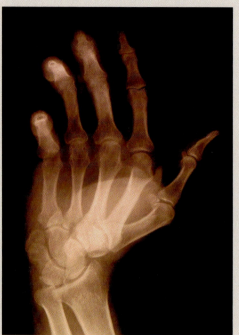

An X-ray of an arthritic hand.

rheumatoid arthritis, and infection. Arthritis is subclassified as site-specified (such as in the hand or shoulder), as site-unspecified, or as occurring in multiple sites. *Rheumatoid arthritis* is a chronic autoimmune disorder and is sometimes confused with the term *rheumatism*, a general term for any condition causing discomfort to the muscles, joints, tendons, or bones.

Injuries

Injuries to the musculoskeletal system are a common result of many traumas, such as automobile accidents. Falls are a leading cause of death for people over sixty-five, usually because of the resulting hip fractures. Other fractures occur over all age groups. A dislocation can occur with or without a fracture and may be further classified as *simple, recurrent, open, closed, subluxation* (partial dislocation), or *articulation* (occurring at a joint). Less traumatic injuries, such as *carpal tunnel syndrome, sprains,* and *strains,* can require medical intervention, including pain management.

Fractures occur at specific or at multiple sites. They are categorized in various ways. First, they are classified based on how they occur: *adduction* (an abnormal turning inward), *abduction* (an abnormal turning outward),

---

> ⚠️ **CODING CAUTION**
>
> **Coding Laboratory and Radiology Services**
>
> Code signs and symptoms for laboratory services that are read by a technician but not confirmed by a physician. Code the definitive diagnosis of the physician-radiologist who reads the films for radiology services.

The information that is available to the coder affects the assignment of ICD-9-CM codes for diagnostic services. If diagnostic tests have been interpreted by a physician and a definitive diagnosis has been documented in the final report, the coder may report the condition that has been confirmed. If the final report is not available, the coder may code only for the condition that is certain at the point of coding.

EXAMPLE A patient presents to the hospital outpatient department for a scheduled echocardiogram because of a heart murmur. The results support the presence of mitral valve prolapse based on physician interpretation.

If this fact is available at the time of coding, the first-listed diagnosis is mitral valve prolapse (424.0). However, if results are not

avulsion (a forcible tearing away), *compression* (resulting from a force pressing on a bone), *crush* (caused by a crushing blow), *dislocation* (movement away from a normal location), *oblique* (at an angle), *separation* (with displacement), *open* (with broken skin), or *closed* (covered by unbroken skin). Closed fractures and open fractures are further divided into types. Some closed fractures are *greenstick* (broken on one side only) and *Colles* (characteristic deformity of the wrist as a result of a fracture). Examples of open fractures are *compound* (with the broken bone protruding through the skin) and *missile* (caused by something projected into the bone from an outside source).

Strains and sprains occur in joints, ligaments, muscles, and tendons. Strains result from overstretching or overexertion. Sprains result from overstraining or wrenching (without fracturing).

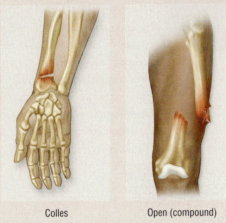

| Colles | Open (compound) |

A Colles fracture and an open fracture.

Degenerative Diseases

Some degenerative diseases are genetically linked (such as Duchenne's muscular dystrophy and some forms of osteoporosis). Others result from other diseases or conditions or have unknown causes. *Osteoporosis* (loss of bone density) is usually categorized as *generalized* (occurring in various parts of the body). It is further divided into types, such as *postmenopausal* and *drug-induced*. *Osteopenia* is a reduction in bone mass that is less severe than osteoporosis. Fractures due to bone disorders such as osteoporosis are *pathologic* fractures rather than traumatic ones.

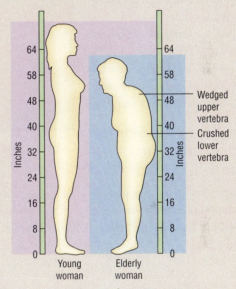

The progression of osteoporosis and its effect on posture.

available at the time of coding, the diagnosis of heart murmur is reported.

EXAMPLE A patient presents to the ED after sustaining an injury to her wrist, and her wrist is X-rayed. Before the radiologist interprets the X-ray, the patient is discharged from the ED with the diagnosis of wrist sprain. After review of the X-ray results, the radiologist documents a diagnosis of wrist fracture.

In this case, the ED coder must assign the code for the condition that was known at the time of discharge. Therefore, the facility reports wrist sprain (842.00). Note that many visits—both outpatient and inpatient–involve conditions of the musculoskeletal system, so coders must be familiar with the key terms and processes that are documented. The basics are presented in the Pathophysiology Refresher above.

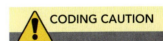

CODING CAUTION

Do Not Code Signs and Symptoms Related to a Definitive Diagnosis

Related signs and symptom should not be coded as additional diagnoses when the underlying condition is documented in physician-interpreted diagnostic test results.

The Integumentary System

The skin shows symptoms of many diseases, such as measles. Often, such diseases are caused by infections or parasites that do not originate in the integumentary system. Some viruses cause disorders of the integumentary system—for example, *warts*.

Diseases of the skin can be categorized as *infections of the skin and subcutaneous tissue, other inflammations and conditions,* and *diseases of specific parts of the integumentary system*. In addition, there are other categories, such as *ulcers* and *urticaria*, that list particular types of skin disorders. Skin lesions may be indicative of a disease process (such as cancer) or may be from an injury (such as burns and scars).

Infections of the Skin and Subcutaneous Tissue

Infections of the skin—especially a *carbuncle* (localized inflammation of subcutaneous tissue with suppuration), a *furuncle* (pus-filled staphylococcal infection), and *cellulitis*

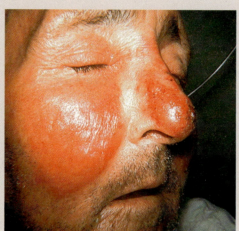

Cellulitis of the face.

(inflammation of the deep subcutaneous tissue)—are usually categorized by location (for example, cellulitis of the face or trunk or a carbuncle of the neck). Localized bacterial infections of tissue are called *abscesses*. Abscesses occur in the skin or elsewhere in the body. *Impetigo* is an infectious skin disease categorized as *bullous* (having blisters), *circinate* (having circular lesions), *contagiosa* (acutely contagious), *neonatorum* (occurring in a newborn), or *simplex* (common and localized). *Pyoderma* is a bacterial skin infection with pus-filled lesions.

Other Skin Inflammations and Conditions

Dermatitis is a general term for inflammation of the skin. It is categorized in many ways, including *allergic* (caused by an allergy), *contact* (caused by contact with something, such as a chemical), *occupational* (work-related), or *venenata* (caused by something poisonous). Dermatitis is further subdivided into specific causes or locations, such as *due to solar radiation* (sunburn) or *diaper rash* (located

---

CODING ALERTS

Inpatient Versus Outpatient Diagnostic Services

Coding from physician-interpreted diagnostic services applies in the outpatient setting only. This differs from the coding practice regarding abnormal findings on test results in hospital inpatient settings.

Code After Pathology Results

Best practice is to code after the pathology results are reposted.

THERAPEUTIC SERVICES

Patients may receive only **therapeutic services**—the many procedures done to treat conditions and injuries—during outpatient visits. For these visits, as for diagnostic services, the ICD-9-CM code reported first represents the diagnosis, condition, problem, or other reason for the encounter that the medical record shows is chiefly responsible for the outpatient services provided.

EXAMPLE A patient presents to the dermatologist's office to have a skin lesion removed from her back. Following removal, the lesion is sent for analysis. The pathology report is returned with a diagnosis of squamous cell carcinoma of the back. The first-listed diagnosis is squamous cell carcinoma of the back (173.3).

In this example, the therapeutic service of skin lesion removal was performed. By waiting for pathologist's interpretation, the coder was able to report the diagnosis of squamous cell carcinoma. If the diagnosis was reported before receipt of the pathology findings, the diagnosis of skin lesion would have been reported (709.9). There is no code to report admission for surgery; rather, the reason

underneath a diaper). It can also be due to allergies (as to food or drugs). Some serious types of dermatitis, such as *pemphigus* (a chronic, blistering skin disease), can be fatal. *Erythematous conditions* (redness of the skin) may be *generalized* or may be due to specific conditions such as *lupus* or *rosacea. Psoriasis,* a chronic inflammatory skin disease, is sometimes associated with inflammatory arthritis.

Pruritus is a general term for itching. Pruritus may be categorized according to location, such as the ear or genital area. *Eczema* is an inflammation of the skin accompanied by itching. It is classified in a number of ways, including *acute, chronic,* and *allergic.* It may also be categorized by location (*external ear*), cause (*contact*), or other (*infantile*).

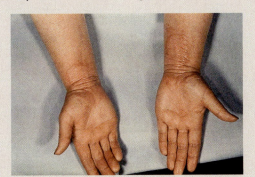
Dermatitis of the hands.

Skin Diseases of Specific Parts of the Integumentary System

Diseases of the hair commonly include *alopecia* (baldness) and *hirsutism* (excess hair growth). Diseases of the nails include *ingrowing nail, onychia* (inflammation of the matrix of the nail), and *paronychia* (inflammation of the skin bordering the nail). The *sebaceous glands* (oil-producing glands) are responsible for *acne,* the most common variety of which is *acne vulgaris.* They also produce *sebaceous cysts, seborrhea* (an excessive discharge of sebum), and *seborrheic dermatitis* or *dandruff.* Disorders of the sweat glands include *anhidrosis* (lack of the ability to sweat), *prickly heat* (a rash produced by sweating), and *hyperhidrosis* (overproduction of sweat).

Ulcers and Urticaria

Ulcers of the skin can occur on any part of the body. *Decubitus ulcers, pressure sores,* or *bedsores* are divided into stages depending on the severity of the skin damage. In stage 1, the skin is warm, firm, or stretched. The other stages indicate the depth of the ulcer; in the last stage the ulcer has reached the bone. Other skin ulcers are categorized by location, such as *ulcer of ankle.* These ulcers may be caused by other underlying conditions, such as arteriosclerosis.

Urticaria are commonly known as *hives.* They are categorized by type (for example, *giant*) or cause (for example, *allergic urticaria*). They may also be *unspecified.*

for the therapeutic services should be reported first. Note that many skin conditions are the target of both outpatient and inpatient visits. Coders must be familiar with the major problems associated with the integumentary system, as discussed in the Pathophysiology Refresher above.

There is an exception to the general rule for sequencing therapeutic services. When the primary reason for the visit is a specialized service of chemotherapy, radiation therapy, renal dialysis, or rehabilitation, the appropriate V code for the service is the first-listed ICD-9-CM code. The diagnosis or problem for which the patient requires the specialized service is reported as a secondary diagnosis.

> **EXAMPLE** A patient presents to the hospital outpatient unit for chemotherapy. He is receiving chemotherapy for his sigmoid colon cancer. The first-listed diagnosis is encounter for chemotherapy (V58.11), followed by the code for sigmoid colon cancer (153.3).

In this example, the patient presented for a specialized service (chemotherapy). Therefore, the V code is sequenced first, followed by the code that represents the problem (sigmoid colon cancer) that required the service.

COMPLIANCE GUIDELINE

High-Volume Medicare Outpatient Procedures

High-volume Medicare-reimbursed outpatient procedures include cataract extraction with intraocular lens (IOL) implant, upper gastrointestinal (GI) endoscopy, and colonoscopy.

PREOPERATIVE EVALUATIONS

Some outpatient encounters occur because the patient needs to be cleared for surgery. When a patient receives a preoperative evaluation only, a code from category V72.8 (other specified examinations) is sequenced first. The coder also assigns additional codes that describe the reason for the surgery along with any findings related to the preoperative evaluation.

> **EXAMPLE** A patient presents to his primary doctor for a preoperative evaluation prior to his scheduled inguinal hernia repair. During the exam, the physician also notes hypertension. The first-listed code is V72.83 (preoperative examination), followed by the secondary diagnosis codes of 550.90 (inguinal hernia) and 401.9 (hypertension).

ROUTINE OUTPATIENT PRENATAL VISITS

The guideline for prenatal visits applies when the prenatal visit occurs and the patient has no complications present. Under these circumstances, the first-listed diagnosis is reported using either V22.0, supervision of normal first pregnancy, or V22.1, supervision of other normal pregnancy. If the patient has a complication of pregnancy, the codes V22.0 or V22.1 are not reported.

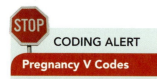

> **EXAMPLE** A female patient presents to her obstetrician's practice for her routine fourth-month prenatal visit. This is her first pregnancy. The first-listed diagnosis is V22.0.

> **EXAMPLE** A female patient who is pregnant with twins presents to her obstetrician's practice for a prenatal visit. The first-listed diagnosis is 651.03 (twin pregnancy, antepartum).

UNCERTAIN DIAGNOSES

In the outpatient setting, uncertain diagnoses—those documented as probable, suspected, questionable, rule out, or working diagnoses—are not coded. Only the condition to the highest degree of certainty for that visit is assigned a code. The code may represent a symptom, sign, abnormal test result, or other reason for the visit.

> **EXAMPLE** A patient presents to the physician office due to cough and fever. The physician documents possible pneumonia. Only the sign (fever, code 780.6) and symptom (cough, code 786.2) are coded because the diagnosis of pneumonia is uncertain.

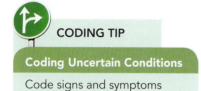

CODING TIP

Coding Uncertain Conditions

Code signs and symptoms unless a physician confirms a definitive diagnosis.

> **EXAMPLE** A patient visits a cardiologist for the first time because of chest pain. Prior to the visit, the patient also had an abnormal electrocardiogram (ECG). After the visit, the cardiologist sends the patient for additional testing and documents the diagnosis as chest pain, rule out coronary artery disease, and abnormal ECG. The codes reported are 786.50 (chest pain) and 794.31 (abnormal ECG). The code for coronary artery disease is not reported because this condition was not confirmed at the time of the office visit.

EMERGENCY DEPARTMENT VISITS

The guidelines for first-listed diagnosis apply to ED visits. The first-listed diagnosis is the diagnosis, condition, problem, or other reason for the encounter shown in the medical record to be chiefly responsible for the services provided. However, ED visits are unscheduled outpatient visits.

Thus, the *Patient's Reason for Visit* codes should also be reported. Reporting both diagnosis codes provides a clear picture of the presenting problems and of the medical necessity of the procedures that were performed.

For example, a patient may present with chest pain (patient's reason for visit), yet after ECG, chest X-ray, and laboratory studies, the ED physician documents the diagnosis of gastroesophageal reflux. If the patient's reason for visit of chest pain (786.50) is not reported, the medical necessity of the ECG, chest X-ray, and blood work may not be met.

Thus the first-listed diagnosis code in this case is the physician's diagnosis after evaluation and management of the patient Also reported are the patient's reason for visit diagnosis codes to reflect the condition of the patient.

Note that the reporting of the chest pain does *not* contradict previous explanations, for two reasons. First, chest pain is not integral to gastroesophageal reflux, which is often diagnosed in patients who do not have that symptom. Second, without the listing of chest pain, the medical necessity of the ED visit is not correctly presented to the third-party payer.

> **EXAMPLE** A patient with chest pain and diaphoresis presents to the ED, yet after ED physician evaluation, the first-listed diagnosis is anxiety attack. The reason for visit codes would be chest pain and diaphoresis, yet the first-listed diagnosis would be anxiety.

Checkpoint 5.3

Code the diagnoses for the following outpatient case scenarios. Sequence the first-listed diagnosis code first, using the outpatient coding guidelines.

1. A patient presents to the outpatient department for a cholecystogram with the diagnosis of possible gallstone. The radiologist interprets the cholecystogram and lists the diagnosis of cholelithiasis. _____

2. At the time of the visit to the physician office, the documented diagnosis is epigastric pain, nausea, and vomiting, rule out gastritis. _____

3. A patient presents to the outpatient department for a screening colonoscopy for malignancy. The colonoscopy reveals the finding of external hemorrhoids. _____

4. A patient has had shoulder pain for months. His physician documents the presence of a chronic rotator cuff tear. The patient now presents for rotator cuff repair in the hospital ambulatory surgery department. After surgery, he requires observation services for chest pain. _____

5. A patient presents at the emergency department with chest pain, fever, and shortness of breath. After ECG, blood work, and chest X-ray, the ED physician documents the diagnosis of pneumonia.

   a. Which code or codes are reported as the reason for the visit? _____

   b. Which code is reported as the first-listed condition? _____

6. A patient presents for coronary angiography due to an abnormal stress test. After the angiography, postoperative documentation supports coronary artery disease of the native coronary arteries. What is the code for the first-listed condition? _____

(Continued)

7. A patient visits her obstetrician for prenatal care. This is her second pregnancy with no complications. _____

8. A patient presents to the hospital outpatient department for a barium enema due to lower gastrointestinal bleeding. The barium enema is normal. _____

9. A patient presents to the hospital outpatient laboratory for thyroid hormone levels. The patient has hypothyroidism, according to the physician order. _____

10. A patient presents to the outpatient surgery center for treatment of ureteral calculus. After preparation for surgery, he develops noncardiac chest pain, which requires the cancellation of surgery. _____

CODING TIP

Chronic/Coexisting Conditions

Code all documented conditions that also exist at the time of the visit and require or affect patient care, treatment, or management.

Reporting Secondary Diagnoses and E Codes in Outpatient Settings

Not only must the coder identify the first-listed diagnosis for an outpatient visit, but other diagnoses (secondary diagnoses) should also be reported as appropriate. The following guidelines cover which chronic conditions and **coexisting conditions** should be reported in addition to the first-listed diagnosis. Information about E codes, also required to be reported if applicable in the hospital facility outpatient setting, is also provided.

CHRONIC DISEASES

Chronic diseases, such as hypertension, diabetes mellitus, and osteoarthritis, persist over a long period of time. Chronic diseases that are treated on an ongoing basis may be coded and reported as many times as the patient receives treatment and care for them. For example, a patient may require regular fingerstick glucose testing for diabetes mellitus, so diabetes mellitus would be reported for each visit in which the patient receives the treatment or care.

COEXISTING CONDITIONS

All documented conditions that coexist at the time of the encounter *and* require or affect patient care, treatment, or management should be coded. Conditions that were previously treated and no longer exist or no longer affect treatment or patient management should not be reported. **History codes** (codes V10–V19) may be used as secondary codes if the historical condition or family history has an effect on current care or influences treatment. For example, a patient may present for a screening colonoscopy (V76.51) due to family history of colon cancer (V176.0). In this case, the secondary diagnosis of family history of colon cancer affects the patient care as this is the reason for the patient screening. Other V codes reflecting a patient's status may also be reported if that status has an effect on current care or influences treatment.

> **EXAMPLES**
> - A patient visits his doctor for evaluation of cough, fever, and shortness of breath. He has previously been diagnosed with hypertension and diabetes. During the office visit, his blood pressure is measured, and his fingerstick glucose is normal. The diagnosis of acute

Table 5.2 Comparison of Coding, billing, and Payment Methods

	Hospital Inpatient	Hospital Outpatient	All Physician Services
Diagnosis Codes	ICD-9-CM	ICD-9-CM	ICD-9-CM
E Codes	Required	Required	Optional
Procedure Codes	ICD-9-CM	CPT/HCPCS ICD-9-CM (optional)	CPT/HCPCS
Billing Form	837I or UB-04	837I or UB-04	837P or CMS-1500
Medicare Payment	MS-DRG	Ambulatory Payment Classification (APC)	Resource-Based Relative Value Scale (RBRVS)

bronchitis is documented along with the diagnoses of diabetes mellitus (Type II) and hypertension. The codes reported are 466.0 (acute bronchitis), 250.00 (diabetes mellitus), and 401.9 (hypertension).

- A patient presents to her doctor for evaluation of ear pain. She was treated for urinary tract infection three months earlier. Physician documentation for this visit states the diagnoses as acute otitis media and history of urinary tract infection (UTI). The correct code is 382.9 (acute otitis media) only. The code for UTI is not reported because the UTI is no longer present and does not affect the current care and treatment.

E CODES

As in inpatient ICD-9-CM coding, in the facility outpatient setting E codes are required; Table 5.2 summarizes this requirement as well as providing an overview of the differences in procedural coding, billing, and Medicare payment system for hospital inpatient, hospital outpatient, and physician services.

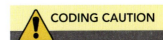

CODING CAUTION

Previously Treated Conditions

Do not code conditions that were previously treated and no longer exist or that do not affect the patient's care.

NOTE

The RBRVS payment system and the 837P/CMS-1500 billling format are covered in Chapter 6 of your program.

Checkpoint 5.4

Assign the appropriate ICD-9-CM diagnosis codes for the following case scenarios.

1. A patient presents to the hospital for chemotherapy to treat his colon cancer. He has a family history of colon cancer. _____

2. A patient presents to the emergency department and is evaluated and treated for acute cystitis. She is also currently being treated for gout. _____

3. A patient sees the dermatologist due to a painful scar. Complete exam also reveals rosacea and seborrheic keratosis. Medications are ordered, and the patient is to return for excision of the scar the next week. _____

4. A patient visits his physician every three months due to his diabetic peripheral neuropathy. During each visit, his other chronic conditions are evaluated. These include osteoarthritis of the lumbar spine, benign hypertension, and asthma. _____

5. A patient sees her cardiologist for preoperative clearance for laparoscopic vaginal hysterectomy due to menometrorrhagia. The cardiologist examines the patient and clears her for surgery. Documentation supports the presence of native coronary artery disease and congestive heart failure as cardiac conditions. _____

1. An outpatient is a patient who is not admitted to an acute care facility, short-term hospital or any other inpatient setting; outpatients receive care from a facility and typically return home the same day. Examples of outpatient encounters are visits to the Emergency Room, Ambulatory Surgery Center, Urgent Care Center, physician office, Radiology Center, Physical Therapist, etc.

2. The first-listed diagnosis refers to the diagnosis code that is listed first for outpatient encounters. The rules and definition for principal diagnosis for the inpatient setting *do not apply to outpatients*. In the outpatient setting, the first-listed diagnosis is the reason for the visit, whether it is for a medical condition, screening, well-visit, routine testing, immunization, or other reason. Uncertain or ill-defined conditions—those that are possible, probable, or suspected—are never coded; instead, the signs and symptoms are the basis for code assignment, because often at the time of the encounter a definitive diagnosis is not yet known.

3. Sequencing of the first-listed diagnosis in the outpatient setting encompasses many different scenarios. An ambulatory surgery visit or an observation stay often has a documented diagnosis of a disease or injury. Other outpatient visits require the use of V codes for reporting the first-listed diagnosis.

4. Conditions that are documented as uncertain (possible, probable, suspected or rule out) should not be reported in the outpatient setting. Instead, the condition(s) reported should be the condition that is known at the time of the visit. Remember that the opposite is true in the inpatient setting, where these uncertain conditions are coded.

5. Chronic or coexisting conditions are also reported for outpatient encounters when these conditions impact the outpatient care. These conditions may impact outpatient care in many ways, such as requiring evaluation or treatment in addition to the first-listed diagnosis (i.e. diabetes, hypertension) or these conditions may influence care (i.e. family history of cancer). Conditions which are not currently present or do not impact care should not be reported.

6. When a patient presents as an outpatient and receives special diagnostic services, therapeutic services, pre-operative exams, or routine prenatal visits, a V code may be the principal diagnosis. In these cases a special diagnostic service such as a screening colonoscopy (V76.51) may be the first listed diagnosis. Other examples include a well-child visit (V20.2) or routine chest x-ray (V72.5).

7. Emergency Department (ED) visits are considered unscheduled visits. Therefore, the reason for visit codes on the UB-04 should be reported in addition to the first-listed diagnosis.

8. The first listed diagnosis reported for routine prenatal visits should be either V22.0 or V22.1. These codes are used only if there are NO pregnancy complications. In the presence of

complications, the complication codes would be assigned and codes V22.0 or V22.1 would not be reported.

9. Additional diagnoses (i.e., secondary diagnoses) should be reported in the outpatient setting. These additional diagnoses represent chronic diseases and coexisting conditions that require or affect patient care treatment or management. E codes are also reported as applicable.

10. The outpatient coding process is similar to inpatient coding, with two major exceptions: The selection of the first-listed diagnosis is based on the reason for the patient's visit, and ill-defined or uncertain conditions are not coded— instead, signs and symptoms are assigned codes.

Review Questions: Chapter 5

Match the key terms with their definitions.

a. OPPS APC status indicator _____

b. ambulatory surgery _____

c. APC _____

d. Patient's Reason for Visit _____

e. visit _____

f. freestanding facility _____

g. history codes _____

h. therapeutic services _____

i. coexisting condition _____

j. hospital-based facility _____

1. The payment group in the Medicare Outpatient Prospective Payment System

2. A facility not owned or managed by a hospital

3. Codes representing factors influencing health status

4. A facility owned or managed by a hospital

5. ICD-9-CM code assigned to the patient's chief complaint

6. Letter connected to a code that shows whether the procedure is payable under the OPPS APC system

7. Services performed for an outpatient in an operating room

8. Another term for encounter

9. Special services provided to treat a patient

10. Documented conditions that are present at the time of the visit that require or affect patient care, treatment, or management

Decide whether each statement is true or false.

1. The UHDDS definition of *principal diagnosis* applies to the outpatient setting. **T or F**

2. An interpretation by a radiologist of an X-ray can be used to assign an outpatient-setting diagnosis code. **T or F**

3. Signs and symptoms codes are never used in the outpatient setting. **T or F**

4. A patient goes to get a lab test. This is considered an outpatient visit. **T or F**

5. A visit to an observation unit in a hospital is always reported with a V code as the first-listed diagnosis. **T or F**

6. In the outpatient diagnostic statement "chest pain due to suspected coronary artery disease," the principal diagnosis is coronary artery disease. **T or F**

7. Chronic conditions that have no bearing on the current outpatient visit should not be reported. **T or F**

8. When a patient presents to the physician office for an annual physical, the diagnosis code of V70.0 is reported. **T or F**

9. There is no difference in coding rules for a hospital inpatient visit and for an hospital outpatient visit. **T or F**

10. The hospital completes a 837P or CMS-1500 form when providing services to a patient who undergoes an upper endoscopy in the outpatient unit. **T or F**

Select the letter that best completes the statement or answers the question.

1. Which of the following is considered an outpatient visit?
   a. a two-day stay in a hospital intensive care unit
   b. a hospital emergency room visit
   c. a baby born in the hospital
   d. all of the above

2. Which is an example of a diagnostic procedure in the outpatient setting?
   a. colonoscopy
   b. appendectomy
   c. cataract extraction
   d. coronary stent insertion

3. Which of the following represents a symptom?
   a. pneumonia
   b. syncope
   c. diverticulosis
   d. peripheral vascular disease

4. Which of the following would be reported for a patient visit to the physician office with a diagnosis of abdominal pain probably due to gastroenteritis?
   a. 789.00
   b. 558.9
   c. 008.8, 789.00
   d. 558.9, 789.00

5. A patient presents to the ambulatory surgery unit for inguinal hernia repair. After surgery, the patient goes to observation for postoperative pain due to surgery. Which codes would be reported?
   a. 550.90 338.18, 780.96.
   b. 550.91, 780.96
   c. 550.90, 338.18
   d. 780.96, 550.90

6. A patient presents to the physician office for an influenza vaccination. Which of the following would be reported?
   a. V06.6
   b. V06.6, V04.81
   c. V70.0, V06.6
   d. V06.6

7. For the visit in question 6, which coding system would be used to report the flu shot?
   a. ICD-9-CM
   b. CPT
   c. UB-04
   d. APC

8. What should the coder do when documentation in an ED record states injury to the wrist, rule out fracture, and the radiologist interprets the X-ray with the diagnosis of wrist fracture?
   a. Code only the wrist fracture.
   b. Query the ED physician to seek clarification.
   c. Code the wrist injury.
   d. Report both the wrist injury and wrist fracture codes.

9. If a patient who is pregnant with her third child presents to the physician office for a routine obstetrical exam in the twentieth week, what code would be reported?
   a. V22.0
   b. V22.1
   c. 650
   d. none of the above

10. If a child presents to the pediatrician's office for evaluation of obesity and the physician documents obesity with body mass index of the ninetieth percentile, which codes would be reported?
   a. 278.00, V85.4
   b. 278.01, V85.4
   c. 278.01, V85.53
   d. 278.00, V85.53

1. Define first-listed diagnosis. _____

2. Differentiate between the 837I/UB-04 and 837P/CMS-1500 billing forms as they pertain to outpatient services. _____

3. Can chronic conditions be reported in the outpatient setting? Explain. _____
_____

4. Differentiate between hospital-based and freestanding facilities. _____
_____

5. Under which circumstances can an uncertain diagnosis (a possible, probable, or suspected condition) be reported in the outpatient setting? _____

6. If a Medicare patient is seen at the hospital clinic for chemotherapy services to treat breast cancer, which code or codes would be reported by the hospital? Which payment system would be used to determine hospital Medicare payment? _____

7. A patient undergoes a colonoscopy for follow-up of colon surgery due to a history of colon cancer. No cancer is found during the exam. Which codes would be reported? (Hint: Look for *follow-up, surgery*).
_____

8. A patient presents for a preoperative examination by his family practice physician prior to outpatient surgery for an old bucket handle tear of the medial meniscus. This patient has COPD and hypertension, which are followed by this physician. Which code or codes would be reported for the preoperative exam? _____

9. This patient presents to the ED in cardiac arrest and is resuscitated and intubated prior to admission as an inpatient. What diagnosis code or codes would be reported by the emergency department physician? _____

10. A patient visits the dermatologist due to a mole on her back. The dermatologist removes the mole. The pathology report states the diagnosis of compound nevus of the back. What diagnosis code or codes would be reported? _____

BUILDING CODING SKILLS

Case 5.1

> Chris Anderson
> 4/2/08
>
> **SUBJECTIVE:** Suture removal. Patient returns for removal of stitches placed about eight days ago.
>
> **OBJECTIVE:** Wound at lateral aspect of the left eye looks well healed. The 5-0 nylon sutures were removed without difficulty.
>
> **ASSESSMENT:** Laceration, healed.
>
> **PLAN:** I advised him to use vitamin E for scar prophylaxis.

1. Would the laceration be coded even though it is healed?

2. Assign the appropriate diagnosis code or codes for this removal of sutures visit.

Case 5.2

> Amy Becker
> 4/2/08
>
> **CHIEF COMPLAINT:** Routine health maintenance.
>
> **HISTORY:** Patient is a 62-year-old married, white female who was here for a yearly exam. She states she has been feeling well and has no specific concerns.
>
> **SOCIAL HISTORY:** She is currently not working out of the home.
>
> **PAST MEDICAL HISTORY: ALLERGIC TO PENICILLIN.** Nonsmoker. Denies any major illnesses. She had a hysterectomy.
>
> **FAMILY HISTORY:** Maternal grandmother had diabetes; mother had breast cancer.
>
> **REVIEW OF SYSTEMS:** No complaints.
>
> **PHYSICAL EXAMINATION: HEENT:** Negative. **NECK:** Thyroid is normal. **HEART, LUNGS, AND ABDOMEN:** Within normal limits. **BREASTS:** Soft bilaterally; no masses are felt. She states she does monthly breast self-exams. **PELVIC EXAM:** External genitalia are normal. Vagina is clear. Cervix is negative. Pap smear was not done.
>
> **IMPRESSION:** Normal annual routine examination.
>
> **PLAN:** Return to see our practice one year, sooner PRN.

1. Assign the diagnosis code or codes for this routine visit.

2. If a paper billing form were used to bill services provided, which form would it be?

Case 5.3

Matthew Wittman
4/2/08

SUBJECTIVE: Matthew comes in today for a 15-month examination. Mother has no complaints. He is feeding himself and putting two words together when talking. He is actually in motor and growth development at the 22-month level.

Most recent hemoglobin was 12.3. He is above the 95th percentile for height; at the 95th percentile for weight.

OBJECTIVE: Head is normal. Ears are clear. Eyes are clear. Pupils are equal, round, and reactive to light and accommodation. Throat is clear. Nose is clear. Neck has good range of motion without nodes. Lungs are clear. Heart has regular heart rate and rhythm. Abdomen is soft without masses. Testicles are descended. Back is straight. He is walking well. He has good muscle tone. See developmental forms in chart.

ASSESSMENT: Normal well-baby examination.

PLAN: Continue present diet and advance as tolerated. Immunizations were given; see form. Recheck in three months, sooner if needed.

---

1. Assign the diagnosis code or codes for this visit.

Case 5.4

Richard Glassman
4/5/08

SUBJECTIVE: Patient is a 15-year-old male with increasing acne over the last one to two years. He has been using soap and Oxy-10 without improvement.

OBJECTIVE: On the face, neck, and upper back, there is mild to moderate acne. Lesions consist of macules, papules, mild oily comedos, and an occasional nodule, but no cysts or boils.

ASSESSMENT: Acne vulgaris, mild to moderate.

PLAN: Oxy-10. Retin A 0.25 mg cream applied sparingly to facial lessons. E.E.S. 400 mg TID x 3 months. Recheck in three months.

---

1. Assign the diagnosis code or codes for this visit.

Case 5.5

Stephanie Miller
4/19/08

SUBJECTIVE: Patient is complaining of vaginal discharge without pruritus. She had unprotected sexual activity but has had no known exposure to AIDS. She wants testing to be sure that she is not infected. She has had vaginosis in the past.

OBJECTIVE: ABDOMEN: Soft and nontender. **PELVIC EXAMINATION:** BSU are normal. Vagina is normal. There is scanty discharge. Wet prep is negative for Trichomonas, yeast, and bacteria. Cervical cultures were done for GC, chlamydia, and herpes. Bimanual examination shows uterus to be normal. There is a small mass about 3–4 cm on the left side, which is tender. This could be a tubo-ovarian abscess, or she could have residual pelvic inflammatory disease.

ASSESSMENT: Pelvis mass; rule out PID or sexually transmitted disease.

PLAN: 1. HIV testing was done.
      2. Doxycycline 100 mg BID x 10 days.
      3. Will await test results.
      4. Methods for prevention of STDs as well as contraception were discussed.

---

1. Which diagnosis would the provider list first?

2. Assign the diagnosis code or codes for this visit.

Case 5.6

Sarah Thompson
4/17/08

SUBJECTIVE: Patient presents with mild urinary frequency and some lower abdominal pelvic cramping. She has no vaginal symptoms.

OBJECTIVE: There is mild suprapubic tenderness; otherwise, exam is unremarkable.

LAB: Urinalysis is negative, but quite dilute from increased fluid intake.

ASSESSMENT: Suspect urethritis.

PLAN: Placed on three-day course of Macrodantin. Recheck if not improving.

1. What are the patient's signs and symptoms?

2. Assign the diagnosis code or codes for this visit.

Case 5.7

Ronald Blackwood
4/15/08

SUBJECTIVE: Ronald is here for diabetes recheck. He rarely checks his blood for sugar—has done so only two to three times in the last two weeks—and he is noncompliant with medical therapy. It has been in the 140s two hours postprandial. He is off all medications for blood pressure and diabetes. He lost 6 pounds before the last visit and lost another 7½ pounds by today's visit due to dietary changes. He does get some heartburn. Two months ago he had chest pain for a half a day with some shortness of breath, which totally resolved. By history, it really doesn't sound cardiac. Discussed multiple related aspects of diabetes monitoring and lifestyle interventions.

OBJECTIVE: BP, 140/98. Comfortable. Funduscopic eye exam is negative. Nose, mouth, neck, and thyroid are negative. Heart is without murmurs. Good pulses. Lungs are clear. Obese abdomen; otherwise unremarkable. Feet are clear.

LAB: ECG shows nonspecific ST changes only. Random Accu-Chek, 267; hemoglobin A1c, pending. Chest X-ray is unremarkable.

ASSESSMENT: 1. Type II diabetes, suboptimal control
2. Overweight but improving
3. Elevated blood pressure
4. Noncompliance with medical therapy
5. Chest pain

PLAN: Await hemoglobin A1c. Redouble efforts in diabetes monitoring. Recheck blood pressure in two weeks. The patient was instructed to call immediately if chest pain returns, but no further workup at this time. Patient to return in three months when we will check kidney status again, earlier PRN.

1. What was this patient's reason for the encounter?

2. What additional chronic problems are documented?

3. Assign the ICD-9-CM diagnosis code or codes for this visit.

Case 5.8

Brian Norwich
4/15/08

Outpatient X-Ray

INDICATION: Abdominal pain and constipation.

X-RAY: Flat plate of abdomen. Patient complains of abdominal pain and constipation.

INTERPRETATION: The intestinal gas pattern is normal. There is no evidence for obstruction or ileus. No masses or abnormal calcifications identified at this time.

ASSESSMENT: Normal flat plate of abdomen.

---

1.   Assign the appropriate diagnosis code or codes.

Case 5.9

Mitchell Herberger
4/10/08

Office Note

SUBJECTIVE: Patient presents with general malaise, fever to 103, and cough occasionally productive of blood-tinged sputum for one day. He denies nausea or vomiting.

OBJECTIVE: Temperature, 102.7. He is in mild distress. **HEENT:** Nares are patent. Pharynx is markedly erythematous without exudates or ulcerations. **NECK:** Supple with shotty anterior cervical lymphadenopathy bilaterally. **CHEST:** Examination reveals rare scattered rhonchi, which clear with cough.

LAB: Chest X-ray reveals no discrete infiltrates.

ASSESSMENT: 1. Viral syndrome
                             2. Acute bronchitis with bronchospasm

PLAN: Push fluids. Tylenol for fever. E.E.S. 400 mg QID x 10 days. Robitussin DM PRN cough. Follow up three days if symptoms do not improve.

---

1.   What are the patient's signs and symptoms?

2.   Assign the diagnosis code or codes for this office visit.

Case 5.10

Jillian Underwood
4/22/08

Office Note

SUBJECTIVE: This 5-year-old female suffered an injury to her left hand in when she fell off playground equipment at home. She was splinted by her parents and brought to the office for evaluation.

OBJECTIVE: She has diffuse swelling and ecchymosis over the dorsal aspect of her right hand in the third and fourth metatarsal midshaft region. She has full range of motion of her fingers. Neurosensory exam is normal. Peripheral circulation is normal.

X-ray shows evidence of nondisplaced oblique shaft fractures of metacarpals without involvement of the articulating structures.

ASSESSMENT: Right third and fourth metacarpal fractures, nondisplaced.

PLAN: She was taped for immobilization and placed in a short-arm splint. She will keep it elevated and use Advil or aspirin. Follow-up will be with Orthopedics in the next three to seven days.

---

1. Which diagnosis code or codes would be reported for this office visit?

2. Would E codes be reported? If yes, assign those codes.

USING CODING TERMS

Case 5.11

These questions are based on the coding principles covered in this chapter and on the disease processes defined in the chapter's Pathophysiology Refreshers. Assign all ICD-9-CM diagnoses codes to the following outpatient vists (do not report procedure codes). Remember to assign E codes if the patient is a hospital outpatient.

1. Knee pain due to possible fractured patella

2. Osteoarthritis of the lumbar spine

3. Admitted to observation for acute post-operative abdominal pain (left lower quadrant) following inguinal hernia repair.

4. Aftercare for healing traumatic fracture of the hip

5. Pruritus, possible poison ivy

6. Carbuncle of the buttock

7. Stage II decubitus ulcers of the hip and heel

8. Seen at the Hospital Emergency Room: Fracture of the navicular bone with foreign body (BB), accidentally shot by a BB gun at home.

9. Seen at the Physician Office: Second degree burn of back of the hand. The patient spilled boiling water at the restaurant where he works.

10. Seen at the Hospital Based Ambulatory Surgery Center: Laceration of the finger with tendon involvement. The patient cut his finger on a kitchen knife at work.

Researching the Internet

1. Access the Uniform Ambulatory Care Data Set (UACDS) list of data elements using the website below. Determine which data elements pertain to diagnosis and procedure coding. Background: The UACDS is a core data set for ambulatory encounters developed by NCVHS in late 1970's and revised by NCVHS and Department of Health and Human Services. This data set has never officially promulgated but is widely disseminated.
http://mchneighborhood.ichp.edu/eds/901027902.html

2. Discover the details of undergoing ambulatory surgery by linking to:
http://www.emedicinehealth.com/outpatient_surgery/article_em.htm

At this website, read an article about Ambulatory Surgery preparation, the surgery itself, after surgery and the synonyms used to reference ambulatory surgery. Identify the documents found in the medical record of an ambulatory surgery patient.

3. An Emergency Room (ER) or Emergency Department (ED) visit is one type of outpatient visit. Access the link below to determine how many ER visits there are per year. What is one of the primary reasons for these visits? Imagine coding each visit! http://www.livescience.com/strangenews/050526_emergency_visits.html

4. Many outpatient tests or procedures are covered by Medicare. Policies called National and Local Coverage Determinations (NCD and LCD's) are available at the Medicare website. These policies provide information for specific tests or services regarding whether or not these services are paid by insurance. Also listed are the ICD-9-CM diagnosis codes that indicate medical necessity for a particular test or service. Access the Medicare Coverage Database website: http://cms.hhs.gov/mcd/overview.asp.

   Click Reports and then click LMRP/LCD Service Indication Report. Complete the screen by entering 93000 in Step 1 (the CPT code for an electrocardiogram) on 394.0 in Step 2 (the ICD-9-CM code for mitral stenosis).

   Click Submit Report. What are the results for a location you select? Can you locate the list of ICD-9-CM codes that support medical necessity in the report? (Note: Click the report number and accept the CPT license agreement if it appears. Then scroll down through the body of the report.)

5. There are numerous Internet newsletters available for many outpatient settings. Access the website of HCPRO (see link below) and look at the latest information for the physician office setting. Sign up to receive the free e-mail newsletter if available. http://www.hcpro.com

Introduction to CPT

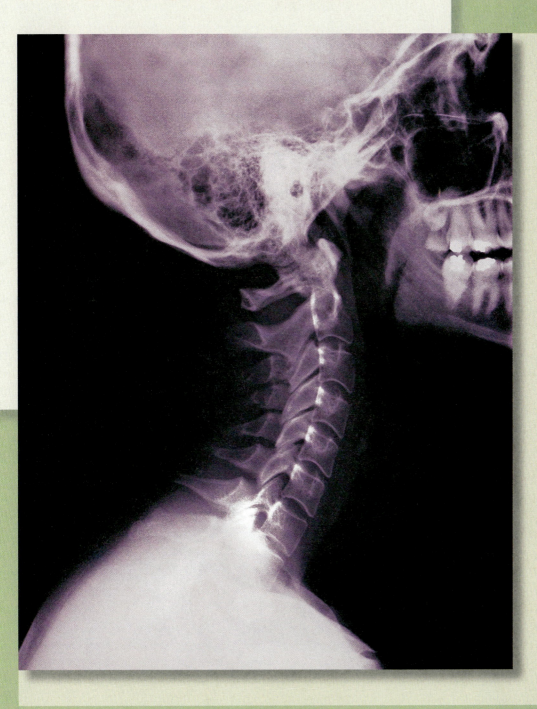

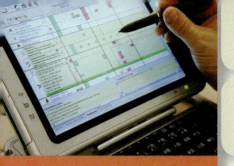

CPT Basics

LEARNING OUTCOMES

After studying this chapter, you should be able to:

1. Explain the purpose of the CPT code set.

2. Identify the medical settings in which CPT is used.

3. Describe the content and organization of CPT.

4. Identify the meaning of the symbols, format, and punctuation used in CPT.

5. Discuss the purpose and use of CPT modifiers, distinguishing among CPT professional, HCPCS, and facility modifiers.

6. Recognize the importance of using current codes, and discuss ways to stay up to date.

7. Compare and contrast the ICD-9-CM and CPT code sets.

8. List CPT coding resources and references.

9. Recognize when an unlisted code is needed, and identify the purpose and parts of a special report.

10. List the nine steps to properly assign CPT codes and to correctly select and append modifiers.

Key Terms

add-on code

837P

American Medical Association

capitation

Category I code

Category II code

Category III code

CMS-1500

code range

crosswalk

Current Procedural Terminology (CPT)

CPT modifier

descriptor

facility modifier

fee-for-service

fee schedule

HCPCS Level I code

HCPCS Level II code

HCPCS modifier

Healthcare Common Procedure Coding System (HCPCS)

modifier

payment-for-performance (P4P)

postoperative period

primary procedure

professional services

resource-based relative value system (RBRVS)

secondary procedure

section guidelines

semicolon

separate procedure

significant procedure

special report

surgical package

unlisted code

usual fee

Chapter Outline

History and Purpose of CPT

Organization and Content of CPT

CPT Punctuation and Symbols

Modifiers

CPT Updates

A Review: ICD-9-CM and CPT Comparison

How to Assign CPT Codes and Modifiers

CPT Coding Resources

Procedural coding is a process that must be performed by both physicians and facilities to receive proper reimbursement for services provided. Procedure codes are used by physicians and facilities to account for outpatient medical, surgical, and diagnostic services. These codes, along with diagnosis codes that show why the procedures were medically necessary, are reported on health care claims that are submitted to payers for reimbursement.

Procedure codes are also used to establish guidelines for the delivery of the best possible care for patients. Medical researchers track various treatment plans for patients with similar diagnoses and evaluate patient outcomes. The results are shared with physicians and payers so that best practices can be implemented. For example, this type of analysis has shown that a patient who has had a heart attack can reduce the risk of another attack by taking a class of drugs called beta blockers.

In practices, physicians, medical coders, or outside companies assign procedure codes. Some practices employ coders who also perform the billing function and are titled medical billing or insurance specialists. Some medical offices share the coding function; physicians assign procedure codes, and the coding staff assigns diagnosis codes. In facilities, the health information management (HIM) department (also called the medical record department) employs coders who specialize in medical coding.

Regardless of the medical setting, accurate coding and adherence to coding guidelines are paramount. A thorough understanding of the organization of the CPT code set and of the printed manual in which it appears is a logical starting point. This chapter establishes a foundation in CPT coding by introducing the format and organization of CPT and explaining procedural coding fundamentals and guidelines.

History and Purpose of CPT

Current Procedural Terminology (CPT) is a coding nomenclature or catalog system that allows descriptions of medical procedures to be translated from words to numbers. The CPT code set is based on the various types of **professional services** performed by physicians and other health care professionals such as physician's assistants; nurses; physical, occupational, and speech therapists; and dieticians. CPT codes cover thousands of professional services, from office visits to surgery, radiology, laboratory and pathology, anesthesiology, and other medical procedures.

CPT BACKGROUND

CPT was developed in 1966 and is currently maintained by the **American Medical Association** (AMA). According to the AMA, "the purpose of a CPT coding system is to provide a uniform language that accurately describes medical, surgical and diagnostic services and provides a means for reliable nationwide communication among physicians, patients, and insurance carriers." CPT was first widely used in 1983 when the Centers for Medicare and Medicaid Services (CMS) (then called HCFA, or Health Care Financing Administration) decided to require it for Medicare and Medicaid claims.

CMS next combined CPT with the **Healthcare Common Procedure Coding System** (HCPCS; pronounced hick-picks)—usually referred to as *supply codes*—to make a multilevel coding system for reporting services, procedures, and supplies to Medicare, Medicaid, and other government insurance beneficiaries. Now, under HIPAA, all these codes are used for reporting these services to all payers.

HCPCS Level I is the CPT code set printed in the AMA's CPT manual. **HCPCS Level II** codes are maintained by the federal government and are printed in commercial printers' HCPCS books. Level II codes are used to report supplies, drugs, and some services that are not in CPT. Officially, then, CPT is the first part of HCPCS, and the supply codes are the second part. Most people, though, refer to the codes in the CPT manual as *CPT codes* and the Level II codes as *HCPCS codes*.

CPT TODAY

CPT codes provide a way to precisely report procedures that have been performed without sending lengthy operative reports or written

---

STOP

CODING ALERT

CPT Only for Professional Services

CPT codes are used for professional services only. They are used in all outpatient settings by doctors and hospitals to report services, but never by facilities to report facility charges for inpatient services.

INTERNET RESOURCE

AMA

www.ama-assn.org

NOTE

HCPCS codes are covered in Chapter 10 of your program.

HIPAA TIP

Mandated Code Sets

- CPT is the mandated code set for physician procedures under HIPAA.
- HCPCS is the mandated code set for supplies under HIPAA.

COMPLIANCE GUIDELINE

Use Current Codes

Compliant coding under HIPAA requires using codes that are current as of the *date of service*.

descriptions to payers. Since health care claims are usually electronically sent and processed for payment decisions, using CPT codes reduces the need for payers to manually process claims and so increases administrative efficiency. For this reason, CPT was designated by the federal Department of Health and Human Services (HHS) as the nationally accepted HIPAA standard code set for physician and other health care professional services.

The information represented by CPT codes is used for many purposes, including:

- Reimbursing physicians' professional services at all types of locations (office, inpatient, nursing home) and for outpatient facility services
- Trending services provided to patients nationally
- Future planning from many perspectives, such as budgeting, policies, and resource allocation by payers, providers, and the government
- Benchmarking against similar facilities, practices, and geographic locations on cost of providing services, availability of services, and the like
- Measuring patient outcomes and quality of care by providers nationwide

To be included in the CPT code set, a procedure or service must meet the following conditions:

- It must be commonly performed by many physicians across the country.
- It must be consistent with mainstream medical practice.
- It must be approved by the AMA CPT Editorial Panel. The panel is made up of physicians and representatives from several organizations, such as CMS, the American Health Information Management Association (AHIMA), and the American Hospital Association (AHA). They decide whether to implement additions, deletions, or changes submitted by payers, medical associations, and physicians. The AMA CPT Advisory Committee consists of individuals chosen by their peers (nominated) to represent each clinical specialty. Their responsibility is to answer questions from the Editorial Panel about a code and/or revisions to a code. They serve as the technical and specialty experts working in the field.

Organization and Content of CPT

Each CPT code is a unique code followed by a **descriptor** of the service. There are more than eight thousand CPT codes, and no two are the same. At times one descriptor may be very close in wording to another, but there are always clear differences in definitions, so each code descriptor must be read in its entirety. One word or a punctuation mark can change the meaning of the entire code.

As you read the following description of CPT entries, look at the sample CPT entries in Figure 6.1. Every CPT code is five digits long. Symbols and notes in parenthesis, called parenthetical notes, are clues and instructions for the coder to follow when assigning codes from the

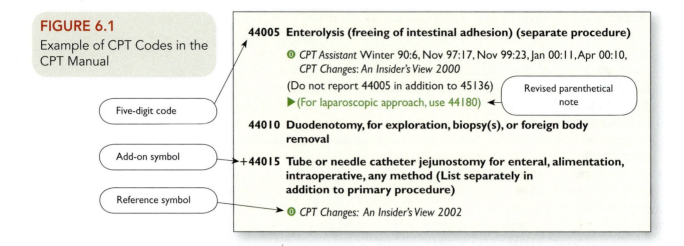

FIGURE 6.1

Example of CPT Codes in the CPT Manual

Five-digit code

Add-on symbol

Reference symbol

44005 Enterolysis (freeing of intestinal adhesion) (separate procedure)

⓪ *CPT Assistant* Winter 90:6, Nov 97:17, Nov 99:23, Jan 00:11, Apr 00:10, *CPT Changes: An Insider's View 2000*

(Do not report 44005 in addition to 45136)

▶ (For laparoscopic approach, use 44180) ◀   Revised parenthetical note

44010 Duodenotomy, for exploration, biopsy(s), or foreign body removal

+44015 Tube or needle catheter jejunostomy for enteral, alimentation, intraoperative, any method (List separately in addition to primary procedure)

⓪ *CPT Changes: An Insider's View 2002*

manual. References are made under particular codes, as in 44005, to provide resources for the coder to read before proceeding with code assignment. (The meaning of the symbols is discussed later in this chapter.)

The printed CPT code set in the CPT manual is arranged, with the exception of the Evaluation and Management (E/M) section, in numerical order. As shown in Table 6.1, the manual begins with an introduction followed by six sections of **Category I codes,** which are the major part of the manual, one section each of Category II and Category III codes, and the appendixes. The index, located at the back of CPT, lists terms and abbreviations in alphabetical order.

INTRODUCTION TO CPT

The introductory information at the beginning of CPT gives insights and rules used in the CPT code set. It also gives instructions on using the CPT manual, explanations of key terms, editorial notations, and information on tapes and disks available as resources. This information should be read carefully, as it supplies useful background.

Table 6.1 Parts of the CPT Manual

Introduction	Appendix A: Modifiers
Evaluation and Management (99201–99499)	Appendix B: Summary of Additions, Deletions, Revisions
Anesthesia (00100–01999)	Appendix C: Clinical Examples
Surgery (10021–69990)	Appendix D: Summary of Add-on Codes
Radiology (70010–79999)	Appendix E: Summary of −51 Exempt Codes
Pathology and Laboratory (80047–89356)	Appendix F: Summary of −63 Exempt Codes
Medicine (90281–99607)	Appendix G: Summary of Codes Include Moderate Sedation
Category II Codes	Appendix H: Index of Performance Measures by Condition
Category III Codes	Appendix I: Genetic Testing Code Modifiers
	Appendix J: Electrodiagnostic Medicine Listing of Nerves
	Appendix K: Product Pending FDA Approval
	Appendix L: Vascular Families
	Appendix M: Summary of Crosswalked Deleted CPT Codes

CATEGORY I CODES: SIX SECTIONS

Category I codes are permanent CPT codes. There are six sections of Category I codes in the CPT manual: Evaluation and Management, Anesthesia, Surgery, Radiology, Pathology and Laboratory, and Medicine. Each of these sections has its own **section guidelines** that appear in the beginning with definitions of terms, explanation of notes that appear around codes, and other related information. Each section also has subheadings and subsections with special instructions throughout. For example, at the end of each subsection there is a code called an **unlisted code** that can be used when there is no CPT code to reflect the exact procedure performed. See Table 6.2 for an overview of these six sections.

Evaluation and Management Section The codes in the Evaluation and Management (E/M) section cover physician services that are performed to determine the best course for patient care. Although the numbers are out of order—ranging from 99201 through 99499—the E/M codes are listed first in CPT because they are used so often by all types of physicians. Often called the *cognitive* codes, the E/M codes cover the complex process a physician uses to gather and analyze information about a patient's illness and to make decisions about the patient's condition and the best treatment or course of management. The actual treatments—such as surgical procedures and vaccines—are covered in the CPT sections that follow the E/M codes, such as the Surgery and Medicine sections.

> **NOTE**
>
> E/M codes are covered in Chapter 7 of your program.

Table 6.2 CPT Category I Code Sections

Section	Definition of Codes	Structure	Key Guidelines
Evaluation and Management	Physician services that are performed to determine the best course for patient care	Organized by place and/or type of service	New/established patients; other definitions Unlisted services, special reports Selecting an E/M service level
Anesthesia	Anesthesia services by or supervised by a physician; includes general, regional, and local anesthesia	Organized by body site	Time-based Services covered (bundled) in codes Unlisted services; special reports Qualifying circumstances codes
Surgery	Surgical procedures performed by physicians	Organized by body system and then body site, followed by procedural groups	Surgical package definition Follow-up care definition Add-on codes Separate procedures Subsection notes Unlisted services; special reports
Radiology	Radiology services by or supervised by a physician	Organized by type of procedure, followed by body site	Unlisted services; special reports Supervision and interpretation (professional and technical components)
Pathology and Laboratory	Pathology and laboratory services by physicians or by physician-supervised technicians	Organized by type of procedure	Complete procedure Panels Unlisted services; special reports
Medicine	Evaluation, therapeutic, and diagnostic procedures by or supervised by a physician	Organized by type of service or procedure	Subsection notes Multiple procedures reported separately Add-on codes Separate procedures Unlisted services; special reports

Anesthesia Section The codes in the Anesthesia section are used to report anesthesia services performed or supervised by a physician. These services include general and regional anesthesia as well as supplementation of local anesthesia. Each anesthesia code includes the complete usual services of an anesthesiologist:

- Usual preoperative visits for evaluation and planning
- Care during the procedure, such as administering fluid or blood, placing monitoring devices or IV lines, laryngoscopy, interpreting lab data, and nerve stimulation
- Routine postoperative care

Surgery Section The Surgery section is divided into each of the body systems (Integumentary, Musculoskeletal, Respiratory, Digestive, Cardiology, Urinary, Male/Female, Nervous, Ocular/Auditory). Surgery section codes are used for the many hundreds of surgical procedures performed by physicians. This is the largest procedure code section, with codes ranging from 10021 to 69990. The Surgery section has codes for **significant procedures,** such as incision, excision, repair, manipulation, amputation, endoscopy, destruction, suturing, and introductions.

In each body system subsection, codes are grouped to make locating them easier, such as under related anatomic, procedural, condition, or descriptor subheadings (see Figure 6.2). The AMA tries to maintain the same order in each of the body system subsections to promote consistency. Headings are arranged from head to toe and from least invasive to most invasive, for example, moving from incision, excision, introduction, removal of foreign body, and repair to destruction.

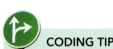

CODING TIP

Eponyms

CPT has procedures that carry the name of the person who developed the particular surgical approach or service, such as a McBride bunionectomy.

Surgical Package As defined in CPT, surgical codes include all the usual services in addition to the operation itself:

- After the decision for surgery, one related evaluation and management encounter on the day before or on the day of the procedure
- The operation: preparing the patient for surgery, including injection of anesthesia by the surgeon (local infiltration, metacarpal/metatarsal/digital block, or topical anesthesia), and performing the operation, including normal additional procedures, such as debridement (cleansing of a wound)
- Immediate postoperative care, including dictating operative notes and talking with the family and other physicians
- Writing orders
- Evaluating the patient in the postanesthesia recovery area
- Typical postoperative follow-up care

FIGURE 6.2

Example of Subsection Format in the Surgery Section

Section: Surgery
   Subsection/Category: Musculoskeletal
      Subcategory: Leg and Ankle Joint
         Heading: Incision
            Procedure: Incision and drainage, leg or ankle; deep abscess or hematoma

Procedural statement: Procedure conducted two weeks ago in office to correct hallux valgus (bunions) on left foot; local nerve block administered, correction by simple exostectomy. Saw patient in office today for routine follow-up; complete healing.
Code: **28290** Bunion correction

In the Surgery section, this grouping of related work under a single procedure code is called a **surgical package.** This is a payment concept; payers assign a fee to a surgical package code that reimburses all the services provided under it for a specified period of time called the **postoperative period.** Visits relating to the surgery are not paid in addition to the fee for the surgical package. Typically, the postoperative period is ten days for minor procedures and ninety days for major surgery.

Two types of services are not included in surgical package codes. These services are billed separately and are reimbursed in addition to the surgical package fee:

1. Complications or recurrences that arise after therapeutic surgical procedures.
2. Care for the condition for which a diagnostic surgical procedure is performed. Routine follow-up care included in the code refers only to care related to recovery from the diagnostic procedure itself, not the condition. For example, a diagnostic colonoscopy was performed to examine a growth in the patient's colon. An office visit after the surgery to evaluate the patient for chemotherapy because the tumor is cancerous is billed separately; it is not included as a postoperative visit.

Separate Procedures In some cases, the phrase *separate procedure* follows a code descriptor. If a procedure is labeled a **separate procedure,** CPT explains that it can be reported if it was performed alone, for a specific purpose, and independent of any other related service provided. If it was performed as a component part of a larger procedure, it is not billed separately.

Radiology Section
The codes in the Radiology section are used to report radiological services performed by or supervised by a physician. Radiology codes follow the same types of guidelines noted in the Surgery section. For example, some radiology codes are identified as separate procedure codes. These codes are usually part of a larger, more complex procedure and should not be reported as separate codes unless the procedure was done independently.

Most radiology services are performed and billed by radiologists working in hospital or clinic settings. Most medical practices do not have radiology equipment and instead refer patients to these specialists. In many cases, the radiologist performs both the technical (capturing the image) and the professional (interpreting the image) components. Codes are selected based on body part and the number and type of views.

Pathology and Laboratory Section
The codes in the Pathology and Laboratory section cover services provided by

> **NOTE**
>
> Radiology, pathology and laboratory, and medicine codes are covered in Chapter 9 of your program.

physicians or by technicians under the supervision of physicians. A complete procedure includes:

- Ordering the test
- Taking and handling the sample
- Performing the actual test
- Analyzing and reporting on the test results

Medicine Section   The Medicine section contains codes for the many types of evaluation, therapeutic, and diagnostic procedures that physicians and other health care professionals perform. (Codes for the Evaluation and Management section described earlier in the chapter, 99201 to 99499, actually fall at the end of this section numerically, but the AMA puts them first in CPT because they are the most frequently used codes.) Medicine codes may be used for procedures and services done or supervised by a physician of any specialty. They include many procedures and services provided by family practice physicians, such as immunizations and injections. The services of many specialists, such as allergists, cardiologists, and psychiatrists, are also covered in the Medicine section. Some Medicine section codes are for services that are used to support diagnosis and treatment, like rehabilitation, occupational therapy, and nutrition therapy.

Checkpoint 6.1

Selecting correct CPT codes begins with locating procedural terms in the index of CPT. Locate each term in the index. Write the type of term—either an abbreviation, an anatomical site, or a procedure. Then indicate the codes that are listed for it.

1. Epstein-Barr Virus   _Eponym_   _86663–86665_
2. Evisceration   _____   _____
3. ETOH   _____   _____
4. Nasolacrimal Duct   _____   _____
5. Myringotomy   _____   _____

CATEGORY II CODES

Category II codes were created by the American Medical Association (AMA) to track physician performance in measuring and monitoring patient care. These alphanumeric codes (four digits and one alpha character) are reported for services such as prenatal care, counseling to stop smoking tobacco, and keeping track of chronic conditions. This type of service, while not directly billable, improves the quality of care and treatment of patients. For example, a number of services are related to watching for problems due to a patient's diabetes mellitus or coronary artery disease (CAD). Category II codes are a quick way to note that these important services were done; they take the place of a lengthy documentation process. An appendix to CPT describes the meanings of the codes.

EXAMPLE
2001F Weight recorded

These codes are optional—that is, they are not required for correct coding. They are not directly reimbursed, but if the insurance carrier has **payment-for-performance (P4P)** measures that reward physicians for providing such care, they can be integral to receiving a higher level of payment under insurance participation contracts.

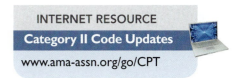

CATEGORY III CODES

Category III codes were introduced in CPT in 2002. These alphanumeric codes (four digits and a *T)* are located immediately after the Category II codes and before the appendixes. They are used to report emerging technology, services, and procedures that do not have CPT codes assigned.

These codes allow researchers to track emerging technology services. In order to be assigned a Category III code, a new procedure must be FDA-approved and performed by many health care professionals in clinical practice in multiple locations. If a Category III code is being widely used, the AMA may advance it to the permanent CPT Category I level. In this case CPT will contain a cross-reference pointing to the location of the advanced code.

Category III codes are added by the AMA twice a year and are published on the AMA's Website. If a Category III code has not been used after five years, it will be archived.

BILLING TIP
Category III Codes

Not all payers accept these codes, and freestanding ASCs are not permitted to use them. Check first, and if a payer does not accept these codes, report the appropriate unlisted procedure code instead.

> **EXAMPLE**
> *0155T* Laparoscopy, clinical; implantation or replacement of gastric stimulation electrodes, less curvature (i.e., morbid obesity)

APPENDIXES

Appendixes, located after the Category III codes, supply extremely important information. The content of the appendixes can answer many coding questions.

CODING TIP

CPT Appendixes: A Helpful Tool

Become familiar with the appendixes, which can assist you in all CPT coding situations.

- *Appendix A—Modifiers:* A listing of modifiers (defined on page 218) with descriptions and, in some cases, examples of usage.
- *Appendix B—Summary of Additions, Deletions, and Revisions:* A summary of the codes added, revised, and deleted in the current version. It is useful as a snapshot of changes from the prior year's book. This appendix, along with Appendix M, is a helpful quick reference when updating office computer systems and billing forms.
- *Appendix C—Clinical Examples:* Case examples of the proper use of the codes in the Evaluation and Management section. This is a tool to help coders and physicians gauge E/M code level assignment by comparing their current coding situation with similar circumstances and levels.
- *Appendix D—Summary of CPT Add-on Codes:* List of supplemental codes used for procedures that are commonly done in addition to the primary procedure. These codes are also located throughout the CPT manual and are indicated by the "+" symbol. Offices can use this valuable tool to flag the add-on codes in their computer systems to ensure that they will not be reported alone or listed first on claims.

- *Appendix E—Summary of CPT Codes Exempt from Modifier −51:* Codes to which the modifier showing multiple procedures cannot be attached because they already include a multiple descriptor. These appear throughout the CPT codebook and are indicated by the "⊘" symbol. Offices can also use this appendix to flag these codes in their computer systems to alert staff members that a modifier is not appropriate.

- *Appendix F—Summary of CPT Codes Exempt from Modifier −63:* This appendix is helpful to specialists who perform surgery on infants. The codes are located throughout the CPT codebook and have parenthetical notes beneath them warning not to assign the −63 modifier to the code.

- *Appendix G—Summary of CPT Codes Which Include Conscious Sedation:* These codes are also located throughout the code set with the "⊙" symbol. Surgical practices refer to this list and flag their computer systems to not permit the assignment of conscious sedation for these surgical procedures.

- *Appendix H—Alphabetic Index of Performance Measures by Clinical Condition or Topic:* A listing of all Category II codes with the criteria of performance measuring.

- *Appendix I—Genetic Testing Code Modifiers:* Notice that none of these modifiers are located on the inside cover of CPT. They are reported by molecular laboratories that perform genetic testing and mutation procedures.

- *Appendix J—Electrodiagnostic Medicine Listing of Sensory, Motor, and Mixed Nerves:* This appendix lists sensory, motor, and mixed nerves and is referenced when coding nerve conduction studies from the Medicine section.

- *Appendix K—Product Pending FDA Approval:* These codes are located in the Medicine section and are denoted by the "✗" symbol.

- *Appendix L—Vascular Families:* This appendix is helpful for coding interventional radiology procedures and catheterizations.

- *Appendix M—Crosswalk to Deleted CPT Codes:* This provides a **crosswalk** (a comparison connecting two sets of items) between deleted codes and the current year's correct codes that replace them.

Checkpoint 6.2

List the name of the CPT section in which each of the following codes is located.

1. 99212 _____
2. 90389 _____
3. 75630 _____
4. 00820 _____
5. 80055 _____
6. 0065T _____
7. 35180 _____
8. 4000F _____

CPT Punctuation and Symbols

The semicolon and various symbols are important to assigning the correct code.

SEMICOLON ;

The **semicolon** (;) is used in CPT to conserve space and to divide the common portion of a code descriptor from the unique portion. It is a way of sorting a long list of procedures that are related. Use of the semicolon avoids repeating the entire code description for each of a related group of codes. The common portion or the main entry (the *root code)* is separated by a semicolon (;) from a unique portion that is indented to make it easier to see. This format indicates that the main entry applies to and is part of all indented entry codes that follow.

The semicolon in CPT reads like the word *and*. Code descriptions should be read carefully, noting where the semicolon is placed. Both the common portion (before the semicolon) and the descriptor after the semicolon are needed for a complete code description.

> **EXAMPLE**
> 33533 Coronary artery bypass, using arterial graft(s); single arterial graft
> 33534   two coronary arterial grafts

The common portion of CPT code 33533, "Coronary artery bypass, using arterial graft(s)," should be considered part of CPT code 33534. The unique portion is "two coronary arterial grafts." Therefore, the full procedure represented by code 33534 is read as "33534 Coronary artery bypass, using arterial graft(s); two coronary arterial grafts."

As a general rule, the farther down an indented listing a code is, the more complex it is. At times, more than one code from the related group is reported; most often, however, just one appropriate code is selected.

Several coding symbols and characters are used to direct the coder. It is extremely important to understand what each of the symbols means. The characters are located inside the front cover of the CPT code as well as along the bottom of each two-page layout.

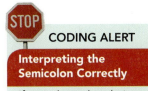

CODING ALERT

Interpreting the Semicolon Correctly

If an indented code is selected, only that code must be assigned, not the root code too.

BULLET ●

The bullet designates a new code for that year. The bullet precedes the code and is found in the left margin. Bullets appear for one year only, because they denote new procedures for that year.

TRIANGLE ▲

The triangle signifies a revised code, meaning that the descriptor is revised in some way. Some changes may not seem great, but the impact on reimbursement may be significant. Approximately 7 percent of the CPT book changes from year to year. Appendix B lists these changed codes. Like bullets, triangles appear in one year's CPT manual only, because they denote that the procedure before which they appear has been revised or changed in some way for the new volume of CPT.

PLUS SYMBOL +

The plus symbol identifies an **add-on code.** Add-on codes are considered "additional" codes for procedures carried out along with a primary procedure. The **primary procedure** is the main procedure performed. It is the most comprehensive, complex in nature, and resource-intensive procedure and is listed first, before all other procedures. **Secondary procedures** are less extensive or resource-intensive and are listed in addition to the primary procedure.

Add-on codes are considered secondary procedures. They cannot be reported alone and must be used with the related base code. (Appendix D lists all add-on codes in CPT. Add-on codes often are described with phrases in the code description like "each additional" or "(List separately in addition to primary procedure)." In Figure 6.1 on page 206, 44010 is the primary procedure and 44015 is the add-on code.

EXAMPLE

11200 Removal of skin tags, multiple fibrocutaneous tags, any area, up to and including 15 lesions

+11201   each additional ten lesions (List separately in addition to code for primary procedure)

In parentheses under code 11201, CPT states to use 11201 in conjunction with 11200. Based on this instruction, if more than 15 skin tags were removed, two codes must be reported, 11200 and 11201, in that order.

MODIFIER −51 EXEMPT ⊘

The symbol ⊘ indicates that a code cannot be assigned a −51 modifier (modifiers are described on pages 218–229). These CPT codes do not fall under the same payment scheme as other codes that allow the modifier (although other modifiers may be appropriate). Appendix E lists these in their entirety.

EXAMPLE

⊘ 20660 Application of cranial tongs, caliper or stereotactic frame, including removal (Separate procedure)

FACING TRIANGLES ▶◀

The facing triangle symbol before a code indicates that text is new or has been revised from the prior year's edition. The triangles mark the beginning and ending of the new and/or revised text in the guidelines and instruction notes. There are many cross-references and additional instructions located within these symbols. Coders should read this information to ensure proper code assignment.

CIRCLED BULLET ⊙

A circled bullet before a code indicates that conscious sedation is included in the service or procedure. Conscious sedation is a moderate, drug-induced depression of consciousness during which patients can respond to verbal commands. This type of sedation is typically used with scope procedures such as bronchoscopies. Since it is an inherent part of providing these procedures, it is incorrect to code and bill for the conscious sedation separately if the physician providing the sedation is the physician who is performing the procedure. Appendix G lists these codes.

EXAMPLE
⊙ 43202 Esophagoscopy, rigid or flexible; with biopsy, single or multiple

LIGHTNING BOLT ⚡

The lightning bolt symbol (⚡) signifies that the code is for a vaccine that is pending FDA approval; all codes with the symbol are located in the Medicine section. When a vaccine is approved, the symbol is removed from the CPT code listing. Coders cannot report a code that has the symbol; when approved, the symbol is deleted and the code can be used.

CPT ASSISTANT OR CPT CHANGES: AN INSIDER'S VIEW

➲ This symbol appears only in the Professional Edition of CPT books below the code description. It means that the coder may refer to a specific issue of *CPT Assistant* or *CPT Changes: An Insider's View* for guidance on the code use.

CPT Assistant is designated under HIPAA as required guidance for the use of CPT codes and is published monthly by the AMA. *CPT Changes: An Insider's View* is published annually by the AMA as a tool for understanding changes made to the text from the previous year.

EXAMPLE
90705 Measles virus vaccine, live, for subcutaneous use
➲ *CPT Assistant* Apr 97:10, Nov 98:31–33, Jan 99:2, Oct 99:9, *CPT Changes: An Insider's View* 2004

Checkpoint 6.3

Answer the following questions.

1. What is the common portion of code 46760? _____

2. What is the unique portion of code 46942? _____

3. What is the complete code description of 54326? _____

4. If a diagnostic flexible colonoscopy is performed in a physician's endoscopy suite and the physician supplies the IV sedation, is it appropriate to report both code 45378 and code 99144? _____

5. In the CPT manual you are using, identify three new codes (indicated by a bullet), three revised codes (indicated with a triangle), and three codes with new or revised text (indicated by facing triangles). _____

CPT and Professional Fees

Physicians and other health care professionals bill for their services based on fee schedules covering their commonly performed services. For example, in physician practices, physicians establish a list of their **usual fees** for the CPT codes they frequently perform. The usual fees on the physician's **fee schedule** are defined as those that they charge to most of their patients most of the time under typical conditions. The typical ranges of physicians' fees nationwide are published in commercial databases, and can be analyzed by physicians and practice managers.

If a physician bills and is paid the full amount on the fee schedule, this payment is called a **fee-for-service.** Payers, though, do not necessarily pay physicians based on the physician's usual fee. Private payers and government payers alike usually negotiate some kind of payment schedule that reduces these amounts. Here are examples:

- If the payer is a health management organization (HMO), it may pay the physician a salary, or may pay on a *capitation* basis. HMO creates a network of physicians, hospitals, and other providers by employing or negotiating contracts with them. **Capitation** (from *capit*, Latin for *head*) is a fixed prepayment to a medical provider for all necessary contracted services provided to each patient who is a plan member. The capitated rate, which is called *per member per month*, is a prospective payment—it is paid *before* the patient visit. It covers a specific period of time. The health plan makes the payment whether the patient receives many or no medical services during that specified period. The capitated rate of prepayment, however, covers only services listed on the schedule of benefits for the plan. The provider may bill the patient for any other services.

- If the payer is another type of health plan called a preferred provider organization (PPO), it usually pays physicians discounted fees under a contract.

Modifiers

Modifiers are two-digit characters that may be appended to (added to the end of) most CPT codes. Modifiers are used to communicate special circumstances involved with services, telling the payer that the physician considers the service noted in the code's descriptor to have been changed in some way, but not enough to assign a different CPT code.

Modifier use is described in each of the six major section's guidelines. Some modifiers are associated with a particular medical specialty, such as coding for a physician office, surgical practice, facility, or anesthesia practice. A modifier often increases or decreases the normal payment for the code to which it is attached. For example, the modifier –76, repeat procedure by same physician, is used when the reporting physician repeats a procedure or service after doing the first one.

EXAMPLE

Procedural statement: Physician performed chest X-rays before placing a chest tube and then, after the chest tube was placed, performed a second set of X-rays to verify its position.

Code: **71020–76** Radiologic examination, chest, two views, frontal and lateral; repeat procedure or service by same physician

In this case, since more work was done, the modifier tells the payer that more than the regular reimbursement should be paid.

If CPT codes are verbs (such as *examine*, *evaluate*, and *operate*), modifiers can be thought of as adverbs. They further describe an action taken or service provided and the circumstances surrounding

Physicians, hospitals and clinics, and pharmacies contract with the PPO plan to provide care to its insured people. These medical providers accept the PPO plan's fee schedule and guidelines for its managed medical care. PPOs generally pay participating providers based on a discount from their physician fee schedules, called *discounted fee-for-service*.

- The major government health plan, Medicare, pays most of its participating providers—those who agree to accept its fees in exchange for the benefit of acquiring Medicare beneficiaries as patients—on the basis of a **resource-based relative value system (RBRVS),** which is a way of assigning a relative weight to each procedure in a group of related CPT codes that can be converted to a fee. There are three parts to an RBRVS fee:
  1. *The nationally uniform RVU:* The relative value is based on three cost elements—the physician's work, the practice cost (overhead), and the cost of malpractice insurance.
  2. *A geographic adjustment factor:* A geographic adjustment factor is a number that is used to multiply each relative value element so that it better reflects a geographical area's relative costs.
  3. *A nationally uniform conversion factor:* A uniform conversion factor is a dollar amount used to multiply the relative values to produce a payment amount. It is used by Medicare to make adjustments according to changes in the cost of living index.

- Workers' compensation patients often must be charged according to a state-mandated fee schedule.

Whatever payment method is applied, coders assist physicians and other outpatient providers by correctly assigning CPT codes that accurately reflect the services that were provided. Assignment of correct ICD-9-CM codes, of course, is also essential to demonstrate the medical necessity of the procedures.

that service. Modifiers are used to indicate:

- That a procedure was performed bilaterally
- That more than one procedure was performed at the same time
- That a service was performed by more than one physician or in more than one location, such as that an assistant surgeon participated
- That a service or procedure was increased or decreased
- That only part of a service was performed
- That unusual events occurred during a procedure or service
- That a service has two parts or components—a technical component and a professional component
- The physical status of a patient for anesthesia administration

TYPES OF MODIFIERS

Three basic types of modifiers are used with CPT codes:

1. *CPT modifiers* for *professional services*
2. *Facility modifiers* approved for hospital outpatient use
3. *HCPCS modifiers*

These three types, plus the special physical status modifiers that are used only with anesthesia codes, are described below.

CPT Modifiers   Thirty-one **CPT modifiers** are approved for use with CPT codes reported for physician services and procedures. Modifiers are listed on the inside front cover of the CPT codebook in the left column. Refer to Table 6.3, which provides an overview of all modifiers. Modifiers highlighted in yellow are considered professional modifiers.

Table 6.3 Modifiers: Description and Common Use in Main Text Sections

Modifier Quick Reference Guide

Legend	Financial Impact of Modifier Use	Directions for Use
🗐 = Bundling/CCI related	↑ = Reimbursement increases	Find the modifier you are considering assigning. Check to see whether the modifier is appropriate to use in your setting. Also check to see whether the modifier can be appended to the code you are submitting by checking the symbols on the left.
☆ = Global package	↓ = Reimbursement decreases	
✋ = Physician E/M code	⟶ = Required to get claim paid. No change in reimbursement.	
# = Number of surgeons	⟵ = No change. Explanation only.	Modifiers that affect payment are sequenced first.
⧗ = Anesthesia		
🖱 = Lab		
⌨ = Facility modifier		
▤ = Special report needed		
✂ = Procedure modifier		
☠ = Radiology		
MD = Physician only modifier		

Modifier	Description	☠⧗	MD Only	E/M	Anesthesia	Procedure	Radiology	Path/Lab	Global Package	Facility
−21	Prolonged E/M service	↑ ⟵	MD	✋	✋					
−22	Unusual procedure service	↑	MD	✋ ▤	⧗ ▤	✂ ▤	☠ ▤	🖱		
−23	Unusual anesthesia	⟶	MD		⧗					
−24	Unrelated E/M service during post-op	⟶	MD	✋					☆	
−25	Significant separately identifiable E/M service	⟶		✋					☆ 🗐	⌨
−26	Professional component	↓	MD	✋			☠	🖱	🗐	
−27	Multiple outpatient hospital E/M encounters same day	⟶		✋						⌨
−32	Mandated service	⟶ ⟵	MD	✋	⧗	✂	☠	🖱		
−47	Anesthesia by surgeon	↑ ⟵	MD			Surgeon only				
−50	Bilateral procedure	↑				✂	☠			⌨
−51	Multiple procedure	↓	MD		⧗	✂	☠			
−52	Reduced services	↓		✋		✂	☠	🖱		⌨
−53	Discontinued procedure	↓	MD		⧗	✂	☠	🖱		
−54	Surgical care only	↓	MD			✂			☆	
−55	Post-op management only	↓	MD	✋					☆	

Table 6.3 (Continued)

Modifier	Description	💰	MD Only	E/M	Anesthesia	Procedure	Radiology	Path/Lab	Global Package	Facility
−56	Pre-op management only	↓	MD	hand					☆	
−57	Decision for surgery	→	MD	hand					☆	
−58	Staged or related procedure	→				scissors	skull		☆	keyboard
−59	Distinct procedural service	→			hourglass	scissors / envelope	skull	mouse	documents	keyboard
−62	Two surgeons	↓	MD			scissors # / envelope	skull			
−63	Procedure performed on infants < 4 kg	↑	MD			scissors (not skin)				
−66	Surgical team	↓	MD			envelope scissors #				keyboard
−73	Discontinued outpatient procedure prior anesthesia	↓				scissors				keyboard
−74	Discontinued outpatient procedure after anesthesia	↓				scissors				keyboard
−76	Repeat procedure by same physician	↓ →				scissors	skull		☆	keyboard
−77	Repeat procedure by other physician in practice	→				scissors	skull		☆	keyboard
−78	Return to OR for related procedure during post-op period	→ ↓				scissors	skull		☆	keyboard
−79	Unrelated service by same physician during post-op period	→		hand		scissors	skull		☆	keyboard
−80	Assistant surgeon	↓	MD			scissors # / envelope	skull			
−81	Minimum assistant surgeon	↓	MD			scissors # / envelope				
−82	Assistant surgeon—qualified resident not available	↓	MD			scissors # / envelope				
−90	Reference outside lab	←	MD					mouse		
−91	Repeat clinical diag. lab test	→						mouse		keyboard
−92	Alt. lab. platform testing	→						mouse		
−99	Multiple modifiers	←	MD			scissors	skull			

Source: CPT 2008.

Table 6.4 OP Facility Modifiers

Modifier	Description
−25	Significant, separately identifiable E/M service by the same physician on the same day of the procedure or other service
−27	Multiple outpatient hospital E/M encounters on the same date
−50	Bilateral procedure
−52	Reduced services
−58	Staged or related procedure/service by the same physician during the postoperative period
−59	Distinct procedural service
−73	Discontinued outpatient procedure prior to anesthesia administration
−74	Discontinued outpatient procedure after anesthesia administration
−76	Repeat procedure by same physician
−77	Repeat procedure by another physician
−78	Return to the operating room for a related procedure during the postoperative period
−79	Unrelated procedure/service by the same physician during the postoperative period
−91	Repeat clinical diagnostic laboratory test

BILLING TIP

Reporting Facility Modifiers on Claims

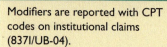

Modifiers are reported with CPT codes on institutional claims (837I/UB-04).

NOTE

HCPCS coding is covered in Chapter 10 of your program.

BILLING TIP

Multiple Modifiers

Sometimes more than one modifier needs to be used with a procedure. When sequencing more than two modifiers, use the −99 modifier first, and then the others, from highest to lowest. Always list the modifier that affects payment first.

Facility Modifiers Approved for Hospital Outpatient Use (Level I CPT)   Thirteen **facility modifiers** are approved for use in coding hospital outpatient services and procedures. Table 6.4 provides an overview of these modifiers. Note that some are the same as the professional modifiers, and some are distinct.

Level II Modifiers (HCPCS/National)   Level II modifiers, which are alphanumeric, are usually called **HCPCS modifiers.** Some HCPCS Level II modifiers are listed in the front of CPT, and the rest are listed in the HCPCS coding book. The HCPCS modifiers are updated annually. They are required specifically when filing claims to government payers such as Medicare. The HCPCS modifiers that are listed in CPT are summarized in Table 6.5.

PROPER USE OF MODIFIERS

A coder needs to clearly understand the meaning of each modifier before using it. Not all circumstances or codes warrant a modifier. Modifiers should not be haphazardly assigned, because reimbursement may be affected. For example, if the goal was to indicate that a procedure was unusual or more difficult and the coder mistakenly put a −52 modifier for reduced service instead of the −22 modifier, the reimbursement will be reduced.

Modifiers are appended to the CPT code by adding a hyphen and the two-character modifier.

EXAMPLE   37720–54 indicates that ligation and division and complete stripping of long or short saphenous veins was the only service provided, not preoperative or postoperative services.

Table 6.5 Selected HCPCS Level II (National) Modifiers

Modifier	Description
−CA	Procedure payable in the inpatient setting only when performed emergently on an outpatient who expires prior to admission
−E1	Upper left eyelid
−E2	Lower left eyelid
−E3	Upper right eyelid
−E4	Lower right eyelid
−FA	Left hand, thumb
−F1	Left hand, second digit
−F2	Left hand, third digit
−F3	Left hand, fourth digit
−F4	Left hand, fifth digit
−F5	Right hand, thumb
−F6	Right hand, second digit
−F7	Right hand, third digit
−F8	Right hand, fourth digit
−F9	Right hand, fifth digit
−GA	Waiver of liability statement on file
−GG	Performance and payment of a screening mammogram and diagnostic mammogram on the same patient, same day
−GH	Diagnostic mammogram converted from screening mammogram on same day
−LC	Left circumflex coronary artery
−LD	Left anterior descending coronary artery
−RC	Right coronary artery
−LT	Left side (identifies procedures performed on the left side of the body)
−RT	Right side (identifies procedures performed on the right side of the body)
−QM	Ambulance service provided under arrangement by a provider of services
−QN	Ambulance service furnished directly by a provider of services
−TA	Left foot, great toe
−T1	Left foot, second digit
−T2	Left foot, third digit
−T3	Left foot, fourth digit
−T4	Left foot, fifth digit
−T5	Right foot, great toe
−T6	Right foot, second digit
−T7	Right foot, third digit
−T8	Right foot, fourth digit
−T9	Right foot, fifth digit
−TC	Technical component

Source: HCPCS 2008.

It is also important to note that, unlike regular CPT codes, not all modifiers are available for use with every section's codes:

- Some modifiers apply only to certain sections. For example, the modifier −21, prolonged evaluation and management services, is used only with codes that are located in the Evaluation and Management section, as its descriptor implies.
- Add-on codes cannot be modified with −51, multiple procedures, because the add-on code is used to add increments to a primary procedure, so the need for multiple procedures is replaced by procedures added on.
- Codes that begin with ⊘ (a circle with a backslash) also cannot be modified with −51, multiple procedures.

Modifier −21, Prolonged Evaluation and Management Services

Modifier −21 is used to describe a situation in which either a face-to-face or a hospital floor or unit service took much longer or was a greater level of service than the highest level of E/M code for that place or type of service. It is not recognized by all payers. Do not use this modifier for a code other than those located in the E/M section of CPT.

Modifier −22, Unusual (Increased) Procedure or Service

Modifier −22 is used to indicate that the procedure is different from that usually included in the code description. For some reason, it was more complex than usual (involved increased risk, difficulty, hemorrhage [blood loss over 600 cc], unusual findings, prolonged cleansing). There may have been a complication that cannot be identified by using another CPT code.

To correctly assign this modifier, work and effort need to have been increased by about 30 to 50 percent. The −22 modifier is not used with E/M; if it is a prolonged E/M service, the −21 modifier is used.

> **EXAMPLE** Excision of a lesion on a morbidly obese patient in the crease of the neck. The obesity makes it more difficult to reach the lesion so it warrants a modifier. In fact, many procedures on the morbidly obese are more difficult to perform because of impaired view and additional tissue to cut through.

Modifier −23, Unusual Anesthesia

Modifier −23 is used when a procedure that normally would not be done under anesthesia required anesthesia. The anesthesiologist is the only physician who would use this modifier. Anesthesia personnel use it occasionally when performing procedures on children and on people with severe anxiety or mental retardation who are uncooperative, making it safer and easier to perform the procedure with IV sedation or general anesthesia.

> **EXAMPLE** Mentally retarded patient required anesthesia to perform a CT scan of the head.

Modifier −24, Unrelated Evaluation and Management Service by the Same Physician During a Postoperative Period

At times a patient is seen for a new problem during the postoperative period. If the reason for the visit is to evaluate a condition that is clearly not related to the reason for the surgery, and if that condition is supported with a different diagnosis code, modifier −24 is used so that the visit will be paid.

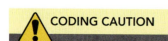

CODING CAUTION

Modifier −22
Documentation must support the amount of and reason for extra work.

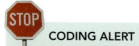

CODING ALERT

Modifier −23
Modifier −23 can be assigned only by anesthesia personnel.

EXAMPLE Patient is three weeks post-op lithotripsy. Patient is now complaining of warts that have appeared on his genital area. Patient is diagnosed with genital herpes. Code: 99212–24.

Modifier −25, Significant, Separately Identifiable E/M Service on the Same Day by the Same Physician on the Same Day of the Procedure or Service

Modifier −25 is frequently misused in a professional practice, often because it seems to be an easy way to be paid for extra work during a patient encounter. It should be used to report an authentic, separately reportable procedure-type service provided at the same time a valid E/M service is rendered.

Note that both the separately identifiable E/M service and the procedure or other service may be related to the same diagnosis. According to CMS, this modifier is assigned for an E/M service that is above and beyond the procedure performed, that is beyond the usual preoperative and postoperative care associated with the procedure, and that requires all the necessary elements of an E/M service.

> **EXAMPLE** A patient presented with an excoriated lesion, and a biopsy was performed along with the services indicative of the E/M code 99214. This would warrant a −25 modifier.

Modifier −26, Professional Component

Modifier −26 is used to report the physicians' professional service or component separately from the facility's services for the technical component of the same service. This modifier alerts the insurance company to pay the physician for his or her professional services separately from the payment to the facility for its costs to provide the technical service, such as the room and the supplies.

Modifier −27, Multiple Outpatient Hospital E/M Encounters on the Same Date

Modifier −27 is used in hospital outpatient coding only, where it indicates more than a single evaluation and management (E/M) encounter for the same patient on the same date of service.

Modifier −32, Mandated Services

Modifier −32 is used when an insurance carrier or outside federal agency requires (*mandates*) that a service be provided. Certain diagnoses may require a second or third opinion from another provider (not a family member's request) before some insurance carriers (not Medicare) will pay for it. This modifier alerts the payer that the claim should be paid at its full amount without any charge to the patient.

> **EXAMPLE** A fifty-three-year-old truck driver is being seen in follow-up from an injury on the job. He fell out of his tractor-trailer and fractured his shoulder, requiring repair with prosthesis. His recent evaluation did not demonstrate total inability to use this shoulder. The workers' compensation carrier is requiring an independent evaluation with an orthopedist who specializes in shoulder joint replacements. Based on this evaluation, the carrier may reduce his benefits. The orthopedist will report this work with an appropriate E/M code and a −32 modifier.

Modifier −47, Anesthesia by Surgeon

Modifier −47 is used when a regional nerve block or general anesthesia is administered by the surgeon, rather than by anesthesia personnel. It is not

CODING ALERT

Use Modifiers −24 and −25 Only with E/M CPT Codes

Modifiers −24 and −25 are never appended to surgical codes. They are strictly used with E/M codes only.

CODING TIP

Modifier −32 for Third-Party-Requested Services

Report modifier −32 when a third party such as a workers' compensation payer is requiring E/M services.

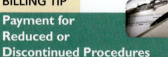
used with anesthesia codes, only by appending it to a CPT code for the procedure. Note that this modifier is not accepted by Medicare.

Modifier −50, Bilateral Procedure   Procedures listed in the CPT book are inherently unilateral unless otherwise stated. The −50 modifier states that the identical procedure was performed bilaterally during the same operative session. The term *bilateral* pertains to paired body organs that are distinctly left or right, such as the left breast and right breast. To use this modifier, the code description may not state "one or both or bilateral" or list the plural form of a body part such as *turbinate(s)*.

> **EXAMPLE**   The description for CPT code 69210 is *removal of impacted cerumen, one or both ears.*

In this example, it would be inappropriate to use −50 because the code description includes "both ears." But in the following example, the −50 modifier is correctly used to mean that foreign bodies were removed from both ears:

> **EXAMPLE**
> 69200–50 Removal of foreign body of the external auditory canal; without anesthesia.

Modifier −51, Multiple Procedures   This modifier is assigned when more than one *surgical* procedure is performed on the *same* day or at the *same operating session* by the *same provider*. The procedures can be performed on the same or different body parts through the same or a different incision.

> **EXAMPLE**   30000 Drainage abscess or hematoma, nasal, internal approach done at the same operative session as 30200 Injection into turbinate(s), therapeutic would be reported as 30000, 30200–51.

Modifier −52, Reduced Services   When a procedure is partially reduced, modifier −52 is used. This alerts the payer that the service was not completed to its full extent, such as when a doctor performs a procedure unilaterally but the code description indicates bilateral. Modifier −52 should be reported when the coder cannot find a procedure code that describes the partially reduced services, when such a code does not exist, or when directed by CPT parenthetical notes.

> **EXAMPLE**   Patient with above-the-knee amputation (AKA) had an extremity arterial study (93923). A −52 modifier would be appropriate here since he does not have an entire leg to study.

Modifier −53, Discontinued Procedure   Modifier −53 indicates that a started procedure was terminated for some reason (threat to patient, instrument failure, or the like). It is not used to report elective cancellations before a procedure is started. The modifier applies to surgical procedures only and would never be applied to E/M codes.

> **EXAMPLE**   Modifier −53 is used for extenuating circumstances such as power outage, fire, arrhythmia, hypotension, equipment failure, physician impairment, and so on.

Global Surgery Modifiers   CPT created a way to submit codes for surgical services in which the same physician did not carry out the entire surgical package. Surgical codes with global periods of greater than ten days where two or three physicians carried out portions of service are submitted with one of three modifiers: −54, −55, or −56.

Modifier −54, Surgical Care Only Modifier −54 is used by the surgeon who actually performed the surgery and did not or will not provide the pre-op or post-op care.

Modifier −55, Postoperative Management Only Modifier −55 is used to reflect care provided by a physician who did not perform the original surgery.

Modifier −56, Preoperative Management Only If a physician performs a preoperative evaluation and determines that surgery is necessary but does not perform the actual surgery and post-op follow-up, it would appropriate to append the −56 modifier to the surgical code.

Modifier −57, Decision for Surgery
If during an E/M visit a physician initially decides that surgery is needed, the visit is reimbursable separately from the global package. Using modifier −57 with the appropriate E/M code notifies the payer of this fact and indicates that a surgical claim will follow.

Modifier −58, Staged or Related Procedure by the Same Physician During the Postoperative Period
For the use of modifier −58, the surgeon's medical record should document that a staged procedure was planned during the specified postoperative period for the first procedure code. This modifier should not be used with codes whose definitions already include the word *staged* or language indicating that the surgery or procedure is usually done in multiple sessions. Instead, it is used when a procedure was planned prospectively, was more extensive than the original procedure, or was for therapy following a diagnostic surgical procedure and each of the stages of the procedure were performed by the original surgeon. This modifier is not used to report a problem or complication resulting from the original surgery that required a return to the operating room.

> **EXAMPLE** A physician performed debridement of a non-healing wound three times and then performed a skin graft. The physician and patient discussed this course of treatment ahead of time.

Modifier −59, Distinct Procedural Service
Modifier −59 states that two codes that are normally paid under one surgical package were performed as two separate procedures. One procedure has been performed independently of the other or is unrelated to the other. Usually one of the codes is a CPT-designated separate procedure, as explained in this instruction from the *CPT Assistant* (July 1999):

> When codes designated as separate procedures are carried out independently or considered unrelated or distinct from other procedures/services provided at the same time, they can be reported in addition to the other procedures by appending a −59 modifier.

Modifier −59 is important for receiving payment for both procedures, rather than a reduced fee for the second procedure. The guideline is that if the procedures were done at different sites or organs, a separate incision was made, a separate excision was done, or the doctor was treating a separate injury or lesion, modifier −59 is correct.

EXAMPLE Excision of a benign 2 cm lesion of the right arm (11402) and a 1.5 cm benign lesion of the back (11402–59).

In this example, the procedures are at different sites, so it is acceptable to report the same code twice, appending the −59 modifier to the second code.

Modifier −62, Two Surgeons

Modifier −62 is applicable when the procedure required 50 percent of each of two surgeons' skill and time if two surgeons were participating in the same procedure. An example is the need for an orthopedist and a neurosurgeon to work together to perform a Harrington rod technique. If two surgeons were operating at the same time but were performing two different procedures, this modifier does not apply.

Modifier −63, Procedure Performed on Infants

Modifier −63 is used to report services on neonates and infants weighing less than four kilograms. Increased complexity and physician work are associated with this type of patient.

Modifier −66, Surgical Team

Modifier −66 is used mainly in transplant procedures or cases of multiple trauma when the skills of several different surgeons were required.

Modifier −73, Discontinued Outpatient Procedure Prior to Anesthesia Administration

Modifier −73 is reported only by hospital outpatient coders to indicate that a procedure was terminated before anesthesia was administered.

Modifier −74, Discontinued Outpatient Procedure After Anesthesia Administration

Modifier −74 is reported only by hospital outpatient coders to indicate that a procedure was terminated after local or general anesthesia was given. This includes situations in which the patient was in the operating room and anesthesia was started and situations in which sedation was given in the holding area.

Modifier −76, Repeat Procedure by Same Physician

Modifier −76 is used to report a second procedure that had been previously performed on the same day. It is usually used to report the exact same service repeated in radiology and the lab, and minor procedures such as repeat blood sugar. Some payers recognize this modifier; others do not.

Modifier −77, Repeat Procedure by Another Physician

At times, a procedure previously performed by another physician must be repeated. For this modifier to be utilized, the exact same CPT code (other than a pathology code) must have been previously submitted on a health claim by another physician. The modifier alerts the insurance company that a procedure was performed again by a different physician and that the claim is not a duplicate claim. Medical necessity must be clear.

EXAMPLE A patient was treated in the ER for epistaxis. The physician performed nasal cautery of the left nostril with packing. He submitted CPT code 30901–LT. Later that day, the patient returned to the

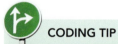

CODING TIP

Familiarity with Anesthesia Administration

Be able to recognize anesthetic drugs and anesthesia types to determine whether a patient was anesthetized before assigning modifiers −73 and −74.

ER and was seen by a different physician who performed the same procedure. He submitted 30901–LT–77 with a procedure note and letter explaining that the patient was seen earlier in the day by another physician who performed the same service.

Modifier −78, Unplanned Return to Operating/Procedure Room by the Same Physician Following the Initial Procedure for a Related Procedure During the Postoperative Period

Modifier −78 is used when the surgeon must perform additional surgery during the postoperative period for a reason related to the original surgery. A complication such as hemorrhaging, a failed flap or graft, or a hematoma that arose from the original procedure requires a return to the operating room (OR). Most payers recognize this as a secondary procedure for a related complication. The patient must be taken back to the OR or procedure room, not to an examining room. For the second procedure, the physician and facility must bill the code that best describes the procedures performed. If one does not exist, an unlisted procedure is filed. The original surgery code is used only if the exact same procedure was carried out a second time.

> **EXAMPLE** A patient returns for removal of internal fixation eighty days after the initial surgery. The patient had a joint replacement and would like the retained screws removed due to persistent pain and swelling. The doctor submits 20680–78 because the original procedure has a postoperative period of ninety days.

Modifier −79, Unrelated Procedure or Service by the Same Physician During the Postoperative Period

A physician may perform surgical or diagnostic services for a patient who had surgery performed by the same doctor within the postoperative period. The −79 modifier alerts the payer that the doctor was aware of the postoperative period restrictions, but that this procedure was unrelated to the previous encounter. Both the diagnosis and the procedure must be unrelated to the reason for the original surgery.

> **EXAMPLE** A patient was treated for ulnar nerve entrapment of the right elbow. Sixty days later the same neurosurgeon also performs a lumbar laminectomy due to a slipped disc The laminectomy code would be submitted with a −79 modifier.

Modifiers −80, −81, and −82, Assistant Surgeons and Minimum Assistant Surgeons

These modifiers are used to indicate that an assistant was required to perform the surgery. Minimum assistants do no hands-on care. It is used when a resident is not available (in teaching hospitals or rural hospitals usually) or there is no adequate training program for the medical specialty.

SUPPORTING DOCUMENTATION

When modifiers −21, −22, −23, −24, −25, −59, −76, −77, and −99 are reported, a claim attachment is submitted to describe the situation to the payer. A **special report** describing the details of the procedure is an example of this documentation; other examples are operative

CODING ALERT

Correct Documentation for Modifier −78

Do not assign this modifier for code descriptions using words like *subsequent*, *staged*, *related*, or *redo*.

BILLING TIP

Resetting Global Periods?

When a code is submitted with the −78 modifier, a new global period does not begin with the date of this service. The global period is determined by the original date of service.

CODING ALERT

Correct Use of Modifiers

Modifiers cannot be appended to Category II codes, Category III codes, unlisted codes, or add-on codes.

CODING ALERT

Medicare Modifier Tips

When reporting services to Medicare, do not use modifiers −32, −47, −63, −81, and −99.

reports and pathology reports. According to CPT, a special report should include:

- Nature, extent, and need for the procedure
- Time and effort and equipment used

The following information may also be included:

- Complexity of symptoms
- Final diagnosis
- Pertinent physical findings (sizes, extent, severity)
- Diagnostic and therapeutic procedures
- Concurrent related or unrelated problems
- Required follow-up

PAYER REQUIREMENTS

It is important to know each payer's requirements regarding modifier use. For example, CPT coding modifier information issued by CMS differs from the AMA's coding advice; therefore, not all modifiers are accepted by Medicare. Many other payer-specific modifiers apply to various coding situations. Coders learn these on the job. Medicaid in particular does not recognize most CPT modifiers and uses its own approved list of modifiers, which are spelled out in the corresponding payer manual or contract.

Accurate reporting of both CPT codes and modifiers is essential for correct coding and maximum appropriate reimbursement, as explained in the Reimbursement Review below.

BILLING TIP

Medicare Modifiers

Medicare periodically issues guidelines or clarification on modifier use and coding issues. Stay up to date with the most recent information via the CMS Website at www.cms.gov

Reimbursement Review

Outpatient Claims: Physician (Professional) Billing

Physicians bill for their professional services. When the place of service is the office or other nonhospital setting, the physician's payment includes an amount that accounts for the provision of the overhead and supplies. When the patient receives outpatient care at a facility or facility-owned place of service, the facility is permitted to bill for its part of the services (the room, and so on), and the physician bills for his or her part (the surgical or other procedural work). For example, a patient visit to a same-day surgery unit for a procedure on a bunion is billed by two entities, (1) the hospital outpatient facility and (2) the physician.

Physicians bill their medical services and procedures on the **837P** or its paper equivalent, the **CMS-1500** claim form. The professional claim format, as shown below, has two major sections. Blanks 1 through 13

are completed with information about the patient, including:

- The patient's health plan and identification number
- The patient's name, address, date of birth, and telephone number
- Data concerning the patient's employer, additional insurance coverage, and whether the claim involves an accident

The second section, made up of blanks 14 through 33, holds the data concerning the particular visit being billed, the dates and services/procedures, and the provider. Note in the illustration that the health plan is Medicare, the place of service is 11 (for office), and the CPT code is 99203. The related ICD-9-CM codes—essential for establishing the medical necessity of the claim—are 780.6 and 785.6. These codes mean that the patient saw the physician for evaluation of his complaints of fever and swollen glands.

1500

HEALTH INSURANCE CLAIM FORM

APPROVED BY NATIONAL UNIFORM CLAIM COMMITTEE 08/05

| | PICA | | | | | | | | | PICA | | |

1. MEDICARE [X] (Medicare #)   MEDICAID [ ] (Medicaid #)   TRICARE CHAMPUS [ ] (Sponsor's SSN)   CHAMPVA [ ] (Member ID#)   GROUP HEALTH PLAN [ ] (SSN or ID)   FECA BLK LUNG [ ] (SSN)   OTHER [ ] (ID)

1a. INSURED'S I.D. NUMBER (For Program in Item 1)
456 22 1234A

2. PATIENT'S NAME (Last Name, First Name, Middle Initial)
NAPJER JOHN D

3. PATIENT'S BIRTH DATE MM DD YY
05 05 1938   SEX M [X] F [ ]

4. INSURED'S NAME (Last Name, First Name, Middle Initial)

5. PATIENT'S ADDRESS (No., Street)
47 CARRIAGE DR

6. PATIENT RELATIONSHIP TO INSURED
Self [X] Spouse [ ] Child [ ] Other [ ]

7. INSURED'S ADDRESS (No., Street)

CITY
CHESHIRE
STATE
CO

8. PATIENT STATUS
Single [ ] Married [X] Other [ ]
Employed [ ] Full-Time Student [ ] Part-Time Student [ ]

CITY   STATE

ZIP CODE
80034
TELEPHONE (Include Area Code)
(720) 123 5555

ZIP CODE   TELEPHONE (INCLUDE AREA CODE)
(   )

9. OTHER INSURED'S NAME (Last Name, First Name, Middle Initial)

10. IS PATIENT'S CONDITION RELATED TO:

11. INSURED'S POLICY GROUP OR FECA NUMBER

a. OTHER INSURED'S POLICY OR GROUP NUMBER

a. EMPLOYMENT? (CURRENT OR PREVIOUS)
[ ] YES [X] NO

a. INSURED'S DATE OF BIRTH MM DD YY   SEX M [ ] F [ ]

b. OTHER INSURED'S DATE OF BIRTH MM DD YY   SEX M [ ] F [ ]

b. AUTO ACCIDENT?
[ ] YES [X] NO   PLACE (State)

b. EMPLOYER'S NAME OR SCHOOL NAME

c. EMPLOYER'S NAME OR SCHOOL NAME

c. OTHER ACCIDENT?
[ ] YES [X] NO

c. INSURANCE PLAN NAME OR PROGRAM NAME

d. INSURANCE PLAN NAME OR PROGRAM NAME

10d. RESERVED FOR LOCAL USE

d. IS THERE ANOTHER HEALTH BENEFIT PLAN?
[ ] YES [ ] NO   *If yes*, return to and complete item 9 a-d.

READ BACK OF FORM BEFORE COMPLETING & SIGNING THIS FORM.

12. PATIENT'S OR AUTHORIZED PERSON'S SIGNATURE I authorize the release of any medical or other information necessary to process this claim. I also request payment of government benefits either to myself or to the party who accepts assignment below.

SIGNED   SOF   DATE

13. INSURED'S OR AUTHORIZED PERSON'S SIGNATURE I authorize payment of medical benefits to the undersigned physician or supplier for services described below.

SIGNED

14. DATE OF CURRENT: MM DD YY   ILLNESS (First symptom) OR INJURY (Accident) OR PREGNANCY(LMP)
10 01 2008

15. IF PATIENT HAS HAD SAME OR SIMILAR ILLNESS. GIVE FIRST DATE MM DD YY

16. DATES PATIENT UNABLE TO WORK IN CURRENT OCCUPATION MM DD YY   FROM   TO

17. NAME OF REFERRING PHYSICIAN OR OTHER SOURCE

17a.
17b. NPI

18. HOSPITALIZATION DATES RELATED TO CURRENT SERVICES MM DD YY   FROM   TO

19. RESERVED FOR LOCAL USE

20. OUTSIDE LAB? $ CHARGES
[ ] YES [X] NO

21. DIAGNOSIS OR NATURE OF ILLNESS OR INJURY. (Relate Items 1,2,3 or 4 to Item 24e by Line)
1. 78.06
2. 78.56
3.
4.

22. MEDICAID RESUBMISSION CODE   ORIGINAL REF. NO.

23. PRIOR AUTHORIZATION NUMBER

24. A. DATE(S) OF SERVICE

	From MM DD YY	To MM DD YY	B. PLACE OF SERVICE	C. EMG	D. PROCEDURES, SERVICES, OR SUPPLIES (Explain Unusual Circumstances) CPT/HCPCS MODIFIER	E. DIAGNOSIS POINTER	F. $ CHARGES	G. DAYS OR UNITS	H. EPSDT Family Plan	I. ID. QUAL.	J. RENDERING PROVIDER ID.#
1	10 02 2008		11		99203	1,2	95 00	1		NPI	8221238999
2										NPI	
3										NPI	
4										NPI	
5										NPI	
6										NPI	

25. FEDERAL TAX I.D. NUMBER   SSN EIN
123 45 9666   [X] [ ]

26. PATIENT'S ACCOUNT NO.
NAP0123

27. ACCEPT ASSIGNMENT? (For govt. claims, see back)
[X] YES [ ] NO

28. TOTAL CHARGE
$ 95 00

29. AMOUNT PAID
$ 0 00

30. BALANCE DUE
$ 95 00

31. SIGNATURE OF PHYSICIAN OR SUPPLIER INCLUDING DEGREES OR CREDENTIALS (I certify that the statements on the reverse apply to this bill and are made a part thereof.)

SIGNED   SOF   DATE

32. SERVICE FACILITY LOCATION INFORMATION
SAME

a. NPI   b.

33. BILLING PROVIDER INFO & PHONE # (720) 554 1222
CENTER CLINIC
3810 EXECUTIVE BLVD
RAYTOWN CO 80033

a. 4455667788   b.

NUCC Instruction Manual available at: www.nucc.org

Checkpoint 6.4

Provide the correct modifier for each of the following descriptions.

1. Multiple modifiers _____
2. Distinct procedural service _____
3. Prolonged Evaluation and Management service _____
4. Staged procedure _____
5. Assistant surgeon _____
6. Discontinued procedure after sedation was started; service is being reported by a hospital outpatient facility _____
7. Repeat procedure by same physician _____
8. Unusual anesthesia _____
9. Mandated services _____
10. Surgical team _____

CPT Updates

INTERNET RESOURCE
AMA CPT Updates
www.ama-assn.org/go/cpt

INTERNET RESOURCE
Category II Codes
www.ama-assn.org/ama/pub/category/10616.html

INTERNET RESOURCE
Category III Codes
www.ama-assn.org/ama/pub/category/3885.html

INTERNET RESOURCE
AMA Website for Errata Data
www.ama-assn.org/ama/pub/category/3896.html

New, deleted, and changed CPT codes are released by the AMA in October of each year and go into effect every January 1. Category II and Category III codes are updated twice a year, on July 1 and January 1. Why is the CPT code set updated so often? Medicine is always changing rapidly; new technology makes new procedures available; and other procedures need to be more accurately described. The AMA CPT Editorial Panel makes CPT changes its members feel best represent medical practices.

Coders must access the current year's codes to guarantee submission of correct codes and to obtain correct and timely reimbursement. If valid codes are not submitted, reimbursement will be delayed or claims will be denied. Coding managers, office managers, and business offices must be sure to update software programs such as practice management programs (PMP) and charge description masters (CDM) with new and revised codes and must remember to delete old codes to ensure submission of the most accurate and current codes.

To stay current, providers access the AMA's CPT website, which has information on updates to the CPT code set.

Each year when the current version of CPT is published, the AMA also publishes errata that list corrections to the manual. Coders can find the errata at the AMA's CPT Website under CPT Code Information and Education. Coders should make notes in their CPT books to fix the errors. This may appear cumbersome, but it takes only a few minutes.

The American Health Information Management Association (AHIMA) along with the American Academy of Professional Coders (AAPC) offer many avenues to stay abreast of CPT changes

232 *Part 3* | Introduction to CPT
CPT only © 2007 American Medical Association. All rights reserved.

and updates. Each organization publishes professional journals and newsletters to notify members of changes. Both also provide educational seminars, administer coding certification exams, and offer a means of networking with coders. AHIMA posts links to the *Federal Register* along with many other helpful resources on its website. Joining these national organizations is paramount and promotes a level of quality and professionalism that cannot be overestimated.

A Review: ICD-9-CM and CPT Comparison

Initially, it is possible to confuse ICD-9-CM and CPT concepts and conventions, but it is important for coders to understand key differences and similarities between the two coding methodologies. In some courses, ICD-9-CM is taught before CPT, while for others, it is the opposite. This review provides an opportunity to confirm the basic differences between the two code sets.

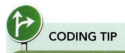

CODING TIP

CPT Crosswalk

Appendix M in CPT lists codes that have been deleted and provides a crosswalk to the current year's correct codes that replace them.

BILLING TIP

Question Whether the Payer's Codes Are Up to Date

Insurance carriers often fall behind in updating their computer systems. Watch for claim denials when submitting new codes during the first quarter of the year.

Table 6.6 ICD-9-CM Compared to CPT

	ICD-9-CM	CPT
Code Length	Diagnoses are three, four, or five digits. E and V codes are made up of the letter and three or four digits. Procedures are three or four digits.	Category I codes are five digits. Category II and Category III codes are four digits and an alphanumeric character.
Decimal Point	Used in diagnosis and procedure codes	Not used
Medical Settings	Volumes 1 and 2 diagnosis codes are used in all settings. Volume 3 procedure codes are used in inpatient hospital facility reporting only.	Used in all outpatient settings. Never used in inpatient facility reporting.
Maintained Primarily by	NCHS (Volumes 1 and 2); CMS (Volume 3)	American Medical Association
Updated	Twice a year; updates take effect each April 1 and October 1.	Category I code updates are released October 1 for use January 1 of the following year. Category II and III codes are prereleased on the AMA website every six months and can be used when they appear.
Official Coding Guideline Source	*Coding Clinic* by the AHA	*CPT Assistant* by the AMA
Modifier Use	None	HCPCS Level I and Level II
Content	Diagnosis and procedure codes	Procedure codes only

How to Assign CPT Codes and Modifiers

To assign CPT codes to procedures or services, follow the process outlined in Figure 6.3 and described below.

STEP 1 REVIEW THE COMPLETE MEDICAL DOCUMENTATION

To code for professional services, the coder first reads the documentation, which is made up primarily of reports created by a physician with other supporting medical documents, and determines where the service took place (the *place of service*) and the health plan (payer) if applicable. For CPT codes to apply, the provider is a physician or other professional practitioner (not an inpatient facility). These points are checked:

- The patient may be cared for as an outpatient or an inpatient. The patient's age and gender should be verified.
- The place of service may be an office, a facility, or another health care setting.
- The payer may be a private or self-funded payer, a government payer (Medicare, Medicaid, TRICARE, or CHAMPVA); or a *self-pay,* the term used when the patient is responsible for the bills.

STEP 2 ABSTRACT THE MEDICAL PROCEDURES THAT SHOULD BE CODED

Based on the documentation, the coder sorts out the procedures and other services the patient received. For medical services, the description is carefully noted; for surgeries, the operative report states the procedure that was performed.

STEP 3 IDENTIFY THE MAIN TERM AND RELATED TERMS

Identify all main terms and related terms for the abstracted procedures. Look for action words or sentences by locating the:

- Procedure or service (such as biopsy, evaluation and management, or laparoscopy)
- Organ or body part (such as intestines, prostate, or bladder)

CODING ALERT

Do Not Code from the Index

Never code directly from the CPT index. The index is just a way of putting you in the approximate area in the appropriate section.

CODING TIP

Read Code Descriptions Carefully

Pay close attention to code descriptions for wording both with and without age-specific notations, the sex of the patient, and punctuation.

- Condition or disease being treated (such as abscess, varicose veins)
- Common abbreviation (such as ECG or CT)
- Eponym (such as McBride operation)
- Symptom (for example, laceration repair, tongue)

STEP 4 LOCATE THE TERMS IN THE CPT INDEX

Locate the procedures in the index at the back of CPT. Locate all main terms (based on the medical terminology in the documentation), accounting for significant procedures or services performed. For each entry, a listing of a code or **code range** directs the coder to the appropriate heading and procedure code(s) in CPT. Some entries have a *See* cross-reference or a *See also* to guide the coder to another index entry.

> **EXAMPLE**
> Code Range Index Entry
> X-RAY
>   Abdomen. 74000–74022

When a code range is listed, read the code descriptions for all codes within the range indicated in the index before assigning a final code. Pay very close attention to punctuation (semicolons, colons, parentheses). The recommended procedure is to also read the description of one code above and one code below the selected code to ensure that the selected code accurately reflects what has been done. The goal is to select the most specific code.

STEP 5 REVIEW THE CODES, DESCRIPTORS, AND NOTES

The next step is to review all possible codes in the CPT section that the index entries points to. Review any notes provided at the beginning of each subsection or the section guidelines, and check for notes directly under the code, within the code description, or after the code description. Parenthetical notes are located immediately above or below a code and apply to that code. They give directions to see other code ranges, use add-on codes, and so on. For example, in Figure 6.1 on page 208, a note below code 44005 directs the coder to 44180 for laparoscopic approach.

STEP 6 VERIFY THE CODE AGAINST THE DOCUMENTATION

Verify that the code description matches what was performed based on the documentation. At this point, choose the most appropriate code based on the service performed and the documentation provided.

STEP 7 ASSIGN CODES FOR ALL SIGNIFICANT SERVICES

If two distinct procedures or services were performed, both can be coded. Continue coding until all components of the procedure or service have been accounted for according to the directions in the CPT book.

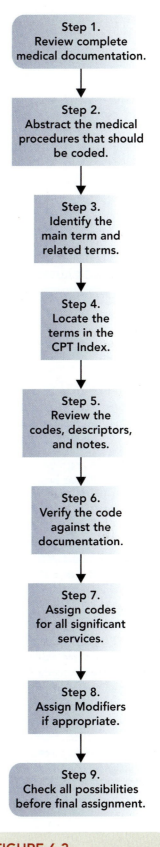

Step 1.
Review complete medical documentation.

Step 2.
Abstract the medical procedures that should be coded.

Step 3.
Identify the main term and related terms.

Step 4.
Locate the terms in the CPT Index.

Step 5.
Review the codes, descriptors, and notes.

Step 6.
Verify the code against the documentation.

Step 7.
Assign codes for all significant services.

Step 8.
Assign Modifiers if appropriate.

Step 9.
Check all possibilities before final assignment.

FIGURE 6.3
CPT Code Assignment Flow Chart

STEP 8 ASSIGN MODIFIERS IF APPROPRIATE

Correct use of modifiers is critical to compliant coding. Coders ask themselves the following questions when determining whether a modifier is required:

- Does the code description for the CPT code I want to assign already include identifiers such as unilateral or bilateral, biopsy(s), staged, or more than one occurrence?
- Will a modifier add more information or clarify any questions regarding the anatomic site (for example, −LT, T5)?
- Does CPT include several body parts in one code description? If so, using anatomic modifiers is incorrect because the code does not identify a specific part or side of the body.
- Will a modifier help eliminate the appearance of duplicate billing? Will it clarify that the same procedure was performed at the same time but on a different site?
- Will a modifier eliminate the appearance of incorrectly reporting multiple procedures? Remember that a separate procedure is typically bundled into a more comprehensive procedure in that subsection if it is performed at the same time as a more complex procedure. In this case, a −59 modifier may apply.
- Will a modifier help explain the time frame within which a service was performed?
- Will a modifier help clarify what portion of a service or procedure was performed by an assistant or other care provider?
- Does the situation require the use of more than one modifier? If so, did I follow the proper sequencing of modifiers?
  - −99 modifier is sequenced first.
  - HCPCS Level I modifier that affects payment is sequenced second (−52, −22, −50, −74, and so on).
  - HCPCS Level II anatomic modifiers are sequenced third (−T1, −E3, −RT, and so on).
  - Remaining HCPCS Level I modifiers that do not affect payment follow.

Not all codes require a modifier. Double-check the code description before assigning −50, −51, or any anatomical modifiers. Look for language in the code description such as "both," "bilateral," "each," "single," "multiple," "each additional," "digit," and so on to assist in making a modifier selection.

STEP 9 CHECK ALL POSSIBILITIES BEFORE FINAL ASSIGNMENT

Coders discover that there is not a designated code in CPT for every procedure or service that may be provided. A procedure's inclusion or exclusion in the book does not indicate whether the AMA supports it. Nor does it mean that a procedure is or is not paid by insurance plans.

Never make a code "fit." If a code cannot be found that matches what was done, check the HCPCS code set, which may have new procedures that are not yet included in CPT. If the HCPCS does not include a code that fits, or if the payer does not accept HCPCS codes, next

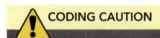

CODING CAUTION

Caution for −51 Assignment
Remember to not assign −51 modifiers to add-on codes, −51 modifier exempt codes, or unlisted procedure codes.

NOTE
HCPCS codes are explained in Chapter 10 of your program.

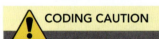

CODING CAUTION

Use Unlisted Code If There Is No Other Appropriate Choice
A code that is *close* to the actual procedure performed should not be used; instead, assign an unlisted procedure code. Before assigning an unlisted code, research the procedure performed and be as specific as possible. Also check HCPCS and Category III codes carefully to avoid assigning unlisted codes if possible.

COMPLIANCE GUIDELINE

Avoid Coding Errors
Trying to make an existing code "fit" is incorrect coding and may be classified as fraud.

check the Category III code section. Finally, if there is not an appropriate code in this section, assign an unlisted procedure code from the appropriate subsection. The guidelines at the beginning of each CPT section include a complete list of unlisted procedure codes available for use. Unlisted procedure codes are easy to identify because they always end in 9, much the same way the NEC code ends in 9 in ICD-9-CM.

CODING EXAMPLE

Using the flow chart in Figure 6.3, what code(s) would you assign to the service described in this example? Assign a modifier also, if needed. Knowing the site of service will enable you to select the correct modifiers, if needed.

EXAMPLE Imagine that you are coding for a physician's work (professional service) at an ambulatory surgery center (ASC). The female patient is fifty-seven years old and has Blue Cross and Blue Shield coverage (a private payer). She was admitted to the ambulatory surgery center for a left breast reconstruction with tissue expander insertion.

First step: Review the documentation and determine the provider, patient, place, and payer. In this example, you are working from a case scenario. The provider is the physician, and the patient is a fifty-seven-year-old female presenting for outpatient surgery. Place of service is an outpatient surgery facility. Blue Cross and Blue Shield is the payer.

Second step: The procedure is left breast reconstruction with tissue expander insertion.

Third step: Identify the main term in the procedural statement. There are actually three main terms to choose from: breast, insertion, and reconstruction.

Fourth step: Go to the index and look up the word *breast*. Scan the subterms for *reconstruction*. You will see many different entries under "reconstruction," with a code range of 19357–19369. You specifically want "reconstruction with tissue expander." Read farther until you find "with tissue expander": 19357.

Fifth step: Look up code 19357, checking all notes.

Sixth step: Double-check that the description of 19357 matches the procedure performed.

Seventh step: No additional procedures were documented.

Eighth step: Since the procedure was done on the left breast, you would assign an −LT modifier to reflect that this breast was operated on.

Ninth step: As a check, use another term to verify the code selection. Look up one of the other main terms, *reconstruction*. In this case, *reconstruction* is the main term and *breast* is the subterm. The code range is 19357–19369. Listed under "breast" are the same methods of reconstruction. You again choose "with tissue expander": 19357. There doesn't appear to be any alternative code to choose; 19357 is a perfect fit.

This scenario is one of many that demonstrate how the same code can be achieved by looking up different words, but always following the correct process.

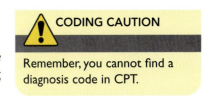

CODING CAUTION

Remember, you cannot find a diagnosis code in CPT.

List all possible index entries for locating the service, and then assign the code.

		Index Entry	Code
1.	Excision of mucous cyst of a finger:	Excision, Mucous cyst	26160
2.	Endoscopic biopsy of the nose:	_____	_____
3.	Laparoscopic meniscectomy of the right knee	_____	_____
4.	Drainage of a salivary gland cyst:	_____	_____
5.	Cystoscopy with fragmentation of ureteral calculus	_____	_____

CPT Coding Resources

The *CPT Professional Edition* is a more complete codebook than the Standard Edition for both beginning and seasoned coders. It has *CPT Assistant* references to expedite researching coding guidelines, along with anatomical and procedural pictures and color coding to assist in proper code assignment. In the *Professional Edition* the edges of the pages are color-coded, and thumb tabs also assist in locating sections of the book. Overall the format of both editions is the same.

Regardless of which specialty or setting a coder works in (physician office, ASC, hospital), there are numerous helpful publications. For example, *Anesthesia & Pain Management Coding Alert,* a newsletter published by The Coding Institute, is helpful in an anesthesia group practice or a pain management facility. Publishers provide references and books geared toward individual specialties For example, Ingenix publishes a *Coding Companion for Ophthalmology* that would be beneficial to an ophthalmologist's practice.

The Office of the Inspector General (OIG) recommends that the following resources be made available and used by coding and billing staff:

- Medical dictionary
- An anatomy and physiology text or atlas
- Current ICD-9-CM codebook
- Current CPT codebook
- Current HCPCS codebook
- *Physician's Desk Reference*
- *Merck Manual*
- Contractor's provider manual
- Up-to-date subscription to the AHA *Coding Clinic*
- Up-to-date subscription to the AMA *CPT Assistant*
- For Medicare billing, the National Correct Coding Initiative (CCI), which can be accessed online at www.cms.hhs.gov/NationalCorrectCodInitEd and coverage information online at http://www.cms.hhs.gov/center/coverage.asp

COMPLIANCE GUIDELINE

Stay Up to Date

Be sure to always use a current edition of any codebook.

You will also want to become familiar with these additional CPT references:

- General Medicare information at www.cms.hhs.gov
- *Coders Desk Reference for Procedures* published by Ingenix, an excellent reference that includes all medical and surgical CPT codes (with the exception of E/M codes) with plain English descriptions of the services provided for each CPT code (information online at www.ingenix.com)
- *Medicare Part B News* on Medicare topics and *Specialty Coder's Pink Sheets* published by Decision Health, which cover coding and billing topics across many specialties; information online at www.decisionhealth.com
- AMA's website (www.ama-assn.org), where coders can submit questions for official direction, read responses to frequently asked questions, and read clinical vignettes with official advice on troublesome or confusing topics

Accurate coding is the first step in obtaining the reimbursement that physicians or facilities have earned. Accurate and consistent coding is achieved through a thorough understanding of CPT. Stay informed of changes and updates by reading recommended periodicals and attending seminars to ensure that your coding is both accurate and consistent.

Summary

1. The CPT code set is used for many purposes. Information gathered from CPT code reporting is used for trending outpatient services, benchmarking services provided, and measuring and improving quality of patient services in addition to being the principal means of communicating with insurance carriers for reimbursement of professional services. CPT provides a system for coding and reporting professional medical and surgical procedures.

2. All outpatient medical and surgical settings are required to report CPT codes for services performed. Facilities report CPT codes for outpatient procedures. CPT codes are submitted by physicians and select allied health professionals to describe professional services rendered regardless of location or type of service.

3. The content and organization of the CPT printed manual are standardized throughout. The CPT codes are listed in three categories: Category I, Category II, and Category III. The book begins with an Introduction followed by six sections of Category I codes, a section of Category II codes, a section of Category III codes, and appendixes. The index is located at the very end of the book. All terms and abbreviations are in alphabetical order.

4. Symbols and punctuation are important features of CPT. Consistently acknowledging symbols and punctuation is important in proper code selection. A legend is located at the bottom of each page with definitions of symbols. Symbols are also described in the Introduction. The lightning bolt symbol (⚡) signifies that the vaccine code is for a product that is pending FDA approval. The bullet (•) designates a new code for that year. The triangle (▲) signifies a revised code, meaning that the descriptor is revised in some way. The semicolon (;) is used to conserve space and to identify and divide the common portion of the code from the unique portion. The plus (+) symbol identifies an add-on code. The symbol ⊘ indicates that a code cannot be assigned a –51 modifier. Facing triangles (►◄) before a code indicate that the text is new or has been revised from the prior year's edition. A circled bullet ⊙ before a code indicates that conscious sedation is included in the service or procedure.

5. Modifiers are reported along with CPT codes to describe events that modified the procedure or service; they do not change the basic meaning of the code. They are located on the inside cover of the CPT codebook. Modifiers are divided into categories for use by hospitals and by physicians. Modifiers for facilities are listed under the heading "Modifiers Approved for Hospital Outpatient Use." Anatomical modifiers or HCPCS modifiers are also located here under the heading "Level II (HCPCS/National)." Not all codes require modifiers. Procedures performed on fingers, toes, eyelids, and coronary vessels require HCPCS Level II anatomical modifiers. Refer to Tables 6.3 and 6.4 for a thorough review.

6. Always use a current edition of a codebook for the most up-to-date codes. Payment will be delayed or claims denied if valid codes are not submitted.

7. Coders must understand the key differences and similarities of ICD-9-CM and CPT in order to correctly assign codes in the appropriate setting. ICD-9-CM diagnosis codes are submitted for inpatient, outpatient, facility, and professional claims alike. ICD-9-CM procedure codes are submitted by the facility for inpatient procedures only. CPT codes are submitted for all outpatient services for both the facility and professional.

8. References are tailored to specialties and work settings. Regardless of work setting, all coders should have access to *CPT Assistant;* the current ICD-9-CM, CPT, and HCPCS code books; a medical dictionary; Medicare Correct Coding Edits; an anatomy book or body atlas; and Medicare Local Coverage Determinations. The *Coding Clinic* and *Merck Manual* are primarily utilized by hospitals and are an absolute necessity for inpatient coders.

9. Do not make a code fit. Assign a HCPCS code, a Category III code, or an unlisted code for services not located in CPT. Unlisted procedure codes are used when a service has no designated Category I, Category II, or Category III code. A special report must be submitted when modifiers that affect payment are assigned.

10. There are nine steps to follow when assigning a CPT code:

    a. Review the complete medical documentation.

    b. Abstract the medical procedures that should be coded.

    c. Identify the main and related terms for the procedures to be coded.

    d. Locate these terms in the CPT Index. Read the descriptions for all codes within the code range.

    e. Review the codes, descriptors, and notes. Follow cross-references located in the index and respective subsection of CPT. Read the guidelines at the beginning of the chapter and section. Read any instructional notes above or below the code.

    f. Verify that the code description matches the services described in documentation.

    g. Assign codes for all significant services and distinct procedures.

    h. Assign applicable modifier(s) based on documentation and code description language.

    i. Check all possible sources for hard-to-locate codes; report HCPCS, Category III, or unlisted codes for services when required by the situation.

Review Questions: Chapter 6

Match the key terms with their definitions.

    a. special report _____

    b. significant procedure _____

    c. separate procedure _____

    d. Category III codes _____

    e. surgical package _____

    f. postoperative period _____

    g. Category II codes _____

    h. add-on code _____

    i. unlisted code _____

    j. modifier _____

1. A major professional service

2. Temporary codes for emerging technology, services, and procedures

3. Procedure code that groups related procedures under a single code

4. A service that is not listed in CPT and requires a special report

5. The period of care following a surgical procedure

6. CPT codes that are used to track performance measures

7. Information that must accompany the reporting of an unlisted code

8. A procedure usually done as an integral part of a surgical package, but that may be reported if performed alone or along with other procedures but for a separate purpose

9. A secondary procedure that is performed with a primary procedure and that is indicated in CPT by a plus sign (+) next to the code

10. A two-character addition to a CPT code indicating that special circumstances were involved with a procedure, such as a reduced service or a discontinued procedure

Decide whether each statement is true or false.

1. Inclusion of a code in CPT indicates that it is covered by insurance. **T or F**

2. Specific guidelines are found at the end of each section of the book. **T or F**

3. CPT codes listed as "(separate procedure)" must be coded separately from the primary procedure. **T or F**

4. The unique portion of the CPT code follows the semicolon. **T or F**

5. Codes that begin with 99 are unlisted Medicine section codes. **T or F**

6. CPT codes cannot be located in the index by looking up a diagnosis as the main term. **T or F**

7. CPT codes are submitted to insurance companies only for services provided by a physician. **T or F**

8. Unlisted procedure codes can never be reported to Medicare. **T or F**

9. It is permissible to code directly from the index in situations where there is only one code choice listed. **T or F**

10. Modifiers are used to indicate when a procedure was modified and the description changed. **T or F**

11. Category III codes are not required for reporting because they are for emerging technology and are considered temporary codes. **T or F**

12. Under HIPAA, HCPCS codes are used for all payers. **T or F**

13. CPT codes are reported for inpatient procedures only. **T or F**

14. All payers recognize all HCPCS Level I and Level II modifiers. **T or F**

15. One of the CPT appendixes contains clinical examples of the codes in the E/M section. **T or F**

Select the letter that best completes the statement or answers the question.

1. Add-on codes can be identified by the following criteria.
   a. They can never stand alone and must be reported with another service.
   b. The code describes additional anatomic sites where the same procedure is performed.
   c. The code is marked with a • in the codebook.
   d. The code can be used with a −51 modifier.
   e. all of the above
   f. a and b only
   g. a, b, and d only

2. Which of the following is the symbol for a new CPT code?
   a. ⊙
   b. ⊃
   c. •
   d. ▲

3. Which of the following contains a complete list of modifier −51 exempt codes?
   a. Appendix F
   b. Appendix A
   c. Index
   d. Appendix E

4. Review the code range 20526–20610. What is the correct code assignment for injection of a carpometacarpal joint?

   a. 20550   c. 20526
   b. 20600   d. 20610

5. Which of the following symbols signifies a revised code?

   a. ⊙   c. •
   b. ➲   d. ▲

6. Which of the following would be considered a Medicine code?

   a. 99212   c. 0123T
   b. 72100   d. 93743

7. What is the correct code assignment for removal of impacted cerumen from both ears?

   a. 69200–50   c. 69210
   b   69210–50   d. 69210–RT, −LT

8. Which modifier would the physician assign to indicate that only a portion of a planned procedure was completed?

   a. −22
   b. −53
   c. −26
   d. −52

9. Additions, deletions, and revisions of codes from the prior year are listed in which appendix?

   a. B   c. G
   b. A   d. H

10. Which modifier is assigned to the code for postoperative care only following right inguinal hernia by another surgeon?

    a. −78   c. −54
    b. −55   d. −24

11. Which of the following identifies codes that are inclusive of conscious sedation?

    a. ⊙   c. ⤢
    b. ➲   d. ▲

12. Anesthesia services are organized by

    a. place of service   c. body site
    b. type of procedure   d. body system

13. A services not included in the surgery package is

    a. separate procedures
    b. routine follow-up from a surgical hysteroscopy
    c. office visit where decision for surgery was made
    d. pre-op appointment the day before the scheduled surgery

14. A patient is on vacation out of state and breaks the left ankle. The patient sees a doctor there who sets the fracture. The patient returns home several days later and will follow up with a local physician. The out-of-state physician will report which modifier?

    a. −55   c. −56
    b. −57   d. −54

15. A special report is required in the following circumstances.

    a. unlisted procedure code
    b. submitting modifier −22
    c. submitting modifier −59
    d. all of the above

1. Which organization developed and maintains CPT codes and guidelines? _____

2. Using CPT, refer to the notes immediately preceding the code 45300 and to the code series 45300–45378. Then answer this question: if a colonoscopy is incomplete, but full preparation for the procedure has been done, which modifier should be used? _____

3. When are updated CPT codes released? As of what annual date do they go into effect? _____

4. The + symbol indicates that this is an _____ code.

5. The ⊘ symbol indicates that the _____ modifier does not apply.

6. When a procedure is marked "separate procedure," you can bill for it if it was _____, for a _____, and _____ of any other related service provided.

7. A(n) _____ procedure code is used when there is no other designated code to describe a procedure or service.

8. A CPT code can be located in the index by looking for the _____ or service performed; _____ for which the patient is being treated; _____, _____, _____ site; or _____.

9. When you see the ▲ symbol in front of a code, what do you know about the code? _____

10. In the following list, label each entry as a section, procedure, heading, subcategory, or subsection.
    Excision _____
    Surgery _____
    Salivary gland and ducts _____
    Excision of submandibular gland _____
    Digestive _____

Applying Your Knowledge

BUILDING CODING SKILLS

Case 6.1

Identify the specific section and heading of CPT where the following codes are located.

1. 21300 _____
2. 81000 _____
3. 1000F _____
4. 12020 _____
5. 99282 _____

Case 6.2

Answer the following questions.

1. List two modifiers (not physical status modifiers) that describe anesthesia services.

2. Name three instances in which the −51 modifier is not appropriate to append.

Case 6.3

Identify the main terms in the following statements.

1. Modified McBride bunionectomy _____

2. Arthroscopic distal claviculectomy _____

3. Sinus endoscopy with concha bullosa resection _____

4. Insertion of tunneled centrally inserted central venous access device

_____

5. Replacement of pacemaker generator _____

Case 6.4

Assign the codes for the following.

1. Percutaneous needle core biopsy of the breast _____

2. Injection carpal tunnel ligament _____

3. Open biopsy, vertebral body, thoracic _____

4. Removal of anal seton _____

Case 6.5

With the use of the CPT section guidelines, identify the following unlisted procedure codes.

1. Medicine: Special dermatological service _____

2. Surgery—Digestive: Unlisted laparoscopy procedure, biliary tract

_____

Case 6.6

Assign the most appropriate modifier to each of the following statements.

1. Surgeon administers a regional Bier block because of ruptured sutures _____

2. Patient hemorrhaged heavily during surgery; procedure took twice as long as is typically required _____

3. Surgeon repairs the flexor tendon of the right foot and excises a ganglion on the right fourth toe _____

4. During an operation, a thoracic surgeon provides surgical access to the spine while an orthopedist performs a spinal fusion _____

_____

5. Surgeon performs part of a procedure _____

6. Patient is returned to the operating room three hours after surgery; service is being billed by a hospital outpatient facility _____

_____

7. Patient fractured his tibia in Vermont while skiing. The surgery to repair the tibia was performed in Vermont. The patient was so anxious to get back home that he left the day after surgery and returned to his own orthopedist, who did all the follow-up care. _____

8. After mammography findings of a density in both breasts, a patient undergoes puncture aspiration of a cyst in each breast. _____

9. A radiologist who is not employed by the hospital provides the reporting function for all X-rays taken at the hospital. What modifier is used to reflect her services? _____

10. During the performance of a left lung lobectomy, a surgeon discontinues the surgery when he realizes the patient is going into shock. _____

11. Elective cancellation of a bunionectomy (28296) prior to prepping the patient's skin and transport to the OR. You are coding for the OP facility in this situation. _____

12. Excision of nail for permanent removal (11750) of the great right toe _____

13. Bilateral nasal endoscopy with anterior ethmoidectomy (31254) _____

14. An orthopedist examines a patient and determines that he has a ruptured C3–C4 intervertebral disk with severe radiating pain to the right arm. The orthopedist fully examines the patient's history and performs X-rays and complete physical. After reviewing the films, the orthopedist requests that a neurologist perform the actual surgery since the orthopedist does not routinely perform surgery on the cervical spine. The orthopedist will submit the surgical code for this procedure along with the _____ modifier.

Researching the Internet

1. Visit the website of the American Medical Association at www.ama-assn.org. Under the banner *CPT Codes and Resources,* read the information on the CPT process, and report on how new CPT codes are approved. Then go to the following site and read more information about the background and development of Category III codes: www.ama-assn.org/ama/pub/category/12886.html

   Assume that you are working as a coder. Based on the update schedule for Category III codes, what advice would you provide about when to update your resources for selecting these codes?

2. Medical societies such as the American Academy of Family Physicians also offer Internet tools to support their coding. Research this site at www.aafp.org, and locate this year's CPT code updates. Prepare a report on other information that you consider valuable from this website.

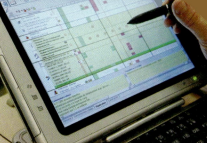
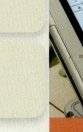

CPT: Evaluation and Management Codes

LEARNING OUTCOMES

After studying this chapter, you should be able to:

1. Describe the organization of the CPT Evaluation and Management (E/M) section.

2. Discuss the use of the section guidelines as a resource for E/M coding.

3. List five questions that are used to select appropriate E/M code ranges and assign correct codes.

4. State the difference between new and established patients in CPT terms.

5. Discuss the three key components that determine the level of service, listing the four levels of each.

6. Describe the process used to determine the level of service for E/M coding, including the part played by the contributing components.

7. Compare and contrast consultations and new patient (referral) E/M services.

8. Discuss the factors that are important in assigning critical care codes.

9. Define observation and standby services.

10. Assign CPT E/M codes, correctly applying the rules and exceptions for each category of service.

Key Terms

category

chief complaint (CC)

consultation

consulting physician

contributory components

coordination of care

counseling

critical care

direct care

E/M components

established patient

evaluation and management (E/M) codes

examination

face-to-face time

family history

history

history of present illness

key components

level of service (LOS)

medical decision making (MDM)

new patient

1995 Documentation Guidelines

1997 Documentation Guidelines

observation

past history

place of service (POS)

presenting problem

preventive medicine

problem-oriented

professional services

referral

referring physician

review of systems

roll-up rule

social history

standby

time

unit/floortime

Chapter Outline

Introduction to E/M Codes

Determining the Level of Service

E/M Flow Chart and Matrix

Office or Other Outpatient Services

Hospital Observation Services

Hospital Inpatient Services

Consultations

Emergency Department (ED) Services

Critical Care Services

Nursing Facility Services

Domiciliary, Rest Home, or Custodial Care Services

Domiciliary, Rest Home, or Home Care Plan Oversight Services

Home Services

Prolonged Services

Physician Standby Services

Case Management Services

Care Plan Oversight Services

Preventive Medicine Services

Newborn Care

Non-Face-to-Face Physician Services

Special Evaluation and Management Services

Modifier −25

This chapter covers coding services that are a core responsibility of physicians: services to assess the nature of the patient's condition and to devise a plan to treat it. This work is done by all medical specialties in the multitude of settings where patients are seen, from the practice office to every type of health care facility. Although these medical services have in common the formal name *evaluation and management,* the time, effort, and training required to perform them varies widely according to the situation. Compare, for example, diagnosing and casting a broken bone of a young, healthy child with handling multiple fractures after an accident for an elderly, frail patient. Because they do vary so widely, many of these services are paid on a scale that reflects time, effort, and complexity. Medical coders who know the guidelines and payer regulations for accurate, complete, and compliant coding of these services are valuable to their employers. They can improve coding accuracy, reimbursement, and compliance through their coding efforts.

Introduction to E/M Codes

Evaluation and management (E/M) codes represent the physician's *evaluation* of a patient's condition and *management* of a patient's care. First developed in 1992 by the American Medical Association (AMA), E/M codes are used by every type of physician to report patients' encounters for health-related problems. They are considered the *cognitive* codes because physicians must gather and analyze information regarding each patient to make a decision about the condition and determine how to manage it. Because they are used so often and so widely, the E/M codes and section guidelines are listed first in CPT.

EVALUATION AND MANAGEMENT CODE ORGANIZATION

The E/M section of CPT is divided into **categories** and subcategories that specifically define the services provided and reported by the physician, as shown in Table 7.1.

BASIC SELECTION PROCESS

Working with E/M codes requires an understanding of the structure of the E/M section. This is best learned by studying a standard set of five questions the coder answers to locate the correct code range in the E/M categories and then to pick the correct code:

1. Who is the patient?
2. What is the place of service?
3. What is the patient's status?
4. What type of service is being provided?
5. What level of service is being provided?

1. Who Is the Patient? In the first step in the E/M coding process, the coder identifies and categorizes the patient. Reviewing the column of subcategories in Table 7.1, the terms *new patient* and *established patient* recur, as do various terms that describe a patient's age and other characteristics.

Table 7.1 E/M Categories and Subcategories

Category	Subcategory	Code Range
Office or outpatient services	New patient	99201–99205
	Established patient	99211–99215
Hospital observation services	Discharge services	99217
	Initial services	99218–99220
Hospital inpatient services	Initial hospital care	99221–99223
	Subsequent hospital care	99231–99233
	Same-day admission and discharge	99234–99236
	Discharge services	99238–99239
Office or outpatient consultations	Initial consultations	99241–99245
Hospital consultations	Initial consultations	99251–99255
Emergency department services		99281–99288
Pediatric patient transport		99289–99290
Critical care services	Adult	99291–99292
	Pediatric	99293–99294
	Neonatal	99295–99296
Continuing intensive care services		99298–99300
Nursing facility services	Initial care	99304–99306
	Subsequent care	99307–99310
	Discharge services	99315–99316
	Other	99318
Domiciliary, rest home, custodial	New patient	99324–99328
	Established patient	99334–99337
	Oversight services	99339–99340
Home services	New patient	99341–99345
	Established patient	99347–99350
Prolonged services	Direct patient contact	99354–99357
	Without direct patient contact	99358–99359
Standby services		99360
Case management services	Anticoagulant management	99363–99364
	Medical team conferences	99366–99368
Care plan oversight		99374–99380
Preventive medicine	New patient	99381–99387
	Established patient	99391–99397
	Individual counseling	99401–99404
	Group counseling	99411–99412
	Other	99420–99429
Newborn care		99431–99440
Non-Face-to-Face Physician Services	Telephone services	99441–99443
	Online medical evaluation	99444
Special E/M services		99450–99456
Other E/M services		99477–99499

New Versus Established Patients Figure 7.1 is a flow chart for distinguishing between a new and an established patient for purposes of E/M coding. A **new patient:**

- Has not received any professional services from the physician within three years

    EXAMPLE Ms. Jones saw Dr. Abbot four years ago and schedules an appointment to be seen by him again. Dr. Jones will report a new patient code from 99201–99205.

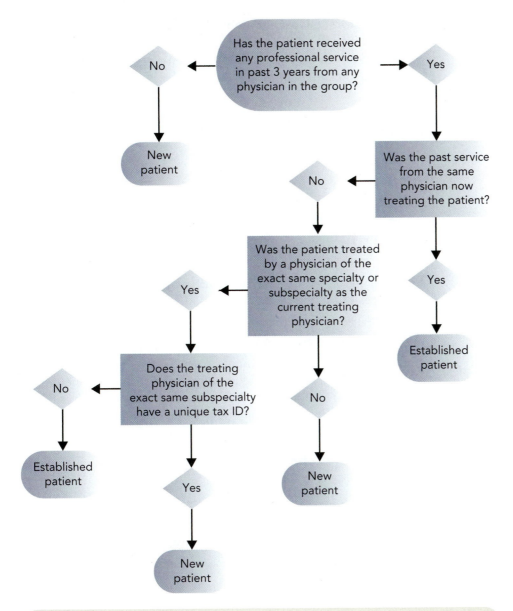

FIGURE 7.1
New Patient (99201–99205) Versus Established Patient (99211–99215) Flow Chart

- Has not received any professional services from another physician of the same specialty in the same group practice within three years

   EXAMPLE Ms. Jones saw Dr. Abbot's partner two years ago and makes an appointment to see Dr. Abbot. Dr. Abbot's partner is in the same specialty as Dr. Abbot. Dr. Abbot will report an established patient code from 99211–99215.

- May have received professional services from another physician in the same group who is in a different specialty within three years

   EXAMPLE Ms. Jones saw Dr. Abbot's partner, a cardiologist, two years ago and makes an appointment to see Dr. Abbot, a gastroenterologist, whom she has not seen in four years. Dr. Abbot will report a new patient code from 99201–99205.

In contrast to a new patient is an **established patient,** a person who either has received professional services from the physician within the past three years or has received professional services from another physician of the same specialty in the same group practice within three years.

Patients Categorized by Age Often different age categories are important, such as:

- Neonate (birth to twenty-eight days)
- Pediatric (twenty-nine days to twenty-four months)
- Adult
- Specific age ranges, such as forty to sixty-four years in preventive medicine coding

NOTE

Appendix A lists the places of service that are generally recognized and the codes that represent them on health claims.

2. What Is the Place of Service (POS?)

The coder next determines the **place of service (POS),** which may be a physician office, hospital, nursing facility, or outpatient department of a facility such as an emergency department or an observation room.

3. What Is the Patient's Status?

The patient's status also points to the correct E/M code range by category or subcategory. Is the patient ill or injured? Is the patient critically ill? Does the patient need to be hospitalized? Is the patient presenting for an annual physical? Is the patient being cared for by an outside agency under supervision of the physician?

4. What Type of Service Is Being Provided?

The major types of care shown in Table 7.1 are:

- Initial care for a first visit for a particular problem
- Subsequent care for follow-up visits for a particular problem
- Prolonged care, meaning care provided for extended time periods
- Standby services, during which a physician is ready to provide services as needed

The coder identifies the type of service (care) that the physician provided to further narrow the possible code range options.

5. What Is the Level of Service?

Questions 1 through 4 help the coder select the correct range of E/M codes. The final step is to determine the **level of service (LOS)** that was provided to the patient, which permits choosing the specific code when a range is offered.

The possible levels are:

- Problem-focused (PF)
- Expanded problem-focused (EPF)
- Detailed (DET)
- Comprehensive (COMP)

The level of service is indicated in each of the code descriptions in the CPT E/M section.

EXAMPLE OF CODE SELECTION

The following example shows how to use the coder's E/M questions to narrow the options and select the correct code.

EXAMPLE A fifty-six-year-old male patient who has never been seen before by the physician has an office visit for left ankle pain caused by a fall.

The coder selects code range 99201–99205 to represent the services provided in *evaluating* the patient's left ankle pain and in determining how to *manage* the patient's condition. The factors used to decide the code range are:

Who is the patient?	New patient, adult
What is the place of service (POS)?	Office
What is the patient's status?	Injured, in pain
What type of service is being provided?	New, or initial care

The answers to questions 1 through 4 point to the range of codes from which a code will be picked. This was a *new* (question 1) *adult* (question 1) patient seen in the physician's *office* (question 2) for an *injury* (question 3). The care was *initial*, or new (question 4), because the visit was for a new injury. The next section explains how to follow a specific process to choose the level of service. If, in the example above, the level of service is determined to be detailed, the appropriate code from the new patient code range of 99201–99205 would be 99203.

Checkpoint 7.1

1. A forty-seven-year old patient was seen last month in the physician office for intermittent chest pain. He is seen today in the office to follow up on the results of medication prescribed during last month's visit and to follow up on his chest pain complaint which resolved with medication.
   - Who is the patient? _____
   - What is the place of service? _____
   - What is the patient's status? _____
   - What type of service is being provided? _____

2. A family with a three-year-old child has moved two hundred miles to a new home. The child became ill with a fever, and the parents have contacted a pediatrician so that the child can be evaluated and treated.
   - Who is the patient? _____
   - What is the place of service? _____
   - What is the patient's status? _____
   - What type of service is being provided? _____

Determining the Level of Service

Evaluation and management services are considered the foundation of physician services because they are provided by almost every specialty in the medical field. E/M codes represent approximately one-third of all charges reported to third-party payers. Because of the importance of E/M codes, third-party payers, auditors, and government agencies pay close attention to how physicians report them. Each E/M code has its own descriptor and key component requirements. Coders must understand the code distinctions to appropriately report E/M services. Determining the level of service is an essential responsibility of coders.

Selection of the level of service for E/M codes is based on the following factors, known as **E/M components** of the level of service:

- History
- Examination
- Medical decision making
- Counseling
- Coordination of care
- Nature of the presenting problem
- Time

The first three of these components (history, examination, and medical decision making, abbreviated H/E/MDM)) are considered the **key components** in selecting a level of service. The next four components (counseling, coordination of care, nature of presenting problem, and time) are considered **contributory components.**

The example in the previous section indicated a code range of 99201–99205 with a detailed level of service (99203). The physician and/or coder determines the LOS by examining the documentation of the key components of E/M coding (history, examination, and medical decision making) and applying the E/M coding guidelines to select a code. For example, the guidelines state that a detailed LOS for a new patient requires a detailed history, a detailed examination, and low medical decision making (MDM).

The information needed to determine the LOS appears in the code descriptions:

CODING TIP

Apply Key Components to Appropriate E/M Code Ranges

The process for identifying key components described here applies to all E/M code ranges that offer the choice of a level of service.

New Patient Codes

99201	Problem-focused history, problem-focused exam, straightforward MDM
99202	Expanded problem-focused history, expanded problem-focused exam, straightforward MDM
99203	Detailed history, detailed exam, low MDM
99204	Comprehensive history, comprehensive exam, moderate MDM
99205	Comprehensive history, comprehensive exam, high MDM

Established Patient Codes

99211	No key components required (code is described later in this chapter)
99212	Problem-focused history, problem-focused exam, straightforward MDM
99213	Expanded problem-focused history, expanded problem-focused exam, low MDM (note the difference from 99202)
99214	Detailed history, detailed exam, moderate MDM (note the difference from 99203)
99215	Comprehensive history, comprehensive exam, high MDM

Note that the three key component requirements for 99204 and 99205 differ only in the MDM.

STEP 1 DETERMINE THE HISTORY LEVEL

The term **history** describes the information that patients communicate to the physician both to explain their illnesses, injuries, and/or symptoms and in response to the physician's questions. History is considered *subjective* information that is provided in the patient's own words, and it is called the patient's **chief complaint (CC).** To determine the level of the history that is documented, the following information is required.

Required for problem-focused:
Chief complaint
Brief history of the present illness or problem

Required for expanded problem-focused:
Chief complaint
Brief history of the present illness or problem
Problem-pertinent system review

Required for detailed:
Chief complaint
Extended **history of present illness** or problem
Extended system review (more than just problem-pertinent)
Pertinent **past history, family history,** and/or **social history** directly related to the patient's problem

Required for comprehensive:
Chief complaint
Extended history of present illness or problem
Review of all body systems
Complete past, family, and social history (all three)

CODING TIP

PFSH

The history is often referred to as PFSH, for past, family, and social history. The patient's past history relates to the personal medical history. The family history reviews the medical events in the patient's family. It includes the health status or cause of death of parents, brothers and sisters, and children; specific diseases that are related to the patient's chief complaint or the patient's diagnosis; and the presence of any known hereditary diseases. The facts gathered in the social history, which depend on the patient's age, include marital status, employment, and other factors.

Checkpoint 7.2

What differentiates an expanded problem-focused history from a detailed history? List each element, and indicate whether it is different or the same.

_____

_____

_____

STEP 2 DETERMINE THE EXAMINATION LEVEL

The term **examination** describes the information a physician collects from examining the patient. The examination is considered *objective:* it is not based on feelings or the patient's interpretation; it is based on factual findings. To determine the level of the examination, the following information is required.

Required for problem-focused:
Limited exam of affected body area or organ system

Required for expanded problem-focused:
Limited exam of affected body area or organ system and other symptomatic or related organ systems

Required for detailed:
Extended exam of affected body area or organ system and other symptomatic or related organ systems

Required for comprehensive:
General multisystem exam or complete examination of a single organ system

STEP 3 DETERMINE THE MEDICAL DECISION-MAKING LEVEL

Medical decision making encompasses the complex process of establishing a diagnosis and determining how to treat or manage the diagnosed condition. Patients present to their physicians with symptoms. It is the physician's role to assess and evaluate those symptoms to determine the correct diagnosis and treatment.

> **EXAMPLE** A patient presents with a three-day history of red eye in the left eye. There is no trauma or foreign body irritation. The patient also complains of itching and discharge from the left eye. There is no evidence of any changes in the patient's vision.

At this point the physician reviews the patient's history, examines the patient, and then makes a decision about what is wrong with the patient.

For **medical decision making (MDM),** CPT departs from the range of problem-focused through comprehensive. Instead, the *level* of MDM can be straightforward, low complexity, moderate complexity, or high complexity. MDM rates how the physician puts all the patient encounter information together to assess the patient's condition and to plan the treatment of that condition. MDM is often referred to as the *assessment and plan*.

To rate the level of MDM, three measurements are considered:

1. The number of diagnoses or management options
2. The amount of and/or complexity of medical records, tests, and other information (data)
3. The risk of complications, morbidity, and/or mortality (overall risk)

Each of the three measurements is assessed and then put into a level as follows:

Straightforward:
1. Minimal diagnoses or management options
2. Minimal or no data
3. Minimal risk

Low complexity:

1. Limited diagnoses or management options
2. Limited data
3. Low risk

Moderate complexity:

1. Multiple diagnoses or management options
2. Moderate data
3. Moderate risk

High complexity:

1. Extensive diagnoses or management options
2. Extensive data
3. High risk

To assign one of the four levels level of MDM, coders will work with three scenarios of medical decision making. First, is the simplest scenario, when all three measurements are at the same level. As indicated in Table 7.2, if all three measurements are at the same level, select the type of decision making shown in that row.

> **EXAMPLE** A limited number of diagnoses, a limited amount of data reviewed, and low risk equal low-complexity decision making.

Second, when two of the three measurements are at the same level and one is at a lower level, disregard the lowest measurement, and base the level of decision making on the remaining two.

> **EXAMPLE** Multiple diagnoses, limited data review, and moderate medical decision making equal moderate complexity. The lowest measure is disregarded, and the decision-making level is based on the remaining two levels.

Third, when all three measurements are at different levels, disregard the lowest measurement, and base the level of decision making on the remaining two measurements. In this scenario, the lowest of the remaining two measurements controls the level of decision making.

> **EXAMPLE** Multiple diagnoses, extensive data review, and low risk equal moderate complexity. The lowest measure is disregarded, and the level of decision making is based on the lowest level of the remaining two measures.

The rule is that two of the three measurements must be at or above that particular level. This is usually phrased as "two of the three must meet or exceed that level." Table 7.2 lays out the MDM measurements and, in the fourth column, the type of decision making.

Table 7.2 Medical Decision Making

Number of Diagnoses or Management Options	Amount and/or Complexity of Data to Be Reviewed	Risk of Complications and/or Morbidity or Mortality	Type of Decision Making
Minimal	Minimal or none	Minimal	Straightforward
Limited	Limited	Low	Low complexity
Multiple	Moderate	Moderate	Moderate complexity
Extensive	Extensive	High	High complexity

EXAMPLE After assessing the patient, the physician determines that there are a *limited* number of diagnoses, which puts a check mark in the low MDM row. The physician has evaluated a *minimal* amount of data, which puts a check mark in the straightforward MDM row, and the overall risk for this patient's problem is *low*, putting another check mark in the low MDM row. The level of MDM that is assigned is low, since the guideline is "two out of three."

Similarly, the number of diagnoses might be *multiple*, the amount of data might be *limited*, and the overall risk might be *high*. With this not-uncommon scenario and using the criterion of "meet or exceed two of the three elements," the level of MDM is moderate.

In a case like this, the step-by-step process to assign an MDM level is as follows:

1. Analyze the MDM measurements, and record their levels:
   - Number of diagnoses is *multiple:* moderate MDM
   - Amount of data is *limited:* low MDM
   - Overall risk is *high:* high MDM

2. Drop the lowest measure of MDM, in this case the amount of data (low), and base the overall level of MDM on the remaining two measures, using the criterion that the lower of the two measures controls the level of MDM. The MDM is moderate.

Continuing the example of the patient with a red eye:

EXAMPLE After reviewing the patient's history and examining the patient, the physician determined that the patient had conjunctivitis of the left eye. The patient is to apply an over-the-counter ophthalmic solution twice a day for one week and also apply warm, moist compresses each morning.

The number of diagnoses or management options: *limited*

Amount and/or complexity of data: *none*

The risk of complications, morbidity, mortality: *low*

The MDM level: *low complexity*

Checkpoint 7.3

1. The physician determines that there are multiple diagnoses, limited data, and low risk based on the review of the history and performance of the examination. What is the level of MDM?

   _____

   _____

2. A patient who suffered a hip dislocation presents with leg and hip pain and chronic abdominal pain radiating into the chest. After obtaining the patient's history and performing an examination, the physician reviews an X-ray and blood work that was ordered and determines that the femur was injured in the course of treating the hip dislocation. The patient has been taking too much ibuprofen for the pain and now has gastroesophageal reflux. The physician prescribes physical therapy for the leg problem and medication for the reflux problem. Assess the three measurements of MDM, and give the level of MDM.

   _____

   _____

In summary, follow these steps to select a level of service:

1. Identify the category and subcategory.
2. Review the guidelines for that category and subcategory.
3. Review the code descriptions specific to that category and subcategory.
4. Determine the extent of history documented.
5. Determine the extent of examination documented.
6. Determine the extent of medical decision making documented.
7. Select the appropriate code based on the three key components.

EXAMPLE A new patient is being seen by a family practitioner. He mentions that he has begun to develop acne and is very self-conscious. He also has a rash on his leg. His physician obtains an expanded problem-focused (EPF) history, an EPF exam, and straightforward MDM.

How does a coder determine the LOS? Utilizing the instructions above:

1. New patient, adult
2. Patient has not been seen within three years
3. Requires three of three key components
4. EPF
5. EPF
6. Straightforward
7. Code that meets the requirements:
   - 99202: EPF history
   - 99202: EPF exam
   - 99202: Straightforward MDM

WORKING WITH THE LEVEL OF SERVICE REQUIREMENTS

To work with the level of service, coders need to know not only the three key components of E/M services but also which codes require all three key components and which require just two of the three key components:

Three Components	Two of Three Components
New patient: 99201–99205 Observation care: 99218–99220	Established patient: 99212–99215
Initial hospital care: 99221–99223	Subsequent hospital care: 99231–99233
Consultations: 99241–99255	
Emergency department: 99281–99285	
Nursing facility initial: 99304–99306	Nursing facility subsequent: 99307–99310
Domiciliary new patient: 99307–99310	Domiciliary established patient: 99334–99337
Home new patient: 99341–99345	Home established patient: 99347–99350

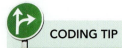

CODING TIP

Lowest Key Component Rule

In determining the LOS, the lowest key component controls the level that is assigned. In other words, the LOS can be no higher than the lowest key component.

The list appears both in the E/M guidelines in the CPT book and in each code descriptor in the E/M section.

For a code that requires all three key components, the key component at the lowest level controls the level of service. For example, if a physician examining a new patient documented a detailed history, a detailed exam, and straightforward medical decision making, the codes for each key component would be as follows:

EXAMPLE
99203: Detailed history
99203: Detailed exam
99202: Straightforward MDM

The component at the lowest level—the one that controls the level of service—is MDM, so the coder would report 99202 as the LOS. For the service to have been coded as 99203, the MDM complexity level would have had to be low.

If a code requires only two of the three key components to be used in determining the level of service, disregard the lowest key component, and base the level of service on the remaining two key components, still following the rule that the lowest key component of the remaining two controls the level of service. If the physician documented a detailed history, a detailed exam, and straightforward MDM for an established patient, the codes for the key components would be:

EXAMPLE
99214: Detailed history
99214: Detailed exam
99212: Straightforward MDM

The MDM level is disregarded because it is the lowest key component. Both of the remaining two key components are at the same level, and the service will be reported as 99214.

If, however, the three key components were at different levels for an established patient, the documentation might look like this:

EXAMPLE
99214: Detailed history
99213: Expanded problem-focused exam
99212: Straightforward MDM

The MDM level is disregarded because it is the lowest key component. Of the remaining two key components, the lowest, the exam, controls the level of service, and the service will be reported as 99213.

Checkpoint 7.4

Determine the level of service in the following scenario using both the new patient and the established patient criteria.

Key Components	New Patient LOS	Established Patient LOS
Expanded problem-focused history	_____	_____
Detailed exam	_____	_____
Moderate MDM	_____	_____

THE CONTRIBUTORY E/M COMPONENTS

Counseling, coordination of care, and the nature of the presenting problem are considered *contributory* factors in E/M coding. While they are important, these services do not have to be provided at every patient encounter.

Counseling The contributory component of **counseling** is a discussion with a patient and/or family about:

- Diagnostic results, impressions, and/or recommended diagnostic studies
- The prognosis
- The risks and benefits of management (treatment) options
- Instructions for management (treatment) and/or follow up
- The importance of compliance with chosen management (treatment) options
- Risk-factor reduction
- Patient and family education

Coordination of Care The **coordination of care** component involves a physician's work to coordinate a patient's care with other providers or agencies. For example, a patient may need to be set up with nursing care at home or may need to see other providers for more specific care (for example, a surgeon or physical therapist), or laboratory studies may need to be arranged.

Nature of the Presenting Problem The nature of the **presenting problem** is generally the reason for the patient's encounter with a physician. It can be a disease, a condition, an illness, an injury, a symptom, a sign, a finding, or a complaint. There are five types of presenting problems:

1. *Minimal:* The problem may not require the presence of a physician but is provided under a physician's supervision, such as a blood pressure check.
2. *Self-limited or minor:* The problem is transient, will not permanently alter a patient's health status, or has a good prognosis.
3. *Low severity:* The risk of becoming seriously ill (morbidity) without treatment is low; there is little or no risk of mortality (death) without treatment.
4. *Moderate severity:* The risk of morbidity and/or mortality without treatment is moderate.
5. *High severity:* The risk of morbidity without treatment is high, and the risk of mortality without treatment is moderate.

TIME

There are two measures of **time** in E/M coding: (1) **face-to-face time,** also referred to as direct time, and (2) **unit/floortime.** Direct time is associated with outpatient services and represents the time a physician spends with the patient obtaining history, providing the examination, and discussing the findings and plan. Unit/floortime represents care provided to the patient in a facility setting (such as a hospital or nursing home) and includes both care given at the bedside and services on the unit or floor where the patient is located, such as reviewing the patient's medical record, writing orders, or reviewing films or test results.

As a general guideline, neither face-to-face time nor unit/floortime should be considered a determining E/M component. Time is indicated in the code descriptors merely to represent averages or estimates of time associated with the levels of service. There is, however, one exception, which is discussed in the following section.

EXCEPTION TO THE KEY COMPONENT RULE: USING TIME AS THE DETERMINING FACTOR

Counseling and/or coordination of care are contributory components of E/M services. When one (or both) of them dominates (is more than 50 percent of) the physician-patient and/or physician-family encounter, time is the key or controlling factor in determining the level of service. The extent of the counseling and/or coordination of care must be documented in the medical record.

> **EXAMPLE** For more than a year, a patient has been treated by his nephrologist for kidney disease. At the current E/M encounter, the physician informs the patient that, based on previous examinations, lab results, and diagnostic tests, kidney transplant surgery is inevitable and recommends placing the patient's name on the transplant list. The patient is upset, and the physician spends 30 minutes of the 40-minute visit talking with the patient about the consequences, lifestyle impact, and family issues associated with transplant surgery.

Based on the physician's documentation:

- The encounter involved a problem-focused history, a problem-focused exam, and high MDM.
- Based on the key components only, the reportable code would be 99212.
- Based on the facts that the visit took 40 minutes and that 30 minutes were spent in counseling, the reportable code would be 99215.

CODING TIP

Time and LOS

The time for each E/M code is listed in the paragraphs below each code description.

Checkpoint 7.5

What is the correct established patient code for the following scenario? _____ Explain how you determined that level of service. _____

A patient has been treated for diabetes for four years and was most recently seen two weeks ago. During today's visit, after reviewing lab results and examining the patient, the physician determines that the patient will have to start insulin treatment immediately. The patient is upset because her mother was severely affected by long-term insulin use. The physician discusses the effects of insulin and its impact on lifestyle and health. The exam is expanded problem-focused, and the medical decision making is moderate. The physician spends 15 minutes of the 25-minute visit counseling the patient.

E/M Flow Chart and Matrix

In order to apply the E/M selection process, coders need to be familiar with the major categories and subcategories of E/M coding, which are discussed in the balance of this chapter. Figure 7.2 presents an E/M code selection flow chart. Coders should refer also to the E/M matrix in Table 7.3 to review the most common E/M services.

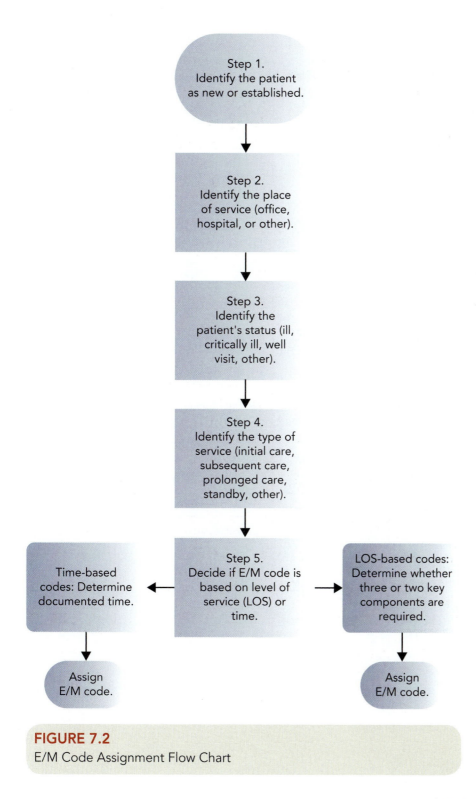

FIGURE 7.2

E/M Code Assignment Flow Chart

Table 7.3 | E/M Matrix

Codes	History	Exam	Medical Decision Making	Comments
Office/Outpatient ***New patient visits: requires 3 key components***				
99201 Problem-focused	Brief HPI* (1–3 elements)	1 body area and/or organ system	Straightforward	
99202 Expanded problem-focused	Brief HPI, review of 1 system	2–4 body areas and/or organ systems	Straightforward	
99203 Detailed	Extended HPI, review 2–9 systems, 1 of the 3 PFSH**	5–7 body areas and/or organ systems	Low complexity	
99204 Comprehensive	Extended HPI, review 10+ systems, 3 of the 3 PFSH	8 or more organ systems	Moderate complexity	
99205 Comprehensive	Extended HPI, review 10+ systems, 3 of the 3 PFSH	8 or more organ systems	High complexity	Level of medical decision making defines the difference between 99204 and 99205.
Established patient visits: requires 2 key components				
99211 Minimal				Visits that include physician involvement are not usually coded with 99211.
99212 Problem-focused	Brief HPI (1–3 elements)	1 body area and/or organ system	Straightforward	
99213 Expanded problem-focused	Brief HPI, review of 1 system	2–4 body areas and/or organ systems	Low complexity	
99214 Detailed	Extended HPI, review 2–9 systems, 1 of the 3 PFSH	5–7 body areas and/or organ systems	Moderate complexity	
99215 Comprehensive	Extended HPI, review 10+ systems, 2 of the 3 PFSH	8 or more organ systems	High complexity	
Consultations, new or established patients: requires 3 key components				
99241 Problem-focused	Brief HPI (1–3 elements)	1 body area and/or organ system	Straightforward	
99242 Expanded problem-focused	Brief HPI, review of 1 system	2–4 body areas and/or organ systems	Straightforward	
99243 Detailed	Extended HPI, review 2–9 systems, 1 of the 3 PFSH	5–7 body areas and/or organ systems	Low complexity	
99244 Comprehensive	Extended HPI, review 10+ systems, 3 of the 3 PFSH	8 or more organ systems	Moderate complexity	

*HPI: history of the present illness
**PFSH: past medical history, family history, and social history

Table 7.3 *(Continued)*

Codes	History	Exam	Medical Decision Making	Comments
99245 Comprehensive	Extended HPI, review 10+ systems, 3 of the 3 PFSH	8 or more organ systems	High complexity	Level of medical decision making defines the difference between 99244 and 99245.
Hospital *Initial care codes: requires 3 key components*				
99221 Detailed	Extended HPI, review 2–9 systems, 1 of the 3 PFSH	5–7 body areas and/or organ systems	Low complexity	
99222 Comprehensive	Extended HPI, review 10+ systems, 3 of the 3 PFSH	8 or more organ systems	Moderate complexity	
99223 Comprehensive	Extended HPI, review 10+ systems, 3 of the 3 PFSH	8 or more organ systems	High complexity	Level of medical decision making defines the difference between 99222 and 99223.
Subsequent care: requires 2 key components				
99231 Problem-focused	Brief HPI	1 body area and/or organ system	Straightforward or low complexity	
99232 Expanded problem-focused	Brief HPI, problem-pertinent ROS***	2–4 body areas and/or organ systems	Moderate complexity	
99233 Detailed	Extended HPI, review 2–9 systems, 1 of the 3 PFSH	5–7 body areas and/or organ systems	High complexity	
Initial consultations: requires 3 key components *New or established*				
99251 Problem-focused	Brief HPI (1–3 elements)	1 body area and/or organ system	Straightforward	
99252 Expanded problem-focused	Brief HPI, review of 1 system	2–4 body areas and/or organ systems	Straightforward	
99253 Detailed	Extended HPI, review 2–9 systems, 1 of the 3 PFSH	5–7 body areas and/or organ systems	Low complexity	
99254 Comprehensive	Extended HPI, review 10+ systems, 3 of the 3 PFSH	8 or more organ systems	Moderate complexity	
99255 Comprehensive	Extended HPI, review 10+ systems, 3 of the 3 PFSH	8 or more organ systems	High complexity	Level of medical decision making defines the difference between 99254 and 99255.

***ROS: *review of systems*

Office or Other Outpatient Services

99201–99205	New patient	Requires all 3 key components
99211–99215	Established patient	Requires 2 of 3 key components

Office or other outpatient services E/M codes represent the services provided to evaluate and manage the care of new or established patients in the physician office or other outpatient facility, such as an emergency department or an ambulatory surgical center. Tables 7.4 and 7.5 provide information on the key component requirements for using these codes.

> **EXAMPLE** Ms. Jones recently moved to Detroit and has not yet established herself with a new physician. When her pancreatitis flares up, she makes an appointment with Dr. Abbot. Dr. Abbot obtains a detailed history, does a detailed examination, and, after his assessment of the patient's condition, provides low medical decision making. Dr. Abbot will report code 99203.

PROFESSIONAL SERVICES AND NEW OR ESTABLISHED PATIENTS

As part of the definition of new and established patients, the AMA has specified that **professional services** are face-to-face services. Why? Review the example:

> **EXAMPLE** A patient with recurrent chest pain is hospitalized by his internist, and electrocardiograms (ECGs) are taken. The hospital contracts with a private cardiologist to review all hospital ECGs. The cardiologist reports the correct CPT for the work of interpreting the tests, but has never seen the patient. This patient later makes an appointment to see this cardiologist—within three years of the hospital stay.

Because professional services are defined as face-to-face services, the cardiologist can report a new patient E/M code for the visit. If the definition did not specify a face-to-face service, the record would show that the cardiologist provided a service to the patient, and the E/M service would have to be reported as an established patient E/M code. This would not be appropriate because the cardiologist had not

Table 7.4 Key Component Requirements, 99201–99215

	History	Exam	MDM
99201	PF	PF	Straightforward
99202	EPF	EPF	Straightforward
99203	DET	DET	Low
99204	COMP	COMP	Moderate
99205	COMP	COMP	High
99211	N/A	N/A	N/A
99212	PF	PF	Straightforward
99213	EPF	EPF	Low
99214	DET	DET	Moderate
99215	COMP	COMP	High

Table 7.5 Evaluation and Management Code Selection Tool: Office Visits

CPT Codes	New Patients					Established Patients				
	99201 NP level 1	99202 NP level 2	99203 NP level 3	99204 NP level 4	99205 NP level 5	99211 EP level 1	99212 EP level 2	99213 EP level 3	99214 EP level 4	99215 EP level 5
Key Components										
History						Minimal				
Problem-focused	Y						Y			
Expanded problem-focused		Y						Y		
Detailed			Y						Y	
Comprehensive				Y	Y					Y
Examination						Minimal				
Problem-focused	Y						Y			
Expanded problem-focused		Y						Y		
Detailed			Y						Y	
Comprehensive				Y	Y					Y
Medical decision making						Minimal				
Straightforward	Y	Y					Y			
Low complexity			Y					Y		
Moderate complexity				Y					Y	
High complexity					Y					Y
Number of key components required	3	3	3	3	3	2	2	2	2	2

provided any type of E/M service to the patient and consequently does not know anything about him.

CRITERIA

To report the new patient codes 99201–99205, a physician's documentation must meet the criteria for all three key components for the level of service reported. To report the established patient codes 99212–99215, a physician's documentation must meet the criteria for two of the three key components for the level of service reported.

BILLING TIP

New and Established Visit Allowed Amounts

Payers reimburse a higher amount for new patient visits than for established patient visits.

Checkpoint 7.6

A patient with long-term hypertension sees her internist. Her previous visit was two years ago, and the patient is concerned that her hypertension has escalated since her last visit. The history is detailed; the exam is detailed; and the medical decision making is low. The physician submits a claim for code 99213. Is the claim correct? Explain your answer.

_____

_____

Brief Comparison of the 1995 Documentation Guidelines and the 1997 Documentation Guidelines

1995 Guidelines
Original guidelines.
Developed in response to specialty physicians' concerns that the 1995 guidelines were inappropriate for their services.

1997 Guidelines
History and medical decision-making criteria are the same for both the 1995 and the 1997 guidelines. The examination criteria differentiate the two sets of guidelines.

1995 Exam Requirements
Problem-focused

Limited exam of affected body area or organ system

Expanded problem-focused

Limited exam of affected body area or organ system and any other symptomatic or related body area(s)

Detailed

Extended exam of affected body area(s) or organ system(s) and any other symptomatic or related body area(s) or organ system(s)

Comprehensive

General multisystem exam or complete examination of a single organ system and other symptomatic or related area(s) or system(s)

1997 General Multisystem Exam Requirements
Problem-focused

1–5 elements identified by a bullet

Expanded problem-focused

At least 6 elements identified by a bullet

Detailed

At least 2 elements identified by a bulled from each of 6 areas or systems, or at least 12 elements identified by a bullet in 2 or more areas or systems

Comprehensive

At least 2 elements identified by a bullet from each of 9 areas or systems

The explanations under the printed 1997 guidelines make reference to bullets or bulleted items.

There are specialty-specific 1997 guidelines in addition to the general multisystem requirements listed above, and these can also be reviewed at the website.

INTERNET RESOURCE

1995 and 1997 E/M Documentation Guidelines

www.cms.hhs.gov/MLNEdWeb Guide/25_EMDOC.asp

DOCUMENTATION GUIDELINES

In 1992 the American Medical Association (AMA) first issued the evaluation and management codes presented in this chapter for determining the level of work associated with E/M services. Before this time, E/M coding was based on conflicting methodologies, like using time rather than clinical content to determine the level of service. Subsequently, to make the assignment of the new E/M codes more consistent, the AMA and the Health Care Financing Administration (HCFA, now CMS) developed code selection guidelines that are now known as the **1995 Documentation Guidelines.**

After the guidelines were used for some time, physicians from the various medical specialties requested a refinement of the guidelines to more appropriately reflect specialty E/M services. In 1997 the E/M guidelines were refined for single-specialty and multisystem exams. This new refinement is referred to as the **1997 Documentation Guidelines.** The Reimbursement Review above provides a brief overview of the differences between the two sets of guidelines.

COMPLIANCE GUIDELINE

Which Guidelines?

Either the 1995 or the 1997 guidelines can be selected for E/M coding and reporting.

CODE 99211: THE EXCEPTION

As defined in CPT, code 99211 is used for

> the evaluation and management of an established patient, which may or may not require the presence of a physician. Usually, the presenting problem(s) are minimal. Typically, 5 minutes are spent performing or supervising these services.

Coders will note that no key components are listed as required, making it difficult to know when it is appropriate to report this code. As indicated in the description, a physician does not necessarily have to directly (face-to-face) provide the service, but the physician must *supervise* the service.

To report 99211, the encounter must be face-to-face:

- Do not use the code for telephone calls.
- The code may be used for a blood pressure check.
- The code may be used by a nurse providing a dressing change or removing sutures.
- The code may be used when a patient comes into the office to have a tuberculin test result read.

Some portion of an E/M service must be provided. The code may not be used for patients who come in to pick up prescriptions, nor may it be used when a nurse takes vital signs before the patient's visit with the physician, since those services are included in the physician visit. It also is inappropriate to use the code for services that are represented more accurately by other codes. Blood draw services should be billed with 36415, for example, a CPT code from the medicine section.

Checkpoint 7.7

A patient is seen by an internal medicine physician for stomach pain. The physician documents a brief history and low medical decision making. The physician examined the gastrointestinal system, the respiratory system, and the cardiovascular system. Based on the 1995 guidelines, which system is the symptomatic system and which are the related systems? What is the level of service for the exam?

_____

_____

Hospital Observation Services

| 99217 | Observation care discharge | |
| 99218–99220 | Initial observation care | Require all 3 key components |

Hospital observation codes represent the E/M services provided to patients who are in observation status at the hospital but who have *not* gone through the hospital admission process. If a patient is in another place of service for observation, such as a clinic or a physician's office, these codes cannot be reported. **Observation** care is initiated because the patient needs further evaluation to determine the necessity for additional treatment or admission to the hospital, or because the

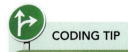

CODING TIP

New or Established Does Not Apply

Observation codes do not differentiate new and established patients.

patient has not improved and is not well enough to be released. The physician who placed the patient in observation status is responsible for the patient during the observation period.

EXAMPLE A physician sees an established patient in the office for stomach pain and rectal bleeding. On examination the physician is not sure the patient is well enough to be at home and sends the patient to the hospital for observation. Later in the day the physician will see the patient at the hospital to determine whether the patient needs to be admitted, to stay under observation, or to be discharged.

OBSERVATION CARE DISCHARGE

Code 99217 represents the services provided when a physician discharges a patient from observation care. These services include final examination of the patient, discussion of the hospital stay, instructions for continuing care, and preparation of discharge records.

INITIAL OBSERVATION CARE

As shown in Figure 7.3, an observation care code assignment flow chart, codes 99218, 99219, and 99220 represent the initiation of observation status, the supervision of the care plan for observation, and the performance of required periodic assessments of the patient while in observation care. Level of service is determined according to the criteria in Table 7.6.

Observation status is usually initiated in the physician office or the emergency department. The patient has not been admitted to the

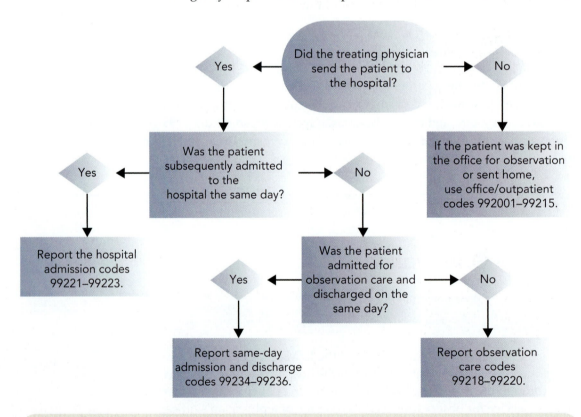

FIGURE 7.3
Observation Care Code Assignment Flow Chart

Table 7.6 Key Component Requirements, 99218–99220

	History	Exam	MDM
99218	DET or COMP	DET or COMP	Straightforward or low
99219	COMP	COMP	Moderate
99220	COMP	COMP	High

hospital, but has instead been sent to or admitted to observation status at the hospital. The patient does not have to be in a specific observation room or area in order for these codes to be used.

ROLL-UP RULE

Observation care codes provide an example of the **roll-up rule** in coding. According to the roll-up rule, if a patient is seen in the office by the physician and is then sent to the hospital for observation on the same day, the only reportable code is an initial observation care code. That code represents all the accumulated services provided to the patient on that day. These codes start at higher levels of service than most of the E/M codes for exactly that reason.

> **EXAMPLE** A patient is seen in the office for chest pain. The physician is not certain that the patient is well enough to go home, but neither is he ill enough to be admitted to the hospital. The patient is sent to the hospital for observation. The physician sees the patient at the hospital later in the day and evaluates his condition, deciding to keep the patient under observation care until the next day. The combined documentation from the office visit and observation care indicates a comprehensive history, a comprehensive examination, and moderate medical decision making. In effect, the services provided in the office roll up into the observation codes.

The initial observation care code, 99219, is assigned for the services provided to the patient on the first day. If the patient is discharged from observation care on the second day, the observation care discharge code, 99217, is assigned for that day.

If, after observing the patient at the hospital, the physician determines that he should be admitted to the hospital, all E/M services provided to the patient on the first day will *roll up* into the codes for initial hospital care, 99231–99233, which are covered in the next section.

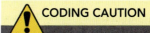

CODING CAUTION

Exceptions

- If a patient is sent for and discharged from observation care on the same day, do not report the observation care codes. Instead, use same-day admission and discharge codes 99234–99236.
- Do not use the observation care codes to report postoperative recovery services for any surgery that has a specified postoperative period. The postoperative recovery visits are part of the surgical package and are not separately reportable.

Checkpoint 7.8

A patient sees her cardiologist for follow up on her hypertension and coronary artery disease. The patient reports intermittent chest pain and some dizziness. The cardiologist is not comfortable sending the patient home, but, based on the examination and blood work, the patient's condition is not severe enough for admission to the hospital. The physician sends the patient to the hospital for observation. The cardiologist reports a code from the 99212–99215 category and another code from the 99218–99220 category of codes. Is this correct? Explain your answer.

_____

_____

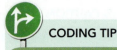

Hospital Inpatient Services

99221–99223	Initial hospital care	Requires all 3 key components
99231–99233	Subsequent hospital care	Requires 2 of 3 key components
99234–99236	Same-day admission and discharge	Requires all 3 key components
99238–99239	Hospital discharge services	Time-based

Hospital inpatient services codes represent E/M services to patients who are admitted to the hospital and are seen by physicians during their hospital stays.

INITIAL HOSPITAL CARE

Initial hospital care codes 99221, 99222, and 99223 (see Table 7.7) are used to report the *first* hospital inpatient encounter by the admitting physician. Only the admitting physician can report these codes.

In using these codes, the date of service (DOS) is the date of *service*, not the date of admission if they differ. This may seem redundant, but there is often confusion about which date should be reported for initial hospital care.

> **EXAMPLE** After discussing the circumstances with a patient's physician over the phone, a resident admits the patient to the hospital on Tuesday evening. The date of admission is Tuesday. The patient's physician visits his patient on Wednesday morning and obtains a history and performs an examination and medical decision making (the three key components).

The physician reports an initial hospital care code from 99221–99223, listing the date of service as Wednesday. The fact that the admission date is different from the initial hospital care date is not relevant.

Other physicians may also see the patient on Wednesday, but they must use either a subsequent hospital care code (99231–99233) or a hospital consultation code (99251–99255), depending on whether they meet the consultation criteria or are providing additional services to the patient.

SUBSEQUENT HOSPITAL CARE

Subsequent hospital care codes 99231, 99232, and 99233 (see Table 7.7) are used to report visits by the admitting physician to the patient after

Table 7.7 Key Component Requirements, 99221–99233

	History	Exam	MDM
99221	DET or COMP	DET or COMP	Straightforward
99222	COMP	COMP	Moderate
99223	COMP	COMP	High
99231	PF	PF	Straightforward or low
99232	EPF	EPF	Moderate
99233	DET	DET	High

Table 7.8 Key Component Requirements, 99234–99236

	History	Exam	MDM
99234	DET or COMP	DET or COMP	Straightforward or low
99235	COMP	COMP	Moderate
99236	COMP	COMP	High

the first day. Other physicians may also use these codes for their visits to the patient during a hospital stay.

EXAMPLE   The patient is admitted by the endocrinologist for uncontrolled diabetes. During the hospital stay, it is determined that the patient also needs to be followed for cardiac disease, and the patient's cardiologist sees the patient. Both the endocrinologist and the cardiologist will report subsequent hospital care codes.

SAME-DAY ADMISSION AND DISCHARGE

The codes 99234, 99235, and 99236 represent the services provided to patients who are in observation care or have been admitted to the hospital *and* are discharged on the same date as they were admitted and received the services. These codes require all three key components to select a level of service (see Table 7.8).

HOSPITAL DISCHARGE SERVICES

Hospital discharge services are the services provided by the admitting or attending physician on the date of discharge. The codes represent the total amount of time spent by the physician for the patient's final discharge, whether the time is continuous or not. The codes are time-based and do not have key component requirements:

99238: 30 minutes or less

99239: More than 30 minutes

The services include final examination of the patient, discussion of the hospital stay, instructions for continuing care with the patient and/or other caregivers, and preparation of discharge records, prescriptions, and referral forms.

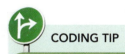

CODING TIP

Remember the Roll-up Rule

The roll-up rule applies to same-day services.

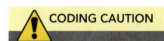

CODING CAUTION

Time Needed for Discharge Codes

Physicians must document time if they intend to report 99239. Without that documentation, the services are considered 99238.

Checkpoint 7.9

What code range would be reported if the patient is seen in the physician office, is sent to the hospital for observation, and is discharged from observation care on the same day? Explain why you chose that range of codes.

_____

_____

_____

_____

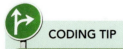

Consultations

| 99241–99245 | Office/outpatient codes | Requires all 3 key components |
| 99251–99255 | Hospital codes | Requires all 3 key components |

Consultation codes (see Table 7.9) represent the services of a physician who has been asked to give an opinion or advice on a patient (the **consulting physician**). The request comes from another physician (the requesting physician) or another appropriate source, such as a physician's assistant, a nurse-practitioner, a doctor of chiropractic, a physical therapist, an occupational therapist, a speech-language therapist, a psychologist, a social worker, a lawyer, or an insurance company.

EXAMPLE A patient has had ongoing chest pain for three months. Her family practitioner cannot determine the cause of the pain and is concerned that it may be caused by a cardiac condition that is not appearing on the ECG or other tests. He indicates that the patient should see a particular cardiologist for an opinion. The cardiologist will report the office consultation codes.

If the family practitioner had decided that the chest pain was cardiac-related and had referred his patient to the cardiologist for care, rather than for an opinion, the cardiologist would report the new patient codes 99201–99205 in place of the consultation codes.

CRITERIA FOR CODING A CONSULTATION

The following criteria are required for coding a consultation:

- The patient encounter is for an opinion or advice about a specific problem.
- The request is made by a physician or another appropriate source.
- The requesting physician or other appropriate source retains responsibility for managing the care of the patient at the time of the consultation.
- The consultant may initiate diagnostic and/or therapeutic services (for example, a cardiologist may schedule a stress test).
- The written or verbal request for the consultation is documented in the patient's medical record. (Both the physician requesting the

Table 7.9 Key Component Requirements, 99241–99255

	History	Exam	MDM
Office Consults			
99241	PF	PF	Straightforward
99242	EPF	EPF	Straightforward
99243	DET	DET	Low
99244	COMP	COMP	Moderate
99245	COMP	COMP	High
Hospital Consults			
99251	PF	PF	Straightforward
99252	EPF	EPF	Straightforward
99253	DET	DET	Low
99254	COMP	COMP	Moderate
99255	COMP	COMP	High

consultation and the consulting physician should document the consultation request in the patient's chart.)

- The consultant's findings is in writing and is sent to the requesting physician. For outpatient consultations, this means a letter to the requesting physician. For inpatient consultations, this means a note in the patient's chart.

- If, after the initial consultation in the office, the patient is again seen by the consulting physician, that physician will report an established patient code from the 99211–99215 E/M codes.

- If, after the initial consultation in the hospital, the patient is again seen by the consultant, the consultant will report a code from the subsequent hospital case range 99231–99233.

- If a consultation is requested by the patient and/or family member, the consultant must use either a new patient code from 99201–99205 or an established patient code from 99211–99215 for the office or outpatient setting, or a subsequent hospital care code from 99231–99233 in the hospital setting.

Referral or Consultation A consultation is reimbursed at a higher rate than a new patient visit. For this reason, payers demand documentation that supports assigning a consultation code. Distinguishing between a new patient **referral** and a consultation is problematic for most physicians and coders. Under a referral, the care of the patient is being passed by the **referring physician** to the provider to whom he or she is referred. Consultants provide an opinion and then return the patient to the requesting doctor's care.

The decision rests with the intention of the requesting physician. Is the requesting physician asking for an opinion about a patient's problem, or is the requesting physician turning the patient over to a new physician to take care of the problem? Often the requesting physician's intention is not known when the appointment is made. Physicians often say to their patients, "I want you to see this cardiologist so we can get a handle on what's going on." When the patient makes the appointment, his or her status is not clear. Because the second physician must have documentation to support the use of the consultation code, that physician needs to be clear on what service is performed. Often, the two physicians have discussed the patient on the phone, and it is clear that the patient is to be seen in consultation, not as a new patient, but documentation is the key.

Coders may want to use a chart to assist in the determination of whether a patient is being seen as a new patient on referral or for consultation. Figure 7.4, a flow chart for consultations, is a useful tool.

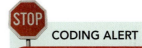

CODING ALERT

Consult Codes

Consultation codes must not be reported for second opinions or for services requested by a patient or by a patient's family member.

Consultation	Referral of a New Patient
Patient with unresolved lethargy and stomach pain is sent to a gastroenterologist for an opinion on treatment and/or diagnosis.	The internist determines the problem and sends the patient to a gastroenterologist for care of the problem.
Gastroenterologist renders an opinion on the patient's diagnosis after doing tests in the office, prescribes medication, and sends a letter to the internist giving her opinion and advice. The patient's care is still in the hands of the internist.	Gastroenterologist takes over the treatment and care of the patient.

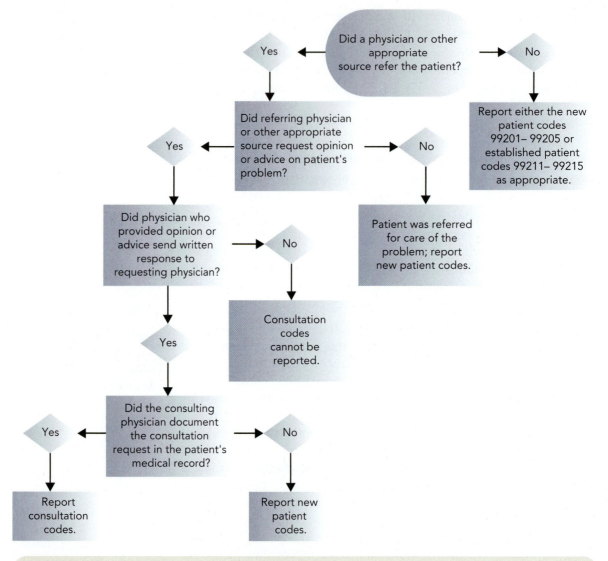

FIGURE 7.4
Consultation Code Assignment Flow Chart

Myths Several consultation myths cause confusion for physicians and coders. The following are the most prevalent false assumptions:

- A consultant cannot bill a consultation if he or she provides treatment during the visit.
- A physician cannot request a consultation from another physician in the same group.
- A nonphysician practitioner cannot request a consultation.
- If the diagnosis is known, a consultation cannot be reported.
- Consultation codes cannot be used for established patients.

These are some of the myths about consultation codes.

PREOPERATIVE CONSULTATIONS

Preoperative consultations are a particular type of consultation service. For example, a patient scheduled for surgery may require preoperative clearance before the surgery is performed. Commonly, a surgeon will

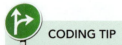

CODING TIP

Three Rs for Consultation Documentation

Think of the three Rs when determining whether to use a consultation code: request, rendering, and response. These three words summarize the consultation criteria: a request from a physician, a rendering of the service to the patient, and a response by the consultant to the requesting physician.

send the patient to the internist, a cardiologist, or another specialist, depending on the planned surgery and the underlying condition that needs evaluation. When a surgeon sends the patient to another physician for preoperative evaluation and clearance, the stage is set for a consultation service. The consultant will see the patient for evaluation before surgery and will provide the surgeon with an opinion about the patient's condition and ability to withstand the surgical procedure, fulfilling the requirement for the three Rs.

EXAMPLE After performing a cardiac exam for an established patient who is diabetic and hypertensive, the internist sends the patient to a cardiologist. Two months later, after performing several tests, the cardiologist determines that the patient needs an angioplasty to clear a blockage in his coronary artery. The cardiologist asks the internist to see the patient for preoperative clearance for the procedure. The internist sees the patient, updates a history on the patient, examines him, and determines whether he can proceed with surgery. The internist sends his findings to the cardiologist.

Is this a consultation for the internist or an established patient visit? To answer, review the following points:

Did the cardiologist ask for the internist's opinion about whether to proceed with the angioplasty procedure?	Yes
Did the internist provide the key components?	Yes
Did the internist send her findings to the cardiologist?	Yes
Does the fact that the patient is already an established patient with the internist mean that a consultation cannot be provided?	No

The internist provided a preoperative consultation and may report a code from the range 99241–99245.

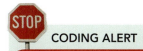

CODING ALERT

Clinical Pathology Consultations

Clinical pathology consultations requested by the attending physician that do not involve the pathologist's examining the patient are coded to the Pathology and Laboratory section, CPT codes 80500 and 80502. An interpretation of clinically abnormal findings and a written report are required.

Checkpoint 7.10

Are the following cases correctly described as consultations?

1. A family physician has been treating a patient with diabetes and is concerned that the patient may develop diabetic retinopathy. The patient is sent to an ophthalmologist for his opinion about whether this condition has developed or may develop. The ophthalmologist examines the patient and sends an opinion on the potential for diabetic retinopathy to the family physician.

   _____

2. An internist has been treating a patient for many years. The patient now presents with urinary difficulties, and the physician is concerned that the problem may be related to an enlarged prostate. The internist sends the patient to an urologist to determine whether the condition is appropriate for surgery or other medical treatment.

   _____

3. A patient goes to the emergency department (ED) with severe leg pain. He is seen and evaluated by the ED physician, who suspects a fracture but also notes muscle deterioration that cannot be explained. The ED calls an orthopedist to come to the ED to advise on the muscle deterioration.

   _____

4. In the above case, if the orthopedist decides that the patient should be admitted, which code should be billed, the consultation code or the admission code? Can both be billed?

   _____

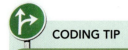
Emergency Department (ED) Services

| 99281–99285 | Emergency department services | Requires all 3 key components |
| 99288 | Physician direction of emergency medical systems | |

Emergency department codes 99281–99285 represent services provided in the emergency department. CPT specifically defines an emergency department as "an organized hospital-based facility for the provision of unscheduled episodic services to patients who present for immediate medical attention. The facility must be available 24 hours a day." The American College of Emergency Physicians defines emergency services as:

> Those health care services provided in a hospital emergency department to treat medical conditions of acute onset and sufficient severity that would lead a prudent lay person possessing an average knowledge of medicine and health care to believe that urgent medical care is required to reduce the level of pain, prevent the deterioration of one's condition, and prevent disability and/or death.

ED codes have five levels of service; to select a level requires all three key components (see Table 7.10). There is no time factor associated with these codes. Generally ED services are related to unexpected health issues or events that call for prompt, if not immediate, medical attention.

CRITERIA

These codes are normally reported by the physicians who are assigned to the ED. This does not preclude other physicians from using the ED codes, but they must be aware of the circumstances that will prevent them from doing so.

> **EXAMPLE** A patient is brought to the ED for evaluation of his injuries after a motor vehicle accident. The ED physician obtains a history, does an examination, and determines that the patient may have internal bleeding in the abdomen. A general surgeon is then asked to see the patient.

In this case, the ED physician will report one of the ED codes (99281–99285). The general surgeon, depending on the circumstances, will report either an office or outpatient consultation code (99241–99245) or an office or outpatient visit code (99211–99215). Because the ED physician provided E/M services to the patient, the general surgeon would not use the same ED codes.

Table 7.10 Key Component Requirements, 99281–99285

	History	Exam	MDM
99281	PF	PF	Straightforward
99282	EPF	EPF	Low
99283	EPF	EPF	Moderate
99284	DET	DET	Moderate
99285	COMP	COMP	High

ED codes are not reported for emergency conditions in the office or other outpatient areas. The codes are based on services performed in the specific location of an emergency department, not just on the patient's condition.

Physicians providing critical care (discussed in the next section) in the ED may report both the ED and the critical care codes, appending modifier −25 to either code. Note that this is an exception to the roll-up rule.

PHYSICIAN DIRECTION OF EMERGENCY MEDICAL SYSTEMS (EMS)

Code 99288 represents the services of a physician located in the hospital emergency department or in the critical care department. This physician, who is in two-way voice communication with ambulance or rescue personnel who are *outside* the hospital, directs the ambulance or rescue personnel in providing medical procedures, including but not limited to the following:

- Telemetry of cardiac rhythm
- Cardiac and/or pulmonary resuscitation
- Endotracheal or esophageal airway intubation
- Administration of intravenous fluids
- Administration of intramuscular, intratracheal, or subcutaneous drugs
- Electrical conversion of arrhythmia

Critical Care Services

99289–99290	Pediatric critical care transport	Time-based
99291–99292	Critical care services	Time-based
99293–99294	Inpatient pediatric critical care	Per day
99295–99296	Inpatient neonatal critical care	Per day
99298–99300	Continuing intensive care services	Per day

Critical care is the provision of medical care to a critically ill or critically injured patient. Medical care qualifies as critical care only if *both* the illness or injury *and* the treatment being provided meet the critical care requirements. Critical illness or injury impairs one or more vital organ systems, causing a high probability of imminent or life-threatening deterioration in a patient's condition.

Critical care involves high-complexity decision making to assess, manipulate, and support vital system functions, treatment of single or multiple vital organ system failure, and/or prevention of further life-threatening deterioration of a patient's condition. Examples of vital organ system failure include but are not limited to:

- Central nervous system
- Circulatory system
- Renal system
- Hepatic system
- Metabolic system

- Respiratory system
- Shock

There are five categories of critical care (and related) services to consider:

1. Pediatric critical care transport
2. Critical care services
3. Inpatient pediatric critical care
4. Inpatient neonatal critical care
5. Continuing intensive care services

CODING ALERT

Add-on Codes

Remember that an add-on code (+) is never reported without its parent code.

PEDIATRIC CRITICAL CARE TRANSPORT

Two codes cover pediatric critical care transport:

99289: Critical care services during transport, first 30 to 74 minutes

+99290: Critical care services during transport, each additional 30 minutes

These codes represent the services of a physician who accompanies a critically ill or critically injured *pediatric* patient during interfacility transport and provides face-to-face services. The face-to-face care begins when the physician assumes the responsibility for the pediatric patient at the referring hospital or facility, and it ends when the receiving hospital or facility accepts responsibility for the patient's care. The patient must be 24 months of age or younger; the service must be face-to-face; and the transport must involve 30 minutes or more of service. Critical care services of less than 30 minutes should be reported with another appropriate E/M code.

Pediatric critical care patient transport includes the following services, so none of the listed items are reported in addition to the transport code:

- Routine monitoring evaluations (for example, heart rate, respiratory rate, blood pressure, pulse oximetry)
- Interpretation of cardiac output measurements (CPT codes 93561 and 93562)
- Chest X-rays (CPT codes 71010, 71015, and 71020)
- Pulse oximetry (CPT codes 94760–94762)
- Blood gases
- Information stored in computers
  - ECGs
  - Blood pressure readings
  - Hematologic data
- Gastric intubation (CPT codes 43752 and 91105)
- Temporary transcutaneous pacing (CPT code 92953)
- Ventilatory management (CPT codes 94002–94004, and 94662)
- Vascular access procedures (CPT codes 36000, 36400, 36405, 36406, 36410, 36415, 36540, and 36600)

Any services not listed above should be reported in addition to the critical care transport services.

CRITICAL CARE SERVICES

Critical care service codes are:

99291: Critical care evaluation and management, first 30 to 74 minutes

+99292: Critical care evaluation and management, each additional 30 minutes

These codes represent critical care services provided to patients beyond the pediatric age criterion of 24 months who are critically ill or critically injured. Figure 7.5 presents a flow chart for code selection. The criteria for selection are as follows:

- Critical care may be provided on multiple days, even if no changes are made in the treatment rendered, provided that the patient's condition continues to require critical care.
- Critical care codes reflect the total amount of time spent by the physician in providing critical care, even if the time spent is not continuous.
- The physician must devote full attention to the patient and cannot provide services to other patients during the same time period.
- Critical care may be provided in any setting; the patient does not have to be in a specific critical care unit of the hospital. Location does not define critical care services.
- The fact that a patient is in some type of critical care unit does not mean that services are critical care services. Physicians may provide routine care in a critical care unit, in which case they would report the subsequent hospital care codes.

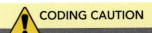

CODING CAUTION

Coding for Outpatient POS

If critical care is provided to a critically ill or injured neonate or pediatric patient in the outpatient setting, use the 99291–99292 category of codes. The neonate and pediatric critical care codes are for the inpatient setting only.

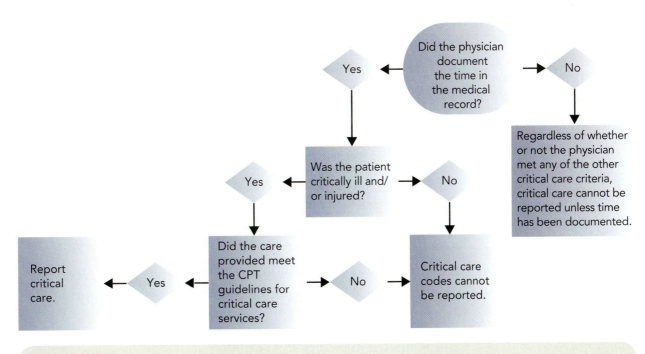

FIGURE 7.5

Adult Critical Care Code Assignment Flow Chart

- Services not listed above are separately reportable. Reportable services include bronchoscopy, Swan Ganz catheter, and cardio-pulmonary resuscitation, among others.
- Physicians may report other E/M codes in addition to the critical care codes.

EXAMPLE A physician sees a heart patient for follow-up care (99231–99232) in the morning. Later in the day, the patient goes into complete heart block, and the physician is called in to stabilize and treat the patient, which is critical care. Both the subsequent hospital care code and the critical care code can be reported using modifier –25 on the subsequent hospital care code.

Physician Work Time for Critical Care Time must be documented to qualify for reporting critical care; doing so is an essential requirement. The following physician work may be included in reporting critical care:

- Caring for the patient at the bedside
- Reviewing test results or studies on the unit or floor
- Discussing the patient's care with other medical staff
- Documenting critical care services in the medical record
- Documenting the patient's clinical condition (an essential requirement)
- Discussing care directly related to the management of the patient on the unit or floor with family members or other decision makers of a patient who cannot participate in discussions

The following physician work may *not* be included in reporting critical care:

- Work that occurs outside the unit or off the floor
- Unrelated work or work that does not directly contribute to the patient's critical care treatment
- Services that are separately reportable from critical care (see above)
- Provision of critical care services that takes less than 30 minutes (use the subsequent hospital care codes 99231–99233 instead)

EXAMPLE The physician spends 1 hour 10 minutes providing critical care at the patient's bedside. He also spends 20 minutes reviewing films in the radiology department on a separate floor and then 15 minutes documenting the care he provided. The physician would report 99291 and 99292 for 1 hour 25 minutes of critical care. The 20 minutes in the radiology department is not reported as critical care because the physician is not immediately available to the patient.

How to Calculate Critical Care Time Code 99291 represents the first 30 to 74 minutes.

- If less than 30 minutes is spent, do not report critical care codes.
- In effect, this code represents the first hour of critical plus an additional 14 minutes.
- If the critical care goes beyond 74 minutes (1 hour plus 14 minutes), then report 99291 and 99292.

Code 99292 represents each additional 30 minutes beyond the first hour. Code 99292 includes the additional 30 minutes plus 14 minutes.

For example, it the physician spent 2 hours providing critical care, report 99291 for the first 60 minutes, and 99292x2 for the additional 60 minutes. If the physician spent 80 minutes providing critical care, report 99291 for the first 60 minutes and 99292 for the additional 20 minutes.

The 15-Minute Rule   According to the 15-minute rule, after the first hour (99291), the time spent must exceed 14 minutes for 99292 to be reported. After the first hour and a half (99291, 99292), the time spent must exceed 14 minutes to report 99292 again.

Time Spent	Description	Code
30–74 minutes	First 30 minutes through first hour plus 14 minutes	99291
74–104 minutes	First hour plus 14 minutes through additional half hour	99291, 99292
104–134 minutes	First hour and a half plus 14 minutes through additional half hour	99291, 99292x2

Critical Care Documentation   When a patient is admitted to a cardiac care unit (CCU), such as for respiratory failure after an acute myocardial infarction with possible renal failure, the physician does a **review of systems** and a medical history (as obtainable). The three key components (H/E/MDM) are not critical care code requirements, so the physician's documentation must focus on the details of clinically appropriate services. The physician is likely to document the:

- Neurological status
- Peripheral pulses
- Skin examination
- Heart and lung examination
- ECG interpretation
- Cardiac enzymes
- Respiratory examination
- Ventilation management
- Lab results
- Gastrointestinal system examination
- Physician's assessment and plan

INPATIENT PEDIATRIC CRITICAL CARE

Inpatient pediatric critical care codes represent critical care provided to critically ill or injured children who are 29 days through 24 months of age. They start with the date of admission and go through the subsequent day or days:

99293: Initial day of pediatric critical care

99294: Each subsequent day of pediatric critical care

Note that these are inpatient-only services.

The same definitions and criteria for critical care apply to adult, pediatric, and neonatal patients. These are *per-day* codes; they are not time-based. Use the same critical care guidelines indicated above, but

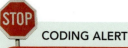
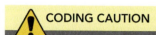
also note that both pediatric and neonate critical care include other CPT codes:

- Umbilical venous and arterial catheters (CPT codes 36510 and 36660)
- Arterial catheterization/cannulation (CPT code 36620)
- Vascular access procedures (CPT codes 36400, 36405, and 36406)
- Vascular puncture (CPT code 36420)
- Endotracheal intubation (CPT code 31500)
- Lumbar puncture (CPT code 62270)
- Suprapubic bladder aspiration (CPT code 51000)
- Bladder catheterization (CPT codes 51701 and 51702)

Any services not listed above are separately reportable in addition to 99293–99294.

INPATIENT NEONATAL CRITICAL CARE

Inpatient neonatal critical care codes represent critical care provided to children twenty-eight days of age or less, and they too start with the date of admission and go through the subsequent day or days:

99295: Initial day of neonatal critical care

99296 Each subsequent day of neonatal critical care

Note that these are also inpatient-only services. The same definitions and criteria for critical care apply for adult, pediatric, and neonatal patients. These are per-day codes; they are not time-based.

If a neonate requires an intensive care setting but is not critically ill, use the initial hospital care codes 99221–99223 rather than the initial critical care code 99295. If the neonate requires an intensive care setting but is not critically ill, use the intensive low-birth-weight codes 99298–99300 or the subsequent hospital care codes 99231–99233 instead of the subsequent critical care code 99296.

The neonatal codes are reportable with the following other newborn care codes if these services are performed:

- Physician standby (99360); for example, if the pediatrician is asked by the obstetrician to stand by during a difficult delivery
- Physician attendance (99436); for example, if the pediatrician is asked by the obstetrician to attend the delivery and to stabilize the newborn
- Newborn resuscitation (99440); for example, if the pediatrician is called into the delivery room to resuscitate a newborn
- Endotracheal intubation (31500) and other resuscitation procedures if they are performed as part of the preadmission delivery room care, are a necessary component of the resuscitation, and are not performed in the delivery room as a convenience before admission to the neonatal intensive care unit

CONTINUING INTENSIVE CARE SERVICES

Continuing intensive care codes represent services provided after the day of admission. Although the infants do not meet the definition of critically ill, they continue to require intensive observation, frequent interventions, and other intensive services. The reporting physician is the physician who directs the continuing intensive care of these patients.

99298: Subsequent intensive care of a recovering very-low-birth-weight infant (less than 1,500 grams)

99299: Subsequent intensive care of a recovering low-birth-weight infant (1,500–2,500 grams)

99300: Subsequent intensive care of a recovering infant (2,501–5,000 grams)

These are per-day codes, and the types of services that are typically provided are management, monitoring and treatment of:

- Circulatory and respiratory systems
- Metabolism
- Hematologic maintenance
- Heat maintenance
- Enteral and/or parenteral nutritional adjustments
- Supervision of the health care team
- Parent/family counseling
- Case management

EXAMPLE A 2,550 gram neonate who was suffering from respiratory distress, shock, and cardiac arrhythmia is now recovering but still requires oxygen and is maintained on his central venous catheter, pending full recovery. His pediatrician will attend to and monitor his cardiovascular stability, pulmonary status, and gastrointestinal function. This will require comprehensive evaluations of these organ systems with particular attention to possible infection and atelectasis in the lungs. The child will be visited throughout the day and evening to ensure that he continues to recover. The code is 99300.

Checkpoint 7.11

Provide codes for the following cases.

1. The physician spent 1 hour 10 minutes at the patient's bedside providing critical care. He also spent 20 minutes reviewing films on the unit and documenting the care he provided. What code(s) would the physician report? _____

2. The physician also performed cardiopulmonary resuscitation (CPR) just before the 1 hour 10 minutes of critical care. May the physician report the CPR in addition to the critical care? _____

3. A three-day-old infant became critically ill. The physician admitted the child to the critical care unit and spent 2 hours with the child, including a discussion with the family regarding the child's prognosis. What code(s) would be reported? _____

Nursing Facility Services

99304–99306	Initial nursing facility care, per day	Requires all 3 key components
99307–99310	Subsequent nursing facility care, per day	Requires 2 of 3 key components
99315–99316	Nursing facility discharge services	Time-based
99318	Annual nursing facility assessment	Requires all 3 key components

CODING TIP

New or Established Does Not Apply

Initial and subsequent nursing facility care codes do not differentiate new and established patients.

CODING TIP

Reporting Services for a Patient Who Dies

According to the May 2002 *CPT Assistant*, the discharge codes can also be used to report services when a physician must pronounce a patient's death as long as the physician performs any of the discharge criteria.

E/M codes for nursing facilities, which are organized like other IP codes, are reported for the evaluation and management of patients in nursing facilities, such as a skilled nursing facility (SNF), an intermediate care facility (ICF), or a long-term care facility (LTCF). They are also used for patients in a psychiatric residential treatment center that provides twenty-four-hour group living and that has been therapeutically planned and is professionally staffed. Table 7.11 shows the key component requirements for these E/M codes.

Physicians who report the nursing facility codes have a central role in ensuring that all residents receive thorough assessments and that medical plans of care for them have been instituted or revised. Nursing facilities are required to use resident assessment instruments (RAI), which include the minimum data set (MDS) and resident assessment protocols (RAPs). The MDS is the primary screening and assessment tool, and the RAPs provide identification of potential problems and guidelines for follow-up assessments.

The *roll-up* rule applies to these codes with one exception. If the patient was discharged from a hospital (99238 or 99239) or from observation care (99217) on the same date as admission to the nursing facility, both services are separately reportable.

Nursing facility codes are per-day codes. The subsequent nursing facility care codes 99307–99310 always include reviewing the results of diagnostic studies and changes in the patient's status.

Table 7.11 Key Component Requirements, 99304–99318

	History	Exam	MDM
99304	DET or COMP	DET or COMP	Straightforward or low
99305	COMP	COMP	Moderate
99306	COMP	COMP	High
99307	PF	PF	Straightforward
99308	EPF	EPF	Low
99309	DET	DET	Moderate
99310	COMP	COMP	High
99315, 99316	Guidelines for these discharge codes are consistent with those for the hospital discharge services codes 99238 and 99239.		
99318	Represents the annual nursing facility assessment service and is not reported in addition to initial or subsequent nursing facility care codes 99304–99316. The annual assessment is a separate service.		

Table 7.12 Key Component Requirements, 99324–99337

	History	Exam	MDM
New Patient			
99324	PF	PF	Straightforward
99325	EPF	EPF	Low
99326	DET	DET	Moderate
99327	COMP	COMP	Moderate
99328	COMP	COMP	High
Established Patient			
99334	PF	PF	Straightforward
99335	EPF	EPF	Low
99336	DET	DET	Moderate
99337	COMP	COMP	Moderate to high

Domiciliary, Rest Home, or Custodial Care Services

99324–99328	New patient	Requires all 3 key components
99334–99337	Established patient	Requires 2 of 3 key components

These codes represent the E/M services provided to patients located in a "facility that provides room, board and other personal assistance services, generally on a long-term basis." AMA also includes assisted-living facilities in this definition; however, to qualify for these codes none of the facilities can include a medical component in their services.

The codes are organized exactly like the new patient and established patient codes for office or other outpatient services. The levels of service of the new patient and established patient codes differ slightly, as shown in Table 7.12.

Domiciliary, Rest Home, or Home Care Plan Oversight Services

99339	Within a calendar month, 15–29 minutes
99340	Within a calendar month, 30 minutes or more

Care plan oversight codes represent the services that physicians provide to patients who are at home or in domiciliary or rest homes (assisted-living facilities), *without* face-to-face contact. These services are comparable to the care plan oversight services in codes 99374–99380 (described later in this chapter), but the patients are not under the care of a home health agency or hospice program. The codes represent the services of the supervising physician who oversees the care of a patient by taking calls or coordinating care with other medical and nonmedical service providers and the patient's family members. The physician is also responsible for developing and/or revising care plans, reviewing reports of patient status, and reviewing laboratory and other studies.

These codes are reported separately from any face-to-face services—such as home, domiciliary, or rest home visits—the physician provides to the patient during the reporting period. They also include the physician's oversight of work or school programs where therapy is provided. The codes are reported per calendar month and represent the services provided during that month.

> **EXAMPLE** An eighty-year-old patient has lived with his children since suffering a stroke two years ago. He is now in the early stages of Alzheimer's disease, is increasingly dependent on his children for all aspects of daily living, and has started to become agitated and uncooperative. His children are unable to get him to the physician's office for visits. A home visit is made by the physician. Over the next month, the physician speaks with the family about the patient's care, assessing progress or lack of progress. The oversight of this patient's care by the physician is necessary to support the caregivers, to avoid hospitalization, and to diminish the patient's potential for delirium.

The selection criteria are:

- Only one physician reports these codes—the supervising physician.
- These codes are reported per calendar month and represent the services provided during that month.
- Do not report these codes unless the patient requires recurrent supervision of their therapy/treatment.
- The physician supervision is such that it requires complex and multidisciplinary care modalities, involving regular physician development and/or revision of care plans, review of reports on patient status, laboratory and other studies.
- The physician supervision will also require communication for the purpose of assessment of the patient, care decisions with health care professional(s), family member(s), surrogate decision maker(s).
- The supervising physician will integrate new information into the patient's medical treatment plan, and/or make adjustments to that plan.
- Do not report these codes for patients under the care of a home health agency, in a hospice program, or for nursing facility assessments (assign those services codes 99374–99380).

Home Services

| 99341–99345 | New patient | Requires all 3 key components |
| 99347–99350 | Established patient | Requires 2 of 3 key components. |

These codes, shown in Table 7.13, represent E/M services provided to patients in their homes. The criteria are the same as those for new and established patients 99201–99215.

Table 7.13 Key Component Requirements, 99341–99350

	History	Exam	MDM
New Patient			
99341	PF	PF	Straightforward
99342	EPF	EPF	Low
99343	DET	DET	Moderate
99344	COMP	COMP	Moderate
99345	COMP	COMP	High
Established Patient			
99347	PF	PF	Straightforward
99348	EPF	EPF	Low
99349	DET	DET	Moderate
99350	COMP	COMP	Moderate to high

Prolonged Services

+99354	Face-to-face services in office or outpatient setting	Use with 99201–99215, 99241–99245, 99304–99350
+99355	Each additional 30 minutes	Use with 99354
+99356	Face-to-face services in inpatient setting	Use with 99221–99223, 99251–99255
+99357	Each additional 30 minutes	Use with 99356
+99358	Non-face-to-face services in office, outpatient, or inpatient setting	Use in addition to other physician service, including E/M services
+99359	Each additional 30 minutes	Use with 99358

The range of prolonged services codes represent services that go beyond typical service in either the inpatient or outpatient setting. They are all add-on codes and therefore are always reported in addition to other E/M codes. The codes are not based on the three key components; instead, they are time-based. They are divided into **direct care** services, meaning those provided face-to-face, and *nondirect care,* which refers to services that are not face-to-face and are provided either before or after face-to-face patient care provided on the same day. Prolonged services can be provided in the physician office or outpatient location or in the hospital (inpatient) unit or floor where the patient is located.

EXAMPLE
Direct prolonged service: An established patient comes into the physician's office reporting chest pain. The patient asks whether the spicy food he has been eating lately could be the cause of the chest pain. An ECG is done, with results comparable to an ECG done two months ago. No problem is found. The physician provides a problem-focused history, a detailed exam, and moderate MDM. The patient then mentions some left arm pain. The physician is not comfortable letting the patient go home, so she allows him to remain in one of the examining rooms for the next four hours; during that time she evaluates the patient's vital signs and examines him to look for conditions that might indicate the underlying problem. The physician spends 40 minutes providing face-to-face care to the patient in addition to the time spent on the key components. Assign codes 99214 and +99354.

Nondirect prolonged service: An eighty-year-old patient with a long history of several complex systemic health problems moves to a new area to be closer to her family. Before the patient's visit, her new physician spends an hour reviewing the medical records sent to him by the patient's previous physician. Assign a new patient code from the 99201–99205 range and +**99358**.

CRITERIA

Prolonged service codes are reported once per day, but the time the physician spends with the patient need not be continuous on that day. However, the physician must exceed the typical primary E/M code time by at least an additional 30 minutes (see Table 7.14 for E/M code times). Additional time less than 30 minutes would be included in the primary E/M code and would not be separately reported.

EXAMPLE   The typical time assigned to code 99214 is 25 minutes. If the physician spends a total of 45 minutes in direct care of the patient, the prolonged care codes are not reported (45 minutes − 25 minutes = 20 minutes). The remaining time of 20 minutes does not meet the minimum 30-minute requirement.

Physicians and coders may want to consider the counseling and coordination of care time rule if applicable. When counseling or coordination of care dominates (uses more than 50 percent of the time of) the physician and patient and/or family encounter, time *is* the key or controlling factor to determine the level of service. The extent of the counseling or coordination of care must be documented in the medical record.

The following services are reportable with prolonged service codes 99354 and 99355:

99201–99205: New patient

99211–99215: Established patient

Table 7.14 Typical Primary E/M Code Times

Code	Typical Time	Code	Typical Time	Code	Typical Time
99201	10	99231	15	99255	110
99202	20	99232	25	99341	20
99203	30	99233	35	99342	30
99204	45	99241	15	99343	45
99205	60	99242	30	99344	60
99212	10	99243	40	99345	75
99213	15	99244	60	99347	15
99214	25	99245	80	99348	25
99215	40	99251	20	99349	40
99221	30	99252	40	99350	60
99222	50	99253	55		
99223	70	99254	80		

At this time, according to the AMA, the nursing facility codes 99304–99310 do not have typical times listed.

99241–99245: Office/outpatient consultations

99304–99350: Nursing facility services

The following services are reportable with the prolonged service codes 99356 and 99357:

99221–99223: Initial hospital care

99231–99233: Subsequent hospital care

99251–99255: Hospital consultations

Some services are not reportable with any prolonged service codes. Services that do not have typical times associated with them and are not reportable are:

99217–99221: Hospital observation care

99281–99285: Emergency department

99289–99300: Critical care

The time-based codes for same-day admission and discharge, 99234–99236, are also not reportable. All the services would be represented by the admission and discharge provided on the same day.

BILLING TIP

Modifier −21

According to CMS, modifier −21 is used when the time spent with the patient is 30 minutes more than the time stated in the code description, but be cautious: the CPT description of modifier −21 specifically states that this modifier may be used with only "the highest level of evaluation and management service within a given category." Examples of the highest level are 99205, 99215, 99223, 99233, 99245, and 99255.

CALCULATING TIME

Use the 15-minute rule to calculate the amount of time to bill for time-based prolonged services:

- After the first hour (99354), 14 minutes must be exceeded to use 99355.
- After the first 1.5 hours (99354, 99355), 14 minutes must be exceeded to use 99355 again.

Time Spent	Description	Code
30–74 minutes	First 30 minutes through first hour plus 14 minutes	99354
75–104 minutes	First hour plus 15 minutes through 1.5 hours plus 14 minutes	99354, 99355
105–134 minutes	First 1.5 hours plus 15 minutes through 2 hours plus 14 minutes	99354, 99355x2

Checkpoint 7.12

Indicate whether the following statements are true or false, and explain why.

1. Prolonged services codes are the only codes reported when counseling and coordination of care are greater than 50 percent of the patient services provided on that day. _____

2. Prolonged services codes are never billed alone. _____

3. Modifier −21 can be reported with codes 99354–99359. _____

4. The difference between direct and nondirect services is the place of service. _____

Physician Standby Services

99360	Physician standby service, requiring prolonged physician attendance, each 30 minutes

CPT code 99360 is used for **standby** services, which are services provided when a physician asks another physician to stand by during treatment of a patient. In effect, the standby physician is required to be available in the location of the patient's treatment, immediately ready to provide services that may be needed. For example, the standby physician reports code 99360 when asked to stand by for possible surgery (a surgeon), to analyze a frozen section (a pathologist), to help with a cesarean or high-risk delivery (a pediatrician), or to monitor an electroencephalogram (a neurologist).

EXAMPLE A cardiologist has scheduled a percutaneous (through the skin) cardiac procedure that may require immediate open-heart surgery if the patient does not respond well. The cardiologist asks a cardiothoracic surgeon to stand by during the cardiac procedure in case her services are required.

The following criteria must be met to use this code:

- The standby physician has no face-to-face contact with the patient.
- The standby physician does not provide care or services to other patients during the standby period; for example, the standby physician does not see other patients who are in the hospital.
- The standby physician is not proctoring another physician (in other words, the physician is not overseeing or monitoring another physician during a procedure).
- If the standby service results in the performance of a procedure subject to a surgical package, the standby physician reports the procedure only, not the standby code.

EXAMPLE In the example, if the standby physician has to perform open-heart surgery such as a coronary artery bypass (CABG), she will report only the CABG code, not the standby code.

- The standby service time must be 30 minutes or longer. Standby service of less than thirty minutes is not reportable.
- To report 99360 more than once, the physician must stand by for a full thirty minutes in addition to the first 30 minutes.

EXAMPLE If the cardiothoracic surgeon stands by for 1 hour during the cardiologist's procedure, she will report 99360x2. If she stands by for 40 minutes during the cardiologist's procedure, she will report 99360 only.

STOP CODING ALERT

Standby Services

Code 99360 is not reported in addition to code 99436, the physician attendance code for newborn care (see the Newborn Care section).

Checkpoint 7.13

A neurologist asks a neurosurgeon to stand by during neurological testing performed in the operating room because there is concern about the stability of the patient to withstand the brain testing, and surgery might be required on an emergency basis. The neurosurgeon stands by for 35 minutes. Code for this service. _____

_____

_____

Case Management Services

| 99363–99364 | Anticoagulant Management | Per days of therapy |
| 99366–99368 | Medical Team conferences | Time-based |

Case management codes represent the services of a physician or non-physician qualified health care professional who is responsible for the direct care of a patient, and for coordinating managing access to, initiating, and/or supervising other health care services for the patient.

ANTICOAGULANT MANAGEMENT

These codes represent the outpatient services provided for anticoagulation therapy, including management of the warfarin drug that keeps the patient's blood at a therapeutic level. Once a patient has been hospitalized and subsequently discharged, the anticoagulation therapy is continued and reported with 99363 and 99364. CPT code 99363 is reported for the initial 90 days of therapy and must include a minimum of 8 INR measurements. CPT code 99364 is for each subsequent 90 days of therapy and must include a minimum of 3 INR measurements during that time.

MEDICAL TEAM CONFERENCES

The team conference codes are used for meetings with interdisciplinary health care professionals to coordinate the care of a patient. The codes are organized by whether or not the patient/family is present and if the participation is by a physician or a non-physician provider.

> **EXAMPLE** A mentally ill patient needs to have a brain aneurysm excised. The patient's neurosurgeon meets with his psychiatrist and radiologist to discuss his care.

The services include physician review and interpretation of the international normalized ratio (INR) results, patient instructions, dosage adjustment, and ordering of additional tests. Also included are communication of the findings to the patient and adjustment of the warfarin dosage. The INR levels can vary over time, so the levels must be monitored and the patient's dosage carefully adjusted.

Most commonly, these services are provided when a patient has had a heart valve replaced or open-heart surgery in general or when a patient has vascular disease. Anticoagulation therapy is required so that the patient's blood does not clot too easily or get too thin (in which case the patient bleeds too easily). Prior to the development of these codes in 2007, coding such services was problematic.

Do not include these services in care plan oversight time (99374–99380), telephone calls (99371–99373), or observation care (99217–99220).

> **EXAMPLE** A patient's aortic valve was replaced. If the patient's blood is too thin or too thick, the replacement aortic valve will be impaired. The patient is required have blood drawn at the physician office or a laboratory to have it tested. The results are evaluated, and the patient's dosage of the anticoagulation medication is adjusted accordingly.

CODING ALERT

Outpatient Only and a Minimum of Sixty Days

Do not use these codes for inpatient services; they are for outpatient services only. A period of fewer than sixty continuous outpatient days is not reported.

CODING ALERT

Inpatient Anticoagulation Services Affect Code Selection

Therapy initiated or continued in the inpatient setting starts a new treatment period. Once the patient is discharged, use 99364 for each subsequent ninety days of therapy.

Care Plan Oversight Services

99374	Home health agency patient, 15–29 minutes
99375	Home health agency patient, 30 minutes or more
99377	Hospice patient, 15–29 minutes
99378	Hospice patient, 30 minutes or more
99379	Nursing facility patient, 15–29 minutes
99380	Nursing facility patient, 30 minutes or more

Care plan oversight codes represent the services that physicians provide to patients who are under the care of a home health agency, a hospice, or a nursing facility without face-to-face contact. These services involve overseeing the care of a patient by taking calls from the nurse or agency handling the patient and by reviewing and revising care plans. The codes are reported separately from face-to-face services, such as office or nursing home visits, provided during the reporting period.

EXAMPLE Ms. Jones is homebound because of uncontrolled diabetes, hypertension, and resulting claudication, making walking far difficult, if not impossible. Her home health agency nurse visits every two days to be sure she is taking care of herself, taking the appropriate medications, exercising correctly, and eating the right foods. At least once every two weeks, the agency needs to call her physician to discuss complications caused by noncompliance. The physician reviews the agency's latest written report, her notes from previous phone calls, and the plan of care, and she revises previous orders based on the latest information. The physician reports 99374 if she spends 15 to 29 minutes on these activities in a calendar month or 99375 for 30 minutes or more.

Selection criteria are:

- Only one physician reports these codes—the supervising physician.
- These codes are reported per calendar month and represent the services provided during that month.
- Do not report these codes unless the patient requires recurrent supervision of the therapy/treatment.
- The supervision requires complex and multidisciplinary care modalities, involving regular physician development and/or revi-

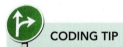

CODING TIP

Care Plan Oversight Not Involving an Agency, a Hospice, or a Nursing Facility

For care plan oversight for patients who are at home, in a domiciliary environment, or in a rest home, but not under the care of a home health agency or hospice, use 99339 and 99340.

Checkpoint 7.14

A physician is responsible for the care of an eighty-four-year old man with many complex health care issues who is currently in a nursing facility. She has seen this patient at the nursing home, and she also takes the calls from the nursing home for required changes in care plans and about lab studies and tests that are required to maintain the patient's health, as well from the patient's daughter, who visits her father daily. The physician discusses treatment with the nurses in charge of her patient's care at the facility on a regular basis. Her office documentation indicates that she has spent 40 minutes on such oversight this month What code should be reported for this month's time?

_____

_____

sion of care plans, review of reports on patient status, laboratory and other studies; communication for the purpose of assessment of the patient, care decisions with health care professional(s), family member(s), surrogate decision maker(s); and integrating new information into the patient's medical treatment plan, and/or make adjustments to that plan.

Preventive Medicine Services

99381–99387	New patient codes for the initial comprehensive preventive medicine service, early childhood (age 1–4 years) through 65 years and older	
99391–99397	Established patient codes for the periodic comprehensive preventive medicine service, same age range as the new patient codes	
99401–99404	Individual Counseling Time-based	Time-based
99406–99409	Behavior Change Interventions	Time-based
99411–99412	Group Counseling	Time-based
99420–99429	Other Preventive Services	

Preventive medicine services codes represent services provided to assess patients' health on a regular basis or to promote their health and prevent illness or injury. This code range is separated from the rest of the E/M code categories, which cover **problem-oriented** visits.

INITIAL OR PERIODIC PREVENTIVE MEDICINE

Codes 99381–99397 are used for patients who present for their annual physicals as either new or established patients. These are age-based codes, and the patient's age generally determines the extent of the services provided. The services include counseling, anticipatory guidance, and risk-factor reduction interventions. (Note that 99401–99429 are reported when the counseling and related services are provided during a separate encounter with the patient.) Other work—such as immunizations, labs, studies, and radiology services—is reported in addition to preventive medicine codes when provided.

The preventive medicine codes are used when patients who are not currently ill present for their annual physicals. It is not unusual for the physician to encounter an abnormality or preexisting condition while performing a preventive medicine service. If the abnormality or preexisting condition is significant enough to require additional work in terms of history, examination, and medical decision making (the three key components), a code from the 99201–99215 (E/M codes for OP problem-oriented visits) should be reported in addition to the preventive medicine code, and the modifier −25 should be appended to the problem-oriented E/M code.

EXAMPLES

A patient who is fifty-five years of age is seen for his annual physical. He also has significant pain, soreness, redness, and heat in his right extremity. This condition requires the physician to ask additional questions (history) and do an additional examination and evaluation (medical decision making) to determine whether the patient has phlebitis. Both the preventive service code and the problem-oriented service codes will be reported.

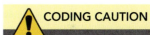

CODING CAUTION

Use of _Comprehensive_
The meaning of _comprehensive_ in this section is not the same as in other key component descriptions. Here it means the normal age- and gender-appropriate history and examination.

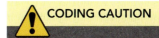

CODING CAUTION

Documentation Required
The record should clearly show that the abnormality or preexisting condition was a significant matter truly requiring additional work by the physician, not something that could easily have been addressed within the confines of the preventive medicine service.

A patient who is forty years of age is seen for her annual physical. She has had a cough for the past week. An evaluation of the respiratory system is part of preventive medicine services. Although the physician may have to ask some additional questions to resolve the cough, this scenario rarely justifies the use of a problem-oriented code in addition to the preventive medicine code.

COUNSELING RISK FACTOR REDUCTION AND BEHAVIOR CHANGE INTERVENTION

These codes represent services provided face-to-face for new or established patients by a physician or other qualified health care professional for promoting health and preventing illness or injury. These services are distinct from other E/M services that may be reported separately when performed. Risk factor reduction services are for persons without a specific illness and address issues such as family problems, diet and exercise, substance use, sexual practices, injury prevention, dental health, and diagnostic/laboratory test results that are available at the time of the encounter.

Newborn Care

99431	History and examination of normal newborn infant
99432	Normal newborn care in other than hospital or birthing room
99433	Subsequent hospital care of normal newborn
99435	History and examination of normal newborn assessed and discharged same day
99436	Attendance at delivery
99440	Newborn resuscitation

Newborn care codes represent various services provided to newborns in different settings and include codes for two types of initial care based on the newborn's delivery location. The code for a newborn delivered in the hospital or birthing room includes initiation of diagnostic and treatment programs and preparation of hospital records. If the child is born in a location other than the hospital or birthing room, the code includes the physical examination of the baby and conferences with the parents.

There is only one code for the subsequent care of a newborn, 99433, which is reported each day the physician provides care to a newborn in the hospital. Code 99435, which represents care provided to a newborn assessed and discharged on the same date, is not commonly used now. It is more likely for a newborn to be delivered and to remain in the hospital for more than one day. However, when the same-date scenario occurs, the code includes preparation of medical records.

A delivering physician sometimes anticipates a problem for the newborn upon delivery and asks a pediatrician to attend the delivery in order to be immediately available to provide care if necessary. The pediatrician will report code 99436, which includes stabilization, including resuscitation, of the newborn. This code may be reported with code 99431 (initial care of newborn), but not with 99440 (resuscitation of newborn) or for standby services (99360, 99361).

A pediatrician who is not asked to attend the delivery may be called in after the child is born if the child is having trouble breathing (acute

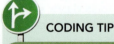

CODING ALERT

Stabilization, Not Standby

Do not confuse stabilization (code 99436) with standby. The pediatrician is actually present in the delivery room, not elsewhere in the delivery suite.

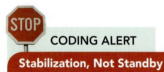

CODING TIP

Discharge After Admission Date

Use hospital discharge code 99238 if the newborn is discharged on a date subsequent to the admission date.

inadequate ventilation) or the child's heart is not pumping correctly (inadequate cardiac output). Under these circumstances, the physician will provide positive pressure ventilation and/or chest compression and will report code 99440.

Non-Face-to-Face Physician Services

TELEPHONE SERVICES

99441-99443	Telephone E/M services	Time-based

These codes represent non-face-to-face services provided to established patients or their guardians only and must be initiated by the patient. They would not be reported for new patients or consultations. The criteria for reporting these services require that the physician has not provided a related E/M service to this patient within the previous 7 days and on the basis of the telephone call service the physician will not provide an E/M service in the next 24 hours or soonest available appointment time.

ON-LINE MEDICAL EVALUATION

99444	Online E/M service Established patient only

These code represents the services provided using internet resources to established patients only, or their guardians in response to an on-line inquiry from the patient or guardian. The criteria for providing this online E/M service is that there was no related E/M service provided to the patient within the previous 7 days and this service is reported only once for the same episode of care during a seven day period by the same physician.

Special Evaluation and Management Services

99450	Basic life and/or disability examination	
99455	Work-related or medical disability	Treating physician
99456	Work-related or medical disability	Other than treating physician
99499	Unlisted E/M service	

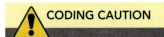

These codes represent services provided to establish baseline information before the issuance of life or disability insurance certificates. They are appropriate for any outpatient setting and for either new or established patients. No active management of the patient's problems occurs during the encounter. Note that code 99455 is for the patient's treating physician, whereas code 99456 is for the service provided by another physician.

Modifier −25

No chapter on E/M coding is complete without reference to modifier −25. This modifier is used to represent an E/M service that is significant and separately identifiable from a procedure or another E/M service provided on the same date.

It is important to understand that all procedures include some E/M services:

- Assessing the site or condition of the problem area
- Explaining the procedure
- Obtaining consent

If the E/M service goes beyond the above criteria, consider using modifier −25 on the E/M service to indicate that the physician has performed a significant and separately identifiable E/M service in addition to what is included in the procedure.

> **EXAMPLE** A new patient is seen by an orthopedist for knee pain. The physician evaluates the patient, determines the cause of the pain, and determines that a knee injection is a possible treatment for the condition.

The E/M service is significant and separately identifiable from the knee injection, and both the E/M code and the knee injection code will be reported. The −25 modifier is placed on the E/M code.

> **EXAMPLE** An established patient who saw his physician for ongoing knee pain returns for a knee injection, as the physician suggested at the last visit, since the patient's knee pain remains the same and no new problems occurred.

At this time, only the knee injection code would be reported. There is no reason for an E/M service that is significant or separately identifiable.

Checkpoint 7.16

A dermatologist has been treating a patient for skin lesions. At the patient's fifth visit, the dermatologist explains that the right arm lesion will need to be incised and drained at the next visit unless it resolves from the application of medication. At the next visit, the lesion is unchanged, and the incision and drainage are performed. However the patient has developed several similar lesions in other body areas. The dermatologist reports an E/M service with modifier −25 and the incision and drainage code. Did the dermatologist report his services correctly? _____ Explain why.

_____

_____

1. The CPT Evaluation and Management (E/M) section is organized by the use of categories and subcategories to delineate a structure of coding. The category identifies the broadest context of services, such as hospital inpatient services. The subcategory identifies the more specific context, such as initial hospital care and subsequent hospital care. This organization allows the coder to identify where the service is provided and the type of service provided.

2. The introductory guidelines for each section (such as Observation Care, Critical Care, and Care Plan Oversight) are the coding instructions specific to each section of E/M coding. They provide the rules that control how the listed codes can be applied and whether other codes in the E/M section affect the use of the codes. They also identify whether codes in that section are time-based and how to determine time. Also included in the guidelines is information on what services may or may not be included in that code set.

3. The five questions to ask in order to select the appropriate E/M category and the correct codes are:

   a. Who is the patient?
   b. What is the place of service?
   c. What is the patient's status?
   d. What type of service is being provided?
   e. What level of service is being provided?

4. To be classified as a new patient, the individual cannot have received a professional service within three years by the physician or another physician of the same specialty in the same group. Established patients have received a professional service within the three-year period. Professional service means that a face-to-face service was provided by the physician. Some code categories in the E/M section do not differentiate new and established patients; the codes are applicable to both. These include codes for consultations, the emergency department, and initial and subsequent hospital care.

5. The three key components are history, examination, and medical decision making. Each key component has a level of service that determines the code to be selected. The levels of service are problem-focused, expanded problem-focused, detailed, and comprehensive. Not all E/M codes have key component requirements.

6. To determine the level of service, first determine the three key component levels: history, examination, and medical decision making. Then review the E/M codes to find out whether they require all three key components to be at the level reported, or if they require only two of the three key components to be at the level reported. The contributory components of counseling and coordination of care will be the determining factors if more than 50 percent of the time spent during the patient encounter was for counseling and/or coordination of care.

7. Consultations require that a physician request an opinion and/or advice from the consultant and that the consultant render the consultation and then respond in writing to the requesting physician. In the new-patient scenario, the referring physician is handing over the care of the patient to a different physician for treatment of a specific condition.

8. To assign critical care codes, coders have to know the meaning of "critically ill and/or injured" and of "critical care." Also, coders must know what services are included in critical care. Critical care codes are time-based, not based on key components, and coders must know what services may and may not be included in the time determination.

9. Observation care coding requires that the patient is in the hospital under "observation status," and it involves periodic reassessments of the patient by the supervising physician. Patients are in observation because their conditions are not severe enough to require admission to the hospital; neither are their conditions stable enough that they can be sent home. To report standby services, the standby is requested by another physician; the service is not face-to-face; at least 30 minutes is spent in standby; and the standby physician is not providing care or services to other patients during the standby period.

10. To correctly assign codes in the E/M section of CPT, close attention must be paid to the extensive rules and exceptions in each category.

    a. Know which codes require all three or only two of the three key components.
    b. Remember that if more than one E/M service is provided by the same physician to the same patient on the same day, only one E/M code is reported (roll-up rule).
    c. Note the exceptions to the roll-up rule.
    d. Know that some codes are based on the level of service and others are based on time.
    e. There are age-based codes.
    f. Certain codes include other services (for example, critical care).
    g. Certain time-based codes are reported on a per-month basis (for example, care plan oversight).

Review Questions: Chapter 7

Match the key terms with their definitions.

a. admitting physician _____
b. category _____
c. chief complaint _____
d. consultation _____
e. contributory component _____
f. direct care _____
g. new patient _____

h. observation care _____

i. preventive medicine _____

j. roll-up rule _____

1. Patient's explanation to the physician of why he or she needs to be seen

2. The situation in which a physician provides an opinion or advice on a patient and does not take over the care of the patient

3. Patient who has not been seen by the physician for three years

4. Nature of the presenting problem in the medical decision-making process

5. The situation in which a patient is sent to the hospital for care, but is not admitted to the hospital

6. Guideline for a coding situation in which, after being treated in the office, the patient is sent to the hospital to be admitted, and an admission code is reported

7. Type of face-to-face care provided by a physician to a pediatric patient in transport from one facility to another

8. Type of E/M grouping called Office or Outpatient Consultations

9. Type of care for a patient who is evaluated by a physician without a specific diagnosis, illness, or condition being reported for that evaluation

10. A physician who is allowed to bill the initial hospital care codes 99221–99223

Decide whether each statement is true or false.

1. Pediatric transport codes 99289 and 99290 represent services provided by nonphysician personnel in emergency situations. **T or F**

2. A physician who treats a patient in the office and also sends the patient for observation will report only the observation care codes and not the office visit codes. **T or F**

3. Time is used as the determining factor for an office visit level of service when time is documented in the medical record. **T or F**

4. If a neonatologist spends 1 hour 30 minutes providing critical care to a critically ill neonate in the intensive care unit, the neonatologist will report codes 99291 and 99292. **T or F**

5. Three key components are required for established patient visits. **T or F**

6. In the emergency department, time is not a determining factor. **T or F**

7. Care plan oversight codes are reported when a physician provides the appropriate key components for a patient who is under the care of a home health agency or hospice or in a nursing facility. **T or F**

8. A patient is seen by the attending physician each day during hospitalization. The physician documents a problem-focused exam and straightforward medical decision making. Because the history key component is not documented, the physician cannot bill for services. **T or F**

9. A patient was admitted by the hospital resident at 11 P.M. on Tuesday. On Wednesday, the patient's own physician comes into the hospital to provide initial hospital care. Even though the patient was admitted on Tuesday, the physician must report the services with Wednesday's date. **T or F**

10. An established patient is one who has received professional services from the physician or another physician of the same specialty in the same group in the previous three years. **T or F**

11. As long as the physician documents how long the visit took, time can be used to determine the level of service. **T or F**

12. If the code description requires two of three key components, you can disregard the lowest key component. **T or F**

13. You cannot determine the level of service until you see documentation of at least one of the contributory components of an E/M service. **T or F**

Select the letter that best completes the statement or answers the question.

1. Which code is used for the initial office visit of a patient with a two-day history of lower abdominal pain and occasional vomiting in which the physician obtains a detailed history and detailed examination and does low MDM?
   a. 99204
   b. 99214
   c. There is not enough information to determine the level of service.
   d. 99203

2. An internist asks an endocrinologist to give an opinion on a diabetic patient's bilateral lower extremity neuropathy. The endocrinologist provides a detailed history, an expanded problem-focused exam, and moderate medical decision making. The endocrinologist writes a letter to the internist indicating his findings. Which code is used?
   a. 99203
   b. 99243
   c. 99242
   d. 99254

3. A patient has diabetes and hypertension and is morbidly obese. The physician provides an expanded problem-focused exam and moderate MDM. Blood work reveals that the patient must start on insulin, and the patient is counseled for 20 minutes regarding the insulin regimen and risks. The total time for the visit is 30 minutes. Which code is used?
   a. 99213
   b. 99214
   c. 99243
   d. 99244

4. An internist sends a patient with long-term back pain to a spine specialist for treatment of the problem. The spine specialist provides an expanded problem-focused history and exam and low MDM. The patient discusses his years of stress-related pain and his dissatisfaction with his previous care. The physician spends 35 minutes with the patient. Which code is used?
   a. 99202
   b. 99243
   c. 99203
   d. 99244

5. A pediatrician examines a two-day-old baby on rounds but is called away during the examination. The pediatrician returns later that day and completes the visit. The total time spent during the two visits is 25 minutes. Which code is used?
   a. 99431
   b. 99231
   c. 99432
   d. 99433

6. A physician provides initial inpatient critical care for a thirty-day-old infant. Which code is used?
   a. 99295
   b. 99293
   c. 99294
   d. 99296

7. An ED physician evaluates a patient in the ED. The patient's internist is called in to admit the patient to the hospital. What service does each physician report?
   a. ED physician reports ED code; internist reports initial hospital care for the admission
   b. ED physician reports initial hospital care; no codes reported by internist
   c. ED physician reports ED code and initial hospital care; no codes reported by internist
   d. ED physician does not report any services; internist reports initial hospital care

8. A fifty-four-year-old established patient is seen for an annual examination. The physician provides a comprehensive physical and spends 15 minutes discussing the patient's anxiety. Which code is used?
   a. 99205
   b. 99386
   c. 99396
   d. 99401

9. A cardiologist asks a surgeon to stand by during a procedure. The surgeon sees patients in the hospital while on standby, but is available via beeper. The procedure takes 1.5 hours. Which code is used?
   a. 99360
   b. 99360x3
   c. This is not a reportable service.
   d. 99360, 99356

10. A patient is in the hospital for a total hip replacement. The patient also has coronary artery disease and develops symptoms. The orthopedic surgeon asks a cardiologist to see the patient and give his opinion on the severity of the problem. What code does the cardiologist use?
    a. consultation code
    b. new patient code
    c. subsequent hospital care code
    d. This is a professional courtesy; no codes are reported.

11. An internal medicine physician asks a local endocrinologist to evaluate a diabetic patient's ongoing bilateral lower extremity neuropathy. He wants to know whether the patient's problem is related to the diabetes or if there is another problem. The endocrinologist performs a detailed history, an expanded problem-focused exam, and moderate medical decision making (MDM). The endocrinologist writes a letter to the requesting physician indicating his findings. Which of the following codes does the endocrinologist use?
    a. 99203
    b. 99243
    c. 99242
    d. 99254

12. An established patient is seen in his physician's office for a chief complaint of persistent cough. The physician performs a brief history and examines the respiratory system. MDM is straightforward. Which code does the physician use?
    a. 99211
    b. 99201
    c. 99213
    d. 99212

13. At an initial office visit with a patient who has a five-day history of leg pain, swelling, and a hot spot, a detailed history is obtained, a detailed exam is done, and MDM is moderate. The patient is concerned about thrombophlebitis because there is a family history of this problem. The physician counsels the patient for 40 minutes. The entire visit takes 65 minutes. Which code does the physician use?
    a. 99203
    b. 99204
    c. 99205
    d. 99203–21

14. A neonatologist attends the delivery of a 1,000 gram infant who is born in respiratory distress. The pediatrician stabilizes the infant while still in the delivery room. What E/M code(s) does the pediatrician report?
    a. 99295
    b. 99436
    c. 99440, 99436
    d. 99440, 99295

15. A pediatrician stood by for 30 minutes during delivery by an obstetrician for a high-risk patient. The obstetrician delivered the baby and the pediatrician performed resuscitation. Which codes would be used for the pediatrician's services?

 a. 99436, 99440

 b. 99436

 c. 99440, 99360

 d. 99360

16. A sixty-year-old patient recently moved to Phoenix and is seeing a new internist there. The patient has a long history of gouty arthropathy but presents today for his annual preventive medicine visit. The physician provides comprehensive H&P, counsels the patient on diet, and orders exercise and blood work. Which code would be used?

 a. 99205

 b. 99386

 c. 99396

 d. 99386, 99402

17. An orthopedic surgeon is called to the ED by an ED doctor to see a patient who was in a motor vehicle accident. The patient has scrapes, contusions, and two dislocations. The orthopedist performs a comprehensive exam, a detailed history, and moderate MDM. Which code is used?

 a. 99243

 b. 99244

 c. 99284

 d. 99283

Answer the following questions.

1. When can time be the dominant factor in determining the level of service? _____

2. Explain the roll-up rule. _____

3. Explain the significance of the statement that "the lowest key component controls the level of service." _____

4. There are two types of care plan oversight services. What differentiates them? _____

5. The statement "a physician cannot report a consultation code if he or she provided treatment to the patient during the visit" represents what consultation concept? _____

6. What is the 15-minute rule, and what codes use this rule? _____

Applying Your Knowledge

BUILDING CODING SKILLS

Case 7.1

1. A seventy-three-year-old woman was seen four years ago by her endocrinologist for diabetes. Her condition is worsening, and today she sees another endocrinologist in the same group to follow up on the diabetes. The endocrinologist does a detailed history, a detailed exam, and moderate medical decision making. Is she a new patient or an established patient, and what code will be reported?

2. The same patient went to the emergency department because she was feeling weak and faint, and she was seen by the ED physician there. Is this an outpatient service that would be reported in the

99201–99215 range of codes, or should this be reported from the emergency department code range 99281–99285? Based on the same key components, what code should be reported for this service?

Case 7.2

A patient with stomach pain and fever is seen in the office. The physician is not convinced that the patient is well enough to go home, but he is also not sick enough to be admitted. The physician sends the patient to the hospital, and later in the day the physician again evaluates the patient and determines whether he is well enough to be sent home.

1. This explains what type of service?

2. What category of codes would be reported?

3. Would the physician report more than one category of codes?

Case 7.3

A patient has been in the hospital for five days and is ready to be discharged. The physician provides all the discharge services and documents them in the hospital chart. He estimates that he spent 40 minutes providing the discharge care. What is the requirement for this physician to be able to report 99239?

Case 7.4

In this case, use the decision steps outlined in this chapter for history, examination, and medical decision making to determine whether the physician adequately documented the key component level, and explain your answer.

1. Patient reports shortness of breath, which has been a problem for the last month, particularly when she climbs stairs. She does not complain of chest pain. E/M key component level reported: expanded problem-focused history.

2. Examination of the mouth is normal; the throat is red and swollen. Abdomen: not tender, no organomegaly, normal bowel sounds. E/M key component level reported: expanded problem-focused exam for a patient who presents with difficulty swallowing.

3.

> **DIAGNOSIS:** The patient has long-term cardiovascular disease but is stable on his medications. His hypertension is also well-controlled, as is his diabetes. I have some concerns regarding his continued problem with leg pain.
>
> **DATA:** I have reviewed his ECG, and it is normal, with no changes from the previous ECG two months ago. I discussed his diabetes with his endocrinologist and ordered additional labs.
>
> **OVERALL RISK:** In all, he is doing well considering his illnesses. E/M key component level reported: moderate MDM.

USING CODING TERMS

Case 7.5

Read the following case study and determine from which code ranges each physician will assign an E/M code.

A fifty-year-old woman developed shortness of breath with mild chest pain. She called her physician. It was 6 P.M., and the physician was making hospital rounds, so he asked her to go to the emergency department to be evaluated and to have the ED contact him if necessary. When she was evaluated by the ED physician, her physician was contacted, and he also evaluated the patient and admitted her to the hospital based on his findings.

Case 7.6

What type(s) of code(s) will the physician report in the following case?

An eighty-year-old man had a total knee replacement. His hip had been replaced six months earlier, and he had developed a hernia as well. He now needs to be discharged from the hospital and admitted to a skilled nursing facility for monitoring of his multiple health issues and for rehabilitation for his knee surgery. His physician will be providing the discharge services and the admission to the nursing facility.

Researching the Internet

1. The Internet can provide insight into coding issues. Here are two links to sites that answer frequently asked questions (FAQs) about E/M coding:
   http://www.kansasmedicare.com/part_B/faqs/evalMgmtCodes.htm
   and
   www.connecticutmedicare.com.
   (On the second site, search the topic of Evaluation and Management (E/M) services.) Visit each site and report on the types of topics that are discussed.

2. As the responsible party for CPT, the AMA issues updates on its website. Visit the AMA CPT website
   www.ama-assn.org/go/cpt
   and search for news about evaluation and management codes.

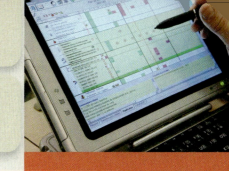

CPT: Anesthesia and Surgery Codes

LEARNING OUTCOMES

After studying this chapter, you should be able to:

1. Define the concept of a complete anesthesia service.

2. Identify documentation necessary to code anesthesia services.

3. Calculate anesthesia time units and fees based on prescribed formulas.

4. Assign CPT anesthesia codes with appropriate HCPCS modifiers and physical status modifiers based on anesthesia procedural statements.

5. Describe the organization, guidelines, and key modifiers for the surgery section in CPT.

6. List the components of a surgical package.

7. Distinguish between the CPT and Medicare definitions of a surgical package.

8. Describe the types of situations in which separate procedure codes are correctly reported.

9. Select appropriate surgical modifiers for physician use and facility (hospital outpatient) use.

10. Assign CPT surgical codes with appropriate modifiers based on surgery procedural statements.

Key Terms

American Society of Anesthesiologists (ASA)

analgesic

anesthesia

anesthesia modifiers

anesthesiologist

anesthesiology

anesthetist

bundled

CCI column 1/column 2 code pair edits

closed procedure

conscious sedation (CS)

Correct Coding Initiative (CCI)

CCI modifier indicators

CCI mutually exclusive code (MEC) edits

diagnostic procedure

edits

endoscope

general anesthesia

global period

global surgery days

incidental procedure

local anesthesia

medically unlikely edits (MUEs)

monitored anesthesia care (MAC)

open procedure

outpatient code editor (OCE)

physical status modifiers

qualifying circumstance

regional anesthesia

Relative Value Guide

therapeutic procedure

time (tm) units

unbundling

Chapter Outline

Anesthesia Background

Anesthesia Coding

Surgery Coding Overview

Surgical Procedure Types

Surgery Modifiers

Integumentary System

Musculoskeletal System

Respiratory System

Cardiovascular System

Hemic and Lymphatic Systems; Mediastinum and Diaphragm

Digestive System

Urinary System

Male Genital System; Intersex Surgery

Female Genital System and Maternity Care and Delivery

Endocrine and Nervous Systems

Eye and Ocular Adnexa; Auditory System; Operating Microscope

Anesthesiologists are active in many aspects of a patient's clinical treatment in addition to providing anesthesia during surgical procedures. They participate in acute and chronic pain management, critical care, ventilation assistance and management, anesthesia for deliveries, and intravascular catheterization procedures. Anesthesia services can be some of the most difficult to code though, especially from a billing perspective. Anesthesiologists are not reimbursed according to the same payment methodology as other physicians, and individual payers have varying rules for coding and billing. Coding for anesthesia services is not routinely done by physician practices or HIM coders; it is considered a coding specialty. However, it is important for all medical coders to have a basic understanding of this important topic.

In contrast, all outpatient coders—whether they code for a physician or for a hospital or other ambulatory facility—must develop proficiency in coding for surgical procedures. The Surgery section of CPT, which contains the greatest number of codes in the CPT code set, is subdivided into surgical specialties and provides codes for all outpatient surgical procedures. To become successful in surgical coding, coders must be familiar with the format and organization of the surgical subsections, have a fundamental understanding of anatomy and medical terminology, master the concepts of the surgical package, correctly apply modifiers, and adhere to payers' rules on billing surgery codes. These skills, with the addition of communication with the provider and adequate documentation, are the formula for accurate surgical coding.

Anesthesia Background

The administration of **anesthesia** causes the loss of the ability to feel pain. The administered drug or other medical intervention causes partial or complete loss of sensation with or without loss of consciousness. According to the American Society of Anesthesiologists, **anesthesiology** is essentially the practice of medicine dealing with:

- The management of procedures for rendering a patient insensible to pain and emotional stress during surgery and obstetrical procedures
- The evaluation and management of life functions under the stress of anesthetic and surgical manipulations
- The clinical management of a patient unconscious from any cause
- The evaluation and management of problems with pain relief
- The management of problems in cardiac and respiratory resuscitation
- The application of specific methods of respiratory therapy
- The clinical management of various fluids, electrolytes, and metabolic disturbances

Anesthesia services are provided by an anesthesiologist or a nurse anesthetist (CRNA). **Anesthesiologists** are physicians specializing in providing anesthesia and pain management services. Nurse **anesthetists** are critical care nurses who have obtained additional training in providing anesthesia. These professionals specialize in anesthesiology and are regulated by the American Board of Anesthesiology, the American Society of Anesthesiology, and state laws. Most anesthesia groups are independent contractors and are not employed by hospitals.

TYPES OF ANESTHESIA

The type of anesthesia the doctor chooses for a procedure depends on the type of procedure being performed as well as the age and health of the patient. The choice is made after the anesthesiologist has interviewed and examined the patient and has obtained consent.

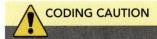

⚠ CODING CAUTION

Only Anesthesiologists Report Anesthesia Codes
Anesthesia services are reported only by the physician who provides or supervises them. The surgeon performing the actual surgical procedure cannot assign separate codes for the anesthesia services.

General Anesthesia Under **general anesthesia,** the patient is rendered unconscious, pain-free, and stable for the entire surgical procedure. Constant attendance of anesthesia personnel and monitoring are required. General anesthesia is performed when procedures are highly invasive, are long in duration, or do not permit patient movement. Some examples of procedures performed under general anesthesia are abdominal surgery such as hysterectomy and cholecystectomy, spine surgery, organ transplants, breast reconstruction, and sinus surgery. Examples of common medications used for general anesthesia are Propofol, Fentanyl, Pentothal, Alfentanil, and Succinylcholine.

The steps involved with administering general anesthesia are:

1. *Preparation:* The anesthesiologist reviews the patient's history (allergies, previous anesthesia experiences, medications, treatments, and so on), performs a physical examination (including oral airway), and determines an anesthesia plan.

2. *Induction:* The anesthesiologist puts the patient to sleep (intubation).

3. *Maintenance:* While the surgeon operates, the anesthesiologist maintains the patient in an anesthetized state and monitors metabolic functions (temperature, pulse, respirations, and neuromuscular function).

4. *Emergence:* The anesthesiologist reverses the anesthetic agents and extubates the patient, who gradually regains consciousness and control of body functions such as breathing.

5. *Recovery:* After the surgeon has turned the patient over to the anesthesiologist, a postanesthesia care unit (PACU) monitors the patient for side effects of anesthesia. The anesthesia provider is responsible for the care of the patient until the patient is stable enough—breathing independently and able to answer questions appropriately—to be discharged to a room or from the facility. The PACU also begins postoperative pain management.

Regional Anesthesia In **regional anesthesia,** the anesthesia numbs a part of the body without inducing unconsciousness. The patient is typically awake enough to respond to stimuli but is sedated and will not recall the procedure. This type of anesthesia is provided for procedures done below the diaphragm or on extremities and for patients for whom general anesthesia is a high risky. With this type of anesthesia, an IV is continuously instilling medication.

There are three types of regional anesthesia:

1. *Spinal anesthesia:* A single injection of the agent is injected into the subarachnoid space between two lumbar vertebrae.

2. *Epidural anesthesia:* Agent is injected by inserting a catheter into the epidural space, numbing the chest and lower body. A catheter is left intact for continuous infusion of anesthetic. This is the approach commonly employed for labor and delivery.

3. *Intravenous regional block:* In this type, which is used for short-term procedures performed on extremities, a tourniquet is placed on the extremity. A common intravenous regional block is a Bier block, which is used for upper extremity procedures.

Peripheral Nerve Blocks Nerve blocks involve injecting an anesthetic solution parallel to or surrounding a peripheral nerve or nerve plexuses such as the brachial plexus. The anesthetic solution diffuses from the outer surface (mantle) toward the center (core) of the nerve. The patient is awake throughout the procedure. This type of anesthesia is also used for controlling postoperative pain, often with trigger point or nerve injections.

Local Anesthesia   **Local anesthesia** affects a specific, small area of the body and is common for procedures on the skin. Administration may be by injection, as a topical anesthesia, or by spray. The patient is not asleep. Procedures performed solely under local anesthesia are performed in a physician office or at the bedside and do not require an operating room (OR) or anesthesia staff. Local anesthesia is commonly used for mole removals, laceration repairs (suturing), catheter insertions, and pin removals. Examples of local anesthesia medications are Lidocaine, Marcaine, Xylocaine, Buvicaine, Nesacaine, and Novacaine.

Monitored Anesthesia Care (MAC)   Under **monitored anesthesia care (MAC),** the patient is not completely anesthetized and can respond to directions and questions. The administration of sedatives, hypnotics, and analgesics as well as anesthetic drugs commonly used for the induction and maintenance of general anesthesia is often a part of MAC. Patients are sedated with a tranquilizer preoperatively. The surgeon may or may not anesthetize the surgical incision site with a local anesthetic.

The patient is monitored throughout the procedure. In some cases, the surgeon may direct the patient to respond to areas of pain or to cough or breathe deeply. Examples of common procedures performed under MAC are podiatry procedures such as hammertoe repair, breast biopsy, carpal tunnel surgery, lesion removals, some hernia repairs, lymph node biopsy, and some gynecological procedures such as conization of the cervix.

Conscious Sedation: Not an Anesthesia Section Service   Conscious sedation (CS) is moderate anesthesia carried out by injecting a sedative and/or analgesic intravenously to relieve pain and anxiety during a medical procedure. **Analgesics,** unlike most anesthesias, relieve pain without the loss of consciousness, though they may have an amnesia effect after the procedure is completed. The patient remains awake and relaxed. Procedures performed under conscious sedation are typically done in an office or clinic setting, not in the operating room.

Instead of an anesthesia provider, conscious sedation is done either by the surgeon or by a specially trained nurse who is supervised by the surgeon. The patient's consciousness and cardiac and respiratory function are monitored and documented throughout the procedure. The physician must be able to recognize deep sedation, manage the consequences, and adjust the level of sedation to a moderate or lesser level.

Differentiation of MAC and IV Sedation/Conscious Sedation
The difference between MAC and conscious sedation is under intense scrutiny by the medical and insurance communities. There are some major differences. MAC anesthesia allows a deeper sedation than does conscious sedation. MAC anesthesia can easily be transitioned into general anesthesia for brief periods of time, permitting the performance of a wider range of invasive procedures. MAC anesthesia requires a CRNA or anesthesiologist with the skill level to distinguish

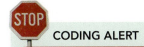

CODING ALERT

Local Anesthesia Not Separately Billable

According to CPT, "local infiltration, metacarpal/ metatarsal/digital block or topical anesthesia" is included in the surgical procedure code and cannot be billed separately.

BILLING TIP

Conscious Sedation

Guidelines and codes for IV conscious sedation (99143–99150) are in the Medicine section, not the Anesthesia section. Codes with the conscious sedation symbol (⊙) in CPT indicate that conscious sedation is not reported separately from the code for the procedure when the physician providing the anesthesia is also performing the procedure. If conscious sedation is provided by another physician or qualified individual, this rule would not apply, since each professional reports his or her services separately.

deep sedation from general anesthesia and to quickly return the patient to deep sedation. It also requires the provider to be prepared to convert to general anesthesia, maintaining the patient's airway, should the procedure require it or if the patient is uncooperative.

To pay for MAC anesthesia, Medicare requires:

- A surgeon's request for MAC
- An anesthesia preoperative examination
- Continuous presence of anesthesia personnel
- Anesthesiologist presence for emergency treatment or diagnosis
- Continuous metabolic monitoring
- Oxygen administration, if indicated
- IV administration of scheduled pharmacologic agents at the discretion of the anesthesia personnel

Anesthesia Coding

Anesthesia codes are located in CPT in the Anesthesia section. The codes are also listed in the **American Society of Anesthesiologists (ASA)** *Relative Value Guide,* which is published annually and contains anesthesia guidelines, modifiers, common procedures performed by anesthesiologists, and elements used in calculating anesthesia fees.

In CPT, anesthesia codes are grouped anatomically by body area, first in the order of the head down to the feet, and then from the shoulder to the hand. The Anesthesia section is divided into nineteen subsections, each covering general, regional, and local anesthesia (see Table 8.1).

Table 8.1 Anesthesia Subsections

Head	00100–00222
Neck	00300–00352
Thorax	00400–00474
Intrathoracic	00500–00580
Spine and Spinal Cord	00600–00670
Upper Abdomen	00700–00797
Lower Abdomen	00800–00882
Perineum	00902–00952
Pelvis (except hip)	01112–01190
Upper Leg (except knee)	01200–01274
Knee and Popliteal Area	01320–01444
Lower Leg (below knee)	01462–01522
Shoulder and Axilla	01610–01682
Upper Arm and Elbow	01710–01782
Forearm, Wrist, and Hand	01810–01860
Radiological Procedures	01916–01936
Burn Excisions or Debridement	01951–01953
Obstetric	01958–01969
Other Procedures	01990–01999

ANESTHESIA SERVICES PACKAGE

Anesthesia services for surgical procedures have one code that pays for the complete anesthesia service, which includes:

- General, regional, supplementation of local anesthesia
- Interpretation of lab values
- Placement of IVs for fluid and medication administration
- Arterial line insertion for blood pressure monitoring or other supportive services to provide the anesthesia care deemed optimal by the anesthesiologist during any procedure
- The usual preoperative and postoperative visits
- The administration of fluids and/or blood
- The usual monitoring services (temperature, blood pressure, oximetry, ECG, capnography, and mass spectrometry)

None of the following CPT codes can be billed in addition to a complete anesthesia service code, since that code includes them: 31500 (intubation), 31505 (laryngoscopy, indirect), 31515 (laryngoscopy, direct), 31527 (laryngoscopy with insertion of obturator), 31622 (bronchoscopy, diagnostic), 31645 (bronchoscopy), 36000 (introduction of needle or intracatheter, vein), 36010 (introduction of catheter, superior or inferior vena cava), 36400–36425 (venipuncture), or 62310–62319 (pain management).

Services Not Included in Routine Anesthesia Services

Some services are not part of a complete anesthesia service package, and if provided they may be billed separately with the −59 modifier:

- Insertion of Swan-Ganz catheter (93503)
- Emergency intubation (31500)
- Central venous pressure line (36555 or 36556 for central venous catheter) through a separate stick
- Unusual forms of monitoring such as placement of central venous lines
- Pain management injections or placement of epidurals for postoperative pain management and not for anesthesia purposes (independent of the anesthesia service)
- Critical care visits (99291–99292)
- Arterial catheter (36620)
- Transesophageal echocardiography (TEE; 93312–93318) if performed for diagnostic purposes and not for monitoring the patient during surgery

> **EXAMPLE**   A patient undergoes a coloproctoscopy for GI bleeding. Because of the patient's condition and chronic illnesses, the anesthesiologist places a central venous pressure line. Report both codes 46614 and 93503–59.

Obstetrical Anesthesia
Two questions must be answered before assigning codes for labor and delivery anesthesia:

1. Did the physician provide anesthesia for labor or only for delivery?
2. Was the delivery vaginal or cesarean?

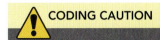

CODING CAUTION

Coding for Surgeon-Administered Anesthesia

Surgeons who render regional or general anesthesia report a code from the Surgery section (code range 10021–69979) with modifier −47. (Modifier −47 is never attached to an anesthesia code.) No additional payment is allowed; anesthesia services are considered part of the procedure.

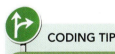

CODING TIP

Anesthesia Requires a Modifier

Anesthesia services are reported using the anesthesia procedure codes 00100–01999 plus an anesthesia modifier.

For obstetrical anesthesia for vaginal delivery, two codes are available—01960 and 01967: CPT code 01960 is used for anesthesia provided for a vaginal delivery, regardless of type (epidural or general); and CPT code 01967 is used if the physician provided anesthesia for labor *and* vaginal delivery. CPT code 01961 is assigned for a cesarean delivery.

Checkpoint 8.1

Use Table 8.1 and the definition of a complete anesthesia service to determine the code(s) that can be reported for this case.

A forty-three-year-old patient requires fusing of the spine due to traumatic injury. The surgeon asks the anesthesiologist to place an epidural for continuous infusion of pain medication for postoperative pain management.

The possible codes are 22612 and 62319.

1. Which code(s) can be assigned? _____
2. What CPT professional services modifier should be appended to indicate that two distinct procedural services were performed? _____

CODING ALERT

Using Anesthesia Modifiers

- Modifier −23 is appended only to anesthesia codes; it is never used with surgery codes or E/M codes.
- Modifier −47, anesthesia by surgeon, is never used by an anesthesiologist for anesthesia procedures.

BILLING TIP

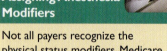

Assigning Anesthesia Modifiers

Not all payers recognize the physical status modifiers. Medicare and Medicaid do not. Check and comply with each payer's rules.

CODING CAUTION

Selecting Medicare MAC Modifiers

Be careful when assigning modifiers for MAC, selecting −QS, −G8, or −G9 based on the patient's condition.

ANESTHESIA MODIFIERS

All anesthesia services are reported using the five-digit CPT Anesthesia section codes along with **anesthesia modifiers,** which are essential to identify who provided the anesthesia services. Three different categories of anesthesia modifiers can be appended to anesthesia codes: physical status modifiers, CPT professional services modifiers, and HCPCS Level II modifiers.

Physical Status Modifiers Physical status modifiers are located on the inside cover of CPT (and in the Anesthesia guidelines) and are shown in Table 8.2. Based on the ranking system used by the American Society of Anesthesiologists, they depict the physical risk to the patient or the complexity of the anesthesia care. The ASA assigns reimbursement units to each modifier, which affects anesthesia fees.

EXAMPLE Non-Medicare patient is a fifty-nine-year-old male with ESRD and CHF undergoing an open reduction with internal fixation (ORIF) of the distal femur. Report 01360–P3.

Table 8.2 Physical Status Modifiers

−P1	Normal, healthy patient
−P2	Patient with mild systemic disease
−P3	Patient with severe systemic disease that is constant threat to life
−P4	Patient with severe systemic disease
−P5	Moribund patient who is not expected to survive without surgery
−P6	Declared brain-dead patient whose organs are being removed for donation

Table 8.3 Applicable CPT Modifiers

−22	Unusual procedural service
−23	Unusual anesthesia reported when anesthesia is administered for a procedure that usually requires local anesthesia or none at all but, because of unusual circumstances, must be done under general anesthesia (For example, the physician requests general anesthesia to perform an examination of the ears and remove impacted cerumen in an autistic child. This procedure typically does not require general anesthesia and is normally performed in the office setting.)
−32	Mandated service
−50	Bilateral procedure
−51	Multiple procedures
−52	Reduced services
−53	Discontinued procedure, used when the physician elects to terminate or discontinue a procedure, usually due to the risk of the patient's well-being, after the surgical preparation of patient or induction of anesthesia (a copy of the operative report should be submitted with the claim)
−59	Distinct procedural service, used to indicate that a procedure or service was independent from other services provided that day only if no other modifier is appropriate
−74	Discontinued outpatient hospital/ambulatory surgery center procedure after the administration of anesthesia because of such circumstances as the threat to the patient's well-being. (For example, the physician encountered massive tumors and adhesions and could not complete the procedure because of extensive bleeding.)

CPT Modifiers   Under certain circumstances, the CPT modifiers listed on the inside of CPT's front cover and shown in Table 8.3 may be used to explain circumstance that arise during surgery or in the operating room. The modifiers (with the exception of modifier −23) can be assigned to procedures anesthesiologists personally perform, not to anesthesia services.

HCPCS Level II Modifiers   HCPCS Level II modifiers, intended for use for Medicare patients, are located in the HCPCS code set; they are not in CPT (see Table 8.4). Documentation to show medical necessity, such as an operative note, may be required for some payers.

> **EXAMPLE**   A sixty-nine-year-old male Medicare patient has a hernia repair under MAC anesthesia. The anesthesiologist is supervising two CRNAs during the procedure. Report 00830–QS–QY.

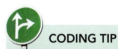

CODING TIP

Reporting Order

If more than one anesthesia modifier is necessary, always list the HCPCS Level II modifier first.

NOTE

HCPCS coding is covered in Chapter 10 of your program.

Table 8.4 HCPCS Level II Anesthesia Modifiers

−AA	Anesthesia personally performed by an anesthesiologist
−AD	Medically directed more than four procedures or CRNAs
−QB	Physician providing anesthesia in a rural health professional shortage area (HPSA)
−QK	Medically directed two, three, and four concurrent procedures involving qualified individuals, used when the anesthesiologist supervised at least two but not more than four CRNAs
−QS	Monitored anesthesia care (MAC)
−QU	Physician providing anesthesia in an urban HPSA
−QY	Medically directed CRNA—two to four CRNAs per one physician
−QX	CRNA service medically directed by a physician—one CRNA to one physician
−QZ	CRNA not medically directed by a physician (no payment reduction occurs when the CRNA is working independent of a physician)
−G8	Monitored anesthesia care (MAC) for deep complex, complicated, or markedly invasive surgical procedure, used in lieu of −QS for Medicare patients with procedures of the face, neck, breast, male genitalia, or for procedures for access to central venous circulation, and appended to anesthesia codes 00100, 00300, 00400, 00160, 00532, and 00920
−G9	Monitored anesthesia care (MAC) for at-risk Medicare patients with history of severe cardiopulmonary condition; chosen over general to avoid potential intraoperative complications

Checkpoint 8.2

Append all modifiers applicable to the anesthesia code in the following case.

A Medicare patient undergoes a radical hysterectomy for cervical cancer. The anesthesiologist is supervising two cases simultaneously. The CRNA provides the general anesthesia.

00846– _____

QUALIFYING CIRCUMSTANCES

Qualifying circumstances (also called *modifying factors*) are particularly difficult situations under which anesthesia must be administered, such as extraordinary condition of the patient, notable operative conditions, and/or unusual risk factors. Four codes, as shown in Table 8.5, are used to report these circumstances. The codes increase the fee due to the complications with the administration of the anesthesia. The qualifying circumstance codes, found in the Medicine section of CPT, can be reported as additional procedure codes. They are also listed in the guidelines at the beginning of the anesthesia section.

Qualifying circumstances codes are add-on codes (+), so they are always listed along with a code for the primary anesthesia procedure and are never used alone. If more that one qualifying circumstance applies, more than one code may be assigned.

EXAMPLE A patient is brought to the ER after a motor vehicle accident in which he was struck while riding his motorcycle. He sustained a near amputation of the right foot and has lost a considerable amount of blood. Report 99140 in addition to the anesthesia code for the surgical repair of the foot due to the nature of the circumstances.

BILLING TIP

QC Codes Are Payer-Specific

Not all payers recognize these qualifying circumstance codes. Medicare and Medicaid do not recognize them. Check with each payer before submitting the codes.

ANESTHESIA DOCUMENTATION

Anesthesia coding is based on the services recorded in the anesthesia documentation. Each facility has a customized anesthesia record to capture anesthesia-specific clinical information. The record contains preoperative notes, intraoperative notes, and postanesthesia care unit documentation. Preoperative notes cover the patient's medical and surgical history, history of anesthetic complications, current medications, and respiratory condition, and the chosen anesthesia. Postanesthesia care unit (PACU) documentation records the monitoring of the patient for immediate postoperative complications.

Intraoperative notes (see Figure 8.1) reflect the close monitoring of the patient during the procedure for any complications. Monitoring is

Table 8.5 Qualifying Circumstances

+99100	Anesthesia for patient of extreme age, under one year and over seventy years of age (list separately in addition to code for primary anesthesia procedure)
+99116	Anesthesia complicated by utilization of total body hypothermia (list separately in addition to code for primary anesthesia procedure)
+99135	Anesthesia complicated by utilization of controlled hypothermia (list separately in addition to code for primary anesthesia procedure)
+99140	Anesthesia complicated by specified emergency condition (list separately in addition to code for primary anesthesia procedure), used when a delay in treatment would lead to a significant increase in the threat to life or body part

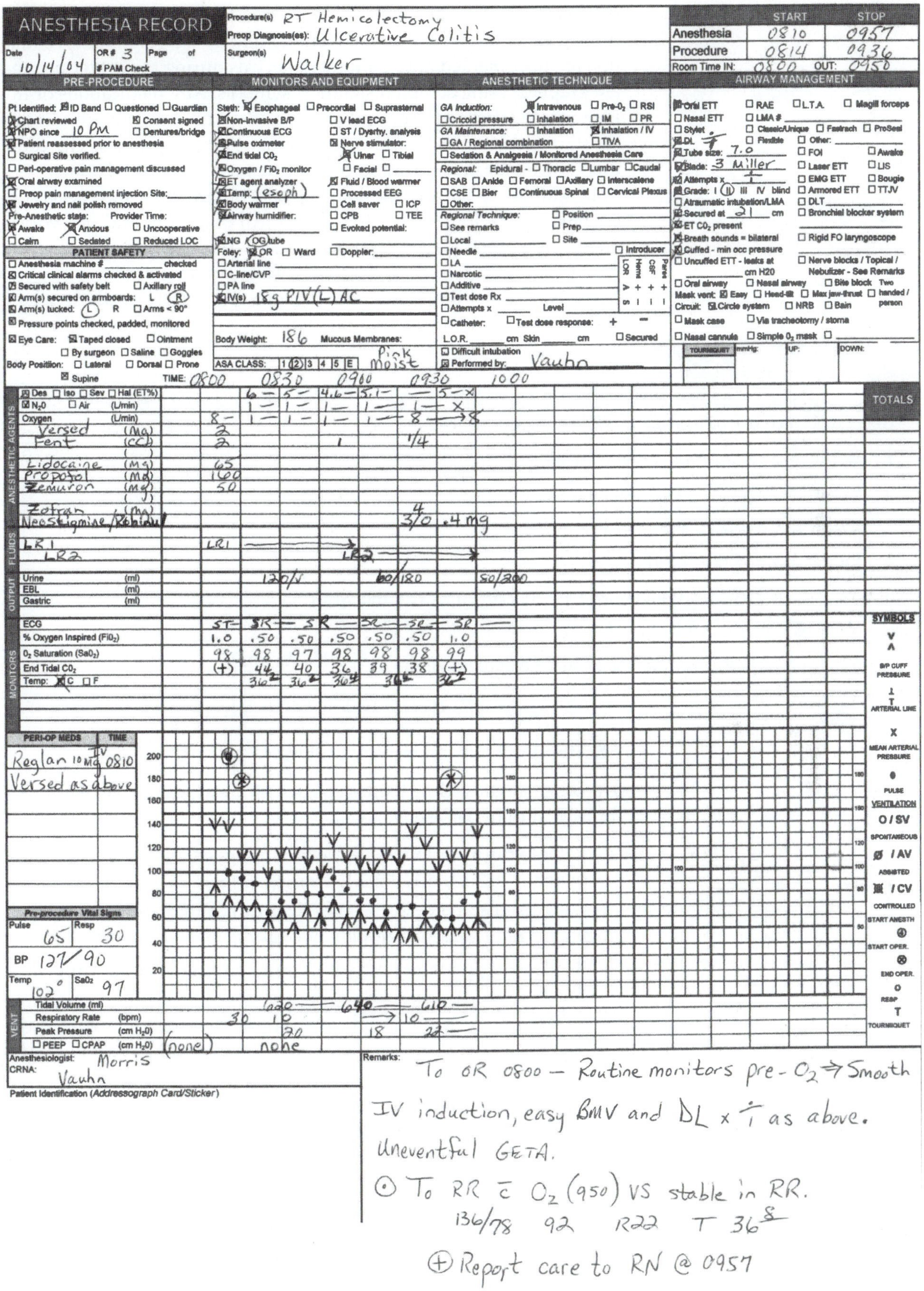

ANESTHESIA RECORD

Procedure(s): RT Hemicolectomy
Preop Diagnosis(es): Ulcerative Colitis
Date: 10/14/04 OR # 3 Page of
PAM Check
Surgeon(s): Walker

	START	STOP
Anesthesia	0810	0957
Procedure	0814	0936
Room Time IN: 0800		OUT: 0950

PRE-PROCEDURE

Pt Identified: ☒ ID Band ☐ Questioned ☐ Guardian
☒ Chart reviewed ☒ Consent signed
☒ NPO since 10 PM ☐ Dentures/bridge
☒ Patient reassessed prior to anesthesia
☐ Surgical Site verified.
☐ Peri-operative pain management discussed
☒ Oral airway examined
☐ Preop pain management injection Site: ______
☒ Jewelry and nail polish removed
Pre-Anesthetic state: Provider Time:
☒ Awake ☒ Anxious ☐ Uncooperative
☐ Calm ☐ Sedated ☐ Reduced LOC

PATIENT SAFETY

☐ Anesthesia machine # ______ checked
☒ Critical clinical alarms checked & activated
☒ Secured with safety belt ☐ Axillary roll
☒ Arm(s) secured on armboards: L (R)
☒ Arm(s) tucked: (L) R ☐ Arms < 90°
☒ Pressure points checked, padded, monitored
☒ Eye Care: ☒ Taped closed ☐ Ointment
☐ By surgeon ☐ Saline ☐ Goggles
Body Position: ☐ Lateral ☐ Dorsal ☐ Prone
☒ Supine

MONITORS AND EQUIPMENT

Steth: ☒ Esophageal ☐ Precordial ☐ Suprasternal
☒ Non-invasive B/P ☐ V lead ECG
☒ Continuous ECG ☐ ST / Dysrhy. analysis
☒ Pulse oximeter ☒ Nerve stimulator:
☒ End tidal CO_2 ☒ Ulnar ☐ Tibial
☒ Oxygen / FiO_2 monitor ☐ Facial ☐ ______
☒ ET agent analyzer ☒ Fluid / Blood warmer
☒ Temp: (esoph) ☐ Processed EEG
☒ Body warmer ☐ Cell saver ☐ ICP
☒ Airway humidifier: ☐ CPB ☐ TEE
☐ Evoked potential:
☒ NG (OG) tube
Foley: ☒ OR ☐ Ward ☐ Doppler: ______
☐ Arterial line
☐ C-line/CVP
☐ PA line
☒ IV(s) 18g PIV (L) AC
Body Weight: 186 Mucous Membranes: Pink Moist
ASA CLASS: 1 (2) 3 4 5 E

ANESTHETIC TECHNIQUE

GA Induction: ☒ Intravenous ☐ Pre-O_2 ☐ RSI
☐ Cricoid pressure ☐ Inhalation ☐ IM ☐ PR
GA Maintenance: ☐ Inhalation ☒ Inhalation / IV
☐ GA / Regional combination ☐ TIVA
☐ Sedation & Analgesia / Monitored Anesthesia Care
Regional: Epidural - ☐ Thoracic ☐ Lumbar ☐ Caudal
☐ SAB ☐ Ankle ☐ Femoral ☐ Axillary ☐ Interscalene
☐ CSE ☐ Bier ☐ Continuous Spinal ☐ Cervical Plexus
☐ Other:
Regional Technique: ☐ Position
☐ See remarks ☐ Prep
☐ Local ☐ Site
☐ Needle ☐ Introducer
☐ LA
☐ Narcotic
☐ Additive
☐ Test dose Rx
☐ Attempts x ______ Level
☐ Catheter: ☐ Test dose response: + −
L.O.R. ____ cm Skin ____ cm ☐ Secured
☒ Difficult intubation
☒ Performed by: Vauhn

AIRWAY MANAGEMENT

☒ Oral ETT ☐ RAE ☐ L.T.A. ☐ Magill forceps
☐ Nasal ETT ☐ LMA #
☐ Stylet ☐ Classic/Unique ☐ Fastrach ☐ ProSeal
☒ DL x 1 ☐ Flexible ☐ Other:
☒ Tube size: 7.0 ☐ FOI ☐ Awake
☒ Blade: 3 Miller ☐ Laser ETT ☐ LIS
☒ Attempts x 1 ☐ EMG ETT ☐ Bougie
☒ Grade: I (II) III IV blind ☐ Armored ETT ☐ TTJV
☐ Atraumatic intubation/LMA ☐ DLT
☒ Secured at 21 cm ☐ Bronchial blocker system
☒ ET CO_2 present
☒ Breath sounds = bilateral ☐ Rigid FO laryngoscope
☒ Cuffed - min occ pressure
☐ Uncuffed ETT - leaks at ____ cm H20 ☐ Nerve blocks / Topical / Nebulizer - See Remarks
☐ Oral airway ☐ Nasal airway ☐ Bite block Two handed / person
Mask vent: ☒ Easy ☐ Head-tilt ☐ Max jaw-thrust
Circuit: ☒ Circle system ☐ NRB ☐ Bain
☐ Mask case ☐ Via tracheostomy / stoma
☐ Nasal cannula ☐ Simple O_2 mask ☐
TOURNIQUET mmHg: UP: DOWN:

TIME:	0800	0830	0900	0930	1000

ANESTHETIC AGENTS

Agent	Entries
☒ Des ☐ Iso ☐ Sev ☐ Hal (ET%)	6 — 5 — 4.6 — 5.1 — — 5 — X
☒ N_2O ☐ Air (L/min)	1 — 1 — 1 — 1 — 1 — X
Oxygen (L/min)	8 — 1 — 1 — 1 — 1 — 8 → 8
Versed (Mg)	2
Fent (cc)	2 1 1/4
Lidocaine (Mg)	65
Propofol (Mg)	160
Zemuron (Mg)	50
Zofran (Mg)	4
Neostigmine/Robinul	3/0 .4 mg

FLUIDS
LR1 — LR1 → LR2 →
LR2

OUTPUT

Urine (ml)	120/V 60/180 50/200
EBL (ml)	
Gastric (ml)	

MONITORS

ECG	ST	SR	SR	SR	SR	SR	
% Oxygen Inspired (FiO_2)	1.0	.50	.50	.50	.50	.50	1.0
O_2 Saturation (SaO_2)	98	98	97	98	98	98	99
End Tidal CO_2	(+)	44	40	36	39	38	(+)
Temp: ☒ C ☐ F		36.2	36.4	36.4	36.6	36.2	

PERI-OP MEDS	TIME
Reglan 10 mg IV	0810
Versed as above	

Pre-procedure Vital Signs
Pulse 65 Resp 30
BP 127/90
Temp 102° SaO_2 97

SYMBOLS: V Λ B/P CUFF PRESSURE; ARTERIAL LINE; X MEAN ARTERIAL PRESSURE; ● PULSE; VENTILATION: O / SV SPONTANEOUS; Ø / AV ASSISTED; ☒ / CV CONTROLLED; ⊕ START ANESTH; ⊗ START OPER.; END OPER.; ○ RESP; T TOURNIQUET

VENT

Tidal Volume (ml)	600 — 640 — 610 —
Respiratory Rate (bpm)	30 10 → 10 —
Peak Pressure (cm H_2O)	20 18 22 —
☐ PEEP ☐ CPAP (cm H_2O)	(none) none

Anesthesiologist: Morris
CRNA: Vauhn
Patient Identification (Addressograph Card/Sticker)

Remarks: To OR 0800 — Routine monitors pre-O_2 ⇒ Smooth IV induction, easy BMV and DL x 1 as above. Uneventful GETA.
⊙ To RR c̄ O_2 (950) VS stable in RR. 136/78 92 R22 T 36.8
⊕ Report care to RN @ 0957

FIGURE 8.1
Anesthesia Record

done with a variety of mechanisms, such as heart monitoring, temperature probes, and pulse oximetry, among others. Vital signs and ventilation are documented at five-minute intervals during the procedure and are graphed using accepted standard symbols. Any medications or fluids provided during the procedure are also documented, as are anesthesia start and stop times and operation start and stop times. The coder must review this document to correctly ascertain anesthesia time.

In addition to the anesthesiologist's documentation, anesthesia coders have access to the operative report. All diagnoses and procedures are captured on this report, allowing the coder to sequence the highest paying procedure first on the claim. If any intraoperative complications required CPR or other unusual anesthesia services, these would also be documented.

Checkpoint 8.3

Refer to Figure 8.1 to answer the following questions.

1. What type of anesthesia was provided? _____
2. What surgical procedure was performed? _____
3. What was the total anesthesia time? _____
4. Who provided the anesthesia care? _____
5. If a CRNA provided the care, did a physician supervise the work? _____
6. What is the anesthesia code for this procedure? _____
7. What physical status modifier should be appended? _____

ASSIGNING ANESTHESIA CODES

The coder should follow these steps, which are also shown in Figure 8.2, for each anesthesia case:

1. Refer to the main term (*anesthesia* or *analgesia*) in the index for most patients, particularly for Medicare patients.
2. Look for the anatomical site of the procedure performed.
3. Locate the code(s) within the Anesthesia section of CPT.
4. Read and apply any notes or cross-references that may appear in the section.
5. Determine the payer (Medicare or other) to ascertain which codes and modifiers to assign. Remember that not all payers recognize qualifying circumstances and physical status modifiers.
6. For Medicare, determine who provided the anesthesia (CRNA or MD). Was an MD in attendance or supervising the CRNA? The answer will determine which HCPCS Level II modifiers apply for Medicare patients.
7. Assign the applicable physical status modifier (non-Medicare).
8. Determine the type of anesthesia that was administered (MAC or general).
9. Assign codes for any qualifying circumstances, if applicable (non-Medicare).
10. Assign any other applicable modifier(s).

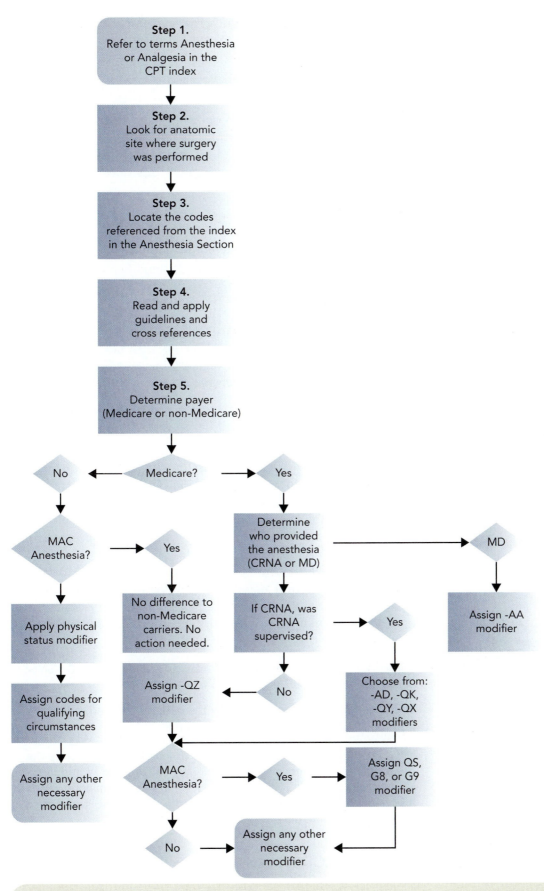

FIGURE 8.2
Anesthesia Code Assignment Flow Chart

EXAMPLE An anesthesiologist provides general anesthesia services to a normal, healthy fifty-six-year-old patient for transurethral resection of the prostate.

1. Under the main term *anesthesia* locate the anatomical site
2. Site is prostate.
3. There are three codes to choose from. Each must be referenced before selecting the most appropriate one: 00865 is not the correct choice because it describes a radical prostatectomy; 00908 describes a perineal approach; 00914 accurately describes the procedure performed.
4. Read and apply guidelines.
5. Patient is non-Medicare.
6. The anesthesiologist administered the anesthesia.
7. Patient is normal and healthy, so a −P1 modifier is appropriate.
8. There were no extenuating or qualifying circumstance. Report 00914–AA–P1.

EXAMPLE General anesthesia services provided to a seventy-year-old Medicare patient with carcinoma of the right breast for radical mastectomy with internal mammary node dissection. Nurse anesthetist provides the anesthesia. She is supervised by an anesthesiologist. The code is 00406–QX.

ANESTHESIA TIME

Anesthesia time begins when the anesthesiologist begins to prepare the patient for the induction of anesthesia. The anesthesia staff must be continuously present in order for time to be calculated. Anesthesia time ends when the anesthesiologist is no longer in personal attendance and the patient may be placed safely under postoperative supervision.

Generally, anesthesia **time (tm) units** are calculated in 15-minute intervals. One time unit equals 15 minutes or a fraction thereof. However, this is determined by the payer's policy; a time unit can range from 10-minute to 30-minute intervals depending on the payer.

EXAMPLE For one payer, 1 to 2 minutes would count as 0.1 units, 3 minutes would be 0.2 units, and so on.

Each preoperative encounter with the patient is added to the procedure time to compile total anesthesia time.

EXAMPLE Surgery was 20 minutes in length. Preoperatively the anesthesia staff member spent 10 minutes starting the IV and interviewing the patient. Total anesthesia time was 30 minutes. Each 15-minute increment was equal to one time unit. Time in this case would be two time units.

ANESTHESIA CODING AND BILLING RESOURCES

The American Society of Anesthesiologists publishes numerous books in addition to *The Relative Value Guide* and a monthly newsletter with helpful information for calculating anesthesia fees, practice

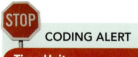

CODING ALERT

Time Units

Time units are not recognized for codes 01995 and 01996.

BILLING TIP

Calculating Time Units

Actual time units are paid. Do not round up to the next 15-minute increment. Instead, round to the tenth place. For example, anesthesia time is 85 minutes ÷ 15 minutes = 5.67. On the health care claim, 5.7 time units are reported.

INTERNET RESOURCE

American Society of Anesthesiologists Publications

www.asahq.org/ publicationsServices.htm

management, and the like. Medicare has a dedicated webpage for anesthesia providers with billing and payment along with educational resources specific to Medicare. Products are available from commercial sources. They include Decision Health's *Anesthesia & Pain Coder's Pink Sheet* and *Anesthesia Answer Book*, the American Academy of Professional Coders' (AAPC) *Coding Edge*, and the American Health Information Management Association's (AHIMA) *Journal of the American Health Information Management Association (JAHIMA)*.

INTERNET RESOURCE

Medicare Anesthesia Webpage

www.cms.hhs.gov/center/anesth.asp

Checkpoint 8.4

Assign the anesthesia code and any applicable modifiers and qualifying circumstances.

1. Radical prostatectomy for a Medicare patient. The anesthesiologist performs the general anesthesia.

   _____

2. Correction of tetralogy of Fallot congenital heart defect with pump oxygenator in a one-year-old girl. _____

3. Emergency appendectomy in a twenty-eight-year-old female who is otherwise healthy. _____

   _____

4. Hammertoe repair in a sixty-six-year-old diabetic female under MAC. The CRNA administered the anesthesia unsupervised. _____

5. A liver biopsy in an ambulatory surgery center under MAC anesthesia of a forty-two-year-old patient with cirrhosis of the liver. _____

Surgery Coding Overview

Codes located in the Surgery section of CPT cover invasive diagnostic or therapeutic procedures performed by surgeons of any specialty in a medical office, clinic, surgery center, or hospital. CPT notes that codes from the Medicine section for noninvasive procedures, services, and reports are also often also used for surgeon reporting.

SURGERY SECTION FORMAT AND ORGANIZATION

The Surgical section, the largest in CPT, has sixteen subsections that cover the various organ systems. A surgical code for one or more organ systems can be identified by its first digit. All surgical CPT codes begin with a 1, 2, 3, 4, 5, or 6 related to the subsection of the Surgical section. For example, the integumentary system makes up the first subsection, and all the codes in this subsection begin with 1. The subsections and their code ranges are presented in Table 8.6.

Most surgical subsections are divided into anatomical sites or organs within each body system, and each anatomical site is further categorized by surgical method:

EXAMPLE
Subsection: Digestive
   Anatomical site: Lip
      Surgical method: Excision

Table 8.6 Surgery Subsections

Subsection	Code Range
Integumentary System	10021–19499
Musculoskeletal System	20000–29999
Respiratory System	30000–32999
Cardiovascular System	33010–39599
Hemic and Lymphatic Systems	38100–37799
Mediastinum and Diaphragm	39000–39599
Digestive System	40490–49999
Urinary System	50010–53899
Male Genital System	54000–55899
Intersex Surgery	55970–55980
Female Genital System	56405–58999
Maternity Care and Delivery	59000–59899
Endocrine System	60000–60699
Nervous System	61000–64999
Eye and Ocular Adnexa	65091–68899
Auditory System	69000–69990

Within a subsection, surgical methods are presented in a typical order:

Incision and Drainage

Biopsy

Excision

Introduction or Removal

Repair

Destruction

Endoscopy/Laparoscopy (if applicable)

Other Procedures

This repeated heading structure helps coders locate the correct surgery code.

The Surgery section guidelines define terms and reporting rules for surgical procedures contained in this section, and coders must carefully read them. Many of the subsections also include instructional notes and definitions, which may be located at the beginning of the subsection, as shown in Figure 8.3, before or after a subheading, or in parentheses below a specific code.

SURGERY GUIDELINES

In the Surgery section, code descriptors are very important. Many coders highlight the semicolon and key words in a code description, like

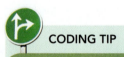

CODING TIP

Check for Notes

Before assigning a code, make a habit of checking for notes at the beginning of the subsection, at the beginning of the surgical method, and above and below the code.

FIGURE 8.3
Subsection Notes Example

**SURGERY
INTEGUMENTARY SYSTEM
DESTRUCTION**
Destruction means the ablation of benign, premalignant or malignant tissues by any method, with or without curettement, including local anesthesia, and not usually requiring closure.

unilateral or *bilateral* or *each, lesions(s),* or *polyp(s)* to hone in on the specificity of the code. These key words indicate how many times a code should be listed and help coders decide whether modifiers are applicable. When both the singular and the plural versions of words appear in the description, the code should be listed once only regardless of number.

EXAMPLE

20550: Injection(s); single tendon sheath, or ligament, aponeurosis
      (e.g., Plantar "fascia").

Because of the term *injection(s),* this code should be reported only once even if several injections were performed in the same tendon sheath, ligament, or aponeurosis.

Other cautionary points include the following:

- Be very careful when assigning the add-on code for a surgical microscope (69990). Some code descriptions include the use of a microscope; assigning this code in addition to such a procedure code would be inappropriate.

- The term *complicated* appears in some code descriptions. If there is infection present, if treatment is delayed, or if the surgery took longer than usual, this code would be appropriate.

- Some codes specify whether they are for one or both of an anatomical pair so the coder can determine whether to use the −50 modifier. For example, 69210 states "one or both ears," so the −50 modifier cannot be used. In contrast, 63030 specifies *one* interspace, and an instructional note below says to append the −50 modifier for a bilateral procedure.

- Add-on codes are never coded independently. They are always reported with their base parent code because they are intended to report a second or third procedure in addition to the primary procedure.

Surgical Package and the Global Period In many cases, the time, effort, and services by a physician performing a surgical procedure are coded with a single surgical package code. In CPT, a complete *surgical* package includes local infiltration of anesthesia, the E/M visits either on the date of surgery or the day before as long as the decision for surgery has already been made, immediate postoperative care, the writing of orders, evaluation of the patient in the recovery area, and any typical uncomplicated follow-up care. CPT also explains that follow-up care for any of these reasons—complications, exacerbations, recurrence, and the presence of other diseases that require additional services—is not included in the surgical package.

Table 8.7 Excerpt from Medicare Global Days

CPT/HCPCS	Description	Global Days
11444	Exc face-mm benign lesion + marg 3.1-4 cm	010
11446	Exc face-mm benign lesion + marg > 4 cm	010
11450	Removal, sweat gland lesion	090
11470	Removal, sweat gland lesion	090
11471	Removal, sweat gland lesion	090

Source: RBRVS Fee Schedule, www.cms.hhs.gov.

Coders need to know what is included in the payer's particular definition of a surgical package, however, to correctly comply with payers' rules. For example, Medicare has its own definition of a surgical package (see Table 8.7). The Medicare approved amount for the procedure includes not only payment for the same services as CPT (when provided by the physician who performs the surgery) but also these items:

- Preoperative visits, beginning with the day before a surgery for major procedures and the day of surgery for minor procedures. Preoperative care includes the H&P (history and physical) and medical decision making that occur before surgery and hospital admission or an office or outpatient visit that occurs before surgery, but it does not include a consultation or new patient office visit where the determination for surgery was made.

- Intraoperative services that are normally a usual and necessary part of a surgical procedure.

- Complications following surgery that do not require additional trips to the operating room.

- Routine postoperative visits (follow-up visits) during the postoperative period of the surgery that are related to recovery from the surgery.

- Postoperative pain management provided by the surgeon.

- Supplies, except for a few specific supplies provided in a physician's office.

- Miscellaneous services such as dressing changes and local incisional care; removal of operative pack; removal of sutures and staples, line wires, tubes, drains, casts and splints, replacement lines, and nasogastric and rectal tubes; and changes or removal of tracheostomy tubes.

The surgical package has a defined time frame for the routine preoperative and postoperative surgical care called the **global period**. The number of days in the global period are referred to as **global surgery days.** The global period is a payer concept under which a set amount is paid for all services furnished by the surgeon before, during, and after a procedure. This is important, because physicians can bill for work done outside—that is, before and after—the start and end of the global period.

The typical global periods are:

- No days for simple procedures
- No days preoperative and ten days postoperative for minor surgery
- One day preoperative and ninety days postoperative for major surgery

An example of a payer's policy is the Medicare rule that a major procedure surgical package includes a preoperative service day (one day before or on the day of surgery) and eighty-nine days after it, totaling ninety consecutive days. A minor procedure surgical package includes a preoperative service (one day before or on the day of surgery) along with up to ten days following surgery, depending on whether the physician saw the patient the day before surgery. If so, nine postoperative days will be included in the global package. If the postoperative period is zero days, postoperative visits are not included in the payment amount for the surgery. Payment is made in this instance if additional treatment is provided on the same day or thereafter as long as it is a covered service. Services by other physicians are not included in the global fee for a minor procedure.

To determine the global period date range for major surgeries, count one day immediately before the day of surgery, the day of surgery, and the eighty-eight days immediately after the day of surgery. For example, for surgery on April 5, the last day of the postoperative period would be July 2. To determine the global period date range for minor procedures, count the day of surgery and the appropriate number of days immediately after it (either zero or ten).

> **EXAMPLE** A patient has axillary hidradenitis, and the physician performs excision of skin and subcutaneous tissue for hidradenitis, axillary; with simple or intermediate repair (11462) on January 2. The patient comes back to the office for a postoperative visit on January 12. CPT 11462 has a global period of ninety days. The visit on January 12 is not charged to the patient or the insurance carrier.

Bundling   Surgical packages are referred to as **bundled,** meaning that each package code contains all the related services. **Unbundling**—taking apart and reporting codes that are included in a bundled or "grouped" code—is a coding error and is possibly fraudulent. Unbundling is also referred to as *fragmenting*. For example, since a single code is available to describe removal of the uterus, ovaries, and fallopian tubes, physicians should not use separate codes to report the removal of the uterus, ovaries, and fallopian tubes individually.

The Medicare policy that explains which codes are bundled in the surgical package is called the **Correct Coding Initiative (CCI).** Its purpose and format are explained in the Reimbursement Review on pages 326–327.

Services Not Included in the Global Surgery Package

Some services are not included in the payment amount for the global surgery and may be coded and paid separately. In many instances, coders need to use appropriate modifiers for these additional services:

- The initial consultation or evaluation of the problem by the surgeon to determine the need for surgery. A −57 modifier would apply in this circumstance.

INTERNET RESOURCE

Medicare Global Days

www.cms.hhs.gov/center/physician.asp,
Click PFS Relative Value file and current year

⚠ **CODING CAUTION**

Bundling Can Include Any CPT Section

Note that codes from any CPT section can be bundled in a surgical package.

Correct Coding Initiative and Medically Unlikely Edits: Compliant Coding for Medicare

Compliant coding for Medicare outpatient claims follows Medicare's national policy on correct coding, the CCI. CCI controls improper coding that would lead to inappropriate payment for Medicare claims. It has coding policies that are based on coding conventions in CPT, Medicare's national coverage and payment policies, national medical societies' coding guidelines, and Medicare's analysis of standard medical and surgical practice.

Updated every quarter, CCI has many thousands of CPT code combinations called CCI edits that are used by computers in the Medicare system to check claims. **Edits** are code combinations that are screened against each other to determine whether the codes in the combination can be reported at the same time. CCI edits apply to claims that bill for more than one procedure performed on the same Medicare beneficiary on the same date of service by the same provider. A claim is denied when codes reported together do not pass an edit.

CCI prevents billing two procedures that, according to Medicare, could not possibly have been performed together, such as reporting the removal of an organ both through an open incision and with laparoscopy or reporting female- and male-specific codes for the same patient.

There are two edits processes—one for physicians and the other for facilities. Physician claim data is processed through CCT edits. Similarly, Medicare's **outpatient code editor (OCE)** checks claims from the outpatient departments of hospitals and other facilities. Because it is possible for a hospital to receive multiple payments (under the APC system, as described in Chapter 5 of your program) for a single outpatient encounter, the CCI edits are applied to prohibit overpayments.

The CCI edits are available on the CMS website. They are organized into three categories: (1) column 1/column 2 code pair edits, (2) mutually exclusive code edits, and (3) modifier indicators.

Column 1/Column 2 Code Pairs

In the **CCI column 1/column 2 code pair edits,** two columns of codes are listed. Most often, the edit is based on one code's being a component of the other. This means that the column 1 code includes all the services described by the column 2 codes, so the column 2 codes cannot be billed together with the column 1 code for the same patient on the same day of service. Medicare pays for the column 1 code only; the column 2 codes are considered bundled into the column 1 code.

Column 1	Column 2
27370	20610, 76000, 76003

If 27370 is billed, neither 20610, 76000, nor 76003 should also be billed because the payment for each of these codes is already included in the column 1 code.

Mutually Exclusive Code Edits

CCI mutually exclusive code (MEC) edits also list codes in two columns. According to CMS regulations, both services represented by these codes could not have reasonably been done during a single patient encounter, so they cannot be billed together. If the provider reports both codes from both columns for a patient on the same day, Medicare pays only the lower-paid code.

Column 1	Column 2
50021	49061, 50020

This means that a coder cannot report either 49061 or 50020 when reporting 50021.

Modifier Indicators

In CPT coding, modifiers show particular circumstances related to a code on a claim. The **CCI modifier indicators** control modifier use to "break," or avoid, CCI edits. CCI modifier indicators appear next to items in both the CCI column 1/column 2 code pair list and the mutually exclusive code list. A CCI modifier indicator of 1 means

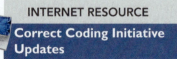

INTERNET RESOURCE

Correct Coding Initiative Updates

www.cms.hhs.gov/
NationalCorrectCodInitEd

- Visits unrelated to the diagnosis for which the surgical procedure is performed, unless the visits occur due to complications of the surgery.
- Treatment for the underlying condition or for an added course of treatment that is not part of the normal recovery from surgery.

that a CPT modifier *may* be used to bypass an edit (if the circumstances are appropriate). A CCI modifier indicator of 0 means that use of a CPT modifier will not change the edit, so the column 2 codes or mutually exclusive code edits will not be bypassed.

Flu vaccine code 90656 includes bundled flu vaccine codes 90655 and 90657–90660. It has a CCI indicator of 0. No modifier will be effective in bypassing these edits, so in every case only CPT 90656 will be paid.

A patient undergoes a biopsy of a salivary gland under general anesthesia. The anesthesia code would be 00100. Below is an excerpt of the Medicare CCI edits for physicians with respect to code 00100. Any code listed in column 2 is considered part of the anesthesia code 00100 and should not be billed separately unless one of the elements above applies. In this case, 36010 can never be coded at the same time as 00100.

Column 1	Column 2	Modifier 0 = not allowed 1 = allowed 9 = not applicable	Column 1	Column 2	Modifier 0 = not allowed 1 = allowed 9 = not applicable
00100	31500	9	00100	36015	1
00100	31505	1	00100	36120	9
00100	31515	1	00100	36405	1
00100	31527	1	00100	36406	1
00100	31622	1	00100	36410	1
00100	31645	1	00100	36420	1
00100	36000	1	00100	36425	1
00100	36005	1	00100	36430	1
00100	36010	0	00100	36440	1
00100	36011	1	00100	36600	1
00100	36012	1	00100	36620	9
00100	36013	1	00100	36625	9
00100	36014	1	00100	36640	1

A patient undergoes excision of tissue and skin for hidradenitis of the right axilla with intermediate closure of the 5.0 cm incision site. Code 11450, excision of skin and subcutaneous tissue for hidradenitis, axillary; with simple or intermediate repair, is reported for the hidradenitis excision and repair of skin. Therefore, code 12032, layer closure of wounds scalp, axillae, trunk and/or extremities (excluding hands and feet); 2.6 cm–7.5 cm is not reported separately because closure of the wound is considered part of the comprehensive procedure.

Medically Unlikely Edits

In 2007 CMS established units of service edits, referred to as **medically unlikely edits (MUEs),** in order to lower the Medicare fee-for-service paid claims error rate. MUEs are intended to reduce the number of health care claims that are sent back simply because of clerical or practice management program (PMP) errors.

MUEs are edits that test a claim for the same beneficiary, CPT code, date of service, and billing provider against Medicare's rules. The initial set of MUEs is based on anatomical considerations. An example is an MUE edit that rejects a claim for a hysterectomy on a male patient. The MUEs also automatically reject claim line items containing units of service billed in excess of Medicare's allowances.

The official method for providers to receive the CCI edits is to purchase them from the National Technical Information Service (NTIS) of the Department of Commerce, the sole distributor of these edits.

- Diagnostic tests and procedures, including diagnostic radiological procedures.
- Distinctly unrelated surgical procedures during the postoperative period. A new postoperative period begins with the subsequent procedure.

INTERNET RESOURCE

CCI Edits

www.ntis.gov/product/correct-coding.htm

- Treatment for postoperative complications that requires a return trip to the operating room or procedure room. An operating room is a place of service equipped and staffed for the sole purpose of performing procedures. It does not include a patient's room, a minor treatment room, a recovery room, or an intensive care unit (unless the patient's condition was so critical there would be insufficient time for transportation to the operating room).

- A more extensive procedure that is required when a less extensive procedure fails.

- For certain services performed in a physician office, a surgical tray. In addition, drugs, splints, and casting supplies are separately payable under the reasonable charge payment methodology.

- Immunosuppressive therapy for organ transplants.

> **EXAMPLE**   A patient complaining of right flank plan, painful urination, nausea, vomiting, and fever is seen in the office. An ultrasound performed in the office shows a staghorn calculus that requires immediate removal from the patient's kidney. The physician schedules surgery for the next day. The physician would report the appropriate level E/M code with a −57 modifier so that this visit will not be bundled into the payment for the surgery.

> **EXAMPLE**   A patient has two lesions of the face that are 3.1 and 3.5 cm, respectively, removed in the office. The patient's wound appears to be red and somewhat infected with fluid collection. The postoperative time for this procedure is ten days, so care related to the lesion removal is included in the payment for this service for the next ten days. On the eighth postoperative day, the patient returns to the office, and the physician incises and drains the fluid collection. The care is directly related to the surgery and therefore is not reported separately.

Let's take the same patient and change the scenario.

> **EXAMPLE**   The patient performs some home improvement tasks and accidentally scrapes his face, rupturing the sutures and dressing. He returns to the office on the ninth day so that the physician can resuture the lesion sites. The physician reports the suturing of the wounds separately, using a −79 modifier to indicate that this service is not related to the primary lesion removal service. Had the patient not been working around his house, this second service would not have been necessary.

Separate Procedure   Reading the words *separate procedure* in parenthesis after a code description is a clue to ask the following question: Is this procedure an integral part of another procedure, and is it more of an incidental procedure than the comprehensive procedure being performed? An **incidental procedure** is performed at the same operative session as a more complex primary procedure. It is clinically related to the procedure being performed and would not usually be reported alone. It is a procedure that is commonly performed as part of standard medical treatment or is part of the package, including the services or supplies that are included in surgical procedures:

- Cleansing, shaving, and prepping of skin
- Draping and positioning of the patient
- Insertion of IV
- Sedative administration by the physician

- Surgical approach (evaluation of surgical field, simple debridement, simple lysis of adhesions, incision of the skin or body part, isolation of nerves and tendons or bone limiting access to surgical field)
- Surgical cultures
- Wound irrigation
- Surgical closure of incision
- Application of dressings and removal of postoperative dressings
- Surgical supplies, unless determined otherwise by payer policy, in which case, HCPCS codes are assigned
- Anesthesia administration (except general)

When a procedure is considered incidental to the primary procedure, it is generally not separately reported. Most of the procedures indicated as separate procedures are considered incidental.

Sometimes a separate procedure can be reported separately with a −59 modifier.

> **EXAMPLE**   CPT 31231 is nasal endoscopy, diagnostic; unilateral or bilateral (separate procedure), and 31233 is nasal/sinus endoscopy, diagnostic with maxillary sinusoscopy. Assigning code 31231 would be accurate if the only procedure is looking in the nose with a scope. However, if this done in addition to looking at the maxillary sinus as in 31233, it would be inappropriate to report 31231; procedure code 31233 already includes what is being described in 31231.

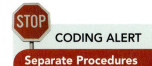

CODING ALERT

Separate Procedures

Do not confuse separate procedures with the note "List separately in addition to the code for the primary procedure."

Modifiers   When reporting more than one procedure or service at a time, modifiers are required to clarify the circumstances surrounding the episode of care. The section guidelines list the modifiers applicable to the Surgery section, and they will be detailed later in this chapter. Not all modifiers are reportable by outpatient facilities, only those on the approved list of modifiers for facilities on the front cover of the CPT manual.

Special Documentation   Any procedure or service that is new, unusual, coded to an unlisted procedure code, or has modifiers −21, −22, −23, −59, −66 −80, −81, −82, and/or −99 requires documentation such as a special report to support the procedure and substantiate its medical necessity. Typically, the history and physical and the operative report will suffice. Essentially the modifier indicates that payment will be positively or negatively affected and that the report will justify that result. The following must be included in a special report:

- Description of the nature, extent, and need for the procedure
- Time and effort
- Equipment necessary
- Complexity of symptoms
- Final diagnosis
- Pertinent physical findings
- Diagnostic and therapeutic procedures
- Concurrent problems
- Follow-up care necessary

Subsection Information   All Surgery subsections are listed in the Surgery section guidelines. Keep in mind that there are important notes located at the beginning of each of these sections. Watch for the ▶◀ symbols for revised or new text, and make sure to review the changes.

Unlisted Procedures Unlisted procedure codes are used for services with no assignable CPT codes—for which no specific code matches the documentation. Each subsection has unlisted procedure codes; the section guidelines list them in numerical order by their location in the Surgery section. Remember to first review HCPCS Level II codes (if the payer accepts them) and CPT Category III codes before assigning the unlisted code for that subsection and anatomical site. Each time an unlisted procedure code is assigned, a special report or documentation supporting the service needs to be submitted with the claim. Refer to the guidelines at the beginning of each section to determine components of the special report.

EXAMPLE The arthroscopic codes available for the metacarpophalangeal joint are 29901 and 29902. Neither is accurate to assign in the case of arthroscopic metacarpophalangeal joint replacement with permanent prosthesis. Code 26531 would be assigned if this procedure was performed with the area opened. Therefore, 29999 is the appropriate code in this situation.

SURGICAL TERMINOLOGY

Coders should refer to a medical dictionary and an anatomy atlas during the surgical coding process to refresh knowledge of anatomy, physiology, and terminology. The terminology can seem overwhelming; medical documents often contain words that coders do not recognize. At a minimum, coders must memorize basic prefixes, suffixes, and root words to be able to break complicated words into smaller parts to decipher meaning. Some key terms are listed in some editions of CPT after the CPT Introduction under the heading Illustrated Anatomical and Procedural Review. Key suffixes are noted in Table 8.8.

STOP

CODING ALERT

Do Not Force a Code Fit

Do not try to make an existing code fit what you are trying to describe! Instead, assign an unlisted procedure code for the appropriate subsection and anatomical site.

STOP

CODING ALERT

Know Your Surgical Terminology

Do not assign codes to technical words and procedures you do not understand. Take the time to look them up in references.

Table 8.8 Common Surgical Suffixes

Suffix	Definition	Example
-otomy	Making an incision or opening into	Laparotomy
-ectomy	Partial or total removal of a body part, bone, or tissue	Colectomy
-ostomy	Creating a hole or opening from the inside to the outside of the body	Colostomy
-lysis	Destruction, breaking down, or freeing	Enterolysis
-plasty	Repair or reconstruct	Mammoplasty
-scopy	Surgical intervention using an endoscope to visualize internal structures without cutting the body open	Laparoscopy
-rrhaphy	suture repair or reduction	Herniorraphy
-graphy	Use of X-ray or fluoroscopy for viewing anatomy during a procedure	Radiography
-desis	Fixation or fusing permanently	Arthrodesis
-centesis	Puncture cavity to remove fluid	Arthrocentesis
-pexy	Surgical fixation of an organ	Mastopexy
-tripsy	Crushing, pulverizing, destroying	Lithotripsy

Using the table of CCI code pair edits in the Reimbursement Review, answer the following questions.

1. Can 36640 be reported separately from 00100? _____

2. Can 36120 be reported separately from 00100? _____

Using Table 8.7 on page 324, answer the following questions.

3. Is code 11471 a major or minor procedure? _____

4. Is 11446 a major or minor procedure? _____

Identify the comprehensive service by underlining it. Circle the incidental or separate procedures that are not reported in addition to the comprehensive service.

5. The surgeon prepped and draped the patient and injected the finger with a digital block. Evacuation of subungual hematoma was performed. _____

Surgical Procedure Types

All significant procedures—such as incisions, excisions, biopsies, repairs, manipulation, amputation, endoscopes, destruction, suturing, and introductions—may be assigned CPT codes for reporting and reimbursement. To correctly assign CPT surgery codes, coders must understand the distinction between the two types of surgical procedures: diagnostic and therapeutic.

DIAGNOSTIC PROCEDURES

Diagnostic procedures, like diagnostic tests, are performed to confirm a physician's working diagnosis or to help determine a best course of treatment. In these cases, patients present with signs or symptoms of illness, and diagnostic procedures are a way of assessing and ruling out potential diagnoses. They involve work such as examining a particular part of the body to identify the cause of the patient's pain, exploring the extent of an injury or disease, and staging an illness such as cancer.

Although done for diagnostic purposes, diagnostic procedures are typically invasive, meaning that instruments are introduced into the body either through a natural orifice or by incising the skin. Many, however, are performed with a minimally invasive technique using an **endoscope,** which is a viewing instrument made up of hundreds of tiny light-transmitting glass fibers bundled tightly together. Diagnostic procedures are usually performed in an operating room or in a special treatment area of a hospital such as the radiology or emergency department.

Invasive diagnostic procedures include:

- *Endoscopy:* The visual inspection of any cavity of the body using an endoscope.

- *Bronchoscopy:* An examination to view the air passages of the lung (the interior of the tracheobronchial tree).

- *Arthroscopy:* An examination of internal structures of a joint space (such as elbow, hip, knee, shoulder, or wrist) via a small incision.

- *Laparoscopy:* A surgical procedure in which a tiny scope is inserted into the abdomen through a small incision, used for a variety of procedures and often to diagnose disease of the fallopian tubes and pelvic cavity.
- *Wound exploration:* An examination of a wound.
- *Biopsy:* A procedure that involves obtaining a tissue specimen for microscopic analysis to establish a precise diagnosis. Biopsies can be accomplished with a biopsy needle (passed through the skin into the organ in question) or by open surgical incision.
- *Angiography:* A radiographic technique in which a contrast material is injected into a blood vessel for the purpose of identifying its anatomy using an X-ray. This technique is used to image arteries in the brain, heart, kidneys, gastrointestinal tract, aorta, neck (carotids), chest, limbs, and pulmonary circuit.

THERAPEUTIC PROCEDURES

Therapeutic procedures involve treating or correcting a confirmed disease, condition, or injury (see Table 8.9). They involve work such as repairing or reconstructing defects or injuries, excising lesions or tumors, removing body parts or organs, and transplanting organs. Examples of specific procedures are hernia repair, appendectomy, polyp removal, hysterectomy, lesion removals, and vessel repairs.

THERAPEUTIC PROCEDURES INCLUDE DIAGNOSTIC PROCEDURES

A diagnostic procedure may be converted to a therapeutic procedure when circumstances warrant. In such a case, the surgeon first performs a diagnostic procedure; upon confirming a condition, the surgeon then moves to a therapeutic procedure to treat it. Surgery coding guidelines state that when a diagnostic and a therapeutic procedure are done at the same operative session on the same anatomical site on the same day for the same patient, only a code for the therapeutic procedure is assigned.

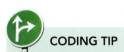

CODING TIP

Therapeutic Procedures Include Diagnostic Procedures

As a general guideline, a therapeutic procedure includes any diagnostic procedure that was also done. When a diagnostic procedure is the only service, it is coded. When the diagnostic procedure is followed by a therapeutic surgical procedure, the diagnostic service is not coded. Surgical or therapeutic procedures during the same session always include the diagnostic procedure.

Table 8.9 Surgical Terms Reflecting Therapeutic Procedures	
Anastomosis	Manipulation
Arthrodesis	Reconstruction
Debridement	Reduction
Destruction	Release
Dilation	Removal
Excision	Repair
Extraction	Resection
Incision and drainage	Revision
Introduction	Suture
Lysis	Transplant

EXAMPLE A biopsy of a suspicious lesion is followed by excising the entire lesion. The biopsy represents part of the overall procedure to remove the lesion and is not assigned a separate code.

Surgery Modifiers

Modifiers are used with Surgery section codes to indicate various situations, such as the following:

- A procedure performed bilaterally
- More than one procedure performed at the same time
- Assistant surgeon participation
- An increased or decreased service or procedure
- Performance of part of a service
- Unusual events during a procedure or service
- A specific anatomical location
- A service that has two parts or components—a technical component and a professional component
- More than one procedure or service performed on the same day or within the global period (described in the Surgery section guidelines)

PROPER USE

Coders become familiar with the modifiers that are available for use in their medical setting. For reporting the outpatient facility charges of a hospital outpatient department (such as the ED) or an ambulatory surgery clinic, the facility modifiers (Modifiers Approved for Hospital Outpatient Use) can be used with CPT Surgery section codes. Physician practices use the CPT modifiers with the surgery codes. HCPCS Level II anatomical modifiers (see Table 8.10) may also be used.

> **NOTE**
>
> Modifiers are covered in Chapter 6 of your program.

> **CODING ALERT**
>
> **Which Modifiers Are Not Used with Surgery Codes?**
>
> Modifiers −21, −24, −25, −90, and −91 cannot be appended to surgical CPT codes. Likewise, modifiers are not appended to add-on codes or to unlisted procedure codes. Codes that are −51 modifier exempt do not permit the −51 modifier, but an anatomical modifier may be permitted by the payer.

Table 8.10 HCPCS (Level II) Surgery Modifiers

−LT	Left side	−GA	Waiver of liability on file
−RT	Right side	−LC	Left circumflex coronary artery
−E1	Upper left eyelid	−LD	Left anterior descending coronary artery
−E2	Upper right eyelid	−RC	Right coronary artery
−E3	Lower left eyelid	−TA	Left foot great toe
−E4	Lower right eyelid	−T1	Left foot second digit
−FA	Left hand thumb	−T2	Left foot third digit
−F1	Left hand second digit	−T3	Left foot fourth digit
−F2	Left hand third digit	−T4	Left foot fifth digit
−F3	Left hand fourth digit	−T5	Right foot great toe
−F4	Left hand fifth digit	−T6	Right foot second digit
−F5	Right hand thumb	−T7	Right foot third digit
−F6	Right hand second digit	−T8	Right foot fourth digit
−F7	Right hand third digit	−T9	Right foot fifth digit
−F8	Right hand fourth digit	−TC	Technical component
−F9	Right hand fifth digit		

Often modifiers are reported to show that more than a usual amount of work was done; the provider wishes to show that an increased charge is appropriate. However, not all payers accept surgery code modifiers and alter payments for more difficult procedures. Coders analyze each payer's rules and follow them in coding and billing. For Medicare and Medicaid, the CPT modifiers and HCPCS modifiers shown in Table 8.11 are available for reporting surgical procedures.

SURGERY-RELATED MODIFIER DESCRIPTIONS

A number of modifiers are commonly used in reporting surgery codes.

Table 8.11 CMS Surgery Modifier Acceptance

Modifier	Medicare Accept?	Medicaid Accept?
−22	Yes	No
−26	Yes	Yes
−32	No	No
−47	No	No
−50	Yes	Yes
−51	Yes	Yes
−52	Yes	Yes
−53	Yes	Yes
−54	Yes	Yes
−55	Yes	Yes
−56	Yes	No
−58	Yes	No
−59	Yes	Yes
−62	Yes	Yes
−63	No	Yes
−66	Yes	Yes
−73	Yes	Yes
−74	Yes	Yes
−76	Yes	Yes
−77	Yes	No
−78	Yes	Yes
−79	Yes	Yes
−80	Yes, for MDs only	Yes
−81	No	No
−82	Yes	Yes
−99	No	Yes
−SG	Yes	No
−TC	Yes	Yes

CPT Modifier −22, Unusual (Increased) Procedure or Service

Modifier −22 means that the services provided were different from those included in the code description, but not different enough to make another code more appropriate. Usually, the surgery involved extra time or prolonged cleansing or was more complex than usual (increased risk, difficulty, hemorrhage—blood loss over 600 cc—or unusual findings). There may have been a complication that cannot be identified by using another CPT code. To justify the use of this modifier, which requests a higher payment, work and effort should be 30 to 50 percent greater. Additional time alone is not sufficient to use the −22 modifier.

Since this modifier triggers payer review of the claim, it is common to also transmit an operative note or letter explaining the circumstances. When the claim is paid as submitted, reimbursement is typically 20 to 30 percent higher, but often payers reject the −22 modifier.

EXAMPLE Excision of a lesion on an obese patient in the crease of the neck. The obesity makes it more difficult to reach the lesion, so it warrants a modifier. The code is 11422–22.

Facility Modifier −27, Multiple Outpatient Hospital E/M Encounters on the Same Date

Modifier −27 may be reported by the facility when a patient is seen in more than one hospital-based clinic on the same day; used only with E/M codes.

EXAMPLE Patient was seen in the cardiology clinic at 9:00 A.M. and in the diabetes clinic at 1:00 P.M.

CPT Modifier −32, Mandated Service

Modifier −32 means that a procedure was requested by the patient's insurance carrier, perhaps for a second opinion, or by an outside organization such as workers' compensation for disability determinations.

EXAMPLE Nerve conduction study prior to surgical intervention. The code is 95903–32.

CPT Modifier −47, Anesthesia by Surgeon

Modifier −47 is used when regional nerve block or general anesthesia is administered by the surgeon without a CRNA or an anesthesiologist. It is not used in conjunction with anesthesia codes but is appended to the CPT code for the procedure. This modifier is not accepted by Medicare.

EXAMPLE Physician performed a paracervical nerve block for a cervical conization procedure. The code is 57520–47.

CPT/Facility Modifier −50, Bilateral Procedure

Modifier −50 is used when a procedure is performed on both the left and right paired body parts or organs. The paired body parts are eyes, ears, sinuses, nostrils, breasts, lungs, ovaries, kidneys, ureters, arms, legs, feet, hands, testicles, vas deferens, and fallopian tubes. A procedure carried out on only one of the pair is considered unilateral, and the HCPCS −RT or −LT modifier would be more applicable (see Table 8.10). Note that a procedure done on the left and right side of the back is not a bilateral procedure because a person has only one back.

The code description should be checked before the −50 modifier is assigned. Unless otherwise stated in the code description, surgical procedures are unilateral. If the code description is *one or both* or *bilateral*, it indicates bilateral procedures performed at the same operative session.

EXAMPLE Bilateral turbinate reduction is coded 30130–50.

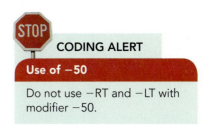

STOP

CODING ALERT

Use of −50

Do not use −RT and −LT with modifier −50.

CPT Modifier −51, Multiple Procedures

Modifier −51 is used when more than one surgical procedure is performed on the same day or at the same operating session by the same provider. The procedures can be performed on the same body part or on different body parts through the same or a different incision.

EXAMPLE Probing of the right nasolacrimal duct and a nasal septoplasty is coded 68811–RT, 30520–51.

CPT Appendix E lists codes that are exempt from −51 modifier use. Modifier −51 exempt code descriptions often use phrases like "each additional" or "list separately in addition to code for X." Note that multiple procedures are not the same as staged procedures, which are planned ahead of time to be done as more than one procedure.

EXAMPLE
⊘ 33517: Coronary artery bypass, using venous grafts and arterial grafts, single vein graft (List separately in addition to code for arterial graft).

CPT/Facility Modifier −52, Reduced Services

When a procedure is partially reduced, modifier −52 is appended to alert the payer that the service was not done to its full extent. The physician may have performed a procedure unilaterally, but the code description indicates bilateral; or no anesthesia was used, but the code specifies its use. Payers have their own policies regarding this modifier, and they usually require documentation. Typically, payers pay half of the allowed amount. Modifier −52 should be reported only when no procedure code describes the partially reduced services actually carried out.

EXAMPLE A patient who previously had a left above-knee amputation had an extremity arterial study. A −52 modifier would be appropriate here since the patient did not have an entire leg to study. The code is 93923–52.

CPT Modifier −53, Discontinued Procedure

Modifier −53 indicates that a procedure that had been started was terminated for some reason, such as a risk to the patient or equipment failure. This modifier is not used to report elective cancellations before the procedure is started. Modifier –53 is similar to the hospital outpatient modifiers –73 and –74, although it is not specific about whether anesthesia was administered, as those are. Typically, payers pay 25 percent of the allowed amount for procedures reported with this modifier.

EXAMPLE A planned colonoscopy was terminated halfway through the procedure due to evacuation of the second floor of the facility because of a possible fire emergency. The codes is 45378–53.

CPT Modifier −54, Surgical Care Only

Modifier −54 indicates that the surgeon who performed the surgery did not or will not provide the preoperative or postoperative care. It is called a *split-care modifier*, indicating that more than one provider is involved. Documentation must record the agreement to transfer care between the physicians.

EXAMPLE A patient who is on vacation is involved in a car accident. She undergoes an open reduction of the fourth left finger and is going to follow up with a physician in her hometown for postoperative care. The surgeon would report 26615–F3–54.

CPT Modifier −55, Postoperative Management Only

Modifier −55 is used by a physician who performed only postoperative management and did not evaluate the patient before the procedure or perform the actual procedure. Payment for the postoperative and postdischarge care is split between two or more physicians when the physicians agree on the transfer of care.

EXAMPLE Three weeks after having a laparoscopic hysterectomy, a woman joins her military husband at his new posting. She follows up with a physician at the military hospital on the new base, who reports 58550–55.

CPT Modifier −56, Preoperative Management Only

Similarly, modifier −56 is appended to the code submitted by the physician who only examined the patient preoperatively and for some reason did not perform the planned procedure. If a physician other than the surgeon provides preoperative care, modifier −56 should be billed with the surgery code.

EXAMPLE A patient is seen by his internal medicine physician for examination and clearance for general anesthesia for laparoscopic gastric banding. This physician reports 43770–56.

CPT/Facility Modifier −58, Staged or Related Procedure by the Same Physician During the Postoperative Period

To use modifier −58, the surgeon should have documented that a staged procedure was planned in advance, that another stage was needed because the work was more extensive than planned, or that surgery for therapy followed a diagnostic surgical procedure (considered a related procedure). All stages of the procedure must be performed by the original surgeon.

This modifier is not needed with codes that already indicate multiple sessions, such as CPT code 67145, prophylaxis of retinal detachment without drainage, one or more operative sessions. It is also not used to report a problem or complication resulting from the original surgery that required a return to the OR (reported with modifier −78).

EXAMPLE A patient has a hysteroscopy with polypectomy. Pathology results indicate carcinoma in situ of the uterus. The patient returns the following week for a hysterectomy. The code is 58150–58.

CPT/Facility Modifier −59, Distinct Procedure
Modifier −59 is used to report that two codes that are not normally reported together are appropriate under the circumstances. One procedure is performed independently of the other or is unrelated to the other. This modifier is often used for separate procedures that are typically bundled into a more comprehensive procedure within that subsection if they are performed at the same time as a more complex procedure. The key to using this modifier is that the procedures are done on different anatomical sites or that a separate incision was required.

EXAMPLE Arthrocentesis of the elbow (20605) and also of the ankle (20605–59) is performed. Since the procedures are done at

CODING TIP

Modifier −58 Resets the Global Period

A new postoperative period begins with each subsequent procedure.

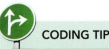

Use of the −59 Modifier

If the procedures were done at different sites or organs, a separate incision was made, or a separate excision was done, or if the physician is treating a separate injury, use the −59 modifier. If a HCPCS anatomical modifier would be a better choice to identify a body site, it should be used instead of the −59 modifier.

BILLING TIP

Reporting More Than One Modifier

Always list the −59 modifier first if more than one modifier is used with a particular code.

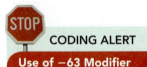

CODING ALERT

Use of −63 Modifier

Modifier −63 is used with Surgery section codes only.

---

different sites, the code is reported twice, with the −59 modifier appended to the second code.

EXAMPLE Excision of a lesion on the right breast is done, and an incision and drainage is done on a separate lesion on the right breast. The second procedure is reported with the −59 modifier.

CPT Modifier −62, Two Surgeons Modifier −62 is applicable when a procedure requires 50 percent of two surgeons' skill and/or time. It applies when the two surgeons are participating in the same procedure, such as when an orthopedist and a neurosurgeon together perform a Harrington rod technique. If two surgeons are operating at the same time but are performing two different procedures, this modifier does not apply.

EXAMPLE A neurosurgeon asks a thoracic surgeon to create the anterior approach through the thoracic cavity for an anterior lumbar diskectomy and arthrodesis. The thoracic surgeon reports 22558–62, and the neurosurgeon reports 22224, 22558–62, and 22845.

CPT Modifier −63, Procedure Performed on Infants Modifier −63 is used for surgical procedures on neonates and infants weighing less than 4 kg. The concept of this modifier is similar to that of modifier −22: the circumstances are more risky or complex, thus warranting extra physician work.

EXAMPLE A premature infant undergoes a procedure to close a patent ductus arteriosus. The code is 33820–63.

CPT Modifier −66, Surgical Team Modifier −66 is used mainly in transplant procedures or multiple trauma procedures when the skills of several different surgeons are required.

Facility Modifier −73, Discontinued Outpatient Procedure Prior to Anesthesia Administration If an intended procedure was discontinued before anesthesia induction, the hospital outpatient clinic or ambulatory surgery center (ASC) uses the −73 modifier.

EXAMPLE A patient is prepped preoperatively and taken to the OR. The anesthesiologist cancels the procedure because of the patient's abnormal heart rate. The facility reports the procedure code for the scheduled procedure with a −73 modifier.

Facility Modifier −74, Discontinued Outpatient Procedure After Anesthesia Administration Modifier −74 is used by facilities to indicate that a procedure was terminated after local or general anesthesia was given. It applies when the patient is actually in the OR and anesthesia has been started as well as when sedation was given in the holding area.

EXAMPLE A planned colonoscopy was terminated halfway through because of an evacuation of the facility when a fire alarm went off. The code is 45378–74.

CPT/Facility Modifier −76, Repeat Procedure by Same Physician Modifier −76 is used to report that the same procedure that was performed for a patient has been repeated on the same day.

The modifier is added to the same CPT code, alerting the payer that it is not a duplicate charge. Some payers recognize this modifier, but others do not. Documentation of the reason for the repeated procedure is required.

CPT/Facility Modifier −77, Repeat Procedure by Another Physician
If a procedure is repeated for the same patient on the same day by a physician other than the original surgeon, modifier −77 is used.

CPT/Facility Modifier −78, Return to the Operating Room for a Related Procedure During the Postoperative Period
Modifier −78 is used when the surgeon must perform additional surgery for a reason related to the original surgery during the global period. This is usually done because of hemorrhage or a failed flap or graft. Most payers recognize this as a secondary procedure for a related complication. In order to use this modifier, the physician must take the patient back to the OR. The global days for the original procedure do not reset.

Both the physician and facility must bill the code that best describes the procedures performed in the second session. If a code does not exist, an unlisted procedure is filed. The original surgery code should not be used unless the exact same procedure was carried out a second time, in which case the −76 or −77 modifier would instead apply.

> **EXAMPLE** An adult patient had a tonsillectomy and adenoidectomy in the morning. Two hours later, the surgeon was called back to the facility for postoperative bleeding that required a return trip to the OR for bleeding control. The code is 42971–78.

CPT Modifier −80, Assistant Surgeon
Modifier −80 is used to indicate that an assistant helped perform the surgery. The modifier is widely used for complex spine and abdominal procedures. The assistant surgeon uses the same CPT code as the primary surgeon and appends the −80 modifier. Payment is usually 20 percent of the allowed amount to the assistant and 80 percent to the head surgeon.

CPT Modifier −81, Minimum Assistant Surgeon
Minimum assistants do no hands-on care, and some payers may not pay for codes reported with this modifier.

CPT Modifier −82, Assistant Surgeon (When Qualified Resident Surgeon Is Not Available)
Modifier −82 is used in teaching hospitals and rural hospitals when a resident is not available or there is no adequate training program locally for the medical specialty needed to perform the procedure. The physician who assists the primary surgeon appends this modifier.

Modifier −99, Multiple Modifiers
Modifier −99 is appended to the primary procedure when two or more modifiers are being reported.

Note on HCPCS (Level II) Modifier −TC (Technical Component)
The −TC modifier is used for charges submitted by

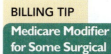

BILLING TIP

Medicare Modifier for Some Surgical Assistants

Medicare requires the use of HCPCS modifier −AS for assistant surgeons who are not physicians, such as nurse-practitioners.

Step 1.
Read all the documentation
necessary to properly determine
the circumstances surrounding
this procedure or service.

Step 2.
Determine whose service is
being coded (i.e., professional
physician component or facility).

Step 3.
Make sure the code description
for the CPT code does not already
include identifiers such as: unilateral
or bilateral, biopsy(s), staged,
or more than one occurrence.

Step 4.
If the CPT code descriptor
includes several body parts in
one code description, do not
assign an anatomic modifier
since it cannot identify any
one part or side of the body.

Step 5.
If a procedure is performed
separately from the complex
procedure, a -59 modifier may
apply to eliminate the appearance
of unbundling a more
comprehensive procedure.

Step 6.
Determine the time frame
within which a service was
performed and consider using
-24, -58, -76, -77, -78, -79.

Step 7.
If an assistant surgeon or other
provider performed a portion
of the procedure consider
using -80, -62, -66, -80, -81. -82.

Step 8.
For Medicare patients, refer to
HCPCS in addition to the CPT book
when coding/ billing for anesthesia
or OT, PT, CRNA,etc. services.

Step 9.
Sequence modifiers: (1) -99
modifier, (2) CPT modifiers that
affect payment, (3) HCPCS level II
anatomic modifiers, (4) CPT
modifiers that do not affect payment

FIGURE 8.4

Surgical Modifier Assignment
Flow Chart

facilities for use of equipment in outpatient cases. The total allowed payment for a procedure requiring use of special equipment is split between the physician, who submits a −26 modifier on the code, and the facility, which adds a −TC to the same code. The −TC is not used by a physician. If a physician submitting charges for use of equipment also owns that equipment and is performing the interpretations, no modifier is necessary. In that case, the physician receives the full allowed payment.

ASSIGNING SURGERY MODIFIERS

Modifier assignment is a skill that must be developed. The coder must make an educated decision after considering all circumstances to determine whether a modifier is required. Remember, not all circumstances or codes warrant modifiers. The coder checks off the list below (these are summarized in Figure 8.4) to determine the need for a modifier.

1. Read all documentation needed to determine the circumstances of the procedure

2. Determine the medical setting and provider (inpatient versus outpatient; facility or physician's professional services)

3. Check the CPT code descriptors for instructional notes that eliminate the need for a modifier, such as *bilateral* and *more than one occurrence.*

4. Consider whether an anatomic modifier (for example, −LT, T5) will provide more information and code accordingly (anatomic modifiers are not used with a CPT code that describes multiple body parts).

5. Consider whether using a modifier will help eliminate
   a. The appearance of duplicate billing (for example, same procedure performed on different body sites).
   b. The appearance of unbundling (for example, a separate procedure performed in addition to a complex procedure requires the use of the −59 modifier). *Separate procedures* are typically bundled into a more comprehensive procedure within that subsection that is performed at the same time.

6. Consider whether using a modifier will help explain the time frame in which a procedure was performed (for example, −24, −58, −76, −77, −78, −79)

7. Consider whether using a modifier will clarify what part of a procedure was provided by an assistant or other provider (for example, −62, −66, −80, −81, −82)

8. For medicare patients, consider HCPCS codes.

9. Correctly sequence multiple modifiers:
   a. −99 is sequenced first to indicate multiple modifiers
   b. CPT modifiers that affect payment are sequenced next (such as −22, −50, −52, −74)
   c. HCPCS anatomic modifiers are sequenced third
   d. CPT modifiers that do not affect payment are sequenced last

Assign the applicable modifiers to the scenarios below.

1. A physician performs cautery of the nose for epistaxis. The patient goes home and comes back six hours later with the nose bleeding again. The physician takes the patient back to the OR to perform further cautery and packing. _____

2. A patient is prepped for surgery and taken to the OR. Anesthesia is administered. The patient's extremity is scrubbed, and the physician notes an infected fingernail and terminates the procedure for fear of infecting the operative site. Select the modifier the facility reports.

   _____

3. A surgeon performs an ectropion repair of the left lower lid. _____

4. A surgeon removes impacted cerumen from the left ear only (69210). _____

5. A child has a speech delay and requires an auditory evoked potentials test of the central nervous system. The child will not sit still and so is taken to an outpatient facility and placed under general anesthesia. What modifier will the anesthesiologist append to the procedure code? _____

   _____

6. A physician performs a tendon procedure on the left hand and administers both local and regional anesthesia. What modifier(s) would be assigned the procedure code? _____

   _____

7. What modifier would be assigned to a bilateral carpal tunnel release procedure? _____

Integumentary System

The integumentary subsection covers procedures performed on the skin and underlying tissues down to the nonmuscle fascia. Procedures include lesion removals, skin grafts, breast procedures, skin biopsies, nail removal, and debridement of wounds and burns. Integumentary system codes are used by dermatologists as well as other medical specialties such as plastic surgeons, family practitioners, and general surgeons.

ORGANIZATION OF THE INTEGUMENTARY SUBSECTION

The integumentary subsection is arranged by anatomical site and by category of procedure. The main headings are Skin, Subcutaneous and Accessory Structures; Nails; Pilonidal Cyst; Introduction; Repair (Closure); Destruction; and Breast. These main headings, which are further divided by surgical method or body part as follows, are used as main terms to locate codes in the index:

Incision and drainage

Excision—debridement

Paring or cutting

Biopsy

Removal of skin tags

Shaving of epidermal or dermal lesions

Excision—benign lesions

Excision—malignant lesions

Repair—simple, intermediate, and complex

Adjacent tissue transfer or rearrangement

Skin replacement surgery and skin substitutes

Flaps

Other flaps, grafts, and procedures

Pressure ulcers

Burns

Destruction, benign or premalignant lesions

Destruction, malignant lesion, any method

Mohs micrographic surgery

Breast repair and/or reconstruction

Under these subheadings, CPT provides specific coding guidelines for differentiating simple, intermediate, and complex skin repairs and skin grafting with various materials and for determining the size of lesions removed and the square surface area of skin repaired or grafted. These guidelines along with any instructional notes or parenthetical notes must be read before assigning an integumentary system surgical code. Begin the coding process by finding action words such as *biopsy*, *excision*, and *repair* and procedure names, and then by finding specific body parts such as breast. Review the code descriptions and instructional notes, paying close attention to the surgical approach to the procedure and technique utilized.

EXAMPLE

11719: Trimming of nondystrophic nails, any number.

The term *trimming* is the action word for the procedure; the body part is *nails*; and the instructional note is *any number*.

SKIN BIOPSY

Biopsy entails removing a portion only of a suspicious lesion or mass. Skin biopsy codes include simple closure of the skin at the biopsy site. Biopsy codes 11100 and 11101 are not the only codes in this section that reflect biopsy services. Always search for a specific code that includes the anatomical site and service performed. For example, for a biopsy of the breast, depending on the technique, the coder must choose a code from the 19100–19103 code range.

LESIONS

The skin lesion size and type determine the mode of removal the surgeon chooses:

- *Excision:* Surgically removing or cutting out part or all of a tumor, lesion, organ, or structure with a scalpel, sharp instrument, laser, loop electrode, or hot knife
- *Paring or cutting:* Trimming or gradually reducing the size by slicing
- *Shaving:* Slicing a raised lesion or mole off at skin level by using a razor or surgical blade
- *Destruction:* Eradicating or exterminating all or a portion of a lesion, growth, or structure by force, chemicals, heat, or freezing, documented as *destruction*, *ablation*, *desiccation*, *fulguration*, and/or *cauterization*

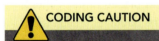

CODING CAUTION

Integumentary or Musculoskeletal Codes?

In the Integumentary subsection, *incision and drainage (I&D)* and *foreign body removal* refer to superficial procedures. Use musculoskeletal surgery codes for procedures that go beyond subcutaneous tissue.

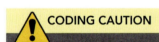

CODING CAUTION

Biopsy Guidelines

- A biopsy is not coded separately from tissue obtained during an excision, shave removal, or destruction of tissue at the same site.
- Multiple biopsies on the same day may be coded and reported from multiple sites on the skin or subcutaneous tissue by using the −59 modifier for each site separately biopsied.

To properly code lesion removal procedures, the coder must know whether the lesion is classified as malignant or benign, the site, the number of lesions, and depth and size of the lesions, including surgical margins.

Base the assignment of lesion-removal codes on the greatest diameter of the lesion itself, not according to the size of the incision necessary to access it. The size of the lesion is taken from the physician's operative report or office procedure note. If there is no documentation of the size, it is permissible to use the excision code with the *smallest size* for that anatomical area, but this is not recommended. Best practice is to query the physician for the information rather than to assume the size of the specimen or lesion.

NAILS

The anatomy of the nail includes the nail bed, nail plate, and matrix. Preventive procedures as well as treatment for traumatic injuries can be performed on nails. Codes in this section are sensitive to the number of nails treated. Some codes specify the number while others simply use the plural *nails*. When *nails* or *nail(s)* is indicated, assign the code only one time no matter how many nails are involved.

INTRODUCTION

The Introduction subheading encompasses services for injecting medications and substances into the skin, introducing implants and devices, and removing these devices. Lesions such as keloids may be injected with drugs to shrink a scar. This does not include injecting lesions with chemotherapy or veins with sclerosing agents. These services are located in other sections of CPT.

The code for intralesional injection (11900–11901) does not include the actual substance injected. A separate HCPCS code for that material must also be submitted. Services that involve placing something into or removing something placed previously from the skin and subcutaneous tissue are located here.

REPAIR (CLOSURE)

Wounds in the skin require closure. Depending on the depth of the wound, one of three types of closure (described in CPT guidelines under the Repair heading) may be performed:

1. *Simple:* Superficial wound repair involves epidermis, dermis, and a minimal amount of subcutaneous tissue requiring one-layer closure. Simple closures include those done with tape, adhesive strips, or glue (Dermabond) and are inherent components of all surgical procedures. Simple closures are not coded separately.

2. *Intermediate:* Closure of one or more of the subcutaneous layers and superficial fascia in addition to the skin are called intermediate repairs. Intermediate closure codes can also be used when the wound has to be extensively cleaned due to contamination or small pieces of foreign material need to be removed before suturing.

3. *Complex:* Complicated repairs include scar revision, debridement (removal of dead tissue), extensive undermining, stents, or retention

CODING TIP

Excision Codes Include Simple Repair or Closure

Excision codes already include the direct, primary, and simple repair or closure of the defect. Any closure other than a simple closure is coded separately.

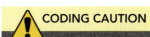

BILLING TIP

Reporting Nail Services

Use HCPCS Level II modifiers from the −FA through −F9 and −TA through −T9 ranges when reporting nail services to Medicare and other payers that accept HCPCS codes.

CODING CAUTION

Suture Types

Pay attention to the type of suture used to close a wound or surgical site. Typically if two different types of suture are used (one absorbable, such as Vicryl, chromic, catgut, or Dexon), an intermediate repair is likely.

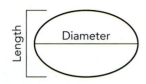

FIGURE 8.5
Lesion or Wound Dimensions

sutures, and more than one-layered closure. Repair of traumatic avulsions or lacerations may fall into this category. Repair of extensive nerve, blood vessel, or tendon damage may be reported in addition when the wound is complex.

Assigning wound repair codes begins with selecting the code range for the level of repair and then considering the site of wound repair and the length of wounds closed in the anatomical site grouping in centimeters (see Figure 8.5). If the size is reported in millimeters, it must be converted to centimeters by moving the decimal point. For example, an 11 mm lesion is 1.1 cm. (Do not confuse the size of the lesion with the size of the specimen or the size of the defect.)

DESTRUCTION

Destruction is the ablation, obliteration, vaporization, or cryosurgery, laser, chemical, or electrosurgical annihilation of a benign, premalignant, or malignant lesion. Codes for destruction from the Integumentary section should not be used if there is a more specific anatomical code from another section of CPT.

Each type of lesion destroyed is reported with a separate code. Codes are determined by the number of lesions destroyed, the size of the lesions prior to destruction, and the type of lesion (benign, premalignant, or malignant). Codes for malignant lesion destruction are also determined by body site.

> **EXAMPLE** The patient has twelve benign and one premalignant lesions across her body. Some are destroyed by chemical means, while others are destroyed by laser. The codes are 17000 and 17110.

BREAST

Breasts are composed of subcutaneous tissue, fat, nerves, blood vessels, and lymph vessels and sit on top of the pectoris muscle; thus they are considered part of the integumentary section. Breasts are categorized into their own subsection with the following subheadings: Incision, Excision, Introduction, and Repair/Reconstruction.

Checkpoint 8.7

Assign CPT codes and applicable modifiers for the following statements.

1. Excision of malignant lesions, 1.1 cm, upper arm; 0.1 cm, foot _____

2. Split graft, 80 sq cm, lower leg, staged procedure on infant _____

3. Surgical removal of excess skin and tissue, upper arm and hand _____

4. Needle core biopsy of both breasts (not using imaging guidance) _____

5. Simple incision and removal of foreign body, subcutaneous tissue _____

6. Laser destruction of four premalignant lesions _____

7. Rhytidectomy of glabellar frown lines _____

8. After observing that a spot on her upper leg had grown bigger, a patient sees her dermatologist. The dermatologist determines that she has a malignant 3.3 cm lesion. He biopsies and excises it, followed by a simple closure. _____

Musculoskeletal System

The musculoskeletal system is the largest subsection of the Surgery section. Many different procedures can be performed on the bones, tendons, soft tissue, and muscles of the body. Common procedures are reduction (manipulation) of fractures and dislocations. It is important to have a good knowledge of all the bones of the body and their locations, tendons, and muscles.

The subsection starts with general codes that apply to the entire body and then goes from the head down to the toes. A consistent arrangement makes finding codes easier: each body site is identified, followed by these headings:

- Incision
- Excision
- Introduction or Removal
- Repair
- Revision and/or Reconstruction
- Fracture and/or Dislocation
- Arthrodesis
- Amputation
- Other Procedures

GENERAL GUIDELINES FOR CODING ORTHOPEDIC PROCEDURES

Orthopedic procedures are coded by the surgical approach to the procedure. The coder should pay close attention to the type and extent of services provided by carefully reading the medical record and then reading the code description in its entirety to identify phrases like *closed, open, with* or *without manipulation or reducton, with traction, with* or *without internal or external fixator*, and *with grafting*. There are also many separate procedures, particularly in the arthroscopic procedure sections, to remain alert for. Note that many procedures can be done using either a traditional open method or an arthroscopic method.

BILLING TIP

Required Documentation

If the term *specify* follows a code description, send an operative note or special report with the claim.

Open Treatment An **open procedure** involves making an incision and surgically opening the body at the site of the injury or ailment. Uncomplicated soft tissue closure may be done. This approach is considered major surgery because large, deep incisions are made, and it involves more risk and most often is performed under general anesthesia. The main term often ends in *-otomy*.

EXAMPLE
23105: Arthrotomy, glenohumeral joint, with synovectomy, with or without biopsy.

Closed Treatment A **closed procedure** does not involve making a large incision and surgically opening the site of injury or area in need of repair or treatment. Closed procedures are primarily performed endoscopically. Clues to look for are words that end in *-oscopy*.

EXAMPLE
29820: Arthroscopy, surgical, shoulder; synovectomy, partial.

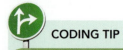

Therapeutic Surgical Procedures Include Biopsies

The general surgery coding guideline applies: a biopsy of a structure—which is a diagnostic procedure—is not coded separately when an excision, destruction, removal, repair, or fixation procedure is also performed at the same operative session (same site, same patient).

In addition to code selection by type of treatment, coders must determine whether the treatment is for a traumatic injury (accident) or a medical condition. For excision, biopsies, and incision and drainage, coders should check both the Integumentary and the Musculoskeletal sections, which may have more codes that are specific to the anatomical part; such codes should be used.

WOUND EXPLORATION

Wound exploration codes are for traumatic wounds that result from acute or penetrating trauma (such as gunshot or stabbing). The codes cover both basic exploration and repair of the area, including dissection to determine depth of penetration of the wound, debridement, removal of foreign body, and ligation or coagulation of minor subcutaneous and/or muscular blood vessels or the subcutaneous tissues, muscle fascia, and muscle.

Wound exploration codes are also used when the repair requires enlargement of the existing wound for cleaning, determination of the extent of the wound, and repair. If the wound does not require enlarging or if deeper structures of the muscle fascia and beyond are not explored, a code from the Integumentary section is appropriate. If the wound is more severe than the wound exploration would encompass or if the repair is done to major structures or major blood vessels, the repair code is selected from the specific area of the Musculoskeletal section.

The following rules apply when coding wound explorations:

- Wound explorations are coded in addition to the E/M service with modifier −25.
- Codes are used for acute and penetrating injuries only.
- Surgical exploration is through the current wound with possible enlargement.
- Muscle fascia and beyond are explored.
- Skin and subcutaneous tissue exploration is coded to the Integumentary section when no enlargement of the wound, extension, dissection, or the like is required.
- Layered closure is expected.
- Drains may or may not be placed.
- Debridement and removal of foreign body is included.
- Ligation of minor subcutaneous tissue and/or muscle blood vessels is included.
- If a thoracotomy or laparotomy is performed, the wound exploration is bundled into these more extensive procedures.

  EXAMPLE   A man stabbed in the thigh comes to the ER with a knife stuck in the wound. The surgeon removes the knife and explores the extent of the penetration. He finds that the femoral artery has been nicked. He proceeds to repair the femoral artery. He does not code and bill for the wound exploration but instead codes for the artery repair.

EXCISION

Excision in this section is similar to excision in the Integumentary section; however, here the excision is typically of deeper structures such as soft tissue, muscle, or bone. An incision is made in the affected area;

the area is inspected and debrided; and the mass or lesion is completely removed. The excision subheading is located in each body area of CPT.

INTRODUCTION OR REMOVAL

Introduction or removal codes include injection of sinus tracts, joints, tendons, and trigger points. The term *arthrocentesis* describes the procedure to aspirate the joint, remove fluid, or insert a therapeutic substance. Codes are grouped according to the size of the joint being injected: small, intermediate, and major. If a more extensive procedure is being done to a joint that is also being injected, the injection is included (bundled) into the more complex procedure. Tendon injections have separate codes. Trigger point injections, usually done for pain management, are coded by the number of muscle groups injected, not the number of times the needle is inserted.

FOREIGN BODY REMOVAL

A foreign body is anything that is "foreign" to the body (such as metal, gravel, a bullet, or an orthopedic device) and embedded in tissue, bone, or a joint, or it could be natural tissue or bone that had broken off (such as bone chip or cartilage). Two factors affect coding for removal of a foreign body: the site and whether the foreign body is superficial or deep. Some of the code sections have a specific code for foreign body removal, and some do not. The codes are usually found under the Introduction or Removal subheading in each body section. When a specific code is unavailable, the coder should refer to the notes in parentheses in the general section of the Musculoskeletal section.

FRACTURES

The following questions must be answered in order to assign the appropriate code for fracture repair:

1. Where was the fracture or dislocation?
2. Was the treatment open or closed?
3. Was a reduction/manipulation of the fracture performed?
4. Was an internal or external fixation device applied?
5. Was percutaneous (through the skin) or skeletal fixation applied?
6. Was infection present, was treatment delayed, or did the surgery take longer than usual?

Open and Closed Treatment of Fractures   Fractures care is coded by the type of treatment (open, closed, percutaneous fixation), not the type of fracture (which is an ICD-9-CM issue). There is no correlation of the type of fracture and the type of treatment; a closed fracture, for example, may require closed treatment or open treatment for adequate repair.

Open treatment of a fracture involves making an incision and surgically opening the site for repair and treatment. Uncomplicated soft tissue closure may be involved. Internal fixation such as screws, a plate, a wire, or a rod may be applied. Closed treatment of a fracture

NOTE

Supply codes (HCPCS) are covered in Chapter 10 of your program.

CODING TIP

Reporting Casting Without a Surgical Procedure

If a cast is placed on a patient and no surgery was performed, code the appropriate level E/M code (outpatient or ER service) plus the codes for any supplies.

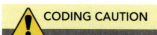 **CODING CAUTION**

Therapeutic Procedures Include Diagnostic Procedures

- A diagnostic arthroscopy should not be coded separately when a surgical arthroscopy is performed.
- Synovectomy of the joint is always included in a more extensive arthroscopic or open procedure unless extensive synovectomy has been performed in more than two compartments.

does not involve surgically opening the site to repair it. Instead, the physician manipulates the fracture (also called reduction) and applies a cast, a splint, a bandage, or a traction, immobilization, or stabilization device.

Casting Guidelines Application or removal of the first cast or traction device is bundled for all orthopedic procedures, so if a cast, splint, or strapping is applied as a result of or during a surgical procedure, it is not assigned a code. In contrast, when the first cast or traction device is replaced, or when the cast or strapping is an initial service performed without a restorative treatment or procedure, codes from the 29000–29799 code range are assigned during the period of follow-up care. These codes can also be used if the physician applying a temporary cast is not the physician performing the fracture reduction. Application of temporary casts, splints, or strapping is not considered part of the preoperative care package and can be reported with modifier −56. Professional component codes for cast removal are assigned only for casts applied by another physician.

FIXATION DEVICES

Fixation devices can be coded only when the device itself is not included in the code description for the procedure. External fixation devices are often adjusted and subsequently removed. Removal of internal fixation devices have separate codes; coders should determine whether there is a more specific code for the particular body site from which the implant is removed. If removal of an internal fixation device is done in conjunction with another procedure at the same site, it is not coded.

ARTHROSCOPY

Many procedures on joints are done using an arthroscope, indicated by terms such as *portals, trocars, cannula,* or *scope.* Arthroscopy codes are located at the end of the Musculoskeletal subsection. When coding these procedures, first locate the word *arthroscopy* in the index, and then find the appropriate site. Note that a code for an open procedure cannot be used for an arthroscopy procedure, even if it appears to closely match the documentation. If no arthroscopy code is provided for the specific site, an unlisted code, 29999, must be used.

ARTHRODESIS

Arthrodesis involves fusing two bones together to prevent movement. Typically arthrodesis is performed on joints such as the ankle, carpals, and spine. The ends of two bones are fused together with screw fixation and possible bone grafting. The bones are aligned in the most functional position, but the joint loses its natural motion. Arthrodesis can be performed alone or with other surgical procedures. If it is performed in addition to fracture care, osteotomy, or spinal laminectomy or corpectomy, the arthrodesis is reported separately with a −51 modifier.

Use the CPT book to assign codes to the following statements, appending modifiers if needed.

1. Humeral osteotomy _____

2. Closed treatment of sesamoid fracture _____

3. Open treatment of right talus fracture _____

4. I&D of left foot bursa _____

5. Right elbow joint arthrodesis _____

6. Synovial biopsy and diagnostic arthroscopy of left hip _____

7. Surgical arthroscopy, left ankle, with removal of foreign body _____

8. Surgical exploration of chest wound with debridement and removal of foreign body _____

    _____

9. Nine months after a right humeral fracture repair, a patient returns to the physician with pain in the fracture area. The patient had not returned before today for fracture care follow-up and now has a nonunion of the humeral fracture. The surgeon does an iliac graft to repair the nonunion.

    _____

10. Late one evening, a patient went to the emergency department for evaluation and treatment after falling off a ladder. He was in extreme pain with intense muscle spasms. The ER physician determined that the patient had wrenched his back, but there was no dislocation or fracture. The ER physician strapped the patient's back and instructed him to see his family physician in the morning for follow-up care. _____

Respiratory System

The respiratory subsection includes many procedures on the sinuses, nose, larynx, trachea, bronchi, lungs, and pleura. Many of them are performed using an endoscope of some kind and are indexed under the terms *endoscopy, laryngoscopy,* or *bronchoscopy.* The surgeon's operative note should state whether the procedures were carried out unilaterally or bilaterally and whether they were open, closed, or endoscopically performed. Codes for nasal and sinus endoscopies are unilateral procedures; those done bilaterally require a –50 modifier.

NASAL PROCEDURES

Procedures done on the nose can be done with an endoscope or through an incision on the face or forehead. Coding is based on whether the approach used was internal or external and was with or without a scope. Common procedures on the nose are septoplasty, removal of polyps, turbinate excisions, and treatment of epistaxis (nose bleeds). Other common nasal procedures, such as control of nasal hemorrhage, ligation of arteries, and fractures of turbinates, are usually bundled with a major procedure if they are not performed alone.

Excision of Nasal Polyps   A *simple* nasal polyp is limited to one polyp or one polyp per side of the nose. Such polyps are usually pedunculated (hanging from a stalk) and are easy to remove. Simple excisions are typically performed in the physician office. Excision of multiple polyps on one side or more than one per side is considered *extensive*, involving sessile polyps (with a thick base) whose removal requires more effort, skill, and time and is usually performed in an outpatient surgical facility.

Excision of Turbinate(s) or Turbinate Reduction   Turbinate excision or reduction is performed for turbinate hypertrophy from chronic inflammation or infection, which can lead to persistent sinus infections. Turbinates can be reduced by removing part of the lining and/or part of the bone itself with cautery, laser, or excision. *Submucosal resection* means that the surgeon performs submucosal removal of the lining of the turbinate, not actually removing part of the bone itself (CPT code 30140). At times turbinates that are enlarged and obstructing the nasal airway may be fractured to reposition them (CPT code 30930).

Rhinoplasty   Rhinoplasty is performed for both cosmetic and therapeutic purposes. This procedure reshapes the external portions of the nose and may involve the cartilage and bone. The extent of this procedure varies. There are two conditional phrases to keep in mind: primary and secondary. The primary procedure is the first rhinoplasty procedure done; *secondary* refers to follow-up or a second rhinoplasty procedure.

Nasal Septal Deviation   When the nasal septum is not midline, or straight, it may obstruct air movement, requiring a septoplasty to fix the alignment. Septoplasty with cartilage graft is included in this code. Surgeons refer to septoplasty as submucous resection. Modifier −50 does not apply to septoplasty procedures.

Nasal Hemorrhage   If bleeding occurs as a late complication and requires a significant separately identifiable service after the patient has been released from an endoscopic procedure, the cautery and packing can be billed with a −78 modifier. To code control of nasal hemorrhage, the coder must decide whether this was an anterior or posterior control. Key words for the anterior approach are *insertion of gauze packing*, *anterior packing*, and *cauterization*. For the posterior approach, terms used are *insertion of nasal stents*, *balloons*, *tampons*, and *catheters* and *posterior nasal packing*.

PROCEDURES ON THE LARYNX: LARYNGOSCOPY

Laryngoscopies are performed for biopsy, removal of foreign bodies, dilation of the larynx, and diagnostic examination of the pharynx and larynx. They can be performed for either diagnostic or surgical purposes and may be direct or indirect surgeries. An indirect laryngoscopy is performed in an office setting with the use of mirrors to view the larynx, pharyngeal walls, oropharynx, and posterior third of the tongue. People with strong gag reflexes and small children have difficulty with this procedure. If so, a direct laryngoscopy may be done in a facility under general anesthesia. It requires a scope to be passed through the mouth and pharynx to the larynx.

PROCEDURES ON THE LUNGS, TRACHEA, AND BRONCHI: BRONCHOSCOPY AND TRACHEOBRONCHOSCOPY

Bronchoscopies are performed for a number of purposes, such as dilation of the trachea; biopsies of the lung, bronchus, and trachea; bronchial lavage; lung brachytherapy; and aspiration. A bronchoscopy is automatically considered a bilateral procedure, so a −50 modifier is not assigned when the procedure is performed on both lungs.

Bronchoscopies can be performed by using a flexible fiberoptic or a rigid right bronchoscope (also known as an open-tube bronchoscope). Fluoroscopy is bundled. The rigid scope is used to remove foreign bodies or to remove a large biopsy sample. The flexible bronchoscopy is more commonly performed and utilizes fiberoptic light to better view the bronchioles.

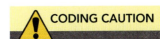

CODING CAUTION

Bronchoscopy vs. Biopsy

When a bronchoscopy is performed with brushings or washings, it is considered a diagnostic bronchoscopy, not a biopsy.

Checkpoint 8.9

Use the CPT book to assign codes to the following statements, appending modifiers if needed. Some of the procedures require two codes. *Hint:* For endoscopic procedures, read the notes before the code group carefully.

1. Surgical thoracoscopy with excisions of pericardial and mediastinal cysts _____

2. Surgical nasal/sinus endoscopy with left maxillary antrostomy _____

3. Planned tracheostomy on infant _____

4. Hematoma drainage from nasal septum _____

5. Laser destruction of two intranasal lesions, internal approach _____

6. Bilateral nasal evaluation using endoscope _____

7. Direct diagnostic laryngoscopy and tracheoscopy with operating microscope _____

8. A CT exam showed that years of chronic sinusitis had created a severe blockage of the patient's ethmoid sinus cavity on the left side. A sinus endoscopy was performed to remove tissue from the ethmoid sinus both anterior and posterior. _____

Cardiovascular System

In the Cardiovascular section, procedures on the heart, veins, and arteries are described. Thousands of procedures are done each year on blood vessels, ranging from heart bypasses to creating access to vessels for chemotherapy and dialysis to varicose vein and hemangioma treatment. This section of the text touches on just a few of the many procedures that are available.

Cardiology coding requires considerable knowledge, skill, and practice. The most difficult part of coding cardiovascular cases is determining the number of codes needed. Codes from three different sections of CPT may be assigned. The Cardiovascular section (33010–37799) houses the surgical codes. The Medicine section (92950–93799) contains codes for the cardiac-related nonsurgical services. Radiology codes (75552–75790) are assigned when imaging is used to perform a service on the heart such as a nuclear study involving angiography, a catheterization, or an angioplasty.

PACEMAKERS AND PACING CARDIOVERTER DEFIBRILLATORS

A pacemaker is installed under the skin to electrically stimulate the myocardium of one or more chambers of the heart to contract when the heart fails to do so on its own. A pacemaker may be permanent or temporary. Another device, an implantable cardioverter defibrillator, may also be installed to regulate the activity of the patient's heartbeat.

A pacemaker has two parts: a pulse generator and leads (electrodes). The pulse generator contains the battery, the electronic circuit, the connector, and the sealed encasement. (A temporary pacemaker does not include an internally placed pulse generator.) To install a pacemaker, the surgeon creates a subcutaneous pocket to house the generator and then places the lead(s) inside a chamber of the heart. The electrodes are either inserted via a vein (transvenous) or placed on the surface of the heart (epicardium). The device can be removed by opening the pocket and disconnecting it. When a battery replacement is necessary, two codes are required—one that describes the removal of the pulse generator and the other for its reinsertion.

To correctly code pacemaker services, the coder must know the answers to the following questions:

- Where were the electrodes (lead) placed: atrium, ventricle, or both?
- Is this initial placement, replacement, or repair of some or all the components of a pacemaker?
- Was the surgical approach transvenous or epicardial?

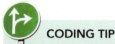

CODING TIP

Coding Checking on Inplantable Cardioverter Defibrillator Operation

Electrophysiological evaluation of the cardioverter defibrillator can be done at the time of initial implantation or replacement or at any time after. Codes from the Medicine section are assigned for this service.

PROCEDURES ON VEINS AND ARTERIES

Codes under the main heading Arteries and Veins describe treatment for aneurysms, angioplasty, bypass surgery, varicose veins, and hemangiomas. Treatment for severe varicose veins involves ligating, dividing, and ultimately stripping the diseased veins. Hemangiomas are benign neoplasms comprised of capillaries and venules in superficial and/or deep dermis that can be treated with laser therapy (codes in the Integumentary section), embolization, or sclerotherapy.

CORONARY ARTERY BYPASS GRAFTS (CABG)

CABG procedures (pronounced like *cabbage*) are performed on the heart to improve blood flow to areas of the heart that were otherwise cut off from blood supply due to an occluded vessel. A blood vessel is typically obtained from the patient's leg or arm and used to surgically reattach healthy vessels (anastomosis) by detouring (bypassing) the clogged or occluded diseased vessels. Coronary artery bypass grafts are coded by type of graft documented in the operative report.

ANGIOPLASTY

Angioplasty is a medical procedure in which a balloon is inserted into a vessel via a catheter to open a narrowed or blocked blood vessel of the heart, kidney, or extremities. A catheter is a thin tube that allows drainage, injection of fluids, or access by surgical instruments into a vessel. Angioplasty can be performed by open or percutaneous approaches. Percutaneous transluminal angioplasty (PTA) involves inserting a balloon catheter into an artery and advancing it to the narrowed portion of the artery (catheterization). A balloon is inflated at this narrowed site to increase the artery's diameter, allowing more blood flow. Angioplasty is commonly performed on the vessels of the heart. Percutaneous transluminal coronary angioplasty (PTCA) codes are located in the Medicine section of CPT.

VENOUS ACCESS DEVICES

Central venous access devices are small, flexible tubes placed in large veins to allow frequent access to the bloodstream for medication administration. When trying to understand which device is being used, the first question is whether it has been placed in a peripheral (superficial) or central (deep) vein.

Catheter Placements   A PICC line (peripherally inserted central venous catheter) is inserted directly into a peripheral vein, but it has a very long catheter that can be fed into a deep vein. Also called a central line, the PICC line is for short-term use.

The most common central venous catheter is the triple lumen. It can be placed percutaneously, whereby the catheter is inserted into vein through a puncture wound, or by cutdown placement—surgical incision made in skin to expose a vein into which the catheter is inserted. A tunneled central venous catheter is placed through a puncture in the skin, then tunneled underneath the skin before being introduced into the vein. Common examples are Hickman, Broviac, and Groshong catheters.

Code 36597 is used for repositioning a previously placed catheter under fluoroscopic guidance.

Generally, removal of a central venous catheter is reflected in the E/M code that is assigned for the patient visit. This usually entails only suture removal and withdrawal of the catheter and should not be coded separately. Should the catheter be embedded and involve more work in removal, use 37799.

Implantable Venous Access Devices   Implantable venous access devices provide easy access to the venous system and avoid repeated venipuncture. The ports are surgically implanted so the device is entirely under the skin. These are for long-term use in chemotherapy and dialysis. Examples are Port-A-Cath, Hemo-Cath, and Perm-A-Cath. Removal of such a catheter is coded to 36589. Declotting of a venous access device is coded to 36593.

Use the CPT book to assign codes to the following statements, appending modifiers if needed. Some of the procedures require two codes. *Hint:* For endoscopic procedures, carefully read the notes before this code group.

1. Subcutaneous removal of pacing cardioverter defibrillator pulse generator, electrodes removed by thoracotomy _____

2. Ligation of secondary varicose veins, left and right legs _____

3. Repair by division of patent ductus arteriosus in ten-year-old _____

4. Ring insertion and valvuloplasty, tricuspid valve _____

5. Excision of infected abdominal graft, surgical care only _____

6. Central venous catheter placed percutaneously in adult _____

7. A patient is placed on heart-lung bypass, and the main pulmonary artery is opened in order to remove the blockage and interior lining of the artery. The artery is then sutured closed, and the pulmonary endarterectomy is accomplished. _____

8. Insertion of transvenous electrode for dual chamber pacing cardioverter defibrillator; initial insertion done twenty days earlier _____

Hemic and Lymphatic Systems; Mediastinum and Diaphragm

Codes in the Hemic (blood-producing) and Lymphatic Systems sections encompass procedures on the spleen, bone marrow, lymph nodes, mediastinum, and diaphragm. Common procedures are splenectomy, lymph node biopsy, and bone marrow transplants.

SPLENECTOMY

A splenectomy is the complete or partial removal of the spleen. Code selection is based on whether the excision is an open procedure or is performed laparoscopically.

BONE MARROW OR STEM CELL WORK

Bone marrow or stem cells must be removed and prepared for implantation or reinfusion in the same patient. The code range includes codes for managing the procedures and for each specific type of transplant preparation.

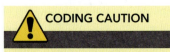

CODING CAUTION

Report Once Daily
Transplant preparation codes are reported on a per diem basis, regardless of the quantity of bone marrow or stem cells that are manipulated.

LYMPH NODE BIOPSY

Lymph node biopsy—performed via a needle, skin incision, or a laparoscope—is removal of part of a lymph node for examination, in contrast to complete removal of the entire node. Although about 30 percent of the body's lymph nodes are located in the head and neck, the rest are throughout the body. Coders must pay attention to the site of the biopsy/excision and the depth (superficial or deep).

LYMPHADENECTOMY

Lymphadenectomy refers to removal of one or more lymph nodes (not simply a biopsy or excision). The term *complete* when describing neck dissection is synonymous with *radical*. When a radical dissection is carried out, all lymph nodes in that area are removed.

Digestive System

The Digestive System section encompasses the digestive flow in the body beginning with the lips and mouth and ending with the anus. Also included are internal organs that aid in digestion, including the pancreas, appendix, gallbladder, and liver. The headings for the code ranges are:

- Lips, vestibule of the mouth, tongue and floor of the mouth, and dentoalveolar structures
- Palate and uvula
- Salivary gland and ducts
- Pharynx, adenoids, and tonsils
- Esophagus
- Stomach
- Intestines (except rectum)
- Meckel's diverticulum and the mesentery
- Appendix
- Rectum
- Anus
- Liver
- Biliary tract
- Pancreas
- Abdomen, peritoneum, and the omentum

GENERAL GUIDELINES FOR ENDOSCOPIC PROCEDURES FOR THE DIGESTIVE SYSTEM

Many procedures performed on the digestive system—such as colonoscopies, cholecystectomies, appendectomies, hernia repairs, and esophagogastroduodenoscopies (EGD)—are done endoscopically. The open procedure codes of a site cannot be assigned to describe a closed (percutaneously performed or done by endoscope) procedure of the same site. Surgical endoscopy always includes diagnostic endoscopy.

> **EXAMPLE** The patient's reducible umbilical hernia is repaired laparoscopically. There is no specific code for a laparoscopic umbilical hernia repair, but there is a code for the traditional open procedure (49585). It is inappropriate to assign this procedure code. Instead, unlisted laparoscopy procedure, hernioplasty, herniorrhaphy, herniotomy (49659) should be assigned.

LIPS

Care is necessary when coding procedures involving lips. If the excision or repair crosses the vermillion (colored portion) border, as is common for cancers of the lip, it is coded using digestive system

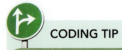

codes. If it does not cross this border, it is classified under procedures on the skin of the lips in the Integumentary section.

TONSILS AND ADENOIDS

Tonsillectomy and adenoidectomy procedures are considered inherently bilateral, so a –50 modifier is not appropriate with these code ranges. Codes are age-specific, and there are codes for tonsils and adenoids together and for tonsils or adenoids separately.

HERNIA REPAIRS

There are several types of hernias, including inguinal, umbilical, and incisional hernias, and each has its own code assignment. Code assignment is based on whether the hernia is initial or recurrent and whether it is incarcerated or reducible. Inguinal hernias can be repaired either open or laparoscopically. Insertion of mesh for any hernia repair other than the incisional or ventral hernia is not coded. CPT 49568 is used in addition to the code for incisional and ventral hernia repairs *only*.

Coders should be familiar with the many terms used to describe types and locations of hernias:

- *Inguinal:* A common hernia of the inguinal canal in the groin
- *Lumbar:* A very rare hernia occurring in the lumbar region of the torso
- *Incisional:* A hernia occurring at the site of a previous incision
- *Femoral:* A common hernia occurring in the femoral canal in the groin
- *Epigastric* (umbilical): A hernia located above the naval or inside the belly button indentation
- *Spigelian:* A hernia usually located above the inferior epigastric vessel along the outer border of the rectus muscle
- *Hiatal:* A hernia that occurs when a part of the stomach slides above the diaphragm
- *Reducible:* A hernia when the organs can be returned to normal position by the surgeon's manipulating the viscera

APPENDECTOMY

An appendectomy can be performed as an open procedure or laparoscopically. An incidental appendectomy—removal of the appendix during another open abdominal procedure—is not coded separately. If the appendix is removed for an indicated purpose, it can be coded separately using 44955 in addition to the other major surgery.

CHOLECYSTECTOMY

A cholecystectomy involves removing the gallbladder; code ranges cover it as an open or a laparoscopic procedure. Removal includes destruction by morcellation, coagulation, or laser technique, so destruction is not coded in addition.

ESOPHAGOSCOPY AND ESOPHAGOGASTRODUODENOSCOPY (EGD)

Code ranges are provided for endoscopic procedures of the pyloric canal to view and treat tumors, lesions, or polyps. An endoscopy of the esophagus (esophagoscopy) or upper gastrointestinal endoscopy passing through the diaphragm into the stomach (esophagogastroscopy), is performed. The most complete procedure is an esophagogastroduodenoscopy (EGD), the inspection of the esophagus through the stomach and the duodenum and/or jejunum with an endoscope. The choice of a code is based on whether the procedure is diagnostic or surgical.

BARIATRIC SURGERY

Bariatric procedures are performed to treat morbid obesity. These code ranges cover various procedures such as gastric banding and gastric bypass.

ENDOSCOPIC PROCEDURES INVOLVING THE COLON

A colonoscopy examines the entire colon, from the rectum to the cecum. A sigmoidoscopy examines the entire rectum, the sigmoid colon, and sometimes part of the descending colon. A proctosigmoidoscopy examines only the rectum and sigmoid colon.

To correctly code colon-related endoscopies, coders must determine how much of the bowel was visualized and where and how the scope was inserted. The scope can be inserted through the rectum or through a colostomy or colotomy. The entrance of the scope determines what the physician views. When the scope is entered through the rectum, the rectum is visualized, followed by the colon and then perhaps the terminal ileum. If the scope is entered through a stoma, as in a colostomy, the scope will require more maneuvering to view the rectum and small intestine.

The coder must also determine whether the procedure was diagnostic or surgical in nature. A diagnostic colonoscopy may collect only specimens and does not entail obtaining biopsies or removal of lesions. In a surgical procedure, some other work is done, such as removing a foreign body or lesion; each of these has a respective code assignment.

> **EXAMPLE** Code 45380, colonoscopy, flexible, proximal to splenic flexure with biopsy, should be reported for the removal of a portion of the polyp by cold biopsy forceps. Code 45385 is used when the entire polyp is removed by cold biopsy forceps (snare technique).

A colonoscopy is coded if the scope is passed beyond the splenic flexure or more than 60 cm of colon. If a patient is scheduled for and fully prepped for a colonoscopy and the scope is not passed beyond the splenic flexure, code 45378 with a −52 modifier.

Colonoscopy with Polyp Removal
Polyp removal is reported when an entire polyp is excised. If different polyps are removed by different techniques or methods, all the techniques used are reported.

> **EXAMPLE** When a polyp is completely removed from the ascending colon by snare technique and a second polyp is removed by hot biopsy forceps, codes 45384 and 45385 (with the −59 modifier) are reported.

CODING TIP

Esophageal or EGD?

Read the procedure to verify that the scope passed through the stomach into the duodenum in order to code an EGD. If not, the procedure is not an EGD and is coded as an upper endoscopy.

BILLING TIP

Medicare Modifier for Colonoscopy

Check with the Medicare payer to determine whether a −53 modifier instead of the −52 modifier should be used.

⚠ CODING CAUTION

Polyp Removal

If several polyps are removed by the same technique, the appropriate code is reported only once. If only a polyp, tumor, or lesion is removed with both the snare and hot biopsy methods, report only the code for the snare technique.

HEMORRHOIDECTOMY

Hemorrhoids are removed by surgically excising them, attaching rubber bands, or using a laser. Complex hemorrhoids are bleeding, prolapsed, or thrombosed or require plastic skin closure (that is, anoplasty). An important note is located beneath code 46262 referring the coder to various codes according to the procedure performed.

Checkpoint 8.11

Use the CPT book to assign codes to the following statements, appending modifiers if needed. Some of the procedures require two codes. *Hint:* For endoscopic procedures, carefully read the notes before the code group.

1. Exploratory laparotomy _____

2. Removal of pancreatic calculus _____

3. Palate resection, repeated procedure by same physician _____

4. Secondary adenoidectomy, ten-year-old patient _____

5. Endoscopic placement of gastrostomy tube with radiological S&I _____

6. Simple ileostomy revision done during same operative session as pharangeal wound suture _____

_____

7. Partial colectomy with ileostomy and creation of mucofistula _____

_____

8. As a result of spasms in the esophagus, the patient is unable to swallow. The physician will need a balloon dilator greater than 35 mm to alleviate the patient's difficulty. Radiologic supervision and interpretation is provided via fluoroscopy using the hospital's equipment. _____

_____

CODING TIP

Removal of Internal Hemorrhoids Only

If the physician excises internal hemorrhoids only, use a −52 modifier with the hemorrhoidectomy code.

CODING TIP

Coding Endoscopies

As with all endoscopic procedures, determine the final destination of the scope before selecting codes.

Urinary System

The urinary system is responsible for maintaining a steady balance in the fluid and chemical composition of the blood and for disposing of waste products from the blood. This system consists of the kidneys, ureters, bladder, and urethra. Urinary surgery codes are organized under those body parts and then follow a format of incision, excision, introduction, repair, and laparoscopy.

Located in this section are many diagnostic procedure codes that evaluate the functionality of the urinary system, such as flow of urine, volume, pressure, and muscle function. Surgical procedures range from minor procedures, such as treatment of ureter and urethral strictures, dilation of the bladder, and biopsy of the bladder, to more complex operations including removal of kidney stones, tumor removal, suspension procedures for urinary incontinence, and kidney transplants. Many of the procedures are carried out through a cystoscope inserted through the urethra.

There are two kidneys and two ureters, so the −50 modifier is appended when procedures are performed on both sides. Coders must also pay close attention to the site where the procedure is being performed. It is easy to confuse urethra and ureter.

ENDOSCOPY

Codes for cystoscopy and urethroscopy are combined under the term *cystourethroscopy*. Many procedures can be done using a cystourethroscope. Coding is based on the site of the cystourethroscopy (for example, the bladder, urethra, or ureter) and on how the scope is inserted—either transurethrally or through an existing stoma.

PROSTATE PROCEDURES

Prostate surgery is commonly performed cystoscopically. Codes are selected by treatment method, such as microwave thermotherapy or laser vaporization. Some of the prostate procedures are carried out endoscopically; others are performed open.

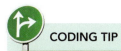

CODING TIP

Foreign Body Removal

Code range 52310–52315 includes any substance not native or natural to the urethra or bladder such as a stone, catheter tip, or stent. A simple procedure usually takes less than 15 minutes. A complicated procedure involves large, numerous calculuses or other difficult factors.

Male Genital System; Intersex Surgery

The male reproductive system consists of the penis, testicles (epididymis, scrotum, vas deferens, spermatic cord, seminal vesicles), and prostate. Procedures located here encompass treatment for undescended testicles, orchiectomy, vasectomy, hydrocele, spermatocele, circumcision, and lesions of the penis. Some of the procedures in this section are differentiated by age. Many procedures on the male anatomy are found in the Urinary section. When coding procedures in male genitourinary, combination coding, assigning codes from both the Urinary and the Male Genital sections, may be necessary.

ORCHIOPEXY

When a testicle does not descend into the scrotum and remains in the pelvis, an orchiopexy is performed to pull the testicle and secure it in the scrotum. Code assignment is based on the surgical technique.

ORCHIECTOMY

An orchiectomy is performed when the testis must be removed because of testicular cancer or prophylactically due to cancer of other parts of the male reproductive system (prostate). Sometimes only a partial orchiectomy is required for other problems associated with the testicle. Orchiectomy can be done as an open procedure or laparoscopically.

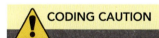

CODING CAUTION

Watching for Similar Terms
Do not confuse the terms *orchiopexy* and *orchiectomy*.

CIRCUMCISION

In performing a circumcision, the surgeon removes the foreskin by excising it. Code assignment is based on the surgical method—either excision or use of clamps. The age of the patient also plays a role in correct code choice (a newborn is a baby up to twenty-eight days old). If the physician performs a dorsal penile nerve block on a newborn while performing the circumcision, code 64450 is reported in addition to the circumcision.

Destruction of Lesions Lesions are typically destroyed by laser. These codes are designated as simple or extensive. If there are more than just a few lesions, if more time is taken, if the lesions are large, if different methods of destruction are used, or if the lesions are on different parts of the penis, the extensive code applies.

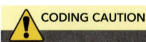

CODING CAUTION

Genital Lesion Destruction
When assigning codes for destruction of lesions on male or female genitals, always code from the Male or Female Genital section, not from the Integumentary section, because the codes are more specific.

Sterilization (Vasectomy) The vas deferens are cut to permanently sterilize the male. In some cases, men change their minds and want to be able to procreate again. A vasovasotomy or vasovasorrhaphy (55400) is performed to reconnect the vas deferens. The −50 modifier is assigned for bilateral procedures.

Checkpoint 8.12

Use the CPT-book to assign codes to the following statements, appending modifiers if needed.

1. EMG studies of urethral sphincter _____

2. Trocar bladder aspiration _____

3. Laparoscopic right nephrectomy _____

4. Percutaneous needle left renal biopsy with radiological S&I (fluoroscopy) _____

5. Discontinued contact laser vaporization of prostate _____

6. Incisional biopsy of testis followed by radical orchiectomy for tumor, inguinal approach

_____

7. Simple electrodesiccation of four lesions on penis _____

8. Radical perineal prostatectomy _____

9. A sixty-five-year old woman with four children who had a hysterectomy performed when she was in her fifties has problems retaining her urine when walking, sneezing, or coughing. Her urologist recommends a sling operation to give her bladder support, and he recommends doing it laparoscopically. Code for the surgery. _____

10. After undergoing a hypospadias repair two months ago, the patient injured his penis during a basketball game and was operated on in order to repair it. _____

Female Genital System and Maternity Care and Delivery

The Female Genital System and Maternity Care and Delivery section covers both the female genital procedures and the procedures for uncomplicated and complicated births.

FEMALE GENITAL SYSTEM

The female genital and reproductive system is complex, consisting of the uterus, ovary, fallopian tubes, vagina, vulva, clitoris, vestibule (urethral meatus and Bartholin's and Skene's glands), and vaginal orifice. This section is subdivided into seven subsections:

1. Vulva, Perineum and Introitus
2. Vagina
3. Cervix Uteri
4. Corpus Uteri
5. Oviduct/Ovary
6. Ovary
7. In Vitro Fertilization

There are two ovaries and two fallopian tubes, so when procedures are performed on both sides, a −50 modifier is appended. The one exception is the code for sterilizations, which is inherently bilateral (that is, it is for unilateral or bilateral procedures).

Some of the procedures in this section are ovarian cystectomy, lysis of pelvic adhesions, hysterectomy, dilation and curettage (D&C), removal of genital lesions, and sterilization. Many procedures performed on the female abdomen can be done laparoscopically, hysteroscopically, or by colposcopy instead of by the traditional open method. Laparoscopic procedures are performed using trocars and cannulas inserted into the abdomen, through which the scope can repair, excise, and evaluate abdominal and pelvic contents. A hysteroscope is used to visualize the uterine contents and perform diagnostic and therapeutic procedures such as D&C and removal of uterine fibroids. It is important for the coder to have a good foundation in the anatomy of the female genital system.

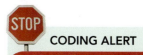

CODING ALERT

Pelvic Exam Bundled

When a pelvic exam is performed in conjunction with a gynecologic procedure, the pelvic exam is not separately coded.

Laser Ablation of the Cervix

Laser ablation of the cervix is performed to destroy precancerous changes in cervical tissue. At times, the dysplasia converts to carcinoma in situ of the cervix. Treatment typically is laser ablation of the cervix (LAC) or cold knife conization (CKC). If conization is done via a loop electrosurgical excision of the cervix (LEEP), code 57522 applies.

Sterilization

Sterilization is more commonly referred to as "tying tubes." It can be done laparoscopically or open by use of varying methods. Sometimes the fallopian tubes are clamped with Hulka clamps or are cut and fulgurated (cauterized). Material may be placed inside the fallopian tube to provide a mechanical occlusion.

Abortion

Codes exist for the treatment of blighted ovum, incomplete abortion (spontaneous miscarriages), and elective abortions. Pay attention to the stage of the pregnancy (first or second trimester, for example) and whether the abortion was missed or incomplete. A missed abortion is the retention of the products of conception after fetal death before twenty-two weeks of gestation. A blighted ovum is considered a missed abortion because the mother did not begin to expel any products of conception. In an incomplete abortion, the woman begins to miscarry but does not expel all the products of conception. Induced abortion is the elective termination of pregnancy before twenty-two weeks of gestation via D&C, D&E, intra-amniotic injections, or vaginal suppositories. Codes 59840–59841 should not be used for the completion of a spontaneous abortion; use 59812 for this service.

Lesion Removal of Vulva

Lesions can be biopsied and/or removed. There are times when destruction of a lesion is appropriate as in condyloma (56501–56515). See the definitions at the beginning of that section to help you determine the extent of the vulvectomy.

MATERNITY CARE AND DELIVERY

Uncomplicated maternity care includes routine antepartum, delivery, and postpartum care. This is called the maternity or OB package, meaning that the physician will be paid for the approximate ten months of care in one payment.

The antepartum care/period includes initial and subsequent H&P; measurement of weight, BP, and fetal heart tones; routine chemical urinalysis; monthly visits up to twenty-eight weeks; biweekly visits up to thirty-six weeks; and weekly visits until delivery. All E/M services pertaining to these services are included. Any other visits during this period are reported separately.

Delivery services include admission to the hospital, admission H&P, management of uncomplicated labor, and vaginal delivery or cesarean delivery (C-section). Delivery of placenta, induction of labor with Pitocin, artificial rupture of membranes (AROM), vacuum extraction, and episiotomy or vaginal repair are all considered part of the delivery package provided by the attending physician and are not coded separately. Episiotomy or vaginal repair performed by a consulting physician is reported with 59300.

If the patient had a previous delivery by C-section, specific codes in the 59610–59622 range must be used for the delivery. These may indicate a vaginal delivery after a previous C-section (VBAC) or an attempted vaginal delivery after a C-section that is completed by C-section.

A physician may provide only one or two of the three phases of obstetric care. In such cases, assign the code as appropriate for the extent of care provided.

EXAMPLE A woman saw Dr. Lee for seven months of her pregnancy until her husband was transferred to an out-of-state job. She saw Dr. Shaw for the remaining two months of the antepartum period, the vaginal delivery, and the postpartum visit. Dr. Lee billed 59426, and Dr. Shaw billed 59425 and 59410.

CODING TIP

Postpartum Coverage

The postpartum care/period includes hospital and office visits following delivery.

Checkpoint 8.13

Use the CPT book to assign codes to the following statements, appending modifiers if needed.

1. Routine obstetric care and vaginal delivery, previous cesarean delivery _____

2. Miscarriage surgically completed in first trimester _____

3. Cesarean delivery, including postpartum care, and total hysterectomy following attempted vaginal delivery; patient had previous cesarean delivery _____

4. D&C, postpartum hemorrhage _____

5. Simple destruction of four lesions, vulva _____

6. Uterine suspension _____

7. Subtotal hysterectomy _____

8. An obstetrician has seen a patient starting with her first visit to determine that she was pregnant. The obstetrician recently performed the vaginal delivery, and the patient is now being seen in the office for her last postpartum visit. How does the obstetrician code for the services?

_____

9. A patient is pregnant with her fourth child and is having contractions that are rapidly coming closer together. The baby is born in the car before she and her husband reach the hospital. Once the baby is secured by emergency medical technicians, the patient is admitted, and her physician delivers the placenta. _____

10. An elderly woman without a prior history of cancer is diagnosed with an extensive malignant vaginal cancer, requiring vaginectomy and complete removal of the vaginal wall.

_____

Endocrine and Nervous Systems

Both the endocrine and nervous systems are needed for regulation of body functions. The Endocrine System section of the surgery codes is brief. By contrast, the Nervous System section is complicated, with three main parts: (1) skull, meninges, and brain, (2) spine and spinal cord, and (3) extracranial nerves, peripheral nerves, and autonomic nervous system. Under these major headings are sections specific to skull-based surgery, neurostimulator insertions, aneurysm repair, shunt insertions, laminectomies, and nerve injections and repairs.

The Nervous System section is dedicated to the subspecialty of neurosurgery. With the exception of nerve injections, epidural injections, and nerve repairs, codes from this section are reported mainly by neurosurgeons. A neurosurgeon often utilizes an assistant surgeon because of the tedious nature of procedures involving the brain and spine, allowing for modifier –80 usage. At times, orthopedic surgeons and neurosurgeons perform complex spinal column procedures in which each carries out specific procedures independently of the other and each reports the –62 modifier.

Nervous system coding is complex, and an entry-level coder would find assigning codes to most procedures difficult. The coder needs both an excellent knowledge of the anatomy of this area and experience with neurological documentation. This presentation touches on a few highlights. One aspect, pain management, is a growing subspecialty of neurology and anesthesia and is widely accepted as treatment for disk herniations, radiculopathy, and intractable pain. Pain management codes encompass epidural steroid injections, nerve injections and destructions, neurostimulator insertion, pain pump insertions, and intricate epidural catheter insertions involving heating the intervertebral disk. As with the cardiovascular section, additional codes may be located in the Medicine section for such services as neurostimulator programming and electromyography.

Many of the procedures performed in this section require the use of a surgical microscope to visualize nerves and intricate anatomy. Some codes include the use of the microscope, while others do not. CPT code 69990 is assigned when microsurgical dissection or microsurgical repair of a nerve is done unless the code description already includes it.

SPINAL INJECTIONS AND PAIN MANAGEMENT

Spinal injections are commonly performed for diagnosis and therapy of patients with chronic back pain. Injections are typically not given unless the pain persists after all conservative measures have been taken. Types of injections include trigger points, hypertonic saline injection for epidural lysis of adhesions, epidural steroid injections, spinal nerve blocks, and facet joint injections.

In order to correctly code spine injections or pain blocks, the coder must determine at least three things: (1) What is being injected (steroid or anesthetic)? (2) Where is the needle inserted (cervical, thoracic, or lumbar)? (3) Is this a single injection or a continuous infusion or regional injection? The names of common steroids and anesthetics are

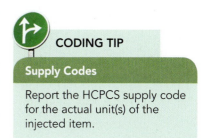

CODING TIP

Supply Codes

Report the HCPCS supply code for the actual unit(s) of the injected item.

Table 8.12 Examples of Anesthetic Agents and Steroids

Anesthetics	Steroids
Lidocaine	Aristocort
Bupivacaine	Kenalog
Sensorcaine	Aristospan
Naropin	Depo-medrol
Duramorph	Solu-Medrol
Marcaine	Methylprednisolone
Xylocaine	Triamcinolone

listed in Table 8.12. The documentation needs to support the codes. See codes 62310 and 62318 for an example.

Nerve Blocks   Peripheral nerves are injected for pain management. For example, the greater occipital nerve is injected for chronic or ongoing headaches. Surgeons commonly inject nerves as a postoperative pain control method. Injections are also performed in the sympathetic nerves (stellate ganglions) for analgesia.

Transcutaneous Electrical Nerve Stimulator (TENS)
Electrodes attached to a battery pack are placed on the skin to stimulate the muscles and nerves for TENS treatment. This is used routinely for sprains and strains of the back and neck and may be used in physical therapy or performed during chiropractic treatment.

Blood Patch   A blood patch is carried out for treatment of spinal fluid leakage following a lumbar puncture or epidural injection. Blood is drawn from the patient's arm and injected into the epidural space. Many patients develop postdural puncture headaches after having myelograms done or epidurals placed for labor and delivery.

Lumbar Puncture   The lumbar puncture procedure is also known as a spinal tap. It is performed for diagnostic purposes when spinal fluid is needed for analysis. A needle is inserted into the subarachnoid space in the lumbar region. The color of the fluid can indicate hemorrhage, infection, and so on.

Sometimes, a therapeutic spinal puncture to drain excess fluid off the spine is required for a condition known as pseudo tumor cerebri.

Chemodenervation   Chemodenervation involves injecting a chemical substance to interrupt nerve function. This code is assigned when Botox or similar chemical injections are performed to block impulses from nerves to the small facial muscles that control expression. The injection relaxes the muscles and reduces the appearance of wrinkles. Chemodenervation is also performed for treatment of neurological disorders such as tics.

It does not matter how many injections are performed or how many muscles are injected; the code is assigned only once per session, along with appropriate supply codes.

NEUROSURGERY

Neurolysis   Neurolysis involves injecting a nerve with a neurolytic agent (alcohol, phenol, iced saline, Ethanol) to destroy the nerve. This is provided to chronic pain patients and to patients with cerebral palsy who have muscle spasms. Coding is based on identifying the targeted nerve and indicating whether a single nerve or a multilevel injection was done. Code descriptions must be examined to see whether they are unilateral or bilateral.

Nerve Decompression   Nerve decompression, transposition, or neuroplasty is the freeing of an intact nerve from scar tissue or entrapment. This procedure can also be called neurolysis. The documentation must be carefully reviewed to determine whether the nerve was moved or injected.

Checkpoint 8.14

Assign the CPT code and applicable modifier to the statements below.

1. Total thyroid lobectomy _____

2. Craniotomy for repair of dural/CSF leak _____

3. Implantation of intrathecal drug infusion programmable pump _____

4. Vertebral corpectomy with decompression of spinal cord, three segments _____

5. Implantation of cranial nerve neurostimulator electrodes _____

6. Laparoscopic adrenalectomy _____

7. After months of back pain, a patient is scheduled for an MRI of the spinal cord. The scan shows a lesion in the thoracic spine near T1 and T2. The physician performs a percutaneous needle biopsy of the spinal cord, using a CT scan for the radiological supervision and interpretation of the needle placement. _____

8. A young patient was born with hydrocephalus due to the accumulation of cerebrospinal fluid (CSF) in the ventricles of his brain. He is now scheduled for surgery to allow the neurosurgeon to create and implant a shunt that will drain the CSF into the peritoneum, thereby relieving the pressure on the brain. _____

Eye and Ocular Adnexa; Auditory System; Operating Microscope

Codes in the Eye and Ocular Adnexa and Auditory sections include procedures on the eyeball, anterior and posterior segment, ocular adnexa, and conjunctiva as well as procedures on the inner and outer ear. The codes are arranged by anatomical part and then by procedure. For the most part, the outline of this section follows the template used in other sections, grouping procedures by incision, excision, repair, and other procedures.

Typical procedures performed on the eye are foreign body removal, cataract removal, glaucoma surgery, laser surgery for vision correction, strabismus surgery on the muscles of the eye, and retinal procedures. Codes for examinations of the eye are located in the Medicine section.

Codes for the auditory system include procedures on the external ear, middle ear, inner ear, and temporal bone. Common procedures are foreign body removal, insertion of ventilation tubes, tympanoplasty, and cochlear implants.

In some circumstances, the microscope code 69990 may be assigned in addition to the procedure codes. Notes located before code 69990 explain that this code should not be assigned in addition to procedures for which use of the microscope is an inclusive component.

EYE AND OCULAR ADNEXA

Procedures and services in this section are performed by an ophthalmologist, never by an optometrist. Some procedure code descriptions specify whether a patient has had prior surgery on the affected eye. Parenthetical notes following codes provide instructions for referring to other sections of CPT if necessary to capture all services and for selecting the most appropriate anatomical code.

When coding procedures for eyes and eyelids, modifier use is important. HCPCS Level II modifiers are required when billing eyelid procedures (E1, E2). The −50 modifier applies when coding procedures on both eyes.

Foreign Body Removal For foreign body removal, codes are differentiated by compartment of the eye and whether a corneal slit lamp is used. Numerous notes located before code 65205 provide instructions on code assignment.

Cataract When coding cataract removal and replacement, the coder must determine what type of procedure is performed. There are three different methods of cataract extraction: intracapsular (ICCE), extracapsular (ECCE), and extracapsular complex requiring devices not routinely used in cataract surgery. Routine cataract surgery involves removing the cataract and replacing the old lens with a new lens. There are times, however, when a new lens is not placed immediately after the cataract extraction. In this case, CPT code 66985 applies when the patient returns for the lens placement. It is not uncommon for patients to require a newly implanted lens to be exchanged (CPT code 66986) due to failure of the implant or to have it repositioned (CPT code 66825).

Lesion Removal If the excision of a lesion from the eye involves only skin of the eyelid, an Integumentary section code should be assigned. If it involves lid margin, tarsus, or otherwise, use codes from the Eye/Adnexa section. Chalazion excision has its own code range.

Glaucoma Surgery Glaucoma is a condition in which the aqueous cannot drain from the anterior segment of the eye. There are two overarching types of glaucoma surgery: laser and incisional. Trabeculoplasty, iridotomy, and iridoplasty are laser treatments.

Trabeculectomy, on the other hand, is an incisional procedure that basically creates a drain for the aqueous and is usually performed *ab externo* (from the outside of the eye). When the trabeculectomy is not indicated, an aqueous shunt may be placed in the anterior chamber between the cornea and the iris.

Vision Correction Surgery   Many patients are taking advantage of the availability of technological advances to eliminate the need for glasses. Two procedures are done frequently to correct vision by altering the surface of the cornea: photorefractive keratectomy (PRK) and laser-assisted in situ keratomileusis (LASIK).

AUDITORY SYSTEM

The ear is a paired body part, requiring the use of the –LT or –RT modifiers with code assignment.

Foreign Body Removal   It is common for children to place such objects as peas, crayons, and beads in their ears and for the objects to become lodged. More often than not, this requires surgical removal under anesthesia.

Ventilation Tube Insertion   Coding the treatment for otitis media (ear infection) depends on whether tubes are used. One treatment involves insertion of tubes in the tympanic membrane to promote drainage. These tubes are often called PET tubes or ventilation tubes. A myringotomy alone may instead be done, in which an incision is made and fluid is suctioned out and/or the eustachian tube is inflated. This does not involve inserting tubes.

Tympanoplasty   Perforation of tympanic membrane can occur from foreign objects being pushed too far into the ear canal and from trauma, infection, and tube placement. When tubes are removed, a tympanic membrane repair is often required to patch the hole left by the tubes. These codes are differentiated by whether the tympanic membrane was repaired or the eardrum was repaired or reconstructed.

OPERATING MICROSCOPE

The operating microscope is utilized for intricate procedures involving the eyes, ears, nerves, and vertebrae. Some payers may consider the microscope to be an inherent portion of the surgical procedure, meaning that it is routinely used and in many cases must be used to carry out the surgery. Instructional notes located prior to this code explicitly list codes for which it is inappropriate to also report the use of a microscope. Surgical code descriptions must be read carefully to verify whether language such as *microsurgical* or *microvascular* is present, indicating that the use of the surgical microscope is already built into the payment for the surgical procedure and should not be reported separately. CPT code 69990 is reported without appending a modifier.

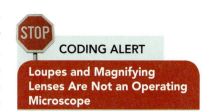

CODING ALERT

Loupes and Magnifying Lenses Are Not an Operating Microscope

Do not assign 69990 unless the operative note specifies the use of a microscope. Loupes and magnifying lenses are not the same as a microscope.

Assign the CPT code and applicable modifier to the statements below.

1. Canthotomy _____

2. Closure of right eyelids by suture, temporary _____

3. Right scleral reinforcement without graft _____

4. Extracapsular cataract removal with insertion of intraocular lens prothesis, mechanical technique, left _____

5. Excision of scleral right lesion _____

6. Chalazion excision right eye during the global period of a strabismus surgery _____

7. Tympanic membrane repair on right with operating microscope _____

8. Biopsy of both external ears _____

9. Impacted cerumen removed from both ears _____

10. Ocular implant removal on left with operating microscope _____

11. A seventy-year-old patient with chronic glaucoma is still suffering from elevated intraocular pressure of the left eye that has not responded to medical therapy. To treat the problem surgically, the surgeon will have to destroy portions of the ciliary body to bring down the intraocular pressure. The surgeon elects to use a freezing probe (cryotherapy) to destroy the ciliary process. _____

12. A senile elderly patient in a nursing home placed an earring into her right ear. The earring is not lodged in the external auditory canal. The patient tends to flail her arms when she is examined, so general anesthesia has to be used to extract the earring. Once the patient has been anesthetized, the physician is able to visualize the earring and extract it with forceps and suction. _____

Summary

1. Anesthesia services are packaged into one payment. Complete anesthesia service includes:

   - General, regional, supplementation of local anesthesia
   - Interpretation of lab values
   - Placement of IVs for fluid and medication administration
   - Arterial line insertion for blood pressure monitoring or other supportive services to afford the anesthesia care deemed optimal by the anesthesiologist during a procedure
   - The usual preoperative and postoperative visits
   - The administration of fluids and/or blood
   - Usual monitoring services (temperature, blood pressure, oximetry, ECG, capnography, and mass spectrometry)
   - Intubation

- Laryngoscopy
- Introduction or insertion of needle or catheter into vein
- Venipuncture

2. If completed properly, the anesthesia record will contain all information necessary to assign anesthesia codes. It should include any preoperative interaction and services and postoperative services received in the recovery area. A copy of the operative report helps anesthesia coders ensure that they have captured all procedures and secondary diagnoses. It is important to determine the payer and the level of CRNA supervision in order to appropriately assign correct codes and modifiers. Coders must read documentation to determine whether the CRNA worked alone and how many rooms the anesthesiologist was responsible for at a given time.

3. Anesthesia coders have to have copies of insurance carrier contracts to determine how each carrier calculates anesthesia time, modifying factors, and base units. The formula for calculating anesthesia charges is (base units + time units + modifying factor units) × conversion factor = total anesthesia administration charge. Coders need a way to validate time and to determine discontinuous time if applicable.

4. Anesthesia coding is a challenge because not all payers have the same requirements for reporting. Check with each payer or read the payer contract to determine how to report anesthesia codes. Most payers require the anesthesia code to be assigned with either a HCPCS modifier or a physical status modifier. Physical status modifiers are appended to anesthesia claims only and coincide with the anesthesia provider's ASA class. Some payers accept modifiers −P3 through −P5 and will reimburse these in addition to the procedure.

5. In general, the organization of each surgical section in CPT follows the same format. Each subsection is divided by body areas working from the head to the feet and then further subdivided as follows: Incision and Drainage, Biopsy, Excision, Introduction or Removal, Repair, Destruction, Endoscopy/Laparoscopy (if applicable), Other Procedures.

6. The surgical package includes local infiltration of anesthesia, the E/M visits either on the date of surgery or the day before as long as the decision for surgery was made, immediate postoperative care, order writing, evaluating the patient in the recovery area, and any typical uncomplicated follow-up care. Follow-up care for complications, exacerbations, recurrence, and the presence of other diseases that require additional services are not included in the surgical package.

7. The major difference between the AMA definition and Medicare's definition of global surgery days is the number of days of preoperative and postoperative care included. In this national global policy for surgical procedures, a single fee is billed and paid for all services furnished by the surgeon before, during, and after the procedure. This can range from zero to ten days for minor surgery and up to ninety days for major surgery.

8. Separate procedure codes are located throughout CPT and should not be assigned if they are performed as part of a more comprehensive procedure.

9. Coders must pay attention to modifiers designated for physician use and those for facility use. Most of these modifiers are identical. They are located on the inside cover of the CPT code book. HCPCS modifiers are required and assigned to all anesthesia codes for claims submitted to government payers. HCPCS modifiers are also assigned when procedures are performed on fingers, toes, eyelids, and paired body parts where either the left side or the right side was affected, and coronary vessels.

10. To correctly assign surgery codes, close attention must be paid to the extensive rules and instructions in each subsection.

Review Questions: Chapter 8

Match the key terms with their definitions.

a. conscious sedation _____

b. unbundling _____

c. open procedure _____

d. physical status modifiers _____

e. incidental procedure _____

f. global period _____

g. analgesic _____

h. therapeutic procedure _____

i. diagnostic procedure _____

j. Correct Coding Initiative (CCI) _____

1. Incorrect billing practice of reporting packaged procedures individually

2. Computerized Medicare system to prevent overpayment for procedures

3. Type of anesthesia that relieves pain without causing loss of consciousness

4. Moderate anesthesia carried out by injecting a sedative and/or analgesic intravenously to relieve pain and anxiety during a medical procedure

5. Type of surgical procedure performed through an incision or other opening

6. Treating or correcting a confirmed disease, condition, or injury

7. Physician's procedure done to confirm a working diagnosis or determine the best course of treatment

8. Procedure performed as part of standard medical treatment or package that would be billed alone

9. Codes used with anesthesia codes to indicate patient's health condition

10. Number of days surrounding a surgical procedure during which related procedures are not billable

Decide whether each statement is true or false.

1. Physical status modifiers are assigned with anesthesia codes. **T or F**

2. An anesthesiologist's history and physical exam is separately reportable with an E/M code in addition to the anesthesia code for the same day of service. **T or F**

3. Qualifying circumstances codes may be assigned for anesthesia services. **T or F**

4. The modifier −50 for bilateral procedures is used to describe bilateral views (X-rays) taken of both knees (see code 73565). **T or F**

5. All HCPCS Level I and II modifiers are appropriate to use for coding in all settings. **T or F**

6. All payers recognize all CPT and HCPCS modifiers. **T or F**

7. It is not appropriate for a physician to assign a −25 modifier when seeing a patient in critical care. **T or F**

8. CPT does not have a way to capture the charges for the technical component of a procedure or service. **T or F**

9. The neurology section of CPT is dedicated solely to neurologists and neurosurgeons, and codes from this section should not be reported by physicians of other specialties. **T or F**

10. If the procedure note indicates that the physician utilized magnifying loupes to visualize blood vessels, 69990 is reported in addition to the procedure code. **T or F**

Select the letter that best completes the statement or answers the question.

1. Which modifier is never used with anesthesia codes?
   a.   −22
   b.   −32
   c.   −47
   d.   −59

2. Surgeons who administer their own anesthesia use which modifier with the surgical code they submit?
   a.   −23
   b.   −47
   c.   −32
   d.   −22

3. Deciding what modifiers to assign for anesthesia services depends on
   a.   the payer
   b.   the patient's age
   c.   the patient's status
   d.   open versus closed procedure

4. Which code is used for removal of both tonsils and adenoids in a twelve-year-old patient?
   a.   42836
   b.   42826
   c.   42825
   d.   42821

5. Which code is used for biopsy of lesion of the earlobe?
   a.   11440
   b.   11100
   c.   69100
   d.   69105

6. Which code is used for removal of a foreign body from the left deep calf muscle?
   a.   20525
   b.   20103
   c.   20520
   d.   11043

7. Which code or codes are used for excision of two nasal polyps in the physician office?
   a.   30300
   b.   30110
   c.   30115
   d.   30110, 30110

8. Which code is used for pericardiotomy with removal of wire from a previous surgery?
   a. 33015
   b. 33020
   c. 33050
   d. 33011

9. Which code is used for drainage of a cervical lymph node abscess?
   a. 38308
   b. 38505
   c. 38300
   d. 38510

10. Which code is used for cystotomy with excision of ureterocele, bilateral?
    a. 51530
    b. 51535–50
    c. 51065
    d. 51535

Answer the following questions.

1. A patient with advanced carcinoma of the esophagus with widespread metastases has anesthesia for a partial esophagectomy. Which code is used? _____

2. A well-conditioned twenty-two-year-old athlete has anesthesia administered for extensive debridement of the shoulder joint by arthroscopy. Which code is used? _____

3. An emergency appendectomy is performed on a sixty-five-year-old patient with insulin-dependent diabetes that is not well controlled. The anesthesiologist begins administration of the general anesthesia at 10:00 A.M. and completes the anesthesia services at 10:45 A.M. List the key elements. Indicate "none" if not applicable.
   a. Anesthesia procedure code _____
   b. Physical status modifier _____
   c. Qualifying circumstances code _____
   d. Anesthesia modifier(s) _____
   e. Calculate time units (15-minute increments) _____

4. A thirty-five-year-old patient in good health has anesthesia services for laparoscopic cholecystectomy with cholangiography for acute cholecystitis. List the key elements. Indicate "none" if not applicable.
   a. Anesthesia code _____
   b. Anesthesia modifier _____
   c. Physical status modifier _____
   d. Qualifying circumstances code _____

5. List four modifiers that describe when services may have occurred more than once. _____

6. List three modifiers that may be reported when a physician helps the primary surgeon in surgery.
   _____

7. List two modifiers (not physical status modifiers) that describe anesthesia services. _____

8. Name three of the services that are not included in the anesthesia code and can be billed separately.
   _____

9. Which anatomical modifier will be assigned for a tendon repair of the left middle finger? _____

10. Which modifier is used by a facility to report the elective cancellation of a hernia repair prior to prepping the patient's skin but after transport to the OR? _____

11. List the modifiers that necessitate a special report to support use and medical necessity. _____
_____

12. What modifier would be appended to the office visit code (E/M) for a patient who is deaf and requires an interpreter? _____

13. Name three instances when the −51 modifier is not appropriate to append. _____

14. What is the ranking or hierarchy of modifier usage? Put the following in order.
CPT (HCPCS) Level I _____
HCPCS Level II _____
CPT (HCPCS) Level I that increases or decreases payment _____

Applying Your Knowledge

BUILDING CODING SKILLS: ANESTHESIA PROCEDURES

Assign the anesthesia procedure code along with any applicable modifiers, including physical status modifiers, like this: 00914–QS. Assume that all patients are on Medicare unless otherwise specified by age. If there is no anesthesia modifier or qualifying circumstance, indicate "none."

1. Biopsy of the clavicle _____

2. Cesarean section of twenty-five-year-old who had no epidural during labor _____

3. Arthroscopic meniscus repair of the knee _____

4. Transurethral resection of the prostate _____

5. Repair of cleft palate _____

6. Nasal septoplasty for deviated septum _____

7. Knee replacement surgery _____

8. Anesthesia provided by anesthesiologist for dressing change of the leg _____

9. Orchiopexy in a three-year-old boy _____

10. Vasectomy in a thirty-five-year-old man _____

11. Insertion of vascular access for chemotherapy drug delivery _____
_____

BUILDING CODING SKILLS: SURGICAL PROCEDURES

Assign the CPT surgical code and any applicable modifier.

1. Hydrocelectomy right testicle _____

2. Revision of an incomplete circumcision _____

3. Ochiectomy of the left testicle with insertion of prosthesis _____
_____

4. Needle biopsy of the prostate _____

5. Cryosurgical ablation of the prostate _____

6. Myringoplasty, left ear _____

7. Revision of pacemaker pocket _____

8. Left oval window fistula repair _____

9. Long and short saphenous vein stripping, right leg _____

10. Excision of deep axillary lymph node, left _____

11. Removal of foreign body of the nose _____

12. Patch closure of ventricular septal defect _____

13. Removal of foreign body, left ear, general anesthesia _____

14. Mastoidectomy, modified radical, right ear _____

15. Bone marrow biopsy, needle _____

16. Tympanoplasty right ear _____

17. Repair of ruptured spleen _____

18. Cochlear implant, left ear _____

19. Vasovasorrhaphy _____

20. Treatment of first trimester missed abortion _____

21. Cardiopulmonary resuscitation for 15 minutes _____

22. Mastoidectomy with labrinthectomy, right _____

23. Bilateral hydrocelectomy _____

24. Hysteroscopy, diagnostic _____

25. Insertion of inflatable penile prosthesis _____

26. Destruction of a 3.5 cm malignant lesion of the back _____

27. Ligation of internal jugular vein _____

28. Laparoscopy with fulguration of oviducts _____

29. Excision of a 4.0 cm lesion of the chest _____

30. Mastopexy, bilateral breasts _____

31. Circumcision, clamp, newborn _____

32. Dilation of salivary duct _____

33. Incision and drainage of perirectal abscess _____

34. Cystourethroscopy with biopsy of the bladder _____

35. Cranioplasty with autograft, 6 cm diameter _____

Researching the Internet

1. The American Academy of Professional Coders (AAPC) certifies medical coders in various medical specialties. Visit www.aapc.com and list the surgery-related specialty coding certifications that are available.

2. Modifier −59 is scrutinized by Medicare and is often found to be abused. Read the excerpt from the *Medicare Carrier Manual* at www.cms.hhs.gov/NationalCorrectCodInitEd/Downloads/modifier59.pdf for a detailed description and examples of proper use.

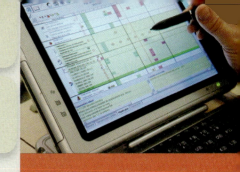

CPT: Radiology, Pathology and Laboratory, and Medicine Codes

LEARNING OUTCOMES

After studying this chapter, you should be able to:

1. Discuss the organization, key guidelines, and common modifiers for the Radiology section of CPT.

2. Discuss the importance of the number of views taken in radiology coding.

3. Explain the difference between the professional and technical components of a procedure.

4. Describe the use of contrast material in assigning radiology codes.

5. Distinguish between screening and diagnostic services.

6. Describe the organization, key guidelines, and common modifiers for the Pathology and Laboratory section of CPT.

7. Recognize common laboratory panels and their associated codes.

8. Describe the organization, key guidelines, and common modifiers for the Medicine section of CPT.

9. Describe the correct coding of immunizations.

10. Assign CPT radiology, pathology and laboratory, and medicine codes with appropriate modifiers based on procedural statements.

Key Terms

administration

analyte

ancillary services

assay

automated

biofeedback

cardiac catheterization

charge capture

charge description master (CDM)

CLIA-waived test

Clinical Laboratory Improvement Amendment (CLIA)

complete blood count (CBC)

complete lab test

computerized axial tomography scan (CT or CAT scan)

continuous positive airway pressure (CPAP)

contrast material (media)

diagnostic procedure

echocardiography

electrocardiogram (ECG/EKG)

encounter form

fluoroscopy

hemodialysis

immunotherapy

magnetic resonance imaging (MRI)

mammography

manual

modality

nuclear medicine

panel

peritoneal dialysis

positron emission tomography (PET)

professional component (PC)

radiation oncology

radiologic examination

radiology

radiology report

red blood cell (RBC) count

screening procedure

single proton emission computerized tomography (SPECT)

spirometry

technical component (TC)

ultrasound

white blood cell (WBC) count

Chapter Outline

Radiology
Pathology and Laboratory
Medicine

This chapter introduces CPT codes for the **ancillary services** that support the diagnosis and treatment of disease or injury. Ancillary services include work such as laboratory tests, radiological studies, pathology studies, physical therapy, and speech therapy. These services are provided for patients at the request of a physician to supplement or enhance medical treatment. They represent various important steps in the process of diagnosing and treating a patient from the onset of symptoms to recovery and maintenance. Some ancillary services are typically provided by hospital departments. Others are done in physician practices, outpatient clinics, or separate facilities. Documentation in the form of physician orders, test requisitions, and ancillary reports is used to assign codes. Ancillary services documentation contains many acronyms and abbreviations; coders become familiar with their meanings as they work with these code sections of CPT.

CODING TIP

Look It Up

Invest in an abbreviation resource (see the list at the back of your text) or use websites to determine the meaning of unfamiliar definitions.

INTERNET RESOURCE

Acronyms

www.AcronymFinder.com

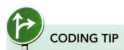

Radiology

The codes in the **Radiology** section of CPT represent a subspecialty of medicine that concentrates on medical imaging to prevent, diagnose, and treat diseases and injuries. Radiologists diagnose diseases by obtaining and interpreting medical images rather than through laboratory testing or conventionally examining a patient. They correlate medical image findings with other examinations and recommend further studies or treatments to the ordering physician. Radiologists not only diagnose conditions but also treat a number of diseases by means of radiation (radiation oncology) or minimally invasive, image-guided surgery (interventional radiology).

Codes in the Radiology section can be used by physicians of any medical specialty to report radiological services performed by the physician or under the physician's supervision. For example, a radiologist supervises a radiology technician (an RT or rad tech), who performs a service such as taking an X-ray and providing the images to the radiologist to interpret. Because of the expense of radiology equipment featuring advanced technology, such as positron emission tomography (PET) scans, many diagnostic services are offered only by hospital radiology departments. However, many physicians, particularly orthopedic physicians, have lower-cost X-ray equipment in their offices. Facilities also have portable X-ray equipment so that X-rays may be taken at the bedside.

ORGANIZATION

The Radiology section has seven subsections, which are organized according to the method or type of radiology and the purpose of the service. The subsections and their code ranges are listed in Table 9.1.

Each subsection is further subdivided by anatomical site and type of service or **modality.** A modality is a method, technique, or protocol used to treat or diagnose a disease or injury. As in other sections of CPT, notes, definitions, and special instructions are extremely important and must be read before assigning a code.

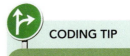

CODING TIP

Radiology Codes Begin with 7

All codes located in the Radiology section begin with the number 7.

RADIOLOGY SECTION GUIDELINES

The section guidelines explain unique terminology and review pertinent common terms such as *separate and unlisted procedures* as they apply to radiology codes. There are also many notes and instructions

Table 9.1 Radiology Subsections

Subsection	Code Range
Diagnostic Radiology (Diagnostic Imaging)	70000–76499
Diagnostic Ultrasound	76500–76999
Radiologic Guidance	77001–77032
Breast, Mammography	77051–77059
Bone/Joint Studies	77071–77084
Radiation Oncology	77261–77999
Nuclear Medicine	78000–79999

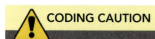
intertwined throughout the section. Unlisted procedure codes are located at the end of the appropriate subsections.

Required Order and Radiology Report A diagnostic radiology service is performed because an ordering physician has sent a patient to the radiologist for a particular procedure and has also sent an order giving the reason for the examination. The order describes the patient's signs or symptoms and provides the radiologist with a working diagnosis.

In response, the radiologist documents the results with a **radiology report,** which is a written report signed by the interpreting physician. After viewing the films, the radiologist dictates this final report, which contains findings, the impression or diagnosis, and at times recommended follow-up care. The dictated report is reviewed and signed by the radiologist.

Administration of Contrast Materials The ordering physician or the radiologist may decide that contrast is indicated to enhance a particular view or tissue of interest. The **contrast material (media)**—a substance that helps provide a clearer image—can be administered, or introduced, with an injection, rectally, or orally. The phrase *with contrast* in the description of a code means contrast material that is administered either intravascularly, directly into a joint (intra-articularly), or into the space under the arachnoid membrane of the brain or spinal cord (intrathecally). Rectal or oral contrast administration alone does not qualify as a study with contrast.

It is common for imaging work to be done in a series—some images with contrast and some without. However, when this is the approach, two codes, one with contrast and the other without contrast, are not both coded for a service. Instead, a code that describes *without contrast followed by with contrast* should be sought. In other words, when a service is done first without contrast material, followed by contrast material and additional images, the coder should report a single code specifying both without and with contrast material. For example, for a CT scan of the head or brain, the coder has three codes:

70450	Computed tomography, head or brain; without contrast material
70460	with contrast material
70470	without contrast material, followed by contrast material(s) and further sections

RADIOLOGICAL BILLING COMPONENTS

A complete radiological service involves both the use of equipment and supplies and the physician's work. Since one code reports both aspects, unless a physician both owns the equipment and does the work, modifiers are used to show who receives payment for each aspect of the service.

The **technical component (TC)** of a radiology service covers the allocation of staff or the technologist's work, equipment, supplies (film and contrast material), and related preinjection and postinjection services. The technical component is the facility's charge for the service provided. When the facility bills, a −TC modifier is appended to the radiology code to designate this portion.

The **professional component (PC)** includes the actual work the physician does in reading and interpreting the radiological test and providing a written report with an opinion, advice, or assessment of findings. If the physician who reports the professional component does not own the equipment, as is usually the case, a −26 CPT modifier is appended to the radiology code. If the physician does own the equipment and provides the complete radiological service, the radiology code alone is reported; no modifiers are needed, since one professional is billing for both components.

EXAMPLES
- A patient has a chest X-ray, two views, taken at the hospital. The radiologist will report 71020–26, and the hospital will report 71020–TC.
- A physician uses fluoroscopy to verify placement of an epidural needle in the epidural space for a pain management procedure. The physician reports code 76005–26, and the facility reports 76005–TC.
- A patient fell while ice-skating. Using the equipment in the office, the orthopedist obtains X-rays, two views, both wrists. The orthopedist reports codes 73100–LT, 73100–RT.

RADIOLOGICAL SUPERVISION AND INTERPRETATION

Many codes in the Radiology section include *radiological supervision and interpretation (S&I)*. These codes describe only the radiological portion of a procedure that two physicians often perform as members of a radiologist—surgeon team. The S&I code does not include the procedure itself, such as an injection; it is used for the professional supervision and interpretation of the results only. In some cases, the radiologist can perform both the radiology interpretation and the injection procedure. The radiological S&I codes are thus used in conjunction with the injection codes from the Surgery section.

RADIOLOGY MODIFIERS

The common radiology modifiers are listed in Table 9.2. For facility reporting, two modifiers often apply—one to distinguish the facility (technical) charges from the physician's (professional) charges, and a second to describe the body part being examined.

EXAMPLE
73020–RT–TC: X-ray of the right shoulder, one view.

Checkpoint 9.1

Assign the correct modifiers to the following, based on whether the code is for the facility or the physician. Do not assign the radiology code.

1. Venography of the right leg _____
2. Intraoperative interpretation of cervical spine CT scan _____
3. Physician use of fluoroscopic guidance for left wrist injection _____
4. Mammography of the right breast, facility charge _____

Table 9.2 Radiology Modifiers

Code	Description
−22	Unusual procedural service
−26	Professional component
−32	Mandated service
−51	Multiple procedure
−52	Reduced service
−53	Discontinued service
−58	Staged or related procedure or service by the same physician during the postoperative period
−59	Distinct procedural service
−62	Two surgeons
−66	Surgical team
−76	Repeat procedure by same physician
−77	Repeat procedure by another physician
−78	Return to operating room for related procedure during the postoperative period
−79	Unrelated procedure or service by the same physician during the postoperative period
−80	Assistant surgeon
−90	Reference outside laboratory
−99	Multiple modifiers
−LT, −RT, −TA to −T9, −FA to −F9, −LC, −LD, −RC	Anatomical modifiers

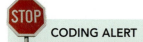

CODING ALERT

Modifier −50 Not Used

Avoid using the −50 modifier with radiology codes. Instead, check with the payer; most require reporting the code twice using the −RT or −LT modifiers.

DIAGNOSTIC RADIOLOGY (DIAGNOSTIC IMAGING)

The Diagnostic Radiology subsection is arranged by anatomical site and then by the modality. Code descriptors are very important in code selection, differentiating between imaging with and without contrast and describing the number of views for radiology studies (X-rays). A descriptor may state a single view, a specified number of views, the word *complete* with the minimum number, or a special view. As long as the minimum criteria are met, views beyond a stated minimum do not change the code selection.

In order to assign a code identified as complete, all views of that area must be taken.

EXAMPLE
73030: Radiologic examination, shoulder; complete, minimum of two views.

Radiologic Examination Radiologic examination refers to X-ray beams sent through the body. X-ray films capture images of hard materials such as bones. Radiologic examination codes refer to standard or conventional plain films of particular sites.

EXAMPLE
73500: Radiologic examination, hip, unilateral.

Computerized Axial Tomography A **computerized axial tomography scan** is more commonly recognized by its abbreviated name, **CT or CAT scan.** This X-ray procedure combines many X-ray images with the aid of computer enhancement. A CT scan can produce cross-sectional views and three-dimensional images of soft tissues such as the internal organs as well as other parts of the body. CT scans are also used to help guide the placement of instruments. CT scans often utilize contrast materials.

The scanner takes X-ray images at many different angles around the body. These images are processed by a computer to produce cross-sectional pictures. In each picture the body is seen as an X-ray "slice" recorded on film. The recorded image is called a *tomogram*. *Computerized axial tomography* refers to the processing of recorded slices at different levels of the body to create a three-dimensional picture of a body structure.

Codes for CT scans of the body are located by body area in the Diagnostic Imaging section. The terms *CT scan* and *CAT scan* are used to locate these codes in the CPT index.

EXAMPLE
72125: CT scan of the cervical spine; without contrast material.

Magnetic Resonance Imaging **Magnetic resonance imaging (MRI)** uses radio frequency waves and a strong magnetic field rather than X-rays to provide detailed pictures of internal organs and tissues. MRI produces clear pictures of soft-tissue structures near and around bones and is therefore the preferred examination for spine and joint problems and sports-related injuries. It also a tool for diagnosing coronary artery disease and heart problems. Physicians can examine the size and thickness of the chambers of the heart and determine the extent of damage caused by a heart attack or observe the flow of blood through vessels.

MRIs can also be done with or without contrast. Gadolinium is a routinely used contrast agent. Codes for MRIs are located by body area in the Diagnostic Imaging section. They are found in the CPT index under the entries *magnetic resonance imaging* and *MRI*.

EXAMPLE
73718: Magnetic resonance imaging, lower extremity other than joint; without contrast material (an MRI of the foot).

Fluoroscopy **Fluoroscopy** uses a continuous, low-level X-ray beam to view the body in motion. Fluoroscopy is used in orthopedic, podiatry, pain management, and gastrointestinal procedures and exams. It is used to follow barium through the intestinal tract to look for ulcers. It can also be used to verify placement of needles and catheters during joint injections, breast biopsies, insertion of venous access devices, and pain management procedures. The time descriptors in the codes apply to the time the technologist or physician is actually using the equipment to assist in a case, not the time the fluoroscopic unit is turned on.

EXAMPLE
77002 Fluoroscopic guidance for needle placement (e.g., biopsy, aspiration, injection, localization device).

DIAGNOSTIC ULTRASOUND

Ultrasound refers to the inaudible ultrahigh-frequency sound waves used for diagnostic scanning. Ultrasound technology is similar to the sonar that submarines use to navigate; the sound waves bounce off the body tissue and produce an echo. Ultrasound waves are emitted by a transducer (the part of the machine that is pressed against the body or placed inside an orifice such as the vagina or esophagus), and a picture of the underlying tissues is built up from the pattern of echo wave feedback that bounces back. Hard surfaces such as bone return a stronger echo than soft tissue and fluids, giving the bony skeleton a white appearance on the screen. There are four different ultrasound approaches in terms of placement: transesophageal, transvaginal, transrectal, and external (placing the transducer on the outer body).

There are four types of ultrasound:

1. *A-mode* refers to a one-dimensional ultrasonic measurement procedure.
2. *M-mode* refers to a one-dimensional ultrasonic measurement procedure with movement of the trace to record amplitude and velocity of moving echo-producing structures.
3. *B-scan* refers to a two-dimensional ultrasonic scanning procedure with a two-dimensional display.
4. *Real-time scan* refers to a two-dimensional ultrasonic scanning procedure with display of both two-dimensional structure and motion with time.

Ultrasounds are routinely performed on the abdomen (liver, gallbladder, kidney, uterus, ovaries) to look for abnormalities or to measure the size of a fetus. They are also performed on the heart and extremities to observe blood flow (Doppler study).

EXAMPLE
76870: Ultrasound, scrotum and contents.

Ultrasound is also often used to guide needle placement and to perform percutaneous procedures and central venous catheter placement. Ultrasound ensures precision in positioning a needle or catheter that is being placed percutaneously through the skin so as to avoid nerves, the spinal cord, a fetus, or other structures. The imaging confirms the needle placement before injecting material, aspirating fluid, or biopsying a site. Palpation or standard X-ray was the approach traditionally used to guide needle placement.

Ultrasound guidance codes 76930–76965 must be reported in addition to codes from the Surgery section that describe the surgical procedure. For example, when a physician performs a needle biopsy of the thyroid using ultrasound guidance, the following codes are reported:

EXAMPLE
76942: Ultrasonic guidance for needle placement, imaging supervision and interpretation.
60100: Biopsy thyroid, percutaneous core needle.

The Ultrasound section is arranged by anatomical site. Codes can be found in the index under the words *ultrasound* and *echography*.

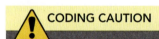

CODING CAUTION

Pregnancy Ultrasounds

A common coding error is coding abdominal ultrasound codes for pregnancy ultrasound. Pregnancy ultrasound codes are located in the Pelvis subsection that refers to a pregnant uterus (CPT code range 76801–76828).

CODING ALERT

Report Either a Diagnostic or a Guidance Ultrasound

Do not report both a diagnostic and a guidance ultrasound code during the same procedure or session.

The Medicine section also contains codes for ultrasound imaging on certain areas:

93303–93350: Ultrasounds of the heart

93875–93893: Cerebrovascular arterial studies

93922–93933: Arterial studies of the extremities

93965–93971: Venous studies of the extremities

93975–93981: Visceral and penile vascular studies

RADIOLOGIC GUIDANCE

Radiologic Guidance is a new subsection for 2007. Guidance is used with a variety of codes, and all except ultrasound were previously scattered in multiple sections.

All the codes in this section pertain to fluoroscopic guidance and localization of needles or placement of catheters. Numerous instructional notes beneath these codes direct the coder to not assign these codes in addition to specific radiological supervision and interpretation procedures. Fluoroscopic guidance codes are not reported with codes that include *arthrography* in the code description. For example, 77002, fluoroscopic guidance for needle placement, cannot be reported with code 73615, radiologic examination, ankle, arthrography, radiological supervision and interpretation. Instructional notes also instruct the coder to assign additional codes for the surgical procedure performed.

BREAST, MAMMOGRAPHY

Mammography, or mammogram, uses a low-dose X-ray system for the examination of breasts. There are two different kinds of mammography, diagnostic and screening, based on the documented reason for the examination. This distinction is important for payers, since some cover the service to assess a suspected condition but not the screening service.

The referring physician's diagnosis on the mammography order determines whether it is a diagnostic or a screening service. A **screening procedure** is performed to detect a disease or condition in the absence of signs and symptoms. A **diagnostic procedure** is performed to assess the extent of an already-diagnosed disease or condition. However, a radiologist (but not a radiologic technologist) who finds an abnormality in a screening can proceed with a diagnostic mammogram even though it was not ordered.

Screening Mammography   A screening mammography is usually limited to two images, craniocaudal and mediolateral oblique views. It is performed to detect unsuspected cancer in an early stage in an asymptomatic woman. CPT code 77057 is inherently bilateral, so the −50 modifier is not required when examining both breasts.

Diagnostic Mammography   A diagnostic mammography (CPT code range 77051–77056) is reported when a suspected mass or abnormality has been found during a physical examination, when the patient has previously had breast surgery, or for follow-up after a related surgery. Diagnostic mammography requires additional work, supervision, and interpretative skills.

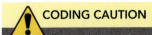

Ultrasound Codes in the Medicine Section

Not all ultrasound codes are located in the Radiology section of CPT. Some are located in the Medicine section as well. It is important to check the index and not to assign codes directly from the Diagnostic Ultrasound section of CPT.

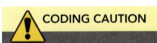

Modifier for Single Breast Service

Pay close attention to the code descriptions for the words *bilateral* and *unilateral*. If only one breast is examined and the description states *bilateral*, a −52 modifier is appended.

BILLING TIP

Medicare Billing of Screening Mammography

A HCPCS G code, rather than the CPT code, is assigned for Medicare.

BONE/JOINT STUDIES

The Bone/Joint studies subheading is new to 2007. This subsection is unique because there are varying methods of study grouped into one subsection. For example, 77084, magnetic resonance imaging, bone marrow blood supply, is not separately listed under a heading or subheading for magnetic resonance imaging and is grouped with codes for traditional X-ray as well as CT scan.

Checkpoint 9.2

Assign the radiology codes for the following procedures. Assign modifiers as needed.

1. Transcranial Doppler study of the intracranial arteries; complete study _____
2. Ultrasound of the gallbladder _____
3. MRI of the heart, complete study for morphology _____
4. Upper GI series with KUB _____
5. Physician uses fluoroscopic guidance for left wrist injection _____
6. Venography of the right leg _____
7. Ultrasound guided thoracentesis _____
8. X-ray ribs, four views (bilateral) _____
9. CT scan of chest, without contrast _____
10. MRI of the brain with contrast _____

RADIATION ONCOLOGY

Radiation oncology is a subspecialty of radiology that utilizes high-energy ionizing radiation to treat malignant neoplasms and certain nonmalignant conditions. Cancers often treated primarily with radiation include those of the larynx, skin, oral cavity, nasopharynx, cervix, and brain and malignant lymphomas. Radiation is an aspect of treatment, along with surgery to remove the tumor and/or chemotherapy, for many other cancers.

Radiation oncology uses several distinct therapeutic modalities, including teletherapy, brachytherapy, hyperthermia, and stereotactic radiation. This range of codes, which begins with notes that should be carefully reviewed, is arranged by type and method of treatment performed.

Radiation oncologists usually see patients for a preliminary consultation or care before starting treatment. This preliminary session should be reported with a code from another appropriate CPT section: E/M, Medicine, or Surgery. The radiologist then provides the oncological services, which include:

- Initial consultation with the radiologist
- Clinical treatment planning with and/or without simulation
- Medical radiation physics, dosimetry (calculating the radiation dose), treatment devices, and special services
- Clinical treatment management procedures
- Normal follow-up care during the patient's treatment and for three months after completion of treatment

NUCLEAR MEDICINE

Nuclear medicine, another subspecialty of radiology, involves the administration of radioisotopes or radiopharmaceuticals for diagnostic imaging and for therapy. It consists of diagnostic examinations of the anatomy that produce images as well as measure organ function. The images are developed based on the detection of energy emitted from a radioactive substance given to the patient either intravenously or orally.

Codes are arranged by the nature of the procedure, meaning whether it was diagnostic or therapeutic, and further subdivided by body system. They are also differentiated by the extent of the area examined (limited area, multiple areas, or the whole body). Nearly a hundred different nuclear medicine procedures are coded, including such common scans as bone scans to determine cancer metastasis and osteomyelitis and cardiac scans to evaluate cardiac output, such as stress tests, and myocardial infarction. Two advanced imaging technologies are PET and SPECT:

Positron emission tomography (PET) exams produce high-energy, three-dimensional computer-reconstructed images of the metabolic function of an organ such as thyroid, liver, spleen, bone, heart, and kidney. PET has been used primarily in cardiology, neurology, and oncology to assess the benefit of coronary artery bypass surgery, to identify causes of childhood seizures and adult dementia, and to detect and grade tumors. It is very sensitive in picking up active tumor tissue but does not measure the size of the tumor.

Single proton emission computerized tomography (SPECT) also provides three-dimensional computer-reconstructed images of an organ. This technology is used to enable in-depth assessment of complex anatomy or functional activity.

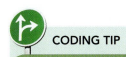

CODING TIP

Coding Nuclear Supplies

The radium or other radiation source is not included in the nuclear medicine service and can be coded separately (CPT codes 78990 and 79900).

Checkpoint 9.3

Assign the radiology codes for the following procedures.

1. PET tumor imaging, whole body _____

2. SPECT myocardial imaging _____

3. Diagnostic nuclear medicine procedure, gastrointestinal, unlisted _____

4. Ten determinations of thyroid uptake _____

5. Brachytherapy, remote afterloading, 11 catheters _____

6. A radiation oncologist provides clinical treatment planning service to patients who are receiving radiation therapy for cancer. Code for the clinical treatment planning that encompasses a single treatment area in a single port with no blocking. _____

ASSIGNING RADIOLOGY CODES

Most coders do not assign radiology imaging and ultrasound codes. When these ancillary services are provided in hospital departments—whether for inpatients or outpatients—codes are assigned automatically

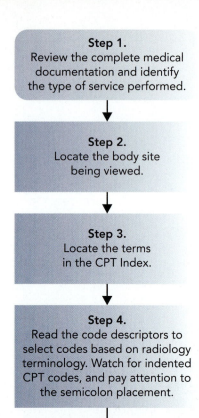

Step 1.
Review the complete medical documentation and identify the type of service performed.

Step 2.
Locate the body site being viewed.

Step 3.
Locate the terms in the CPT Index.

Step 4.
Read the code descriptors to select codes based on radiology terminology. Watch for indented CPT codes, and pay attention to the semicolon placement.

Step 5.
Consider assignment of modifiers, especially for supervision and interpretation variables.

FIGURE 9.1
Radiology Code Assignment Flow Chart

during the coding and billing process. (See the Reimbursement Review on pages 388–389.) However, familiarity with their meanings and selection is required knowledge for coders. Figure 9.1 presents the steps in selecting radiology codes, which are as follows:

1. Review the documentation (X-ray report, imaging study, or other source.), and identify the type of service performed.

2. Locate the body site being viewed

3. Look in the CPT index for the service or the body part. Common words are X-ray, CT scan, magnetic resonance imaging (MRI), magnetic resonance angiography (MRA), ultrasound, echography, mammography, radiology, nuclear medicine, nuclear imaging, and the names of the body sites.

4. Read the code descriptions, paying attention to the code descriptions about complete or limited, obstetric or nonobstetric, bilateral, with or without contrast, *fingers(s)* (meaning more than one), minimum number of views, radiologic supervision and interpretation. Watch for indented CPT codes, and pay attention to the semicolon placement.

5. Consider whether the assignment of modifiers will clarify the code being reported. If the code description does not say *bilateral*, use −LT or −RT. Make note of whether the physician prepares a written report. If the physician reads the X-ray (interprets) but does not provide a written report, a −26 modifier is required.

EXAMPLE A patient is seen in the ER after tripping on a curb and fracturing her right wrist. X-rays were ordered, and two views of the wrist were obtained. The radiologist reviewed the films, dictated a written report, and made a verbal report to the ER physician.

What service would you look up in the index?	X-ray
What is the body site?	Wrist
Based on the documentation, was fluoroscopy used?	No
How many views were obtained?	Two
Based on the documentation, was any contrast used?	No
Is a modifier applicable based on the body part examined?	Yes, −RT
Does the physician own the equipment?	No
Did the physician dictate a formal report?	Yes
What is the correct code?	73100–RT

Pathology and Laboratory

The Pathology and Laboratory section of CPT contains the codes relating to a broad range of services from routine tests performed in a physician office to highly specialized tests performed in sophisticated labs. Laboratory services are done to assess patients' specimens, and pathologists work to identify diseases by studying cells and tissues under a microscope. Common procedures include urinalysis, culturing bacteria, organ and disease panels, microscopic examination of tissue and blood, and dissection of surgical specimens.

Referred to in short as *path and lab,* these services are coded through the charge description master when done in the hospital setting. In a physician office that has an on-site lab, the lab technician identifies the codes for the lab tests. Coders who work for billing services must also be familiar with this type of coding and billing for professional fees. The ability to verify path and lab codes against documentation is an important part of a general background in coding.

Services are performed by physicians or by technologists (such as medical laboratory technicians, or MLTs) under physicians' supervision. Some services combine the professional component (the physician's supervision and interpretation), but most path and lab codes are for the technical component only. The techniques for testing are very complex and involve methods and terminology that must be carefully studied. Good references that explain the tests in layperson's terms include the *Coder's Desk Reference for Procedures*, the *Laboratory Cross Coder*, and the *Coding and Payment Guide for Laboratory Services*, all published by Ingenix.

PATHOLOGY AND LABORATORY GENERAL GUIDELINES

As in all other sections of CPT, guidelines are located before the codes themselves. Notes are also located at the beginning of code ranges or appear as parenthetical notes. It is appropriate to list as many CPT codes from this section as necessary to capture all services performed, whether or not they have been performed on the same date of service. Unlisted procedures are also available for most subsections but should be assigned only after checking for a Category III or HCPCS Level II code.

ORGANIZATION OF THE PATHOLOGY AND LABORATORY SECTION

Table 9.3 lists the subsections in the Path and Lab section. These code ranges are organized by the type of service, not anatomy.

CODING TIP

Code Assignment by Testing Method or Analysis

In the Path and Lab section, identifying the method of testing or analysis performed on a specimen is a key factor in assigning the correct code.

NOTE

HCPCS Level II codes are covered in Chapter 10 of your program.

CODING TIP

Pathology and Laboratory Codes Begin with 8

All codes located in the Path and Lab section begin with the number 8.

Table 9.3 Pathology and Laboratory Subsections

Subsection	Code Range
Organ or Disease Panels	80047–80076
Drug Testing	80100–80103
Therapeutic Drug Assays	80150–80299
Evocative/Suppression Testing	80400–80440
Consultations (Clinical Pathology)	80500–80502
Urinalysis	81000–81099
Chemistry	82000–84999
Hematology and Coagulation	85002–85999
Immunology	86000–86849
Transfusion Medicine	86850–86999
Microbiology	87001–87999
Anatomic Pathology	88000–88099
Cytopathology	88104–88199
Cytogenetic Studies	88230–88299
Surgical Pathology	88300–88399
Transcutaneous Procedures	88400
Other Procedures	89049–89240
Reproductive Medicine Procedures	89250–89356

Charge Capture: Physician and Facility

The medical billing process followed in physician practices and hospitals is aimed at effective **charge capture** to ensure payment for all the medical services and procedures patients receive. The basic steps are similar for offices and facilities:

1. Preregister patients.
2. Establish financial responsibility for visits.
3. Check patients in.
4. Check patients out.
5. Review coding compliance.
6. Check billing compliance.
7. Prepare and transmit claims.
8. Monitor payer adjudication.
9. Generate patient statements.
10. Follow up on patient payments, and handle collections.

Two different tools are used in these environments to help capture the work done.

Charge Description Master

Normally, facilities have tools for charge capture. But since the number of possible services is vastly greater, hospitals use a computerized list of all billable services, procedures, devices, medications, and supplies that can be provided to inpatients and outpatients. This list is called the **charge description master (CDM).**

The typical hospital CDM encompasses thousands of service-line items ranging from drugs, medical supplies, and equipment to ancillary department tests and procedures. For example, the following departments are represented:

- Ambulatory surgery
- Anesthesia
- Cardiac catheterization
- Cardiology/cardiopulmonary
- Chemotherapy
- Clinics (pain, wound)
- Coronary care
- Emergency room
- Intensive care
- Laboratory
- Medical imaging/interventional procedures
- Nursery
- Observation room
- Operating room
- Pharmacy
- Radiology
- Recovery room
- Rehabilitation (physical, speech, occupational, cardiac, and pulmonary therapies)
- Room and board
- Sleep studies/neurology
- Surgery supplies
- Tissue pathology and cytology

The CDM contains the hospital's billing structure for creating claims and bills. Typically, for each item, there is the hospital's own master charge code (digits that stand for the department and the item), a description (the name of the procedure or service), a HCPCS/CPT code if the item is an outpatient procedure, a three-digit revenue code for billing purposes, a quantity or dose indicator, and a price. The facility's finance department has the main responsibility for assigning the numbers and keeping the CDM current; but other departments help as well.

In each hospital department, computer screens in the departmental charge entry system called charge slips (or charge tickets) are used to input the services the patient has received. For example, in the ancillary service departments, to capture charges, the physician or the technician enters data from a requisition form, physician order, or other order into the hospital's charge description master, and those data are translated into CPT/HCPCS codes. Therefore, typically coders do not assign the radiology and the pathology and laboratory codes directly. The health information management (HIM) department assigns codes for diagnoses and major inpatient procedures.

Charge Code	Description	Revenue Code	CPT Code	Units	Charge
55438867	Doxycycline tablet, 200 mg	250		1	$4.52
56637740	Established pt, Level 4	510	99214	1	$235.00
75436610	Wrist, complete	320	73110	1	$112.00
77749348	ICU, per diem	202		1	$1,897.00

Encounter Form

In the professional setting, an **encounter form** (also called a *superbill*) may be completed by the provider after a patient's visit. As shown below, the encounter form contains a summary of the provider's major or frequent services. The provider uses the form to check off procedures done, and the medical coder examines the documentation to verify the code selection. The encounter form is also used by billing staff to update the diagnosis and procedure information for the patient in the practice management program (PMP). The updated data are used to create health care claims and patients' bills.

Encounter form.

VALLEY ASSOCIATES, PC
Christopher M. Connolly, MD - Internal Medicine
555-967-0303
FED I.D. #16-1234567

PATIENT NAME	APPT. DATE/TIME	
Deysenrothe, Mae J.	10/6/2008	9:30 am

PATIENT NO.	DX
DEYSEMA0	1. V70.0 Exam, Adult 2. 3. 4.

DESCRIPTION	✓	CPT	FEE	DESCRIPTION	✓	CPT	FEE
OFFICE VISITS				**PROCEDURES**			
New Patient				Diagnostic Anoscopy		46600	
LI Problem Focused		99201		ECG Complete	✓	93000	70
LII Expanded		99202		I&D, Abscess		10060	
LIII Detailed		99203		Pap Smear		88150	
LIV Comp./Mod.		99204		Removal of Cerumen		69210	
LV Comp./High		99205		Removal 1 Lesion		17000	
Established Patient				Removal 2-14 Lesions		17003	
LI Minimum		99211		Removal 15+ Lesions		17004	
LII Problem Focused		99212		Rhythm ECG w/Report		93040	
LIII Expanded		99213		Rhythm ECG w/Tracing		93041	
LIV Detailed		99214		Sigmoidoscopy, diag.		45330	
LV Comp./High		99215					
				LABORATORY			
PREVENTIVE VISIT				Bacteria Culture		87081	
New Patient				Fungal Culture		87101	
Age 12-17		99384		Glucose Finger Stick		82948	
Age 18-39		99385		Lipid Panel		80061	
Age 40-64	✓	99386	180	Specimen Handling		99000	
Age 65+		99387		Stool/Occult Blood		82270	
Established Patient				Tine Test		85008	
Age 12-17		99394		Tuberculin PPD		85590	
Age 18-39		99395		Urinalysis	✓	81000	17
Age 40-64		99396		Venipuncture		36415	
Age 65+		99397					
				INJECTION/IMMUN.			
CONSULTATION: OFFICE/OP				Immun. Admin.	✓	90471	20
Requested By:				Ea. Add'l.		90472	
LI Problem Focused		99241		Hepatitis A Immun		90632	
LII Expanded		99242		Hepatitis B Immun		90746	
LIII Detailed		99243		Influenza Immun	✓	90659	68
LIV Comp./Mod.		99244		Pneumovax		90732	
LV Comp./High		99245					
				TOTAL FEES			355

PHYSICIAN ORDERS AND TEST REQUISITIONS

If a specimen (for example, urine, blood, sputum, saliva, or tissue) is obtained in the office, it is recorded, and the sample is sent to the lab for analysis or processing. Otherwise, the patient is instructed to go to the outside laboratory. Every laboratory test must be ordered by a physician, a physician's assistant (PA), or a registered nurse-practitioner (RN-P). A test requisition that specifies what tests to perform on the specimen and justifies its medical necessity by supplying a diagnosis or reason for the test, even if it is a sign or symptom, must be sent with every laboratory test ordered, as shown in Figure 9.2, which also illustrates the wide range of possible tests.

COMPLETE LABORATORY CODES

In order to properly code and bill for a physician, the coder must determine whether the physician performed the complete procedure or only a component of that procedure, and whether the procedure was performed on-site or off-site. A **complete lab test** includes ordering the procedure or test, obtaining the sample or specimen, handling the specimen, performing the actual procedure or test, and analyzing and interpreting the results.

Blood can be collected via a vein (venipuncture), capillary (finger) stick, or other device. Some offices have sophisticated equipment and can perform a wider variety of laboratory procedures. In such cases, if the physician sends the sample or specimen to a freestanding lab or a hospital-based lab for testing and analysis, the physician office codes only the collection and handling for preparation of the specimen.

All lab work is regulated by **Clinical Laboratory Improvement Amendments (CLIA)** rules. Most offices do easy-to-administer, low-risk tests (such as ovulation, blood glucose, dipstick or tablet reagent urinalyses, and rapid strep test) that are called **CLIA-waived tests,** meaning they are subject to minimal requirements. A provider who wants to perform these tests files an application and pays a small fee. Offices that handle more complex testing (like CBCs, PSAs, routine chemistry panels, and antibiotic susceptibility tests) must apply for accreditation and be certified and inspected.

The physician may send the patient to a local hospital or freestanding laboratory that obtains the sample or specimen, performs the test or procedure, and analyzes and interprets the results. In the case of a surgical procedure performed at a facility, the surgeon removes a surgical specimen and sends it to the pathology department for examination. In these situations, three sets of services are coded and billed:

1. The surgeon bills for the surgical procedure using a surgical code.
2. The pathologist bills for the professional interpretation of the specimen using a path and lab code with the professional component modifier.
3. The facility bills both the surgery and the path and lab codes with the technical component modifiers for the associated facility fees.

INDIVIDUAL TEST REQUEST FORM

PATIENT'S NAME (LAST)   (FIRST)

BIRTH DATE   SEX   DATE & TIME COLLECTED

ADDRESS

CITY   STATE   ZIP CODE

PHONE (INCLUDE AREA CODE)   SOCIAL SECURITY NO.

DOCTOR'S NAME (LAST)   (FIRST)   UPIN#

ADDRESS

CITY   STATE   ZIP CODE

PHONE NO.   FAX NO.

DIAGNOSIS: 780.6, 780.79

DOCTOR'S SIGNATURE
If signature is not available, please attach doctor's prescription.

BILLING INFORMATION

BILL TO
- ❏ DOCTOR ❏ LAB
  by permission or request

PREPAID
- ❏ CASH ❏ CHECK ❏ MC ❏ VISA

CARDHOLDER'S NAME _____

CREDIT CARD NO. _____

EXPIRATION DATE _____

CARDHOLDER'S SIGNATURE _____

SPECIMENS RECEIVED:
- ❏ RED/SST ❏ LAVENDER ❏ YELLOW ❏ BLUE
- ❏ URINE ❏ SALIVA ❏ SERUM ❏ SPUTUM
- ❏ OTHERS:

COMMENTS _____

DATE RECEIVED: TIME RECEIVED:

PLEASE MARK THE APPROPRIATE BOX BELOW

INDIVIDUAL TESTS

General & Immunological Tests

- ❏ Complete Blood Count (CBC)
- ❏ Complete Blood Chemistry
- ❏ Anti-Nuclear Antibody
- ❏ Apoptosis (Programmed Cell Death)
- ❏ Cell Cycle Analysis
- ❏ Natural Killer Cell Cytotoxic Activity
- ❏ T & B Cell Function
- ❏ Lymphocyte Subpopulation Analysis
- ❏ Lymphocyte T-Helper/T-Suppressor Ratio
- ❏ Immunoglobulins Basic (IgG, IgM, IgA)
- ❏ Immunoglobulins Complete (IgG, IgM, IgA, IgE)
- ❏ Immune Complexes (IgG, IgM, IgA)
- ❏ C3, C4 Complement
- ❏ Saliva Secretory IgA

Bacterial Antibodies

- ❏ Chlamydia Species (IgG, IgM, IgA)
- ❏ Chlamydia pneumoniae (IgG, IgM, IgA)
- ❏ Chlamydia trachomatis (IgG, IgM, IgA)
- ❏ Helicobacter pylori (IgG, IgM, IgA)

- ☑ Lyme Disease (B. burgdorferi) (IgG, IgM)
- ❏ Lyme Disease by Western Blot (IgG, IgM)
- ❏ Mycoplasma fermentans (IgG, IgM, IgA)
- ❏ Mycoplasma genitalium (IgG, IgM, IgA)
- ❏ Mycoplasma hominis (IgG, IgM, IgA)
- ❏ Mycoplasma orale (IgG, IgM, IgA)
- ❏ Mycoplasma penetrans (IgG, IgM, IgA)
- ❏ Mycoplasma pneumoniae (IgG, IgM, IgA)

Viral Antibodies

- ❏ Coxsackie Virus (IgG, IgM)
- ❏ Cytomegalovirus (IgG, IgM)
- ❏ Epstein-Barr Virus (EBV) Ab Complete
- ❏ Herpes Type 1 (IgG, IgM)
- ❏ Herpes Type 2 (IgG, IgM)
- ❏ Herpes Type 6 (IgG, IgM)
- ❏ Herpes Type 7 (IgG, IgM)
- ❏ HTLV (IgG to HTLV-1 and HTLV-2)
- ❏ Human Papillomavirus
- ❏ Measles (Rubeola) (IgG, IgM)
- ❏ Mumps (IgG, IgM)
- ❏ Parvovirus (IgG, IgM)
- ❏ Rubella (IgG, IgM)

- ❏ Smallpox Virus (IgG, IgM)
- ❏ Varicella Zoster (IgG)
- ❏ Western Equine Encephalomyelitis IgG
- ❏ West Nile Virus (IgG, IgM)

PCR for Infectious Diseases

- ❏ Chlamydia Species by PCR
- ❏ Chlamydia pneumoniae by PCR
- ❏ Chlamydia trachomatis by PCR
- ❏ Lyme Disease by PCR
- ❏ Mycoplasma Species by PCR
- ❏ Mycoplasma fermentans by PCR
- ❏ Mycoplasma genitalium by PCR
- ❏ Mycoplasma hominis by PCR
- ❏ Mycoplasma orale by PCR
- ❏ Mycoplasma penetrans by PCR
- ❏ Mycoplasma pneumoniae by PCR
- ❏ Ureaplasma urealiticum by PCR
- ❏ Cytomegalovirus by PCR
- ❏ Epstein-Barr Virus (EBV) by PCR
- ❏ Herpes Type 1 by PCR
- ❏ Herpes Type 2 by PCR
- ❏ Herpes Type 6 by PCR
- ❏ Herpes Type 7 by PCR

FIGURE 9.2

Sample Laboratory Test Requisition Form (Permission granted for Reproduction, Immunosciences Lab., Inc.)

Table 9.4 Pathology and Laboratory Modifiers

Modifier	Description
−22	Unusual procedures
−26	Professional component
−32	Mandated services
−52	Reduced services
−53	Discontinued procedure
−59	Distinct procedural service
−90	Reference (outside) laboratory
−91	Repeat clinical diagnostic lab test
−92	Alternative lab platform testing

BILLING TIP

Medicare Billing for Off-Site Lab Work

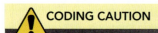

Medicare does not allow a provider who does not perform the test to report the path and lab code. A code for the venipuncture only should be reported (and only once even if more than one specimen is drawn). Other payers do allow physicians to report the lab code with a −90 modifier when specimens are sent off-site for analysis.

⚠ CODING CAUTION

Modifier −51

Modifier −51 (multiple procedures) is not used with laboratory and pathology codes.

EXAMPLE A bone marrow biopsy was performed by a surgeon, and the specimen was sent to a pathologist for review and interpretation. The surgeon reports 85102 for the actual biopsy of the bone marrow. The pathologist reports 88305–26 for the review and interpretation of the specimen. The facility reports both 85102 and 88305–TC for the surgery and the technical component of the specimen processing.

If a physician is requested to review a test result because of abnormalities or is asked to interpret the test or specimen, the −26 modifier is appended to show the professional component. In the example above, the pathologist renders an opinion after examining tissue or cultures, and the −26 modifier is used to capture this professional service.

MODIFIERS

As with every section of CPT, modifiers may be used to further describe a service or circumstances surrounding a procedure. Table 9.4 lists the modifiers commonly used with pathology and laboratory codes.

EXAMPLE A blood sample from a non-Medicare patient was obtained by the internist and was sent to an outside laboratory for testing, analysis, and interpretation. The internist reported 80061–90 to describe the lab test with interpretation and analysis performed at an off-site laboratory.

ORGAN- AND DISEASE-ORIENTED PANELS

A **panel** is a group of lab tests commonly performed together to diagnose organ dysfunction or to monitor a disease. CPT maintains a number of organ- and disease-oriented laboratory panels, shown in Table 9.5, as a convenient way for physicians to order tests and subsequently bill for them. Other tests commonly appear on lab requisition forms under test titles that indicate groups of related procedures. For example, a rheumatologist can group a routine battery of tests under the designation of "arthritis panel," although CPT does not have a panel for arthritis tests.

To bill a panel code, all the listed tests must be performed. No substitutions are permitted. If fewer tests are performed, the individual CPT codes for each test should be reported, not the panel code. In CPT,

Table 9.5 Laboratory Panels

Code	Panel	Components (Individual Tests Included)
80048	Basic metabolic	Calcium, carbon dioxide, chloride, creatinine, glucose, potassium, sodium, blood urea nitrogen (BUN)
80050	General health	Comprehensive metabolic panel, automated CBC with manual differential WBC, automated CBC and platelet count with automated differential WBC count, thyroid-stimulating hormone (TSH)
80051	Electrolyte	Carbon dioxide, chloride, potassium, sodium
80053	Comprehensive metabolic	Albumin, total bilirubin, calcium, carbon dioxide, chloride, creatinine, glucose, phosphatase, alkaline, potassium, total protein, sodium, alanine amino transferase (ALT), SGPT, aspartate amino transferase (AST), SGOT, blood urea nitrogen (BUN)
80055	Obstetric	Automated CBC with manual differential WBC, automated CBC and platelet count with automated differential WBC count, hepatitis B surface antigen (HBsA$_g$), antibody screen, RBC, blood typing ABO, blood typing Rh (D)
80061	Lipid	Total serum cholesterol, HDL, LDL, triglycerides
80069	Renal function	Albumin, calcium, carbon dioxide, chloride, creatinine, glucose, phosphorus, potassium, sodium, blood urea nitrogen (BUN)
80074	Acute hepatitis	Hepatitis A antibody (HAAb), IgM antibody, hepatitis B core antibody (HBcAb), IgM antibody, hepatitis B surface antigen (HBsAg), hepatitis C antibody
80076	Hepatic function	Albumin, bilirubin total, bilirubin direct, alkaline phosphatase, Total protein, ALT, SGPT, AST, SGOT

the individual test codes can be located quickly because the CPT code for each test listed under the panel is next to the test's name.

Typically, a single diagnosis code is sufficient to justify the use of a panel code. Tests ordered in addition to a panel, however, must be justified with a separate diagnosis.

EXAMPLE A physician orders a comprehensive metabolic panel. CPT code 80053 is assigned. If one of the tests included in this panel is not performed, the panel code would not be assigned, and the tests that were performed would be listed individually.

DRUG TESTING

At the beginning of the drug-testing subsection, a list of common drugs and classes of drugs assayed by qualitative screening is provided, followed by confirmation with a second method. *Qualitative* tests detect the presence of a particular analyte, constituent, or condition. An **analyte** is a chemical or substance being measured or analyzed. *Quantitative* testing provides specific numerical amounts of an analyte in a specimen or sample; it tells how much of the drug is in the patient's system. Quantitative tests are usually performed after qualitative studies to identify the specific amount of a particular substance in the sample. Code 80100 is used each time a qualitative test is performed per drug class.

EXAMPLE A patient reeking of alcohol and in a coma is brought to the ER. The ER physician has a drug screen done (multiple class, one procedure), and the presence of barbiturates, opiates, and alcohol is noted. Confirmatory tests for each drug class is run. The notes direct the coder to use 80100 for each screening and 80102 for each procedure necessary for confirmation. In this case, there were three drug classes to confirm, so 80102 is assigned three times: 80100, 80102x3.

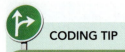
THERAPEUTIC DRUG ASSAYS

Codes in the therapeutic drug assays section describe the quantitative determination of blood levels of various therapeutic compounds. An **assay** tests drug purity or the absorption level of prescribed drugs in the body. These tests are performed to help the clinician monitor the best level of medication for the patient or monitor compliance with a given medication regimen, such as Coumadin (blood thinner) levels.

> **EXAMPLE** A patient diagnosed with bipolar disorder must have his blood drawn every month to measure the lithium level. The codes is 80178.

EVOCATIVE/SUPPRESSION TESTING

Tests in the evocative/suppression code range measure how endocrine glands are working, evaluating a patient's endocrine status and the response to agents that are intended to stimulate or suppress a particular hormone. The physician will administer agents to evoke or provoke a response or production of analytes or to suppress them. The analyte being measured is something that a person must take as a supplement because his or her body does not produce it. Sometimes, it may be a product that is given to suppress production of a different substance.

Each code depicts a panel listing the specific analyte and the number of times it must be tested.

> **EXAMPLE** Code 80430, growth hormone suppression panel (glucose administration), must include glucose (82947x3) and human growth hormone (HGH, 83003x4). This code description means that the glucose must be tested three times on blood samples and the HGH four times.

The administration of the agent is reported with codes from the Medicine section (90780–90784), and the supply of the agent with a HCPCS supply code.

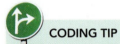
URINALYSIS

In the process of analyzing a patient's urine, the technician observes the sample and notes its specific gravity, opacity, color, and appearance. Code descriptions in the urinalysis code range identify the method of testing (dipstick, automated, nonautomated, with microscopy), the color of the specimen, and the volume of urine.

Urinalysis can be performed either manually or automated and with or without microscopy. **Automated** testing utilizes a machine to analyze the specimen, speeding up the process. **Manual** testing does not use a machine and can be performed by dipstick. The color change on each segment of a dipstick is compared to a color chart. Dipsticks are used to determine the urine's pH (acidity), specific gravity (density), protein content, ketones, nitrite content, and glucose and to estimate the number of white blood cells in the urine.

> **EXAMPLE**
> **81005** Urinalysis; qualitative or semiquantitative, except immunoassays.

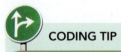

CHEMISTRY

The chemistry code range reports individual chemistry tests that are not performed as part of an automated organ- or disease-oriented panel. They can be performed on any body source. Calculations in reporting the results are included in the code description. The majority of the tests in this section are quantitative because the code descriptions cite the amount of an analyte that is being measured.

> **EXAMPLE** A PA performs a glucose screening by Dextrostix method (reagent strip) using capillary blood. The codes for all components are 82948, 36416.

HEMATOLOGY AND COAGULATION

Tests in this code range are performed on blood and blood components. Hematology, the study of blood, involves counting the cells in blood. Coagulation measures how fast the blood clots. Commonly performed tests are bleeding times, hemograms, blood count, clotting factor analysis, prothrombin time, coagulation time, viscosity, and thromboplastin time. A **complete blood count (CBC)** includes a **white blood cell (WBC) count, red blood cell (RBC)** count, hemoglobin, hematocrit, and platelet count. A hemogram includes a CBC, the differentials, and platelets.

> **EXAMPLE**
> 85009: Blood count; spun microhematocrit.

The code for a blood marrow smear (85097) is located in this section; collection of the bone marrow is reported with a Musculoskeletal section bone biopsy code.

IMMUNOLOGY

Immunology codes represent testing immunity to specific diseases as well as testing for the presence of antigens. The specific organism or disease related to the test must be identified. The coder must then determine whether the procedure was to detect antigens or antibodies, followed by the method used to perform the test.

TRANSFUSION MEDICINE

Many code descriptions in the transfusion medicine code range are reported per each technique, each elution, or each panel. CPT specifies separately identifying each procedure performed in the blood bank: typing blood, screening antibodies, identifying antibodies, and processing blood and blood products.

MICROBIOLOGY

Microbiology covers bacteriology, virology, parasitology, and mycology. The coder must know several important factors about the specimen, including source, method of handling, identification techniques, and stains performed. If a specific agent is not specified, a general methodology code should be used (87299, 87449, 87450, 87797, 87799, 87899).

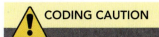

CODING CAUTION

Repeat Tests

If the exact test is performed on two different specimens on the same day, use modifier −91.

BILLING TIP

Medicare Fecal Occult Blood

A frequently reported service is the Medicare-covered fecal occult blood screening test, a colon cancer screen, CPT code range 82270–82274.

CYTOPATHOLOGY

For cytopathology, the study of diseased cells, samples are collected via washings, brushings, fine needle aspiration, or needle biopsy and are examined under a microscope. Code assignment depends on the method of screening and examining the slide. There are professional and technical component services in this code range. Code 88141 reports the physician interpretation of a smear and is used in addition to the technical component. Codes for vaginal or cervical screening are selected by whether the slides were prepared by the Bethesda or non-Bethesda reporting system.

PATHOLOGY CONSULTATIONS

Two types of clinical pathology consultation codes are available in the Clinical Pathology section. As with all consultations in CPT, this service must be requested by an attending physician and requires the interpretive judgment of a specialist, in this case the pathologist. Tests must be outside the clinically significant normal range before the service is requested. The pathologist must prepare a written report of findings and send it to the requesting physician, and the report must be included in the patient's record.

There are also codes for consultations in the Surgical Pathology section (CPT code range 88321–88329). These are used when a physician office sends a specimen for the pathologist to examine and identify. This is different than routine tissue examination from biopsies. In this case, a physician has attempted and failed to treat a disease and needs pathological advice. There are also codes to be used when a pathologist is asked to provide a second opinion and review samples from another lab, or during a surgical procedure (88329).

SURGICAL PATHOLOGY

Surgical pathology codes report tests conducted on specimens submitted from operating rooms as a result of biopsies or removal of abnormal growths or organs. The specimen—the tissue or fluid that requires macroscopic and microscopic examination and pathologic diagnosis—is placed in a container and is sent to the pathology department for examination and analysis. Gross examination involves viewing the specimen with the naked eye and making note of color, appearance, size, weight, texture, and the like. Some specimens can be diagnosed adequately with the use of the naked eye. Microscopic examination involves slicing the specimen, preparing slides, and viewing the slides under a microscope.

Of the six levels of surgical pathology, level I identifies gross examination of tissue only and levels II–VI refer to gross and microscopic examination of tissue. Each level represents a degree of difficulty and interpretation for the physician as well as the type of specimen examination.

Correct coding follows these rules:

- If several specimens are received in the same container without separate identification, bill only one surgical pathology code.
- If several specimens are received in the same container and are identified separately, bill each specimen separately.

- If several specimen bottles are received, one with the uterus, one with the right tube and ovary, and another with left tube and ovary, bill per specimen using applicable codes for each, based on anatomical part.

EXAMPLE A patient undergoes a septoplasty for chronic nasal obstruction and severe septal deformity. The tissue removed was nasal cartilage. Gross description: specimen is labeled with the patient's name and the words *nasal cartilage* and consists of multiple fragments of tan tissue and fragments of bone. Gross diagnosis: nasal septum. Microscopic diagnosis: Nasal cartilage and bone.

To code this, the coder first looks up the pathology in the CPT index. The coder knows that there were a gross exam and a microscopic exam, but not which level. The coder skips level I and begins at 88302, level II. The coder reads through the levels until the tissue type, nasal cartilage, is found. Code 88304 lists bone fragments and cartilage. The pathologist reports 88304–26 for the service, and the facility reports 88304–TC.

ASSIGNING PATHOLOGY AND LABORATORY CODES

To assign laboratory procedure codes, follow the steps shown in Figure 9.3. These are as follows:

1. Identify the services in the CPT index. The main terms may be (1) the specific names of tests, such as urinalysis or fertility test,

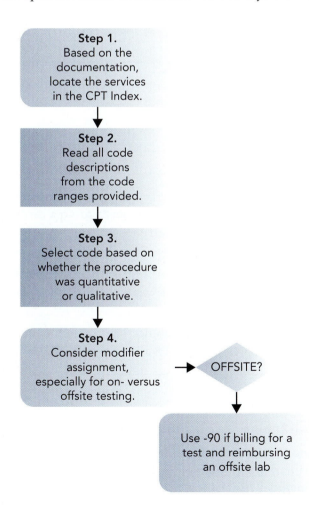

FIGURE 9.3
Pathology and Laboratory Code Assignment Flow Chart

(2) a specific substance, specimen, or sample, such as glucose, insulin, sputum, urine, blood, and stool, or (3) a specific method used to conduct the test, such as culture, microbiology, urinalysis, and fine needle aspiration.

2. Read the code descriptors.

3. Select the appropriate code based on quantitative or qualitative procedures.

4. After selecting the appropriate code, assign modifiers for on- or off-site lab work.

EXAMPLE A company requires one of its employees, a recovering crack cocaine addict, to have random drug tests (screening) performed as part of his drug rehab program. He submits a urine sample at the lab. A qualitative drug test is performed. What code does the lab report?

What test is being performed?	Drug screening
What specimen or substance is being tested?	Cocaine in a urine sample
What method of testing is conducted?	Qualitative drug test
What words can be located in the index?	Drug, screening, or cocaine
Was testing done off-site from where the sample was obtained?	No
What is the code?	80101

Checkpoint 9.4

Assign the pathology and laboratory codes for the following procedures.

1. HCG, quantitative _____

2. Cholesterol, HDL, triglycerides, LDL _____

3. Rubella screen _____

4. Cryopreservation of five cell lines _____

5. HGH antibody _____

6. Comprehensive clinical pathology consultation with report _____

7. Mandated alcohol screen _____

8. A cardiologist suspects a blockage in a patient's coronary arteries and needs to do a cardiac catheterization. One of the tests the hospital will need both before and after surgery is the test that shows how long it takes for the blood to clot (bleeding time). Code for this test.

   _____

9. After her most recent chemotherapy treatment, a patient is quite weakened. Her oncologist orders a complete CBC. _____

10. A patient has chronic edema despite years of treatment with diuretics. The patient's pituitary gland may be secreting excessive amounts of vasopressin, an antidiuretic hormone. Code for the ADH test. _____

Medicine

The Medicine section includes codes for services (called procedures) that are primarily evaluative, diagnostic, and/or therapeutic in nature. It includes codes for noninvasive or minimally invasive services (meaning percutaneous access to a vein through the skin) that are not surgical, pathology, laboratory, or radiology work. Medicine is something of a catchall section that groups diagnostic and therapeutic services for specialties such as allergy, cardiology, pulmonology, and psychiatry.

Physicians commonly provide most of these services in the office, and they typically assign several codes from this section on a given date of service. In some cases, Medicine services are performed along with services or procedures listed in other sections of the book. Code descriptions must be read carefully for correct assignment. Many codes are driven by time (for example, each fifteen minutes), quantity (such as two or more injections), age (for example, seven years and older), and professional component service (with interpretation and report).

ORGANIZATION

Medicine is the sixth major section of CPT and is located immediately before the Category II and III codes. Medicine subsections are arranged by specialty areas or type of service (see Table 9.6). The section is divided into more than thirty subsections. Several have special instructions that are applicable to the code ranges, particularly the Psychiatry, Dialysis, Cardiovascular, and Neurology sections.

As with all sections of CPT, unlisted procedures are reported if no other CPT code, Category II or III code, or supply code fits the situation, and the section also includes add-on codes and separate procedures. Some medical specialty evaluation and management (E/M) services—such as the codes in the Ophthalmology subsection—are located in the Medicine section rather than in the general E/M section.

CODING TIP

Medicine Codes Begin with 9

All codes located in the Medicine section begin with the number 9.

GUIDELINES

Coders must pay close attention to add-on codes and separate procedures when coding multiple procedures to avoid unbundling (also called fragmenting) a comprehensive service. Payer-specific instructions are also very important. Medicare requires—and other payers may recognize—HCPCS Level II codes to be reported for many of the services provided in this section. (This chapter uses the HCPCS Level II codes in examples to illustrate correct usage.)

More than one code is often required, possibly from other CPT sections, for multiple services and procedures for the same patient on the same date of service. For example, for an office visit it is common to assign both an E/M code and a separate code from the Medicine section (for a vaccination, for example).

NOTE

HCPCS Level II codes are covered in Chapter 10 of your program.

> **EXAMPLE** A child being seen by a pediatrician for an annual physical exam receives immunizations. The Medicine code is used for the immunizations in addition to the E/M code for the office visit.

If the patient presents only for the procedure (such as an immunization), an E/M visit is not medically necessary and cannot be coded. Only a significant, separate evaluation and management service justifies reporting an additional E/M code. When this occurs, modifier −25 goes with the E/M code.

Table 9.6 Medicine Subsections

Subsection	Code Range
Immune Globulins	90281–90399
Immunization Administration for Vaccines/Toxoids	90465–90474
Vaccines, Toxoids	90476–90749
Hydration, Therapeutic, Prophylactic, and Diagnostic Injections and Infusions	90760–90779
Psychiatry	90801–90899
Biofeedback	90901–90911
Dialysis	90918–90999
Gastroenterology	91000–91299
Ophthalmology	92002–92499
Special Otorhinolarygologic Services	92502–92700
Cardiovascular	92950–93799
Noninvasive Vascular Diagnostic Studies	93875–93990
Pulmonary	94002–94799
Allergy and Clinical Immunology	95004–95199
Endocrinology	95250–95251
Neurology and Neuromuscular Procedures	95805–96020
Medical Genetics and Genetic Counseling Services	96040
Central Nervous System Assessments/Tests	96101–96120
Health and Behavior Assessment/Intervention	96150–96155
Chemotherapy Administration	96401–96549
Photodynamic Therapy	96567–96571
Special Dermatological Procedures	96900–96999
Physical Medicine and Rehabilitation	97001–97799
Medical Nutrition Therapy	97802–97804
Acupuncture	97810–97814
Osteopathic Manipulative Treatment	98925–98929
Chiropractic Manipulative Treatment	98940–98943
Education and Training for Patient Self-Management	98960–98962
Special Services, Procedures, and Reports	99000–99091
Qualifying Circumstances for Anesthesia	99100–99140
Moderate (Conscious) Sedation	99143–99150
Other Services and Procedures	99170–99199
Home Health Procedures/Services	99500–99602
Non-Face-to-Face Nonphysician Services	98966–98968

MODIFIERS

Table 9.7 lists modifiers commonly used with Medicine section codes.

IMMUNE GLOBULINS

The codes in the first subsection, for immune globulins, are used for the immune globulin product provided as a result of a confirmed exposure to a disease. An immune globulin is a substance (such as an

Table 9.7 Medicine Modifiers

Modifier	Description
−22	Unusual services
−26	Professional component
−51	Multiple procedures
−52	Reduced services
−53	Discontinued procedure
−55	Postoperative management
−56	Preoperative management
−57	Decision for surgery
−58	Staged or related procedure
−59	Distinct procedural service
−76	Repeat procedure by same physician
−77	Repeat procedure by another physician
−78	Return to OR for related procedure
−79	Unrelated procedure or service by same physician
−LC, −LD, −RC	Coronary artery modifiers
−FA to −F9, −TA to −T9, −LT, −RT	Anatomic modifiers

antibody) that has been "manufactured" by another person in response to having a specific disease. When it is obtained from an infected person's blood and injected into patients who were exposed to the disease and are not immune, it quickly provides short-term protection, just as if they had developed the substance on their own. Examples are broad-spectrum and anti-infective immune globulins, antitoxins, and various isoantibodies.

These codes represent the injected substance only; an **administration** code (90765–90768, 90772, 90774, 90775) must also be coded to show the complete service.

IMMUNIZATION ADMINISTRATION FOR VACCINES AND TOXOIDS

As with the injection or infusion of an immune globulin, two codes are always reported for vaccinations. One code from range 90476–90749 is for the vaccine, and a second from range 90465–90474 is for the administration of the shot. The administration codes are organized by the patient's age, the type of injection, and the number of vaccines given.

Some vaccine codes are based on how the product was purchased. For example, vaccines for hepatitis B and *Hemophilus* influenza b (HIB) can be purchased separately or as a combined vaccine. If purchased together, they are coded as 90748. If they were purchased separately, they would be coded as 90743, 90744, or 90746 for the hepatitis B vaccine and 90647 or 90648 for the HIB vaccine, along with 90471 and 90472 to capture the administration of the injections.

> ⚠ CODING CAUTION
>
> **Immunizations Compared to Immune Globulins**
>
> An immunization (vaccination) is given to help the body develop protection against a disease. It is given before exposure to the disease. An immune globulin is given after exposure to a disease.

CPT says that a vaccination is usually done in conjunction with another service (office visit). Code for the service (an E/M code) and the substance injected along with the administration of the injection.

EXAMPLE A child seen by a pediatrician for a twenty-four-month checkup receives the varicella and hepatitis B (second dose) immunizations. The CPT codes are 99392, 90465, 90744, 90716.

HYDRATION, THERAPEUTIC, PROPHYLACTIC, AND DIAGNOSTIC INJECTIONS AND INFUSIONS (EXCLUDES CHEMOTHERAPY)

Infusion codes describe prolonged intravenous infusion requiring the presence or direct supervision of the physician. These codes are based on time. Infusions are not coded when performed during a procedure for which they are part of the standard of care or routine practice.

EXAMPLE The infusion of IV sedation for a colonoscopy procedure is not reported, as it is inherent in the code for the colonoscopy.

Codes from this section should not be used for allergen immunotherapy injections.

The code descriptions include the phrase *specify substance or drug*, requiring reporting the specific substance injected with an additional HCPCS supply code. Additional services performed at the same time as an injection are reported separately.

EXAMPLE A patient sees her gynecologist for her monthly Depo-vera shot. The office bills for the injection (90782) and the HCPCS code for the Depo-vera (J1051).

PSYCHIATRY

Psychiatry services may be provided in outpatient or inpatient settings.

EXAMPLE
90821: Individual psychotherapy, insight oriented, behavior modifying and/or supportive, in an inpatient hospital, partial hospital or residential care setting, approximately seventy-five to eighty minutes face-to-face with the patient; with medical evaluation and management services.

If the description of the code does not include medical evaluation and management or if E/M services are provided along with services from the Psychiatry subsection, both the E/M and psychiatry codes can be assigned.

BIOFEEDBACK

Biofeedback is a treatment modality in which people are trained to improve their current state of health by recognizing signals from their own bodies. Physical therapists use biofeedback to help stroke victims regain movement in paralyzed muscles. Psychologists use it to help teach anxious clients to relax. Code 90901 is used for biofeedback training by any modality. Biofeedback used in conjunction with individual psychophysiologic training is included in code 90875.

DIALYSIS

Dialysis is used to manage end stage renal disease (ESRD) or acute renal failure (ARF) patients whose kidneys fail to work or fail to adequately remove wastes from the body. There are two types of dialysis. In **hemodialysis,** blood is circulated through an artificial kidney machine to clean it. In **peritoneal dialysis,** blood is cleaned inside the body by placing fluid in the periotoneal cavity and cycling or draining it several times a day.

These codes include normal care (not requiring hospitalization during the month): establishment of the patient's dialysis regimen, phone calls, patient management during treatments, and physician services during treatments. ESRD dialysis is reported by assigning one code per month (90918–90921) or per day if less than thirty days (90922–90925). The per-month codes do not include the actual dialysis services. Hemodialysis codes 90935–90940 are used to report inpatient ESRD services and dialysis for non-ESRD. Peritoneal dialysis (90945–90999) is coded for each date of service rather than by month. Pay attention to the age of the patient.

GASTROENTEROLOGY (GI)

GI codes are assigned when studies are performed to assess the functionality of the stomach or esophagus. Many of these tests require the patient to swallow a tube or probe to measure movement of these parts or the level of acid in the stomach. For example, tests are performed for the presence of *H. pylori* and for lactase deficiency. Specimens may be taken and sent to the laboratory. Both 91000 and 91055 are separate procedure codes; if either is performed as part of a larger procedure, it should not be coded separately.

> **EXAMPLE** 91030: Bernstein test for esophagitis. During the Bernstein test, a nasogastric tube is inserted (intubation) through the nose down to the stomach, and samples of acid are taken. Therefore, only 91030 is reported.

OPHTHALMOLOGY

Ophthalmology is the only subsection with its own specific E/M visit codes (92002–92014). Codes are categorized by new or established patient as in the E/M section. These codes are assigned for routine office visits involving vision exams, contact lens and glasses prescriptions and fittings, and very specialized ocular examinations.

Codes from the E/M section are assigned when the patient is being seen for an ocular injury or as part of a medical examination to monitor a disease with ocular involvement, such as diabetes and glaucoma. Codes from the Special Ophthalmological Services section are coded in addition to those from the General Ophthalmological section. Detailed definitions of service levels and examples are located at the beginning of this section.

> **EXAMPLE**
> 92130: Glaucoma water provocation test with tonogram.

SPECIAL OTORHINOLARYNGOLOGIC SERVICES

Much like the Ophthalmology section, the Otorhinolaryngologic section includes specialized examinations of the ears, nose, and throat (ENT) that are performed in the office or procedure room. Services

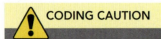
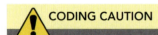

range from audiology exams, hearing aid checks, and speech language communication to swallowing studies. A code from 92601–92604 is assigned and may be used many times during the training period after cochlear implantation. Implants must be programmed after they are placed, and the patient must be taught about the sounds generated.

EXAMPLE

92625: Assessment of tinnitus (includes pitch, loudness matching, and masking).

CARDIOVASCULAR

The extensive Cardiovascular section is subdivided into eight subsections, each with thorough guidelines and instructions for use at the beginning of the code ranges. The subsections are:

1. Therapeutic Services
2. Cardiography
3. Echocardiography
4. Cardiac Catheterization
5. Intracardiac Electrophysiological Procedures/Studies
6. Peripheral Arterial Disease Rehabilitation
7. Noninvasive Physiologic Studies and Procedures
8. Other Procedures

Most of the cardiovascular codes are either noninvasive or diagnostic in nature. The codes are located in the Medicine section because they do not meet surgical criteria: they do not require incisions, replace a body part, or excise or remove anything, and they do not carry an anesthetic risk because only local anesthesia is normally administered. Many of the codes located in this section are performed by an interventional radiologist or cardiologist, not a surgeon.

An **electrocardiogram (ECG or EKG)** is commonly performed in the physician office. CPT code 93000 is used if the physician owns the ECG equipment and interprets and reports the results. If the physician only interprets the report, 93010 is assigned, with a −26 modifier. Event monitors such as Holter monitors are worn for extended periods of time to record ECG activity; the measurments are stored in the devices.

Another common procedure is **echocardiography,** an ultrasound procedure used to examine the cardiac chambers and valves, the great vessels, and the pericardium. The complete procedure includes interpretation, documentation of clinically relevant findings, and a description of any abnormalities.

A **cardiac catheterization** involves passing a catheter into the heart through a vein or artery to withdraw samples of blood, measure pressures within the heart's chambers or great vessels, and inject contrast media. The catheter, a thin, flexible, hollow tube, is first introduced into the femoral artery in the groin. From there, it is advanced under X-ray guidance (fluoroscopy) through the aorta to the heart. The contrast medium injected into the coronary arteries (as they branch off the aorta) will highlight the course of these vessels when an X-ray is performed so that any coronary blockage or narrowing can be detected.

At least three codes are needed to capture all aspects of a cardiac catheterization: a code for the catheterization (inserting and positioning the catheter), a code for the injection, and a code for the imaging (supervision, interpretation, and report). Codes are differentiated by whether a professional fee or a technical fee is being submitted. The professional component is reported with a −26 modifier unless the physician owns the catheterization lab.

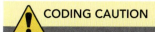

> ### ⚠ CODING CAUTION
>
> **Biopsy with Cardiac Catheterization**
>
> If an endomyocardial biopsy is taken during a cardiac catheterization, it is reported separately in addition to the codes for the cardiac catheterization.

PULMONARY

Physicians as well as respiratory therapists assign codes from the pulmonary section. Pulmonary function tests or studies (PFT) are performed for many reasons: to give preoperative surgical clearance for individuals who are smokers or have histories of breathing problems, to diagnose lung disease, to assess the extent of a patient's pulmonary disability, and to manage or monitor a patient's treatment regimen.

The most common pulmonary test is **spirometry,** which measures the volume of air in the lungs by measuring how much air is expelled from the lung and how quickly it is expelled. Patients are asked to take a deep breath and blow into a machine. Patients with asthma or other problems that obstruct airflow to the lungs require nebulizer treatments, which are commonly performed in the physician office or at home. When a nebulizer treatment is performed in the office, a HCPCS supply code for the medication is also reported.

> **EXAMPLE** A six-year-old boy with reactive airways disease is seen in the pediatrician's office for wheezing and cough. He receives an albuterol nebulizer treatment. The codes are 94640, J7613.

ALLERGY AND CLINICAL IMMUNOLOGY

The Allergy and Clinical Immunology subsection includes many types of allergy testing techniques, such as percutaneous tests, skin end point titrations, patch or application tests, ophthalmic mucous membrane tests, and direct nasal mucous tests. Code selection is based on the type of testing performed and the number of tests (units) performed.

> **EXAMPLE**
> 95024: Intracutaneous (intradermal) tests, sequential and incremental, with allergenic extracts, immediate type reaction, specify number of tests.

Immunotherapy, or immunology, is a process in which an allergic patient can become desensitized to antigens that trigger such allergic responses as rhinitis (nasal congestion), allergic conjunctivitis, asthma, and reactions to insects. Small doses of the allergenic substance are injected weekly. Gradually a protective antibody, also known as immunoglobulin G, is formed to block the allergic reaction. Codes differentiate the physician's both providing and injecting the antigen from his or her simply administering the injection.

NEUROLOGY AND NEUROMUSCULAR PROCEDURES

Codes for sleep studies, nerve conduction studies, and neurostimulator programming are coded with neurology and neuromuscular procedural codes. Selection of codes for the two types of sleep studies—testing

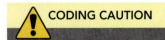
for sleep latency and polysomnography—is based on what stages of sleep are monitored and whether the patient is tested during a full night's rest or during daytime naps. Some of the codes depend on whether **continuous positive airway pressure (CPAP)** is applied. A CPAP device consists of a mask, tubes, and a fan. It uses air pressure to push the tongue forward and open the throat to prevent sleep apnea.

Nerve conduction studies (NCS), electromyography (EMG), electroencephalogram (EEG), and neuromuscular junction (NMJ) are also classified here.

MEDICAL GENETICS AND GENETIC COUNSELING

Genetic testing identifies the likelihood of parents' passing specific genetic diseases or disorders to offspring. Genetic counseling involves interviewing pregnant couples or those considering conceiving about the likelihood of passing genetic disorders such as Down syndrome, cystic fibrosis, and Tay-Sachs disease, to their offspring. In genetic counseling, the family history and family tree are evaluated, medical records are reviewed, genetic tests are ordered, the results are analyzed, and the couple's risk is assessed. Counseling is reported in thirty-minute increments. Only nonphysician genetics counselors may report the codes in this section. If a physician conducts genetic counseling, E/M codes are submitted from the Preventive Medicine section.

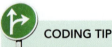

CODING ALERT

CNS Codes Not Used with MMSE

Codes in this section are not used when a physician performs a mini-mental status exam (MMSE). This is part of E/M service provided by the physician and is not reported separately.

CENTRAL NERVOUS SYSTEM ASSESSMENTS AND TESTS

Central nervous system assessments and tests evaluate cognitive function. Cognitive testing is usually performed by a neuropsychologist to measure alertness and level of consciousness, attention, memory, thinking ability, perception, psychomotor behavior, judgment, and speech. Codes in this section are based on total time spent testing, analyzing test results, and preparing a report.

These tests are commonly performed on the elderly and people with Alzheimer's and Parkinson's disease, but they are not limited to these conditions. Code 96110–11 is reported to diagnose developmental delays in children.

CODING TIP

Physician Assessments and Interventions

When a physician performs these services, assign a code from the E/M section, such as a preventive medicine service code.

HEALTH AND BEHAVIOR ASSESSMENT AND INTERVENTION

Health and behavior assessment and intervention codes report procedures used by nonphysicians to identify psychological, behavioral, emotional, cognitive, and social factors relevant to preventing, treating, and managing physical problems. The evaluation is focused on acute or chronic illness, the prevention of future illness or debility, and overall maintenance of health. Codes in this section include evaluation of risk factors and intervention. Services are reported in fifteen-minute increments.

CHEMOTHERAPY ADMINISTRATION

Chemotherapy administration codes are subdivided to describe the method of administration and the technique, whether intramuscular, push intravenous, infusion intravenous, subcutaneous, oral, or push intra-arterial. A separate code is assigned for each method of administration. The CPT guidelines clarify when an E/M service code can be reported in addition to chemotherapy administration and when additional medications can be coded. If medications are administered before or after chemotherapy, they are reported separately using HCPCS supply codes and the appropriate administration code. The catheterization or access to administer chemotherapy is also coded separately.

PHOTODYNAMIC THERAPY

The three photodynamic therapy codes report the application of light for various medical purposes. Note that two of the three are add-on codes.

SPECIAL DERMATOLOGICAL PROCEDURES

Special dermatological procedures are not included in the Integumentary section because they are noninvasive or nonsurgical in nature. These services are usually performed in addition to an E/M service on the same day and therefore require a −25 modifier. Services range from taking pictures of the entire body of a high-risk patient, to monitoring for changes of nevi, to treating skin conditions via photochemotherapy or laser.

PHYSICAL MEDICINE AND REHABILITATION

Physical medicine and rehabilitation services encompass physical therapy, occupational therapy, and wound management. These services are provided by physical therapists and occupational therapists, not by physicians. Before conducting treatment, the therapist first evaluates the patient to determine what mode or modes of therapy are indicated; codes from the evaluation services that begin the code range are reported for this service.

The notation *direct one-on-one contact* means that the therapist must conduct the treatment and be in constant attendance, not treating any other patient at the same time. Some services require constant attendance by the therapist, while others do not.

MEDICAL NUTRITION, ACUPUNCTURE, OSTEOPATHIC MANIPULATIVE TREATMENT, AND CHIROPRACTIC MANIPULATIVE TREATMENT

Codes in these subsections report other medical interventions. Most are either time-based or are selected by the number of body regions treated.

SPECIAL SERVICES AND REPORTS

The procedures coded in the range of 99000–99090 provide the reporting physician with the means of identifying the completion of special reports and services that are adjuncts to the basic services rendered. The specific number assigned indicates the special circumstances under which a basic procedure is performed. For example, when a specimen is obtained in the office and is transferred to the lab that will analyze it, 99000 is assigned in addition to the code for the collection of the specimen. Educational supplies, educational services, medical testimony, travel, and preparation of special letters or reports are also located here.

Payment for these procedures varies among payers. It is important to check with the payer before using the codes. Also, payers may request the use of a more-specific HCPCS Level II code.

OTHER SERVICES AND PROCEDURES

Codes in this subsection include procedures that do not fall naturally into any other category.

- 99170: anogenital exam in child for suspected trauma
- 99173: screening visual acuity test not part of a general ophthalmologic service or E/M
- 99175: administration of ipecac to cause emesis and empty the stomach of poison
- 99183: hyperbaric oxygen therapy supervision

ASSIGNING MEDICINE CODES

As shown in Figure 9.4, medicine codes are located by identifying the key word or main service provided, such as *dialysis* or *immunization*. These are the main terms. Start by determining the type of services provided. If medications are administered, the specific medicine as well as the method of administration must be known.

EXAMPLE   Diabetic nutrition and meal planning education, 1 hour, 5 patients. Following the flow chart, the first step is to determine the type of service. In this example, education is the type of service, so this term is located in the CPT index. Next, based on the index entry, you must determine whether this was a group or individual service. Five patients were instructed. Finally, the code description states that this service is based on thirty-minute increments of time. We must account for one hour or sixty minutes of time. The correct coding is 98961, 98961.

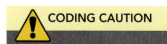

Checkpoint 9.5

Assign the medicine codes for the following procedures.

1. Electroencephalography (EEG) monitoring of greater than one hour _____

2. Active tetanus toxoid immunization _____

3. Professional services and provision of extract for single injection allergen immunotherapy _____ _____

4. Thirty minutes face-to-face with the patient for individual behavior-modifying outpatient psychotherapy _____

5. IV infusion of a dehydrated patient in the doctor's office _____

6. Visual acuity screening _____

7. Nurse visit to a assisted-living facility for colostomy care _____

8. Dialysis training, one session _____

9. Fitting of bifocal lenses _____

10. IM chemotherapy administration _____

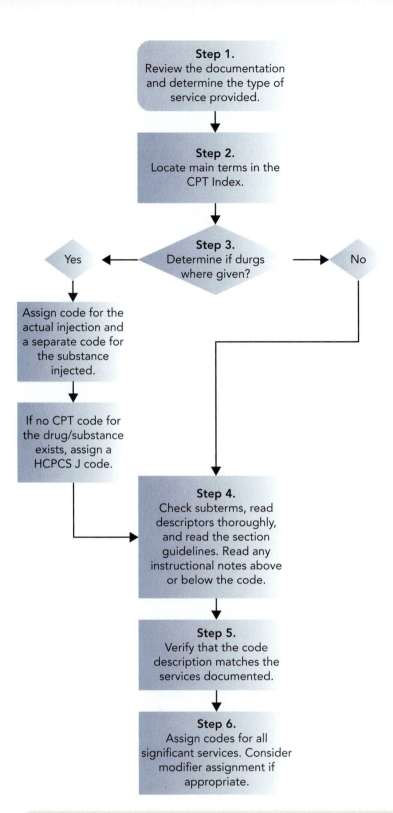

Step 1.
Review the documentation and determine the type of service provided.

Step 2.
Locate main terms in the CPT Index.

Step 3.
Determine if durgs where given?

Yes

No

Assign code for the actual injection and a separate code for the substance injected.

If no CPT code for the drug/substance exists, assign a HCPCS J code.

Step 4.
Check subterms, read descriptors thoroughly, and read the section guidelines. Read any instructional notes above or below the code.

Step 5.
Verify that the code description matches the services documented.

Step 6.
Assign codes for all significant services. Consider modifier assignment if appropriate.

FIGURE 9.4
Medicine Code Assignment Flow Chart

1. The Radiology section has seven subsections organized according to method or type of radiology and its purpose. Codes in this section begin with the number 7. Coders must read key guidelines and notes at the beginning of the section as well as those in the subsections and in parentheses. Many modifiers may be used with radiology procedure codes. For facility reporting, two modifiers commonly apply: one to distinguish the facility (technical) charges from the physician (professional) charges and a second to describe the body part being examined.

2. Coders must identify the number of radiological views taken in order to properly assign the correct code. To assign a code identified as *complete*, all views of that specific area must be taken.

3. A complete code in the Radiology and the Pathology and Laboratory sections often has component parts. The technical component (TC) is the allocation of staff or the technologist, use of equipment, supplies, and related services. The professional component (PC) encompasses the physician's time and skill in reading and interpreting the test and providing a written report rendering an opinion, advice, or assessment of findings.

4. Many radiology codes are selected on the basis of whether contrast was introduced. Oral and rectal contrast administration alone does not qualify as a study *with contrast* because the phrase with contrast represents contrast material administered intravascularly or directly into a joint.

5. A screening service is performed to detect a disease or condition in the absence of signs and symptoms. A diagnostic service is performed to assess the extent of an already-diagnosed disease or condition.

6. Codes in the Pathology and Laboratory section begin with 8. This section is organized by the type of test performed and then alphabetically within each section. Guidelines are located at the beginning of the section, and instructional notes appear in many of the subsections. There are two types of pathology consultation codes: clinical pathology and surgical pathology. Medicare does not allow a provider who does not perform the test to report the pathology and laboratory code. A code for only the venipuncture should be reported (only once, even if more than one specimen is drawn). Other payers allow physicians to report the laboratory code with a −90 modifier when specimens are sent off-site for analysis.

7. When assigning codes for a test associated with an organ or disease panel, all tests included as part of the panel must have been performed. If not, each test must be coded separately rather than submitting the panel code.

8. Medicine is the sixth major section of CPT, located immediately before the Category II and III codes. The section is divided into more than thirty subsections, which are arranged by specialty areas or type of service. Several have special instructions that are applicable to their code ranges, particularly Psychiatry, Dialysis, Cardiovascular, and Neurology. Codes in the Medicine section begin with the number 9 and include some E/M codes.

9. When coding for immunizations, two codes are required: one for the administrative and clinical staff services of the actual injection and a second for the substance injected. Administration can be intradermal, intramuscular, percutaneous, subcutaneous, intranasal, or oral.

10. Correct assignment of CPT radiology, pathology and laboratory, and medicine codes with appropriate modifiers follows the basic code-assignment process of reading the complete documentation, locating main terms in the CPT Index, and selecting the correct code from the range in the CPT section, paying attention to the language, indention, and other instructions provided for correct CPT coding.

Review Questions: Chapter 9

Match the key terms with their definitions.

a. fluoroscopy _____
b. analyte _____
c. biofeedback _____
d. ultrasound _____
e. assay _____
f. administration _____
g. hemodialysis _____
h. charge description master _____
i. technical component _____
j. immunotherapy _____

1. Uses ultrahigh-frequency sound waves for diagnostic scanning

2. Encompasses the allocation of staff or use of equipment

3. Uses a continuous low-level X-ray beam to view the body in motion

4. Method by which a drug or chemical is introduced into the body

5. Process in which an allergic patient can become desensitized to antigens

6. Chemical or substance being measured or analyzed

7. Testing drug purity or absorption level in the body

8. A computerized master list of hospital services with associated fees and codes

9. Circulation of blood through an artificial kidney machine to clean the blood

10. Method in which people are trained to improve their current state of health by recognizing signals from their own bodies

Decide whether each statement is true or false.

1. The diagnostic ultrasound definition of an A-mode implies a one-dimensional ultrasonic measurement procedure. **T or F**

2. The time descriptors for fluoroscopic exam codes apply to the actual time the fluoroscopic unit is turned on. **T or F**

3. X-rays are considered packaged in the service (global) when the physician owns the equipment and provides a report of the results. **T or F**

4. Nuclear medicine involves imaging that uses injection or infusion of radio elements to allow visualization of a specific area. **T or F**

5. The abbreviation *PC* stands for professional charge. **T or F**

6. For situations in which contrast is provided orally, codes with contrast are chosen. **T or F**

7. Unlisted procedure codes are listed under their specific subsections. **T or F**

8. The −26 modifier reports the professional and technical component of a procedure. **T or F**

9. When an additional test is performed with tests specifically indicated for a particular organ or disease panel, the additional test should be reported separately in addition to the panel code. **T or F**

10. Pathology and laboratory services are provided by a physician only. **T or F**

11. The codes in the Surgical Pathology section represent levels of difficulty of the particular specimen examined. **T or F**

12. Pathologists never examine people but rather examine specimens obtained from people. **T or F**

13. Each cardiac catheterization procedure requires at least three codes. **T or F**

14. It is appropriate to report 99213 and 90819 for an ophthalmological office visit. **T or F**

15. Dialysis procedures are determined by age and number of days of service. **T or F**

Select the letter that best completes the statement or answers the question.

1. What does the abbreviation *S&I* mean?
   a. search and intervention
   b. supervision of iodine
   c. supervision and interpretation
   d. supervision of injection

2. Two views of the thumb and two views of the second digit on each hand are coded
   a. 73130–50
   b. 73120–FA, 73120–F5, 73140–F1, 73140–F6
   c. 73120–50, 73140–50
   d. 73120–LT–RT, 71340–LT–RT

3. When a diagnostic mammogram is performed on the same day as a screening mammogram, which modifier is used on the diagnostic mammogram?
   a. −76   c. −22
   b. −GA   d. −GH

4. Ophthalmic ultrasound of the eye with amplitude quantification is coded
   a. 76511   c. 76516
   b. 76513   d. 76519

5. The code for the injection for a shoulder arthrogram with supervision and interpretation is
   a. 73020   c. 73040
   b. 73050   d. 23350

6. A complete cervical X-ray with flexion and oblique views is coded
   a. 72010   c. 72050
   b. 72052   d. 72040

7. An X-ray of the paranasal sinuses, two views is coded
   a. 70160
   b. 70250
   c. 70210
   d. None of the above

8. A CT scan of the lumbar spine without contrast and with contrast is coded
   a. 72131, 72132
   b. 72120
   c. 72100
   d. 72133

9. A hysterosalpingography, S&I is coded
   a. 74740
   b. 58340
   c. 58345
   d. 74742

10. A barium enema with KUB is coded
    a. 74246
    b. 74270
    c. 74280
    d. 74241

11. A lab perfroms a hepatic function panel with the following components: albumin, bilirubin (total and direct), alkaline phosphatase, total protein, SGOT, SGPT, and GGT. How is this coded?
    a. 80076
    b. 80076, 82977
    c. code each test separately
    d. none of the above

12. Code a microscopic examination of urine sediment performed in the office of a physician who has a CLIA waiver on file.
    a. 81000
    b. 81000–26
    c. 81002
    d. 81015

13. The source of the specimen for a chemistry test coded to 82000 through 84999 is
    a. urine
    b. blood
    c. sputum
    d. any source

14. Code a glucose tolerance test performed over a four-hour period, with blood samples taken every thirty minutes.
    a. 82952
    b. 82951
    c. 82950
    d. 82951, 82952, 82952, 82952, 82952, 82952

15. A patient is being tested for crack cocaine abuse. What would the lab report?
    a. 80103
    b. 80801
    c. 82520
    d. 82486

16. A urine pregnancy test performed in the office using Hybritech ICON (visual color comparison) is coded
    a.   84703
    b.   81025, 26415
    c.   84702
    d.   81025

17. A stool culture for Sal*monella* is coded
    a.   87102
    b.   87046
    c.   87045
    d.   86768

18. A Pap smear, screening by automated system with manual rescreening under physician supervision is coded
    a.   88166
    b.   88154
    c.   88175
    d.   88148

19. A pathological gross and microscopic examination of the entire left testicle is coded
    a.   88302
    b.   88304
    c.   88305
    d.   88307

20. For a pathology consultation, the physician reviews complete medical records and provides a written report. Which code is reported?
    a.   88355
    b.   80500
    c.   88321
    d.   80502

21. A patient suffering from asthma presents to the clinic for a pulmonary examination. An evaluation is performed in which the patient exhales and the air is measured. Total time and capacity are recorded. The patient is then given a bronchodilator, and the air is measured again. Select the CPT code for this procedure.
    a.   94150
    b.   94060
    c.   94250
    d.   94010

22. Which of the following identifies antibodies that have been "manufactured" by a person in response to a specific disease and that are injected into someone else who was exposed to the disease but is not immune?
    a.   immunization
    b.   immune globulin
    c.   vaccination
    d.   none of the above

23. A Doppler venous ultrasound, right leg is coded
    a.   93965
    b.   93922
    c.   93965–52
    d.   93922–RT

24. Scratch tests for 5 trees, 3 venom are coded
    a. 95010 x 8
    b. 95010, 95015
    c. 95044 x 8
    d. none of the above

25. A home infusion of peritoneal dialysis, two hours is coded
    a. 90945
    b. 90999
    c. 99601
    d. none of the above

26. A cardiac stress test, tracing only, is coded
    a. 93005
    b. 93041
    c. 93017
    d. 93012

27. The injection of immune globulin, IM is coded
    a. 90283
    b. 90281
    c. 90399, 90772
    d. 90281, 90772

28. The analysis of a dual chamber pacemaker at rest and during activity without reprogramming is coded
    a. 93734
    b. 93733
    c. 93731
    d. 93732

29. An EEG all-night recording is coded
    a. 95950
    b. 95827
    c. 95816
    d. 95822

30. Electromyography, left arm is coded
    a. 95860
    b. 95872
    c. 95870
    d. 95861

Answer the following questions.

1. When a laboratory drug test is qualitative, it measures the _____ of the drug.

2. How many levels of surgical pathology are there? _____

3. Which panel contains the following tests: uric acid, sed rate, FANA, and Rh factor? _____
_____

4. Name the two modes and two scan definitions of diagnostic ultrasound.
   _____   _____

   _____   _____

BUILDING CODING SKILLS: RADIOLOGY

Case 9.1

Assign the appropriate radiology codes.

1. X-ray, left elbow with four views, complete _____

2. Thyroid imaging with vascular flow _____

3. Limited B scan abdominal echography _____

4. Unlisted CPT code for therapeutic radiology clinical treatment planning _____

5. Echography, chest, B-scan and real time with image documentation

    _____

6. Therapeutic radiology simulation-aided field setting; complex

    _____

7. Adrenal imaging, medulla _____

8. Chest X-ray with two views of lateral and frontal with fluoroscopy

    _____

9. Bilateral screening mammography in a forty-eight year old _____

10. CT scan of the head with contrast material by radiology clinic (include modifier) _____

11. AP view of the pelvis and AP and oblique views of the hips _____

12. Ultrasound at twenty-three weeks gestation to determine placental location _____

13. Injection of contrast for ankle arthrography reported by the physician who performed both the procedure and the interpretation

    _____

14. A fifty-year-old post-hysterectomy female taking Prednisone undergoes a dual energy X-ray absorptiometry body composition exam. The patient lies on the exam table, and the central DEXA unit measures bone density of the hips and lower spine. _____

    _____

15. Myelography, cervical; *complete* with injection procedure _____

    _____

16. A patient diagnosed with breast cancer undergoes mastectomy and chemotherapy. She receives radiation treatment delivery to the right breast area at 4 MeV. _____

    _____

17. A patient is diagnosed with inoperable endobronchial tumor. Following localization radiographs, HDR brachytherapy treatment is administered. A remote afterloader guides the iridium-192 source into position. _____

BUILDING CODING SKILLS: PATHOLOGY AND LABORATORY

Case 9.2

Assign the appropriate pathology and laboratory codes.

1. A patient suffers from chronic kidney disease and is experiencing shortness of breath. The physician orders a blood gas measurement along with pH and CO_2 _____

2. Clinical diagnosis: torn meniscus. Tissue submitted: meniscus, left knee. Gross and microscopic examination performed. _____

3. Obstetric panel _____

4. Urinalysis; microscopic only _____

5. Testosterone; total _____

6. Creatinine; blood _____

7. Semen analysis; complete _____

8. Peripheral blood smear interpretation by physician with a written report _____

9. Amniocentesis for alpha-fetoprotein analysis _____

10. Gross and microscopic examination of prostate, radical resection by pathologist _____

11. Examination of bone marrow biopsy _____

12. Gross and microscopic examination of the kidney specimen from a total resection procedure _____

13. A parent brings a child with a sore throat to the pediatrician's office. The physician suspects a strep A infection and performs an analysis using a rapid identification diagnosis kit. _____

14. A patient who is six months post-heart valve replacement is prescribed Coumadin. He presents for his monthly prothrombin time and activated partial thromboplastin time tests. _____

    _____

15. A patient is seen in the ER for rapid heart beat. He is currently taking digoxin, but the patient is a poor historian. The physician orders a test to identify the amount of digoxin in the patient's blood.

    _____

    _____

16. A woman is convicted of vehicular manslaughter and is sentenced to twelve months in prison. Her child must be placed in the custody of the father. The woman indicates that she is unsure of who the father is, and she provides two names to authorities. The judge orders paternity testing on both men. _____

    _____

    _____

17. A patient has been complaining of feeling bloated and suffers from frequent constipation. The patient has a family history of colon polyps. The doctor wants to rule out colorectal disease and performs the guaiac smear fecal occult blood test, two determinations. _____

    _____

    _____

BUILDING CODING SKILLS: MEDICINE

Case 9.3

Assign the appropriate medicine codes.

1. ENT (otolaryngologic) examination under anesthesia _____

2. Hearing, language, and speech evaluation _____

3. A fifty-nine-year-old female presents to her family practitioner's office for her annual flu vaccine. Split virus is injected. _____
_____

4. Postop follow-up visit _____

5. The use of a surgical tray or supplies in the office _____

6. Comprehensive eye examination, new patient _____

7. Intralesional chemotherapy administration; eight lesions injected _____

8. ESRD services for a fifty-five-year-old male consecutively provided over a full month in an outpatient setting _____

9. Physician-supervised cardiovascular stress test on a female with recent ECG changes _____

10. Injection of the MMR virus vaccine, live _____

11. Interactive group psychotherapy for a six-patient group _____

12. Application of hot pack to the neck and knee; manual electrical stimulation, fifteen minutes _____

13. Esophageal intubation and collection of cytology specimens _____

14. Simple pulmonary stress test _____

15. Hemodialysis procedure with one physician evaluation, inpatient _____

16. Intracutaneous tests with allergy extracts, immediate type reaction, five tests _____

17. Nasal function study _____

18. Awake and drowsy EEG and photic stimulation in the clinic _____
_____

19. An office employee hand-delivers a specimen from the physician's office to a lab. _____

20. Individual patient medical nutrition therapy reassessment and intervention, thirty minutes duration _____

21. Nurse visit to patient's home for urinary catheter change _____
_____

22. A war veteran fitted for a below-the-knee prosthesis receives leg prosthetic training by a therapist in the PT department for forty-five minutes. _____

23. School officials ask a psychologist to test a nineteen-year-old to assess his mental stability. The psychologist spends two hours administering the Thematic Apperception Test (TAT), in which the patient tells stories about pictures, and a sentence completion test.

24. A patient visits her audiologist for her six-month binaural hearing aid exam. The audiologist inspects and cleans her hearing aids and checks the power. _____

25. A patient who underwent amputation of the left pinky toe is experiencing slow healing and excoriation. The physician orders wound debridement with abrasion and wet-to-dry dressings of the left foot, three sessions. _____

Researching the Internet

1. Visit the site of the American Society for Therapeutic Radiology and Oncology at www.astro.org/HealthPolicy/RadiationOncologyCoding/CodingFAQ/documents/brxyguide.pdf to learn more about brachytherapy. Read the information, and explain the difference between low-dose and high-dose therapy. What coding tips are provided for coding interstitial brachytherapy. What items does the site note that Medicare does not pay for?

2. Visit the Medical Newswire online newsletter at http://medicalnewswire.com/artman/publish/article_7124.shtml, and report on the varying requirements for reporting more than one radiation treatment per day.

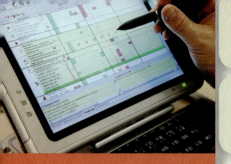

HCPCS

LEARNING OUTCOMES

After studying this chapter, you should be able to:

1. Explain the purpose of the HCPCS code set.

2. Differentiate between HCPCS Level I (CPT) and HCPCS Level II codes.

3. Identify circumstances under which codes from both HCPCS Level I and HCPCS Level II are required.

4. Compare permanent and temporary HCPCS codes.

5. Describe the content and organization of the index, the Table of Drugs, and the main text in HCPCS.

6. Describe the purpose and correct use of HCPCS modifiers, including the ABN modifiers.

7. Choose the correct medication code based on the route of administration and the amount of medication administered.

8. Apply rules for choosing which level of HCPCS codes to assign.

9. Discuss the sources of information to keep up to date on current HCPCS codes.

10. Assign HCPCS codes with appropriate modifiers based on procedural statements.

Key Terms

advance beneficiary notice (ABN)

certificate of medical necessity (CMN)

CMS HCPCS Workgroup

Current Dental Terminology (CDT)

DME Medicare Administrative Contractors (DME MACs)

durable medical equipment (DME)

durable medical equipment, prosthetics, orthotics, and supplies (DMEPOS)

Durable Medical Equipment Regional Carriers (DMERCS)

enterally

Food and Drug Administration (FDA)

inhalant solution (INH)

injection (INJ)

intra-arterial (IA)

intramuscular (IM)

intrathecal (IT)

intravenous (IV)

Level I

Level II

Local Coverage Determinations (LCDs)

Medicare Carrier Manual (MCM)

National Coverage Determinations (NCDs)

Notice of Exclusions from Medicare Benefits (NEMB)

other routes (OTH)

parenterally

permanent codes

Statistical Analysis Durable Medical Equipment Regional Carriers (SADMERC)

subcutaneous (SC)

Table of Drugs

temporary codes

transitional pass-through payments

unclassified HCPCS code

various routes (VAR)

Chapter Outline

History and Purpose of HCPCS

Permanent and Temporary Codes

Features of HCPCS Code Books

HCPCS Code Sections

Modifiers

Assigning HCPCS Codes

HCPCS Coding Resources

The national codes for products, supplies, and those services not included in CPT are in the Healthcare Common Procedure Coding System (HCPCS). Establishing the medical necessity of these items for reimbursement is handled through the correct coding process for assigning HCPCS codes, as explained in this chapter.

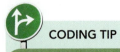

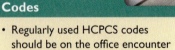
History and Purpose of HCPCS

The HCFA Common Procedure Coding System (HCPCS) was developed in 1983 to standardize codes on health care claims for the Medicare program. The Centers for Medicare and Medicaid Services (CMS), then called the Health Care Finance Administration (HCFA), developed a three-level coding system for services and procedures provided to Medicare patients. In 2002, when HCFA changed its name to the Centers for Medicare and Medicaid Services (CMS), the code set was given its current name, the Healthcare Common Procedure Coding System, abbreviated as HCPCS, which is pronounced hick-picks.

HCPCS has two main parts: Level I and Level II. HCPCS **Level I** is CPT (Current Procedural Terminology), maintained by the American Medical Association (AMA), with codes that are used primarily to identify medical services and procedures furnished by physicians and other health care professionals. CPT does not include codes needed to separately report medical items or services that are regularly billed by suppliers other than physicians. **Level II** of HCPCS fills this need. Level II is a standardized coding system that is used primarily to identify products, supplies, and services not included in the CPT codes, such as ambulance services and durable medical equipment, prosthetics, orthotics, and supplies when used outside a physician office. Physician offices also use the codes for supplies provided to government insurance program beneficiaries, such as Medicare and Medicaid patients.

HCPCS TODAY

In October 2003, the Department of Health and Human Services, acting under HIPAA, authorized CMS to maintain, update, and distribute HCPCS Level II codes. A specific CMS HCPCS Workgroup, made up of representatives from CMS, consultants from federal agencies, and representatives from private insurance agencies, manages this process while also providing input about what is necessary to meet each party's operational needs.

HCPCS codes are submitted to insurance carriers by physicians' offices, facilities, and other providers such as medical supply companies. They are required for reporting services, injections, materials, and supplies to federally funded programs (Medicare, Medicaid, TRICARE, and CHAMPVA). Also, many private insurance carriers accept and at times mandate the use of HCPCS codes for certain services and supplies; the coding rules appear in the contracts between providers and payers.

HCPCS codes can have a significant effect on the financial bottom line for practices and facilities. Revenue is lost each time the health care claim does not show a HCPCS code for a supply that is used or an injection that is given. For example, if Medicare is billed for an injection using only a CPT code, the office will be paid for the injection only, not for the drug administered.

Physicians and facilities most commonly use the HCPCS codes for medical and surgical supplies and injections. Other providers, such as skilled nursing facilities (SNF), use many of the HCPCS codes that describe equipment sold or rented as durable medical equipment and medical appliances provided by supply companies.

Table 10.1 Comparison of HCPCS Levels I and II

Level	Published_by	Code Format	Modifiers	Use	Updated
Level I: CPT	AMA	Five-digit numeric, except for Category II and Category III codes. Codes begin with a number.	Two-digit numerical	Physician procedures and services; facility outpatient procedures and services	Annually; some codes more often
Level II: HCPCS national	CMS (formerly HCFA)	Five-digit alphanumeric codes begin with letter A through V.	Two-digit alphanumeric or alpha	Physician and nonphysician providers; supplies, drugs, DME, ambulance.	Annually

PURPOSE OF HCPCS

HCPCS is a system for identifying medical services and supplies, not a payment methodology. The fact that a HCPCS code is available for assignment does not guarantee payment for the item. Decisions about coverage and allowed amounts are made by carriers and are independent of the decision for adding, deleting, or revising a HCPCS code.

Physicians, facilities, and suppliers select codes for items that they bill to insurance carriers. Most often, the HCPCS code represents the actual supply of an item, not the professional service or procedure for applying or inserting it, for which a code is selected from HCPCS Level I (CPT). Table 10.1 compares these two levels.

There are well over four thousand HCPCS codes for products and supplies. The code descriptions represent the definitions of the items or services provided. The descriptors do not refer to specific products by brand name or trade name; items can be located only by type of product or supply.

Level II codes are used to file for services of physicians and nonphysicians (for example, physician's assistants, nurse-practitioners, audiologists, speech pathologists, and chiropractors), surgical supplies, medications administered, ambulance transports, and durable medical equipment. **Durable medical equipment (DME)** is ordered by a physician, used at home to serve a medical purpose, and designed to withstand repeated use. Examples of DME include hospital beds, walkers, wheelchairs, transfer benches with commode seats, and oxygen tents. An example of a DME listing in the HCPCS book is shown in Figure 10.1. Medicare does not consider medical supplies of an expendable nature, such as bandages, rubber gloves, and irrigating kits, to be DME.

Medicare has four **Durable Medical Equipment Regional Carriers** or **DMERCs,** contractors that process Medicare claims for **durable medical equipment, prosthetics, orthotics, and supplies (DMEPOS).** DMEPOS dealers provide patients with durable medical equipment and supplies, and DMEPOS claims for items provided to patients by dealers or by physicians are sent to regional **DME Medicare Administrative Contractors (DME MACs)** that have contracts with CMS. Each DME MAC covers a specific geographical region of the country and is responsible for processing DMEPOS claims.

When a health care provider treats a patient and provides DME, the provider prepare two claims, each of which must be sent to a different location for processing.

FIGURE 10.1
Sample DME Listing from HCPCS

E0250	Hospital bed, fixed height, with any type side rail, with mattress
E0251	Hospital bed, fixed height, with any type side rail, without mattress
E0255	Hospital bed, variable height, hi-lo, with any type side rail, with mattress
E0256	Hospital bed, variable height, hi-lo, with any type side rail, without mattress
E0260	Hospital bed, semi-electric (head and foot adjustment), with any type side rail, with mattress
E0261	Hospital bed, semi-electric (head and foot adjustment), with any type side rail, without mattress
E0265	Hospital bed, total electric (head, foot, and height adjustment), with any type side rail, with mattress
E0266	Hospital bed, total electric (head, foot, and height adjustment), with any type side rail, without mattress

COMPLIANCE GUIDELINE

Certificate of Medical Necessity

Before billing certain items or services to a DMERC, the supplier must have received a signed **certificate of medical necessity (CMN)** from the treating physician. A CMN communicates required information about medical necessity, and it must be maintained by the supplier and available if the DMERC requests additional documentation to support the claim.

EXAMPLE A patient is seen in the podiatrist's office for diabetic foot care. The physician issues the patient a special diabetic shoe that is directly formed and compression molded to the patient's foot. The claim for the E/M service goes to the local Medicare carrier claims processing center, and a separate claim for the shoe (HCPCS code A5510) is sent to the regional MAC claims processing center for that area.

HCPCS CODE FORMAT

HCPCS Level II codes are five alphanumeric characters in length. Each code begins with a letter from *A* through *V* followed by four numbers.

EXAMPLE J1100 is the code for the injection of dexamethasone acetate, 1 mg.

Like CPT, HCPCS Level II has its own set of codes and a unique set of modifiers. Discontinued (deleted) procedure codes and modifiers appear in the HCPCS file for four years to facilitate claim processing. Following the deletion, a deleted code also appears in the printed HCPCS book with a line drawn through it for one year.

EXAMPLE E0192, low pressure and positioning equalization pad, for wheelchair, was deleted in 2004 but was printed in the 2005 edition of the HCPCS book like this: E0192 Low pressure and positioning equalization pad, for wheelchair.

Checkpoint 10.1

Determine whether the following codes are CPT (HCPCS Level I) or HCPCS (Level II national) codes.

Examples:

28285 CPT

A4649 HCPCS

1. 15000 _____
2. A0430 _____
3. 72040 _____
4. J0550 _____
5. 69990 _____
6. E0992 _____

Permanent and Temporary Codes

HCPCS national Level II codes are categorized depending on the purpose of the codes and on who is responsible for establishing and maintaining them. The **CMS HCPCS Workgroup** is a code advisory committee made up of representatives from CMS and other government agencies. Its role is to identify services for which new codes are needed.

PERMANENT CODES

The CMS HCPCS Workgroup maintains the **permanent codes** that are available for use by all government and private payers. No code changes can be made unless a majority of the group's members agree. This panel is responsible for making decisions about changes to existing permanent codes, including additions, revisions, and deletions of alphanumeric codes.

Advisers from private payers provide input to the CMS HCPCS Workgroup. The **Statistical Analysis Durable Medical Equipment Regional Carriers (SADMERC)** association also participates. SADMERC is responsible for providing suppliers and manufacturers of devices, drugs, and supplies with guidance and assistance in determining the appropriate HCPCS Level II codes for their products.

TEMPORARY CODES

Temporary codes, which begin with C, G, H, K, Q, S, and T, are added, changed, and deleted on a quarterly basis. They serve the purpose of meeting the immediate needs of a particular payer. Once established and approved, temporary codes are usually implemented within ninety days. During this period, instructions for providers are prepared and issued, the new code is entered into CMS's and the contractors' computer systems, and bulletins and newsletters with implementation information and assistance are sent to suppliers. The changes are also posted to the HCPCS website. Coders who regularly use these codes must stay up to date with the new and deleted items. Temporary codes may later be given permanent status if they are widely used; otherwise, they can remain temporary indefinitely.

Features of HCPCS Code Books

HCPCS code books have varying features, such as color coding; general instructions for use; guidelines for each section; symbols to identify deleted codes, new codes, quantity alert, and age and sex edits; and appendixes. At the beginning of each section is a short paragraph with a description of the purpose of the section.

HCPCS INDEX AND TABULAR SECTIONS

The HCPCS index is arranged alphabetically, with the main term in bold print followed by the HCPCS Level II code. The listing of codes— the equivalent of the ICD Tabular List and the CPT sections—is organized alphabetically by the code range.

SPECIAL FEATURES: APPENDIXES

It depends on the publisher, but there are usually several appendixes in the HCPCS book. Most code books include a Table of Drugs that presents drugs in alphabetical order, followed by each drug's dosage, the way it is administered (such as intravenously), and the HCPCS code. Some books include sections listing specific modifiers, abbreviations, and acronyms; payers that accept Level II codes; Medicare coverage issues; and *Medicare Carrier Manual* references. The **Medicare Carrier Manual (MCM)** directs Medicare payers on coverage of services based on the two levels of coverage guidance (as explained in the Reimbursement Review on pages 428–429).

Some publishers, such as the American Medical Association (AMA), use color coding to indicate non-Medicare-covered codes, special coverage instructions, and codes with carrier discretion. Legends explaining the colors and symbols are located at the bottom of the page. For example, Appendix 4 in the AMA's publication has detailed coverage guidelines and instructions for code use. The abbreviation *MED* followed by a number references the web-based *Medicare National Coverage Determinations* manual.

EXAMPLE
E0782 MED: 100-3, 280.14: Infusion pump, implantable, non-programmable.

The words and numbers following the code indicate that a national coverage determination applies and that the coder should read and follow the guideline in publication 100-3, *Medicare National Coverage Determinations*, section 280.14.

SYMBOLS

Symbols in HCPCS are similar to those in CPT, although they can be located to the left of the code as well as to the right of the code description. Coders must pay close attention to the color coding and symbols, using the legends at the bottom of pages to guide their code selection. Table 10.2 lists some common HCPCS symbols.

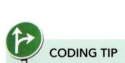

CODING TIP

HCPCS Code Book Selection

Review copies of several HCPCS books from different publishers before selecting the book that is easiest for you to use.

INTERNET RESOURCE

Medicare Carrier Manual and Transmittals on New Coverage Decisions for Part B

www.cms.hhs.gov/manuals

Table 10.2 HCPCS Symbols

Symbol	Description	Example
A	Adult-only service	D1205: Topical application of fluoride—adult
M	Maternity only	E0602: Breast pump, manual, any type
P	Pediatrics	L3214: Benesch boot, pair, junior
I	Infant	L3201: Orthopedic shoe, Oxford with supinator or pronator, infant
▲	Revised code	*Changes annually*
⊘	SNF excluded	E0954: Semi-pneumatic caster, each
MED	Pub 100/NCD reference	E0480: Percussor, electric or pneumatic, home model
♿	DMEPOS paid	E0618: Apnea monitor, without recording feature
☑	Quantity alert	L4205: Repair of orthotic device, labor component, per 15 minutes
●	New code	*Changes annually*
○	Reinstated code	C2622: Prosthesis, penile, non-inflatable
A - Y	APC status indicator	L5684: Addition to lower extremity, below knee, fork strap
♀	Female only	J7303: Contraceptive supply, hormone containing vaginal ring, each
♂	Male only	E0325: Urinal; male, jug-type, any material

Using the current HCPCS book, write the notations that appear for the codes below. Describe the action taken by Medicare in the column titled "Alert/Action" (designating Medicare notification or action since the last publication). If information on coverage is supplied, list it in the column titled "Coverage"). Look at the color coding, symbols, and instructional notes.

Code	Alert/Action	Coverage
Example:		
J9160	K̲ ̲A̲P̲C̲ ̲S̲t̲a̲t̲u̲s̲ ̲i̲n̲d̲i̲c̲a̲t̲o̲r̲ ̲f̲o̲r̲ ̲o̲u̲t̲p̲a̲t̲i̲e̲n̲t̲ ̲ ̲p̲r̲o̲s̲p̲e̲c̲t̲i̲v̲e̲ ̲p̲a̲y̲m̲e̲n̲t̲ ̲s̲y̲s̲t̲e̲m̲ ☑Q̲u̲a̲n̲t̲i̲t̲y̲ ̲a̲l̲e̲r̲t̲	Y̲e̲l̲l̲o̲w̲ ̲h̲i̲g̲h̲l̲i̲g̲h̲t̲:̲ ̲c̲o̲v̲e̲r̲a̲g̲e̲ ̲a̲t̲ ̲c̲a̲r̲r̲i̲e̲r̲ ̲d̲i̲s̲c̲r̲e̲t̲i̲o̲n̲
1. J9390	_____	_____
2. L3217	_____	_____
3. A6206	_____	_____

HCPCS Code Sections

HCPCS Level II classifies medical products and supplies into categories for ease of coding and processing claims. The first character of each alphanumeric code identifies the category. Some categories are easy to remember, such as *D* for dental and *M* for medical services, but the letters used for most sections do not correlate with the first characters in the section titles. For example, *A* identifies the section on medical and surgical supplies.

SECTION A: TRANSPORTATION SERVICES INCLUDING AMBULANCE, MEDICAL AND SURGICAL SUPPLIES (A0000–A9999)

Codes for ambulance services, chiropractic services, and medical and surgical supplies are located in section A. Transportation services include ground and air transportation and ancillary transportation-related fees.

EXAMPLE
A0429: Ambulance service, basic life support, emergency transport (BLS-emergency).

Ambulance transportation services require single-digit origin and destination modifiers, which are listed at the beginning of section A. The first modifier indicates the origin (where patient was transported from) and the second is the destination (where patient was transported to).

HCPCS code A4550 is commonly used for surgical tray use for minor procedures performed in a physician office. If the payer does not recognize HCPCS codes for medical or surgical supplies, CPT code 99070 is used. Facilities typically use A4649 for miscellaneous supplies and L8699 for implants surgically placed.

INTERNET RESOURCE

Notice of Exclusions from Medicare Benefits Form

www.cms.hhs.gov/BNI/ Downloads/CMS20007English.pdf

BILLING TIP

NEMB or ABN?

NEMB	Service not covered under Medicare.
ABN	Medicare does not consider a service reasonable and necessary in this situation.

INTERNET RESOURCE

Advance Beneficiary Notice Form

www.cms.hhs.gov/cmsforms/ downloads/cmsr-131-g.pdf

Medicare Coverage Compliance

The Centers for Medicare and Medicaid Services (CMS) states that it is responsible for promoting healthcare services and delivery for its beneficiaries and maintaining payment processes that pay claims only for covered, medically necessary services, at correct payment amounts, and in a timely manner. Medicare coverage is regulated by federal laws that specify what procedures to treat conditions and illnesses are reimbursed, as well as what screening tests are paid.

For reimbursement, Medicare services must be covered and must meet Medicare's medical necessity criteria. To be considered medically necessary, a treatment must be

- Appropriate for the symptoms or diagnoses of the illness or injury (that is, in line with clinical practice standards)

- Not an elective procedure

- Not an experimental or investigational procedure

- An essential treatment; not performed for the patient's convenience

- Delivered at the most appropriate level that can safely and effectively be administered to the patient

Claims may be denied because the service provided is *excluded* by Medicare or because the service was *not reasonable and necessary* for the specific patient. Excluded services are services that are not covered under any circumstances. The services that are excluded change from year to year. Other services that are not covered are classified as not medically necessary under Medicare guidelines. These services are not covered by Medicare unless certain conditions are met, such as particular diagnoses. For example, a vitamin B12 injection is a covered service only for patients with certain diagnoses, such as pernicious anemia, but not for a diagnosis of fatigue. If the patient does not have one of the specified diagnoses, the B12 injection is categorized as not reasonable and necessary.

Determining Medicare Coverage

There are two coverage policies, National Coverage Determinations (NCD) and Local Coverage Determinations (LCD). **National Coverage Determinations (NCDs)** describe whether specific medical items, services, treatment procedures, or technologies can be paid for under Medicare. The NCD manual is organized by categories, such as medical procedures,

---

COMPLIANCE GUIDELINE

Do Not Use "Blanket" or Blank ABNs

- Medicare prohibits the use of blanket ABNs given routinely to all patients just to be sure of payment.
- Never have a patient sign a blank ABN for the physician to fill in later. The form must be filled in before the patient signs it.

BILLING TIP

Billing Ambulance Services

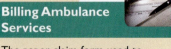

The paper claim form used to bill ambulance services is the CMS-1491.

SECTION B: ENTERAL AND PARENTERAL THERAPY (B4000–B9999)

Section B includes codes for supplies, formulas, nutritional solutions, and infusion pumps. If documentation in the patient's record indicates a brand name that is not listed in HCPCS, the physician should be queried for help in identifying the appropriate code description.

Codes from this section are submitted when patients require tube feedings. Feedings can be administered **enterally** through the intestine, **parenterally** into the body other than through the digestive tract (IV therapy, nasogastric tube) or via percutaneous endoscopic gastrostomy tube (PEG) inserted into the patient's stomach. Some codes include the administration set and some pertain only to the formula given when the supplies and the administration set are not changed with each feeding.

EXAMPLE

B4102: Enteral formula, for adults, used to replace fluids and electrolytes, 500 ml = 1 unit.

If medication was given through a feeding tube or via the parenteral method, an additional J code for the medication should be assigned.

supplies, and diagnostic services. **Local Coverage Determinations (LCDs)** are developed to specify under what clinical circumstances a service is reasonable and necessary. They serve as an administrative and educational tool to assist providers in submitting claims correctly for payment. LCDs are also posted to an online Medicare manual.

Actions Required for Noncovered Services

Generally, providers may bill Medicare beneficiaries for services that are not covered by the Medicare program. Giving a patient written notification that Medicare will not pay for a service before providing it is a good policy, although it is not required. When patients are notified ahead of time, they understand their financial responsibility to pay for the service. CMS Form No. 20007, **Notice of Exclusions from Medicare Benefits (NEMB)** is available for this purpose. Providers use NEMBs on an entirely voluntary basis. Their purpose is to advise beneficiaries, before they receive services that are not Medicare benefits, that Medicare will not pay for them and to provide beneficiaries with an estimate of how much they may have to pay. Providers may also choose to design their own NEMBs based on the services they offer.

Providers also may not bill patients for services that Medicare declares as being not reasonable and necessary unless the patients were informed ahead of time in writing and agreed to pay for the services. If a provider thinks that a procedure will not be covered by Medicare because it is not reasonable and necessary, the patient is notified of this before the treatment by means of a standard **advance beneficiary notice (ABN)** from CMS. A filled-in form is given to the patient for signature. The ABN form is designed to:

- Identify the service or item that Medicare is unlikely to pay for
- State the reason Medicare is unlikely to pay
- Estimate how much the service or item will cost the beneficiary if Medicare does not pay

The ABN for general use is form CMS-R-131-G. Variations of the form for laboratory use (CMS-R-131-L) and home health care (CMS-R-296) are also available.

For inpatient services, a similar form called a *hospital-issued notice of noncoverage (HINN)* is used. This document has a number of formats, rather than one form that is mandated.

SECTION C: OUTPATIENT PPS (C1000–C9999)

Section C lists temporary codes used in hospital-based surgery centers and hospital-based outpatient services. They cannot be used by freestanding ambulatory surgery centers (ASCs) or physician offices. C codes are used according to the Medicare Outpatient Prospective Payment System (OPPS) reimbursement methodology for hospital outpatient services and supplies. Most services are packaged into ambulatory payment classifications (APC) that have predetermined payment amounts. C codes identify **transitional pass-through payments** under OPPS, providing temporary additional payments (over and above the APC payment) for certain medical devices, drugs, and biologicals provided exclusively to Medicare patients.

> **NOTE**
>
> OPPS and APC payments are covered in Chapter 5 of your program.

EXAMPLE
C2625: Stent, non-coronary, temporary, with delivery system.

SECTION D: DENTAL PROCEDURES (D0000–D9999)

D series codes are **Current Dental Terminology codes** that are copyrighted and maintained by the American Dental Association (ADA) and are reported for procedures performed in a dental office. Until 2002, CDT codes were separately printed; after that they were incorporated into the HCPCS code book. Medicare does not cover the procedures and services listed in this section.

EXAMPLE
D0272: Bitewings—two films.

SECTION E: DURABLE MEDICAL EQUIPMENT (E0100–E9999)

E codes are used for DME such as canes, crutches, hospital beds, pacemakers, and dialysis kidney machines.

EXAMPLE
E0148: Walker, heavy duty, without wheels, rigid or folding, any type, each.

SECTION G: PROCEDURES/PROFESSIONAL SERVICES (G0000–G9999)

Section G has temporary codes assigned to services being evaluated and reviewed for inclusion in the CPT book. They may or may not be used by commercial insurance plans. In many cases, G codes are used in lieu of CPT codes for Medicare patients.

EXAMPLES
- G0105, colorectal cancer screening; colonoscopy on individual at high risk, is preferred over CPT code 45378.
- G0289, arthroscopy, knee, surgical for removal of loose body, foreign body, debridement/shaving of articular cartilage (chondroplasty) at the time of other surgical knee arthroscopy in a different compartment of the same knee, is preferred over CPT code 29877.

SECTION H: ALCOHOL AND DRUG ABUSE TREATMENT SERVICES (H0001–H2037)

Codes in section H are used by state Medicaid agencies, some of which are mandated by state law to establish separate codes for mental health services that include alcohol and drug treatment.

EXAMPLE
H0001: Alcohol and/or drug assessment.

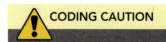

CODING CAUTION

Note the Dosage
Be careful to read documentation closely to determine correct code assignment according to the dosage of the formula given.

NOTE

J codes and the Table of Drugs are discussed later in this chapter.

SECTION J: DRUGS ADMINISTERED OTHER THAN ORAL METHOD (J0000–J9999)

This section is for injectable drugs that are administered subcutaneously, intramuscularly, or intravenously.

EXAMPLE
J0585: Botulinum toxin type A, per unit.

When coding for injectables, the dose must be determined for proper billing as well as for maintaining inventory and tracking waste of unused drugs. Most drugs have a quantity limitation.

Medicare CAP Program

Section 303 (d) of the Medicare Modernization Act requires the implementation of a competitive acquisition program (CAP) for Medicare Part B drugs and biologicals not paid on a cost or prospective payment system basis. Since January 1, 2005, payments for the vast majority of such drugs and biologicals have been based on the average sales price (ASP) methodology. HCPCS codes for drugs are not listed on the Medicare physician fee schedule; determining reimbursement requires finding the Payment Allowance Limits for Medicare Part B Drugs on the CMS website.

The competitive acquisition program is the newest alternative payment method for injectable and infused drugs currently billed under Part B that are administered in a physician office incident to the physician's service. Contracts for acquisition of and payment for categories of competitively biddable drugs and biologicals are awarded within CAP geographic areas. A physician who elects to participate in the program does not submit claims for the drugs and biologicals; instead the claims are submitted by the contractor that supplied them. The contractor is responsible for collection of deductibles and coinsurance, and payment is made to the contractor directly.

To determine allowed amounts and reimbursement for drugs, the coder must access the Medicare Part B Competitive Acquisition Program (CAP) area on the CMS website. HCPCS J codes along with drug descriptions and corresponding NDC (National Drug Classification) codes and reimbursable amounts are located there.

SECTION K: TEMPORARY CODES (K0000–K9999)

These codes are used by MACs when no permanent Level II code is available to implement a MAC coverage policy.

EXAMPLE
K0552: Supplies for external drug infusion pump, syringe type cartridge, sterile, each.

SECTION L: ORTHOTIC PROCEDURES (L0000–L4999)

L codes describe orthotic and prosthetic procedures and devices as well as orthopedic shoes and prosthetic implants.

EXAMPLE
L0120: Cervical, flexible, non-adjustable foam collar.

SECTION M: MEDICAL SERVICES (M0000–M0301)

M codes include office services, cellular therapy, IV chelation therapy, and fabric wrapping of abdominal aneurysms. As of 2007, there are only six codes in this section.

EXAMPLE
M0300: IV chelation therapy.

INTERNET RESOURCE

Medicare Claims Processing Manual, Publication 100-04, Transmittal 1204, on Medicare Part B Drug Pricing and Reporting J Codes

www.cms.hhs.gov/transmittals/downloads/R1204CP.pdf

SECTION P: PATHOLOGY AND LABORATORY SERVICES (P0000–P9999)

P codes include chemistry, toxicology, and microbiology tests and PAP smears. Codes P9612 and P9615 are now reported using CPT codes according to the HCPCS instruction to "see also new CPT catheterization codes 51701–51703."

EXAMPLE
P2031: Hair analysis (excluding arsenic).

SECTION Q: TEMPORARY CODES (Q0000–Q9999)

Section Q codes identify drugs, medical equipment, and services that typically do not receive CPT codes, have not been given CPT codes, and are not identifiable in the permanent Level II codes, but are needed to process a billing claim.

SECTION R: DIAGNOSTIC RADIOLOGY SERVICES (R0000–R5999)

R codes are used for transportation of portable X-ray and/or ECG equipment.

EXAMPLE
R0076: Transportation of portable EKG to facility or location, per patient.

SECTION S: TEMPORARY NATIONAL CODES (NON-MEDICARE) (S0000–S9999)

The codes in section S were developed by Blue Cross and Blue Shield and other commercial payers to report drugs, services, and supplies for which there are no national codes but that are needed to implement policies. These codes can also be used by Medicaid, but they are not reportable to Medicare. It is very important for the coder to review carrier contracts to determine which payers accept these codes.

EXAMPLE For an arthroscopic thermal capsulorrhaphy (capsular shrinkage), code S2300 can be assigned if the payer accepts S codes. Otherwise, CPT code 29999 must be submitted.

SECTION T: NATIONAL T CODES (T1000–T9999)

National T codes are used by state Medicaid agencies when no HCPCS Level II codes are available but codes are needed to administer the Medicaid program. They are not used by Medicare but can be used by private insurers.

SECTION V: VISION AND HEARING SERVICES (V0000–V2999)

V codes are for vision and hearing screenings and supplies, including glasses, contacts, intraocular lenses, audiology services, and prostheses.

EXAMPLE
V2623: Prosthetic eye, plastic, custom.

MISCELLANEOUS/UNCLASSIFIED CODES

Under certain circumstances, a coder must assign an item or service to an **unclassified HCPCS code.** Health care is in a constant state of change. New drugs, devices, and equipment are developed and marketed at various times throughout the year. It is impossible and impractical to revise the HCPCS code sets each time a new item or service is introduced. An item or service that is newly approved by the **Food and Drug Administration (FDA)**—the federal organization that protects against public health hazards by ensuring the safety and in most cases the quality and effectiveness products and services—may not yet have a HCPCS code.

Services or items without specific Level II codes are assigned to an unclassified code until a new code can be implemented. A number of unclassified codes exist in each section of HCPCS. Unclassified and unlisted codes give providers a way to submit claims and carriers a way to process claims for items or services without designated codes.

In CPT, a procedure that does not have a designated code is assigned to an unlisted procedure code in the appropriate body system. Unlike CPT, HCPCS does not use consistent terminology throughout the book. The code description may include any of the following terms: unlisted, NOS (not otherwise specified), unspecified, unclassified, other, and miscellaneous.

EXAMPLE A4649, surgical supply; miscellaneous may be used for an implanted device that does not have a permanent or temporary code that is more specific.

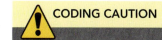

CODING CAUTION

Do Research Before Assigning an Unclassified Code

When assigning an unclassified code, contact the local Medicare carrier in case there is a preferred Level II code.

Checkpoint 10.3

In which sections are the following HCPCS services located?

1. Motorized wheelchair _____

2. Alcohol wipes, box _____

3. Recement crown _____

4. Ambulance waiting time _____

5. Contact lens, gas permeable _____

Modifiers

The nearly three hundred HCPCS Level II modifiers serve the same purpose as the CPT professional modifiers. Level II modifiers do not change the definition of the procedure or service but give more explanation about where the procedure was performed, the type of equipment used, the provider of the service, and so on. Level II modifiers may be used with Level I or Level II codes.

Level II modifiers are two characters in length and are either alphanumeric or alphabetic only. They are listed on the inside covers of the HCPCS code book or in an appendix. A limited number of the commonly used modifiers are listed on the inside front cover of the CPT codebook as well. Frequently used modifiers are discussed below.

EXAMPLE The −AA modifier is appended to an anesthesia code to indicate anesthesia services performed personally by the anesthesiologist.

When both a Level I and a Level II modifier are required, the Level II modifier is sequenced first, followed by the Level I modifier.

EXAMPLE A tarsal tunnel release is performed on the left foot and a hammertoe repair is performed on the fourth toe right foot. The codes are 28035–LT and 28285–T8–51.

ANATOMICAL MODIFIERS

The HCPCS Level II anatomical modifiers show exact body location and help describe exactly which digit received treatment. They are more specific than the CPT modifiers and should be used instead of −LT or −RT with procedures on toes, eyes, and fingers.

Modifiers −TA to −T9 are used for procedures performed on the phalanges, or toes, rather than on the foot. They are specific to individual toes on each foot and are the modifiers of choice when doing multiple procedures on different toes.

Modifiers −E1 to −E4 are used for procedures performed on the eyelids specifically, not the actual eye. These are specific to the upper and lower lids of each eye.

EXAMPLE
67840–E1: Excision of lesion of eyelid without closure or with simple direct closure.

Modifiers −FA to −F9 are used for procedures done on the phalanges, or fingers, rather than on the hand. They are specific to individual fingers on each hand and are the modifiers of choice when doing multiple procedures on different fingers.

MODIFIERS RELATING TO MEDICARE COVERAGE

A series of modifiers relate to coverage for Medicare services (see the Reimbursement Review on pages 428–429 for background information).

Modifier −GA is used when a waiver of liability (advance beneficiary notice (ABN)) for a Medicare patient is on file. This document must be signed when the service will not be covered by Medicare; the modifier notifies Medicare that the patient is aware that he or she is liable for the cost of the service.

Modifier −GZ is used when payment for a service is expected to be denied as not reasonable and necessary and the patient has been given but has not signed an ABN.

Modifier −GY is used when an item or service is statutorily excluded or does not meet the definition of any Medicare benefit. Excluded services, which include cosmetic surgery, dentures, acupuncture, and hearing aids, do not require a signed ABN to be on file. Use of the −GY modifier acknowledges that Medicare will deny the item or service as noncovered but that a secondary insurer may consider coverage following Medicare's denial. The modifier is not used on claims for services that are expected to be denied for medical necessity.

When a diagnostic mammogram is converted from a screening mammogram on the same day, modifier −GH is used. When a patient has both a screening mammogram and a diagnostic mammogram on the same day, modifier −GG is used.

LAB TEST MODIFIER

Modifier −QW is appended to codes for CLIA-waived tests—laboratory tests performed in a physician office that have been deemed safe to perform outside a certified lab.

EXAMPLE
81025–QW: Urine pregnancy test, by visual color comparison methods.

TECHNICAL COMPONENT MODIFIER

Charges submitted by facilities for use of equipment receive the −TC (for technical component) modifiers. The only time a −TC modifier is used by a physician is when the physician owns the equipment and is billing for the facility charge in his or her own office.

EXAMPLE
76005–TC: Fluoroscopic guidance and localization of needle or catheter tip for spine or paraspinous diagnostic or therapeutic injection procedures, including neurolytic agent destruction.

ASC-ONLY MODIFIER

When surgery is performed in an ambulatory surgical center (ASC), the −SG modifier is appended to the CPT surgical procedure code. This modifier indicates that the charge is for the ASC facility service, and it is used to determine the appropriate reimbursement rate for the ASC. The modifier is used in addition to other applicable modifiers. It should not be used on supply codes billed by the ASC. Physicians performing services in the ASC setting should not use the −SG modifier when billing for their services.

In some situations, insurance carriers instruct suppliers and providers to use a modifier to provide information about the service or item, and payment may be denied or reduced if the modifier is missing. Also, although both the alphabetic and alphanumeric modifiers are used across the country, some carriers do not recognize them. The coder must make sure to reference each carrier contract and coverage manual and to submit appropriate documentation with claims that have been questioned.

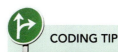
CODING TIP

Multiple Services

Any HCPCS Level II modifier outranks the −59 modifier and is reported first, followed by −59.

Checkpoint 10.4

Indicate which Level II modifier applies to the following:

1. Physician's assistant, nurse-practitioner, or clinical nurse specialist services for assistant at surgery

_____

2. Outpatient occupational therapy service _____

3. Medicare beneficiary election to purchase an item _____

4. Service that is not reasonable and necessary _____

5. Office-performed CLIA-waived test _____

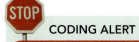
Step 1.
Read the documentation to determine the item, service, or procedure to be coded.

↓

Step 2.
Review all subterms and code ranges.

↓

Step 3.
Read the guidelines for the sections, and read each description.

↓

Step 4.
Pay attention to all color coding and symbols.

↓

Step 5.
Select the code, and assign modifiers if necessary.

FIGURE 10.2
HCPCS Code Assignment Flow Chart

Assigning HCPCS Codes

Looking a code up in the HCPCS index is similar to looking up a code in CPT and ICD-9-CM. Keeping in mind that HCPCS codes are for services and supplies only, look up the medical or surgical supply, the service provided (such as *screening* or *implant*), the orthotic or prosthetic device, or the generic or brand name of the drug. Some codes are indexed by the condition or body part, but this is not the norm.

The index points to the general area of the code listings. The coders must then locate the appropriate code in the appropriate section.

EXAMPLE A podiatrist performs a complex bunionectomy with implant insertion. The CPT code for the procedure is 28293. The code for the supply of the implant itself must be located in HCPCS. If a HCPCS code is not assigned, the physician or facility will not be reimbursed for the implanted device.

CODING STEPS

As illustrated in Figure 10.2 coders follow a series of steps to assign HCPCS codes:

1. Read the documentation, and determine the item, service, or procedure to be coded.
2. Find the terms in the index. Entries may appear under more than one term. Note, though, that not all indexes are the same—those of some publishers are more complete. It may be necessary to research similar entries. Once the main term is located, review all subterms and code ranges to determine the most accurate code. Do not code straight from the index.
3. Read the guidelines for the sections referenced, and read each description.
4. Pay attention to all color coding and symbols to the left and right of the code for coverage directions, quantity alerts, gender edits, and cross-references. An example of a cross-reference is:

    EXAMPLE E0235, paraffin bath unit, portable (see medical supply code A4265 for the paraffin).

5. Select the code or codes, and assign modifiers if necessary.

To find the code for a urinary indwelling catheter, use *urinary* as the main term and *catheter* as the subterm. You see the code ranges A4324–A4325, A4338–A4346, and A4351–A4353. Locate and review each code in these ranges to determine the best one. You could also find the same code by looking up *catheter* and then *indwelling* and reviewing each code in the A4338–A4346 range.

DETERMINING WHETHER TO ASSIGN A HCPCS LEVEL II CODE OR A CPT (HCPCS LEVEL I) CODE

Some CPT codes and HCPCS Level II codes have identical narratives, and a coder must occasionally decide which to choose. Before choosing a code, follow these rules:

- The determination of which code to use varies with the carrier. Check documentation to determine which code the carrier prefers.
- For non-Medicare patients, if the CPT code has the same description as the HCPCS code, use the CPT code.
- For Medicare patients, if there is not a CPT code that describes the procedure or service, use a HCPCS code instead of assigning an unlisted code. Medicare has G codes that supersede any other CPT codes. Examples are screening colonoscopies (G0105, G0121, and so on) and arthroscopy with removal of loose body (G0289).

USING THE TABLE OF DRUGS

HCPCS Level II J codes describe drugs by using their generic and trade names, amounts, and routes of administration. Consulting the **Table of Drugs** is more effective than using the index in most cases. The table is included as an appendix to the HCPCS book. Depending on the publisher, the brand name drugs are capitalized, and the generic drugs are in lowercase letters.

Determining the Mode of Administration   Before assigning a code, the coder must determine the amount of drug given and the mode of administration. Abbreviations used to indicate the mode of administration are summarized in Table 10.3.

Determining the Units of Medication   The dosage of medication administered must be determined from the medical record and correctly matched to the available dosage amount in HCPCS. If the coder has reason to doubt the accuracy of the documentation, the nurse or other provider who administered the medication should be queried. The coder should not calculate actual dosages by converting milliliters (ml) to cubic centimeters (cc) or milligrams (mg) to grams (gm). This is a clinical responsibility. Coders are responsible for choosing the correct units of the drug and the mode of administration based on the nurse's or physician's documentation.

Table 10.3 Modes of Drug Administration

Abbreviation	Term	Description
IA	Intra-arterial	Introduced via an artery
INH	Inhalant solution	Inhaled via the nose
INJ	Injection, not otherwise specified	Injected
IT	Intrathecal	Introduced into the space under the arachnoid membrane of the brain or spinal cord
IV	Intravenous	Introduced via a vein
IM	Intramuscular	Introduced into a muscle
ORAL	Oral	Taken by mouth
OTH	Other routes	Introduced by some other route
SC	Subcutaneous	Introduced under the skin
VAR	Various routes	Introduced by various routes, such as into joint, into cavity tissue, or topical

EXAMPLE   A patient was injected with 40 mg of Elavil. The coder looks up the drug in the Table of Drugs and finds this information:

Drug Name	Unit	Route	Code
Elavil	20 mg	IM	J1320

The dosage in the table is 20 mg. Based on the amount of medication given, the coder calculates the units: a 40 mg dose comes to two units of J1320 (J1320x2). Be careful when reading the code descriptions. Some of them say "up to" a specific amount of medication; anything less than that dosage should be coded by assigning the code one time.

EXAMPLE   A patient was given 80 mg of Phenobarbital.

Drug Name	Unit	Route	Code
Phenobarbital Sodium	120 mg	IM, IV	J2560

The Table of Drugs shows 120 mg as the unit, but only 80 mg was given. The code description for J2560 in the book states "Injection, Phenobarbital sodium, up to 120 mg." So this code is appropriate to assign.

> ⚠️ **CODING CAUTION**
>
> A J code must be verified by looking at the complete description of the code in the J code section of the book. Do not code directly from the Table of Drugs.

Checkpoint 10.5

Assign the HCPCS Level I or II codes for the following, appending any necessary HCPCS Level II modifiers.

1.   Blood glucose monitor with integrated lancing _____
2.   Injection depo-estradiol cypionate 2.5 mg _____
3.   Thoracic Lumbar Sacral Orthosis back brace _____
4.   LPN nursing care in the home, per diem _____
5.   Blood glucose reagent strips for home blood glucose machine _____
6.   Injection of Cordarone IV 45 mg _____
7.   One hour of outpatient speech therapy by a speech pathologist in the office _____
8.   Prostate screening in a sixty-nine-year-old patient _____

HCPCS Coding Resources

As is the case for all code sets, coders must stay up to date with annual changes to HCPCS. Good reference materials and access to Internet-based information are both important.

HCPCS UPDATES

HCPCS Level II codes are updated each January 1, with the exception of the temporary codes that begin with *C, G, H, K, Q, S,* and *T,* which are updated quarterly. Several publishers offer the HCPCS codes in book format with very helpful indexing, color coding, cross-references, and other features. Computer-generated lists of HCPCS codes are also available at no cost from CMS and local Medicare carriers. Unlike CPT codes, which are owned by the AMA, HCPCS codes are in the public domain.

HCPCS codes can be modified at the request of a provider. A document explaining the HCPCS revision process, as well as a format for submitting a request for revision or addition, is available on the HCPCS website. The HCPCS code review process is an ongoing effort. Requests may be submitted any time during the year for inclusion in the next annual update.

Errata (corrections of mistakes) for HCPCS codes are available. The errata list can be located on the AMA and CMS websites.

HCPCS CLEARINGHOUSE

The American Hospital Association (AHA) and CMS have developed a clearinghouse to provide official interpretations of HCPCS codes. The clearinghouse provides information on the proper use of Level I HCPCS (CPT) codes in the facility environment and on certain Level II HCPCS codes for hospitals, physicians, and other health care professionals. The clearinghouse is available to anyone with questions about HCPCS coding. Questions and supporting documentation may be faxed or mailed to the AHA Central Office on HCPCS.

AHA *CODING CLINIC FOR HCPCS*

The quarterly AHA *Coding Clinic for HCPCS* provides information on the use of HCPCS codes related to the payment system for outpatient facility billing. It is arranged much like the *Coding Clinic for ICD-9-CM* that hospitals use.

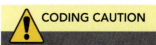

INTERNET RESOURCE

HCPCS Review Process

www.cms.hhs.gov/
MedHCPCSGenInfo

CODING CAUTION

Use Current Codes
Stay current with HCPCS codes by purchasing annual editions of HCPCS books and periodically checking the CMS website for updates.

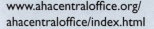

INTERNET RESOURCE

Form for Submitting Questions

www.ahacentraloffice.org/
ahacentraloffice/index.html

Summary

1. The HCPCS code set is the HIPAA-mandated coding system for products, supplies, and services not included in the AMA's CPT code set.

2. HCPCS Level I (CPT) codes are five-digit numeric codes (with the exception of Category II and Category III codes). HCPCS Level II codes are five-digit alphanumeric codes starting with the letters A–V.

3. HCPCS codes are assigned along with CPT codes to identify supplies and drugs used or provided. They are required by federal health insurance programs for claims for services, supplies, and drugs.

4. The HCPCS code set contains both permanent and temporary codes. Permanent codes change just once a year based on the recommendations of the CMS HCPCS Workgroup. Temporary codes are updated quarterly.

5. The HCPCS index is arranged alphabetically, as is the Table of Drugs included in HCPCS code books. The main text is made up of sections of codes arranged numerically according to the initial letter of each, from section A through section V.

6. HCPCS Level II modifiers, like CPT professional and facility modifiers, are used to report that the circumstances of a service changed, but not enough to select another code. The −GA, −GZ, and −GY modifiers are related to the status of the ABN.

7. To correctly assign the J code that accurately reflects the dose provided and method of administration of a drug, it is necessary to pay close attention to the units and route columns in the Table of Drugs.

8. There is a hierarchy for assigning HCPCS codes. Determining the patient's insurance will help the coder determine whether a HCPCS Level I or Level II code is required.

9. Sources for keeping up to date include the HCPCS website, the HCPCS Clearinghouse, and the AHA *Coding Clinic for HCPCS*.

10. Correct assignment of HCPCS codes with appropriate modifiers follows the basic code-assignment process of reading the complete documentation, locating main terms in the HCPCS, and selecting the correct code from the appropriate section, paying attention to the dosage, coverage notes, and other instructions provided for correct coding.

Review Questions: Chapter 10

Match the key terms with their definitions.

a. durable medical equipment (DME) _____
b. HCPCS _____
c. *Medicare Carriers Manual* (MCM) _____
d. permanent national codes _____
e. temporary national codes _____
f. Level II modifiers _____
g. Notice of Exclusion from Medicare Benefits (NEMB) _____
h. CMS HCPCS Workgroup _____

1. HCPCS Level II codes that are maintained for the use of all payers

2. Reference containing guidelines established by Medicare related to covered services in HCPCS Level II

3. HCPCS Level II codes that are used by individual payers for items not covered in permanent national codes

4. Form used to inform patients that Medicare does not cover and will not pay for a planned service

5. Code set providing national codes for supplies, services, and products

6. Reusable medical equipment for use in the home

7. Two-character codes that are assigned to clarify Level II codes

8. Government committee that maintains and advises on HCPCS Level II codes

Decide whether each statement is true or false.

1. HCPCS Level II codes have six digits. **T or F**

2. HCPCS Level II codes are used only by hospitals. **T or F**

3. HIPAA mandates the use of HCPCS codes. **T or F**

4. CPT modifiers and HCPCS Level II modifiers are the same. **T or F**

5. HCPCS permanent national codes can be altered or deleted by a single payer alone. **T or F**

6. HCPCS permanent national codes are issued on January 1 of each year and must be used as of their effective date. **T or F**

7. HCPCS code books use symbols to show new, revised, and deleted codes and descriptors. **T or F**

8. Coding drugs involves paying attention to both the method of administration and the quantity administered. **T or F**

9. DME supplies are located in the K section of the main listing. **T or F**

10. Private payers are not permitted to use HCPCS codes; use is restricted to government programs. **T or F**

11. An ABN is an example of a certificate of medical necessity. **T or F**

12. Prosthetics are assigned from the P category of codes in HCPCS. **T or F**

13. The DME section of HCPCS includes codes for equipment and supplies. **T or F**

14. The route of administration for Foscavir is IV. **T or F**

15. Providers must report HCPCS codes to Medicare when reporting magnetic resonance angiography (MRA) of the chest, head, neck, or vessels of the lower extremities. **T or F**

16. Medicare G codes supersede any other HCPCS code assignment. **T or F**

17. HCPCS is a three-tiered coding system. **T or F**

18. Medicare will not cover code J3535. **T or F**

19. Claims for A4259 must be sent to the regional DME contractor. **T or F**

20. If a code is highlighted in yellow, the coder must contact the carrier to find out whether there is coverage for the service or supply. **T or F**

Select the letter that best completes the statement or answers the question.

1. Transportation services are HCPCS _____ codes.
   a. A
   b. B
   c. C
   d. D

2. Vision and hearing services are HCPCS _____ codes.
   a. D
   b. E
   c. H
   d. V

3. Temporary codes are HCPCS _____ codes.
   a. D
   b. Q
   c. T
   d. V

4. Durable medical equipment (DME) codes are HCPCS _____ codes.

   a. D

   b. E

   c. H

   d. V

5. Prosthetic procedures are HCPCS _____ codes.

   a. D

   b. E

   c. H

   d. L

6. Temporary National Codes for private insurers to identify drugs, services, supplies, and procedures that are not reimbursable under Medicare are HCPCS _____ codes.

   a. D

   b. E

   c. S

   d. V

7. Diagnostic radiology services are HCPCS _____ codes.

   a. R

   b. E

   c. H

   d. V

8. Chemotherapy drugs are HCPCS _____ codes.

   a. D

   b. E

   c. H

   d. J

9. Laboratory and pathology are HCPCS _____ codes.

   a. D

   b. E

   c. P

   d. V

10. Dental codes are listed in HCPCS as _____ codes.

    a. D

    b. E

    c. H

    d. V

11. According to the HCPCS book, transcutaneous electrical nerve stimulation devices are

    a. covered by Medicare

    b. covered for chronic pain only

    c. covered on a trial basis if the therapist or physician tells the patient to rent the unit from a supplier

    d. diagnostic procedures involving needle electrode insertion

12. A patient receives a walking air boot for an Achilles tendon and a pair of below-the-knee 35 mm Hg compression stockings. How is this coded?

    a. 14386, A6534

    b. L4360, A6531x2

    c. L3260, A6531

    d. L4386

13. What modifier is appended to code J9015 when the CAP area contractor does not supply the drug?
    a. −KD
    b. −QV
    c. −J1
    d. −J3

14. What should the coder do when a service has both a CPT code and a HCPCS code?
    a. always report the CPT code
    b. always report the HCPCS code
    c. report the HCPCS code only if the patient is on Medicare
    d. check payer instructions

15. A Medicare patient receives a Vantas implant for treatment of prostate cancer. How is this coded?
    a. J9219
    b. J9225
    c. L8699
    d. J7306

16. A patient is status post left mastectomy and undergoes breast reconstruction with a silicone breast implant. Code for the implant.
    a. L8035
    b. L8600
    c. L8039
    d. L8030

17. When are HCPCS permanent codes updated?
    a. every January 1, with updates as needed
    b. every October 1, with updates as needed
    c. on July 1
    d. every quarter

18. Who publishes and maintains the HCPCS coding system?
    a. AMA
    b. AHA
    c. CMS
    d. OIG

19. What is another name for the CPT codes?
    a. HCPCS Level I
    b. HCPCS Level II
    c. HCPCS Level III
    d. National

20. A patient with glaucoma has an aqueous shunt implanted into his right eye. Code for the implant.
    a. L8670
    b. L8612
    c. V2623
    d. V2629

Define the following abbreviations:

1. MCM _____

2. HCPCS _____

3. DME _____

4. INH _____

5. DMERC _____

6. DMEPOS _____

7. ABN _____

8. NEMB _____

Applying Your Knowledge

BUILDING CODING SKILL

Case 10.1

Supply the correct HCPCS codes.

1. Ocular implant _____

2. Interphalangeal joint implant _____

3. Intradiscal electrothermal therapy, single interspace _____

4. Arthroscopy of the knee with harvesting of cartilage (chondrocyte cells) for a workers compensation patient. _____

5. Urethral stent (urolume) _____

6. Implantable neurostimulator electrodes, per group of four _____
   _____

7. Injection 8 mg Compazine _____

8. Apnea monitor, high-risk infant _____

9. Dorrance hook hand prosthesis, model 6 _____

10. Sterile gloves, one pair _____

11. Preschool screening for language problems _____

12. Evaluation for hearing aid _____

13. Kit for collagen skin test _____

14. Single root canal, right upper incisor _____

15. Injection, 1.2 million units Bicillin C-R _____

16. A patient with osteoarthritis undergoes a metatarsal joint arthroplasty of the right first toe with insertion of a silicone joint
    _____

17. A patient has a cochlear device implanted. _____

Case 10.2

Look up the follow procedures, check the color coding and symbols, and list the notations that appear for each code. Describe the action by Medicare (the notification that Medicare has given or the action taken since the last

publication) in the Action/Alert column. If information on coverage is supplied, list it in the **Coverage** column.

		Action/Alert	Coverage
Examples:			
A7019		<u>Deleted code</u>	<u>Not covered</u>
A6456	<u>Quantity alert</u>	<u>New code,</u>	<u>Carrier discretion</u>

1. A4206: Syringe with needle, sterile 1cc, 1 each _____ _____

2. A4550: Surgical trays _____ _____

3. J2995: Injection, Streptokinase, per 250,000 IU _____ _____

USING CODING TERMS

Read the following Medicare instruction and answer the questions.

HCPCS code G0107 will be retired at the next annual release of the clinical diagnostic laboratory fee schedule effective January 1, 2007, and replaced with Current Procedural Terminology (CPT) code 82270.

Prior to January 1, 2007, use G0107 for billing Medicare for screening FOBT; however, on or after January 1, 2007, use code 82270 for billing Medicare for screening FOBT.

1. What is FOBT? _____

2. What is the correct code for a FOBT service on April 28, 2007?

   _____

Researching the Internet

1. Visit the website at www.cms.hhs.gov/home/Medicare.asp and click HCPCS Release and Code Sets. Report on the most current HCPCS quarterly update. Include any new temporary codes that will go into effect.

2. Visit carrier websites such as Aetna (www.aetna.com) and Blue Cross and Blue Shield (www.bcbsm.com/) and locate their HCPCS payment and reporting policies. Write a brief report.

Coding Case Studies

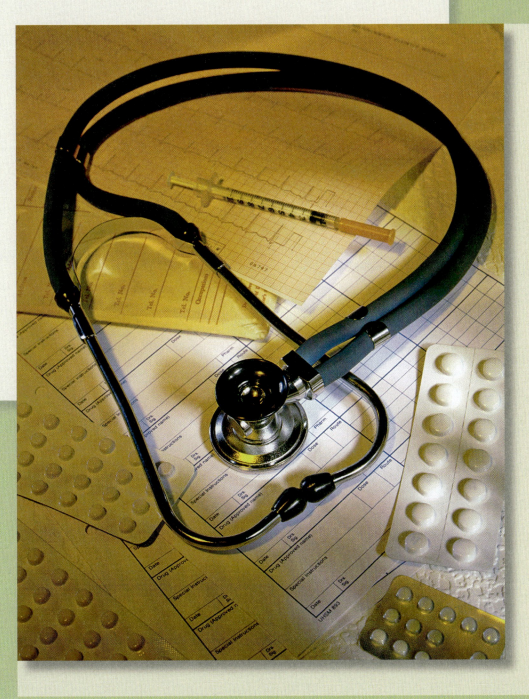

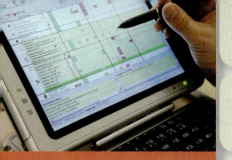

Pulling It All Together: Coding Diagnosis and Procedures

LEARNING OUTCOMES

After studying this chapter, you should be able to:

1. Discuss the role of medical coding in clearly identifying the treatments, services, and procedures that are provided to patients and in demonstrating the medical necessity of the care.

2. Define the code sets that are required for compliant coding in the inpatient versus outpatient settings.

3. Explain the use of an online coding tool.

4. Based on the specified medical environment, assign correct ICD-9-CM and CPT/HCPCS codes to the chapter cases.

Chapter Outline

This chapter discusses the role of coding in clearly identifying the treatments, services, and procedures that are provided to patients and in demonstrating the medical necessity of the care. Connecting procedures and diagnoses helps to ensure that encounters are correctly coded, so that the coding and billing process results in the maximum appropriate payment for the provider. The correct code sets for compliant reporting of those diagnoses and procedures are then presented, "pulling it all together" for the coder.

The second part of the chapter provides an opportunity to combine the diagnosis and procedure coding skills learned in the program and demonstrate correct, compliant assignment of medical codes. Seventy case studies are presented. The groups of case studies provide coding situations for a variety of services in a variety of settings for a variety of providers. Each case describes a common encounter that coders must work with, and provides instructions to the coder for completing the assignment correctly in the particular coding setting.

Relating Coding and Billing

A function of medical coding is to supply the essential and compliant diagnosis and procedure codes for reporting on claims and for generating visit charges. A general coding/billing process is as follows:

VISIT
1. Registration of patients
2. Financial responsibility for visit established
3. Patients admitted (inpatient) or checked in (outpatient)
4. Patients discharged (inpatient) or checked out (outpatient)

CLAIM
5. Documentation assembled and coded
6. Coding and billing compliance verified
7. Claims prepared and transmitted to payers

POST-CLAIM
8. Payer adjudication monitored and payments received
9. Patient billing
10. Monies due from payers and patients are followed up in a collection process

The importance of correct, compliant coding is evident in this figure initially presented in Chapter 1:

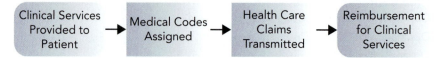

The coding and billing flow demonstrates the central role of medical coding in securing payment for health care services. Correct codes, when transmitted to payers, both explain what was done and demonstrate why it was necessary to be done. The codes for patients' treatments, procedures, and services must be supported by diagnosis codes to establish medical necessity. The diagnosis codes must also support the need for the particular place of service (POS) and the level of care and the frequency of services to pass payers' edits such as medically unlikely edits (MUEs).

Correct and Compliant Code Sets

Under the regulations of HIPAA, providers are required to use multiple coding systems to code single episodes in order to satisfy the data needs for reimbursement, case mix analysis, practice profiling, research, and outcomes measurement. Figure 11.1 reviews the basic steps in the medical coding process and the code sets that are required for the various billing settings.

Facility (institutional) billing refers to charging payers and patients for the costs incurred by the hospital or other entity in the delivery of health care. *Professional billing*, on the other hand, refers to charging for the costs of providing physicians' or other professional providers' services, such as those of a surgeon, a nurse practitioner, or a CRNA. When the physician provides services, treatments, and procedures in the physician's office or other physician-owned setting, the physician's charges incorporate the cost of the "facility." When the physician performs professional work in the hospital, however, the physician is charging for the particular procedures, and the hospital is charging for the facility's part of the costs, such as:

- Room and board
- Medications
- Ancillary tests and procedures
- Equipment/supplied used during surgery or therapy
- The amount of time spent in an operating room, recovery room, or intensive care unit
- Administrative and patient care services

In the *inpatient* setting, for *facility billing*, the medical coder in the Health Information Management (HIM) department assigns both diagnosis and procedure codes based on the ICD-9-CM. Volumes 1 and 2 are used to classify the diagnoses. Volume 3 is the source for inpatient procedure codes, which result in reimbursement to the facility for all the services it provided.

In the *inpatient* setting, for *professional billing*, the medical coder who is employed by the physician practice assigns diagnosis codes based on ICD-9-CM and procedure codes based on CPT/HCPCS.

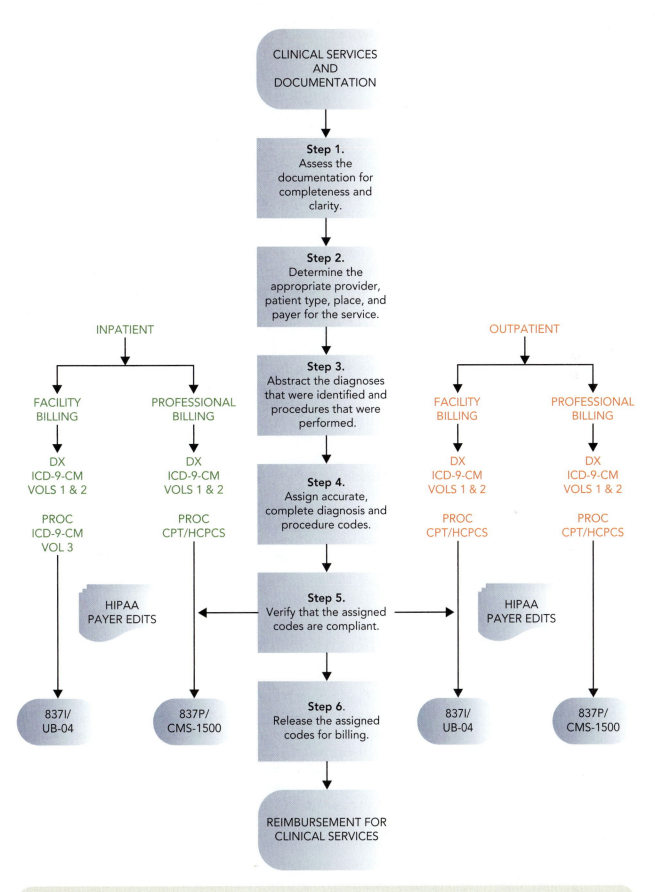

FIGURE 11.1
Code Set Selection Flow Chart

In the *outpatient* setting, for both *facility and professional billing*, the medical coder assigns diagnosis codes again based on volumes 1 and 2 of the ICD-9-CM. Procedures are coded using the CPT/HCPCS code set.

Description of Coding Case Studies

In the cases for this chapter, these four environments and assignments are presented:

- Facility billing, inpatient setting: Code for the patient's diagnosis and the inpatient procedures provided by the *facility*.
- Professional (physician) billing, outpatient setting: Code for the patient's diagnosis and the services provided by the *physician*.
- Combined facility/professional billing, inpatient setting: Code for the patient's diagnosis, the facility inpatient procedures, and the services provided by the physician.
- Combined facility/professional billing, outpatient setting: Code for the patient's diagnosis and the outpatient procedures.

Each case presents the documentation for code assignment. If needed, specific instructions for the case are noted in *italic type*; if there are no specific instructions, the general notes for the group of cases apply. As an example:

CASE EXAMPLE 1
Professional Billing/Outpatient Setting
A 73-year-old female, a new patient, is seen by her endocrinologist in his office for diabetes. The endocrinologist does a detailed history, a detailed exam, and moderate medical decision making. The documentation cites that the patient has Type II diabetes mellitus, which is well-controlled by her recently begun insulin use. *Assign codes for the diagnosis(es) and the evaluation and management services.*

A. Dx: (*ans.* ICD-9-CM 250.00)

B. E/M: (*ans.* CPT 99203)

CodeItRightOnline™: Your Online Coding Tool

Technology has and will continue to change the way medical coders perform coding tasks. Currently, many vendors of health information technology offer software solutions to aid the coding process. The products include (1) *online coding tools* that offer code sets online (often called *encoders*); (2) programs, called *groupers*, that calculate payment classifications such as DRG and APC assignment; and (3) programs that assign codes for coder review, generally referred to as *computer-assisted coding (CAC)*.

ONLINE CODING TOOLS

Typically, online coding tools are sold as subscriptions to physician practices and hospitals. These tools offer a very important advantage: The code sets in use for coding and billing can be rapidly updated and implemented by subscribers. When new codes or edits (such as Medicare's Correct Coding Initiative) are released by the payer, online subscribers can quickly update their code lists, such as encounter forms and charge description masters (CDMs), to reflect the right codes for compliant billing.

GROUPERS

Groupers are computerized inpatient and outpatient record grouping, editing, and reimbursement systems for providers, insurance companies, managed care companies, claims review companies, and other payers of hospital-submitted patient claims. The software is used to assign patient records to inpatient or outpatient groups, evaluate the accuracy and completeness of clinical data, identify potential coding errors, and verify hospital claims for reimbursement.

COMPUTER-ASSISTED CODING

CAC products automate the coding process, beginning with analyzing documentation to identify diagnoses and procedures to be coded. Such automated coding programs replace the totally manual search for codes in printed code sets, permitting coders' skills to be used to verify code assignment. Initial code assignment is done with the aid of software, and the final coding is validated by coders who act as editors, using their critical thinking and communication skills to ensure accurate coding that reflects documentation, whether in printed or electronic form.

CAC products use one of two approaches: structured data input (SDA) or natural language processing (NLP). With SDA, the end-user is the physician. The software presents the physician with a limited set of medical choices used to generate documentation, and then the computer assigns a code based on that documentation. For example, when a physician performs a colonoscopy, the SDA software might prompt for the following information before assigning a code:

- Procedure indication
- Medicine used during the procedure
- What the physician found and performed during the procedure
- Recommended treatment modality or follow-up procedure

When the NLP approach is used, the software requires that the facility or practice have some type of electronic document, even though it does not require a complete electronic health record. It then looks for certain words and the context in which those words were used, and assigns a code along with a degree of certainty for that code. NLP is good for analyzing large amounts of information for relatively straightforward medical cases, and not as good when the nature of the cases varies greatly. For example, specific radiology procedures are documented in similar fashion, so the documentation is relatively predicable and is well suited for NLP.

CODEITRIGHTONLINE™

So that you can gain experience with the use of an online coding tool, you will have access for a 21-day period to CodeItRightOnline, produced by the Medical Management Institute, a Contexo Media Company. You may use this tool, rather than code books, to select the correct ICD-9-CM and CPT/HCPCS codes for the chapter's Case Studies.

Using the Online Coding Tool   CodeItRightOnline is available to you through a portal that is located on the Online Learning Center (OLC) site for this program:

http://www.mhhe.com/JurekIntroMedCoding

Access the OLC. From the left-hand navigation section, select Online **Coding Tool**. This will take you to a second screen with a link to the Web portal for CodeItRightOnline. Click on the Web portal link to complete the steps you need to begin. On the portal screen that appears, locate this YOUR INFORMATION dialog box:

Your Information	
Name: *	
E-mail: *	
Organization: *	
Address: *	
City: *	
State: *	Select one... ▼
Zip: *	
Phone: *	

* Required

Enter your name, email address, the name and address of your school (the school name goes in the Organization box), and a phone number. After you enter your information and click Submit, you will be guided to complete your account profile, a one-time process which optimizes CodeItRightOnline for your particular location. After accepting the AMA Agreement, you may select a specialty if desired. Then, choose your state from the pull-down list.

These actions set up your trial subscription. Now, to use the online coding tool to locate codes, click Code Search and select the appropriate code set. Next, choose the start point—usually the Index—for your code search. For example, select ICD-9-CM, Index, Disease in the Type box, enter the term *fracture*, and click Search. CodeItRightOnline will return a list of the various fracture entries in the Alphabetic Index for your selection. To see how it works, choose Malunion and click the code number to review the Tabular List entry.

Facility Billing/Inpatient Setting:

CASES 11.1–11.15

Assign ICD-9-CM diagnoses codes with a present on admission indicator. Include E codes if appropriate. Also assign ICD-9-CM procedure codes. (Do not assign an admitting diagnosis.) Correctly sequence the codes, listing the principal diagnosis and procedure for each case first.

Case 11.1

A patient with a history of colon cancer is admitted for closure of her colostomy, which was performed under general anesthesia.

A.   Dx: Admission for colostomy closure, history of colon cancer _____

B.   Proc: Closure of colostomy _____

Case 11.2

The patient presented with a cough, fever, and dyspnea. Chest x-ray was positive for a left lower lobe infiltrate. Sputum culture was positive for Hemophilus influenzae (H. influenzae). The patient developed hypokalemia after admission that was treated with KCL.

A.   Dx: H. Influenzae pneumonia, hypokalemia _____

Case 11.3

The patient was treated as an outpatient for cellulitis of the leg. He did not respond to treatment and required inpatient hospitalization for intravenous antibiotics. Culture was positive for methicillin resistant staphylococcus aureus (MRSA). The patient was also treated for chronic obstructive pulmonary disease (COPD) exacerbation that developed on the third day. He has a history of glaucoma, a condition that is currently treated with drops.

A.   Dx: Cellulitis due to MRSA, COPD, glaucoma _____

B.   Proc: Intravenous infusion of antibiotics _____

Case 11.4

Patient presents to the ER with shortness of breath and chest pain. Diagnostic work-up in the ER was positive for congestive heart failure (CHF) with atrial fibrillation, and she required admission, where she was treated with IV medication. Patient has known coronary artery disease of the native vessels with stable angina that requires long-term use of aspirin.

A.   Dx: CHF with atrial fibrillation, CAD with stable angina. Long-term aspirin use. _____

Case 11.5

Patient is 39 weeks pregnant with no complications. She presented to the hospital in active labor. She delivered a single liveborn baby boy after 10 hours of labor. Her delivery was a spontaneous vaginal delivery with required episiotomy. *Remember that you are coding for the patient, who is the mother, rather than for the infant.*

A.   Dx: Normal delivery of single liveborn male _____

B.   Proc: Spontaneous delivery with episiotomy _____

Case 11.6

Patient is a single newborn male delivered via cesarean section. He initially had feeding problems that resolved prior to discharge. Circumcision was performed the day he went home.

A.   Dx: Newborn male, feeding problems _____

B.   Proc: Circumcision _____

Case 11.7

The patient has had left knee pain for years. The pain is now severe and requires a total knee replacement due to her osteoarthritis. Her current comorbidities of seizure disorder and mild mental retardation are monitored during this hospitalization. She underwent total knee replacement successfully. After surgery she developed acute blood loss anemia that was treated with packed blood cell transfusion.

A.   Dx: Osteoarthritis on the left knee, seizure disorder, mental retardation, anemia _____

B.   Proc: Total knee replacement, blood transfusion _____

Case 11.8

Patient presented with difficulty breathing. He was diagnosed with acute asthma exacerbation and hypoxemia (pulse oximetry 89%). Treatment with oxygen, intravenous steroids and intravenous antibiotics resolved his asthma exacerbation. Unfortunately this patient had a prolonged hospital stay due to Clostridum difficile enteritis that developed from the therapuetic use of Rocephin.

A.   Dx: Asthma exacerbation, C. Difficile enterocolitis due to antibiotics _____

B.   Proc: Intravenous antibitoics, intravenous steroids _____

Case 11.9

The patient is an 89-year-old women with Alzheimer's dementia, old cerebrovascular accident with hemiplegia of her dominant side, hypertension, and depression. All of these conditions were monitored during her hospitalization. She now presents to the hospital with upper gastrointestinal (GI) bleeding. Esophagogastroduodenoscopy (EGD) with biopsy was done on the second day which was positive for chronic duodenal ulcer. Patient then required BiCap cautery of her ulcer to control the bleeding on the fourth day, because the ulcer had continued to bleed.

A.   Dx: GI bleeding due to duodenal ulcer, Alzheimers dementia, CVA with resultant hemiplegia, hypertension, depression. _____

B.   EGD with biopsy, EGD with control of bleeding. _____

Case 11.10

Patient presented with chest pain. Further evaluation ruled out myocardial infarction (MI). The cause of noncardiac chest pain was due to either gastroesophageal reflux or anxiety.

A.   Dx: Chest pain due to either GE reflux or anxiety _____

Case 11.11

The patient had a syncopal event and presented to the ER via ambulance. EKG was positive for a third-degree heart block. He required dual chamber pacemaker insertion with transvenous lead insertion into the atrium and ventricle.

A.   Dx: Third-degree heart block _____

B.   Proc: Dual chamber pacemaker and transvenous lead insertion _____

Case 11.12

The patient fell out of her wheelchair at the nursing home. She sustained a head injury with loss of consciousness for 2 minutes. Upon evaluation she also complained of headache, blurred vision and pain in her left leg. She was diagnosed with a concussion and non-displaced fracture of the femoral shaft. Her treatment was complicated by her multiple sclerosis. The facture was treated by cast application.

A.   Dx: Cerebral concussion, femur fracture, multiple sclerosis _____

B.   Proc: Casting _____

Case 11.13

Patient presented with numbness in her legs. She is a known diabetic with rheumatoid arthritis. After admission she developed chest pain and EKG was positive for acute myocardial infarction of the anterior wall. After the initial treatment of her MI she was discharged home. She will require further evaluation of her numbness after complete recovery of her MI.

A.   Dx: Diabetic neuropathy versus rheumatoid arthritis, acute MI _____

Case 11.14

Patient came to hospital because of flank pain and hematuria. Cystoscopy with retrograde pyelogram was positive for ureteral calculus and hydronephrosis. Later he underwent cystourethroscopy with basket extraction of ureteral calculus and insertion of indwelling ureteral stent.

A.   Dx: Ureteral calculus with hydronephrosis _____

B.   Proc: Removal of ureteral calculus with stent insertion, cystoscopy with retrograde pyelogram _____

_____

Case 11.15

Patient had his tonsils taken out two days ago. He now presents with postoperative hemorrhage status post tonsillectomy. He required control of his bleeding. Unfortunately he then developed hives from the use of Demerol for pain.

A. Dx: Postoperative tonsillar hemorrhage, hives due to Demerol _____

B. Proc: Control of tonsillar hemorrhage _____

Professional Billing/Outpatient Setting:

CASES 11.16–11.45

Assign ICD-9-CM diagnoses and CPT/HCPCS procedure codes for the following outpatient cases. Cases 11.16 through 11.30 require codes from the Surgery or Medicine sections; Cases 11.31 through 11.45 will be assigned evaluation and management codes.

Case 11.16

This patient had been in Vermont skiing where he fractured his tibial shaft. Closed treatment with manipulation was performed in Vermont to repair the tibia. The patient was so anxious to get back home that he left the day after surgery and returned to his own orthopedist who did all the follow-up care. *Code for the physician providing the follow-up care (aftercare).*

A. Dx: _____

B. Proc.: _____

Case 11.17

Patient had mammography of both breasts performed three days ago. Mammography findings are masses in both breasts. The patient undergoes puncture aspiration of a cyst in each breast in her general surgeon's office under local anesthesia.

A. Dx: _____

B. Proc.: _____

Case 11.18

After observing that a spot on her upper leg had grown bigger, a patient sees her dermatologist. The dermatologist determined that she had a malignant 3.3-cm skin lesion which he biopsied and excised, followed by a simple closure.

A. Dx: _____

B. Proc.: _____

Case 11.19

Patient is suffering from frequent urination, pressure, and pain in the bladder. Upon examination, the physician found dysplasia of the prostate. An incisional biopsy of the prostate was performed under local anesthesia to determine the nature of the dysplasia.

A. Dx: _____

B. Proc.: _____

Case 11.20

Patient has been complaining of a fullness in her right ear and decreased hearing. Upon examination, the physician discovered impacted cerumen. The physician uses suction and forceps to remove the impaction. Patient is instructed to use Dobrox to prevent impaction in the future.

A. Dx: _____

B. Proc.: _____

Case 11.21

An 11-year-old boy presents to the physician office with a foreign body (piece of wood) in his right calf. He was swinging on a tree branch and accidentally hit his leg, lodging a 4-cm piece of wood into his leg. Physician numbed the area locally using 1% Lidocaine, and the foreign body was removed with forceps. Wound did not require any closure. Patient also received a tetanus vaccination. *Assign the diagnosis code including the E code and the CPT codes for the removal and injection.*

A. Dx: _____

B. Proc.: _____

Case 11.22

This patient suffers from painful urination and blood in his urine. The urologist needs to examine both ureters and the bladder. She inserts a scope into the ureter(s) making an incision in the opening of the ureters to the bladder (meatotomy) and completes the examination.

A. Dx: _____

B. Proc.: _____

Case 11.23

After receiving a report of an abnormal Pap smear two weeks ago, the patient presents in the office today for diagnostic colposcopy with biopsy of the cervix to rule out cervical dysplasia.

A. Dx: _____

B. Proc.: _____

Case 11.24

A chemotherapy patient suffering from anemia secondary to treatment presents to her oncologist's office for her routine B12 injection for vitamin B12 deficiency anemia due to chemotherapy for treatment of breast cancer. While she is there, she also has her CBC drawn, which is sent to an outside lab for processing. *Assign the diagnosis(es) codes, CPT codes for the injection, and the HCPCS code for the supply.*

A.   Dx: _____

B.   Proc.: _____

C.   Supply: _____

Case 11.25

Patient has been experiencing recurring sore throats, hoarseness, and cough. Physician performs a diagnostic indirect laryngoscopy in his office to determine the source of the problem.

A.   Dx: _____

B.   Proc.: _____

Case 11.26

The patient is seen by her primary care doctor. She states she has felt flu-like symptoms, jaw pain, and night sweats. The physician is concerned about possible heart attack and performs an EKG with interpretation. She also attaches a pulse oximeter to the patient's finger to measure her oxygen saturation.

A.   Dx: _____

B.   Proc.: _____

Case 11.27

A 12-year-old boy has been complaining of not feeling well, fever, and severe sore throat for two days. Nurse performs a rapid strep test to rule out strep throat. Test comes back positive for strep pharyngitis. *Assign the diagnosis code and the CPT code for the test.*

A.   Dx: _____

B.   Proc.: _____

Case 11.28

The patient sees her internist after a week of gastroenteritis and fever. Patient is noted to be dehydrated, and the physician orders IV fluids and electrolytes. Patient stays at the office for 2 hours for fluid administration. *Assign the diagnosis(es) codes and CPT code for the fluid administration.*

A.   Dx: _____

B.   Proc.: _____

Case 11.29

A 5-year-old girl has been suffering from an angry red rash all over her back and legs throughout the year and is referred to an allergist for allergy testing to differentiate between contact and allergic dermatitis. The allergist orders patch testing of 20 different allergens.

A. Dx: _____

B. Proc.: _____

Case 11.30

A diabetic patient sees her podiatrist for her quarterly foot check and nail trim. Her nails are very thick with onychomycosis. Physician uses a motorized shaver and trimmers to cut all 10 nails. *Assign the diagnosis(es) codes and the CPT code for the trimming.*

A. Dx: _____

B. Proc.: _____

Case 11.31

The patient was seen 4 years ago for atrial fibrillation by his cardiologist. He has been followed by his internist during that period but now presents to the cardiologist again because the atrial fibrillation has not resolved. The internist feels it is a condition that should be followed by the cardiologist. The history was detailed, the exam was comprehensive and the medical decision making was moderate. *Code for the visit with the cardiologist.*

A. Dx: _____

B. E/M: _____

Case 11.32

After being evaluated in the morning by an internist, the patient is sent to the hospital for observation for her unresolved left upper quadrant abdominal pain. The internist re-evaluates the patient again in the hospital observation area that evening and determines that the patient is able to go home and take over the counter medication but must call if her pain increases. *Assign diagnosis(es) codes and E/M code range, providing a rationale for your E/M code range selection.*

A. Dx: _____

B. E/M Range: _____

C. Rationale: _____

Case 11.33

A patient goes to the emergency department with severe back pain. The emergency department physician determines that the patient has an enlarged prostate with urinary frequency. Due to the extremely high level of protein in the patient's urine (that is, proteinuria), the ED physician admits the patient to the hospital. Will the ED physician report an ED code and the initial hospital care code? *Assign diagnosis(es) codes and E/M code(s), providing a rationale for your E/M assignment.*

A. Dx: _____

B. E/M: _____

C. Rationale: _____

Case 11.34

An internist has treated the patient for ongoing shoulder pain for several weeks. The patient's pain is increasing, and he is now unable to move his shoulder or to carry even a cup of coffee without pain. The internist decides to have the problem treated by an orthopedist and sets up the appointment. The orthopedist provides an expanded problem-focused history and exam, with moderate medical decision making. The diagnosis is localized osteoarthritis of the shoulder. The orthopedist wants to report 99204 because he spent approximately 40 minutes with this patient. The coder states that 99202 is the appropriate codes. Who is correct and why? *Assign diagnosis(es) codes and E/M code(s), providing a rationale for your E/M assignment.*

A. Dx: _____

B. E/M: _____

C. Rationale: _____

Case 11.35

A patient sees her internist because of back pain. Based on the physician's examination, blood work and a CT scan are ordered, and the patient is asked to return one week later for another evaluation. The total time for the return visit is 60 minutes, no history is documented, the exam is problem focused and the medical decision making is high. The physician tells the patient that the scan revealed a small abdominal aortic aneurysm. The patient is very upset, and the physician spends 40 minutes discussing the findings and options with the patient. *Code for the return visit.*

A. Dx: _____

B. E/M: _____

Case 11.36

Using the scenario in Case 11.35, code for the return visit if no key components were provided.

A. Dx: _____

B. E/M: _____

Case 11.37

An elderly patient with congestive heart failure has been in a nursing facility for 3 months. During the last month the physician received two phone calls from the facility's nursing staff to have care orders changed. The physician's documentation indicated 10 minutes were spent providing these services. *Explain your reason for your answer.*

A. Dx: _____

B. E/M: _____

C. Rationale: _____

Case 11.38

A 15-year-old patient comes in for her annual physical. During the exam she discusses her concerns about her family history of breast cancer. After the examination, the physician discusses the potential risk factors and the steps that can be taken to ease the patient's anxiety. The total visit time was 40 minutes, and 15 minutes were spent in discussion.

A. Dx: _____

B. E/M: _____

Case 11.39

An 8-year-old falls and injures his lower left leg on a protruding tree stump in a neighbor's yard. His parents take him to the hospital emergency department, where the ED physician reviews the child's history, noting how long ago the injury occurred, the location and depth of the injury, and other potential health risks based on a review of the patient's respiratory and musculoskeletal systems. The history and exam are expanded problem focused and the medical decision making is moderate due to the depth of the injury and the potential for infection.

A.   Dx: _____

B.   E/M: _____

Case 11.40

A patient has been evaluated for several months by his family physician related to the patient's difficulties with walking and bradykinesis. The family physician cannot determine a specific cause for the problems and refers the patient to a neurologist for an opinion on the problem. The neurologist questions the patient regarding the progress of the symptoms, examines the patient, and does a series of tests. The neurologist's diagnosis is Parkinson's disease, and she prescribes medication to the patient and documents her findings in a letter to the family physician. She also sets up a follow-up appointment for 3 months to evaluate the patient's response to the medication. *Assign the diagnosis(es) codes, select the E/M code range, and state whether the visit with the neurologist is a consultation or a new patient visit.*

A.   Dx: _____

B.   E/M Range: _____

C.   Rationale: _____

Case 11.41

An elderly patient developed arteriosclerotic dementia after a right lower extremity arterial bypass procedure. The patient was discharged from the hospital and admitted to a nursing facility by the same physician. The nursing facility care was needed to deal with both the dementia and generalized muscle weakness. The physician provided a comprehensive history, a comprehensive examination, and low medical decision making. *Code for the nursing facility services, and decide whether the physician would report a hospital discharge code.*

A.   Dx: _____

B.   E/M: _____

C.   Rationale: _____

Case 11.42

The patient was seen by an endocrinologist for three years due to her type II uncontrolled diabetes. She is being seen today by a nephrologist in the same practice because she has developed nephrosis caused by the diabetes. The patient has never seen the nephrologist before but was treated by the endocrinologist three months ago. *Code the diagnosis(es) and state the range of E/M codes from which the nephrologist will assign a code.*

A.   Dx: _____

B.   E/M Code Range.: _____

Case 11.43

A retired nurse has been suffering with right lower quadrant abdominal pain and is diagnosed with a fibroid tumor on the right ovary. The pathology report indicates that the tumor is benign and her physician recommends surgery. The patient is not convinced that she needs surgery, and she makes an appointment with a gynecologist she has not seen before for a second opinion. *Will the gynecologist report a new patient code or a consultation code?*

A. Dx: _____

B. E/M: _____

C. Rationale: _____

Case 11.44

A 22-month-old child falls from a ledge and lands face down. His breathing is impaired, and he develops respiratory distress. He is rushed to his pediatrician's office because it is closer than the emergency department, and the pediatrician provides critical care to restore the child's breathing back to normal. *Will the pediatrician report the 99291-99292 series of codes or the pediatric critical care codes 99293-99294? Explain your answer.*

A. Dx: _____

B. E/M Code Range: _____

C. Rationale: _____

Case 11.45

A patient is seen by the office nurse for painful urination (dysuria). The patient was examined one week ago by the physician and was asked to bring in a urine sample the following week. The nurse questions the patient regarding any changes in the patient's symptoms and packages the specimen.

A. Dx: _____

B. E/M: _____

Combined Facility/Professional Billing/Inpatient Setting:

CASES 11.46 -11.55

First assign ICD-9-CM diagnoses codes and facility procedure codes for the entire hospitalization documented in the following inpatient cases. Include the present on admission indicator for each diagnosis. Include E codes in the diagnoses code assignments if appropriate.

Next, assign ICD-9-CM diagnoses codes followed by CPT procedure codes for the physician's services. Note that often the correct diagnosis code is the same for both facility and professional billing. Be alert, however, for differences such as the assignment of E codes in the facility setting and possible or probable conditions.

Case 11.46

After a prolonged latent phase of labor and attempt to deliver vaginally, the patient agrees to a cesarean section delivery. She had previously delivered her first child by cesarean and had hoped for a vaginal delivery with her second child. Because of the prolonged latent phase, the obstetrician asks that the baby's pediatrician attend the delivery. She delivered a full-term healthy baby boy via low cervical cesarean section.

Hospitalization

A.   Dx: _____

B.   Proc.: _____

Pediatrician's services

C.   Dx: _____

D.   E/M.: _____

Case 11.47

A 4-day-old newborn, born by cesarean section, is in the neonatal intensive care unit (NICU) and is being followed by the NICU attending for her continued tachypnea and jaundice. She has been placed on continued positive airway pressure (CPAP) in order to control the tachypnea. She was evaluated by the attending for 45 minutes in the morning, and he returned again for 15 minutes in the afternoon.

Hospitalization

A.   Dx: _____

B.   Proc.: _____

Pediatrician's services

C.   Dx: _____

D.   E/M: _____

Case 11.48

A long-term Type I diabetic patient has been hospitalized due to the complication of ketoacidosis. He was admitted 2 days ago and is now being seen in follow-up by his physician on the third day. No interval history was documented, but the physician did check the patient's heart, lungs, and extremities for an expanded problem-focused examination and ordered blood work to monitor the diabetes and ketoacidosis. The medical decision making was low. *Code for the hospitalization and the physician follow-up visit.*

Hospitalization

A.   Dx: _____

Physician's services

B.   Dx: _____

C.   E/M: _____

Case 11.49

A patient was admitted to the hospital with a history of bloody diarrhea for 2 days. The admitting physician evaluated the patient and requested that a gastroenterologist see the patient for an opinion on what is causing the problem. As a result of her discussion with the patient, the gastroenterologist obtained an extended history of the present illness, an extended system review and a complete past, family and social history, and documented a detailed history. Her examination of the patient was detailed and the resulting medical decision making was moderate. The diagnosis is acute diverticulitis with hemorrhage. A colonoscopy with biopsy confirmed the diagnosis.

Hospitalization

A. Dx: _____

B. Proc.: _____

Gastroenterologist's services

C. Dx: _____

D. E/M: _____

Case 11.50

Upon admitting a patient to the hospital for severe chest pain, the physician was able to determine that the patient did not have a myocardial infarction. Tests were done and the patient was evaluated by her physician. The results of the tests and the evaluation indicated reflux esophagitis. The admission documentation showed a detailed history, a comprehensive examination, and moderate medical decision making. The attending physician documented the diagnosis of chest pain due to reflux esophagitis

Hospitalization

A. Dx: _____

Physician's services on the day of admission

B. Dx: _____

C. E/M: _____

Case 11.51

After a month of ignoring the bulge in his left abdomen, a patient is seen by his family doctor and admitted to the hospital. Because of the patient's complex personal history of multiple sclerosis, chronic obstructive pulmonary disease, old CVA with residual neurogenic dysphagia, and coronary artery disease, and family history of colon cancer, a surgeon is asked to evaluate the patient and determine if surgery is possible. The surgeon provides a comprehensive history, a comprehensive examination, and high medical decision making. The surgeon's diagnosis is incarcerated left inguinal hernia. The patient then undergoes an indirect hernia repair.

Hospitalization

A. Dx: _____

B. Proc.: _____

Surgeon's visit

C. Dx: _____

D. E/M: _____

Case 11.52

A patient is scheduled for a laparascopically assisted vaginal hysterectomy (LAVH), and the hospital pathologist has been asked to standby for immediate frozen section availability if there is any concern as to whether or not the leiomyoma are cancerous. The surgery took 2 hours; the pathologist was on standby for 40 minutes. The final pathology report and the attending physician confirmed the diagnosis of endometriosis of the uterus.

Hospitalization

A. Dx: _____

B. Proc.: _____

Pathologist's standby services

C. Dx: _____

D. E/M: _____

Case 11.53

After a transurethral resection of the prostate (TURP) was performed for carcinoma of the prostate. The day after surgery, the patient developed acute postoperative respiratory failure and became critically ill. The patient was placed in the intensive care unit (ICU) for recovery. The hospital intensivist treated the patient and restored his respiratory function. This physician also discussed the patient's history and prognosis with the family. The time spent in critical care was 50 minutes; the physician spent 15 minutes documenting the critical care services and 15 minutes with the family.

Hospitalization

A. Dx: _____

B. Proc.: _____

Intensivist's services

C. Dx: _____

D. E/M.: _____

Surgeon's diagnosis code(s)

E. Dx: _____

Case 11.54

A patient is admitted to the hospital by an orthopedic surgeon for an open reduction with internal fixation (ORIF) of a bimalleolar fracture. The patient sustained the fracture when he fell off his rollerblades at home. The surgery is performed and the patient remains in the hospital for three days and is discharged. Each day the patient was seen by the surgeon and evaluated; on the day of discharge the surgeon sees the patient and handles the discharge care.

Hospitalization

A. Dx: _____

B. Proc.: _____

Surgeon's services

C. Dx: _____

D. Services provided after the surgery and on the day of discharge/rationale: _____

_____

Case 11.55

A patient is admitted to the hospital for severe chest pain and shortness of breath. It is determined that the patient suffered an acute non-ST elevation myocardial infarction. In addition to the detailed history, detailed examination, and high complexity medical decision making, the physician spends 20 minutes talking with the patient's family regarding his condition. The physician wants to report the admission code and a prolonged care code. After admission, the patient developed atrial fibrillation. This was treated along with the patient's chronic hypertension and Type II diabetes mellitus. The patient had a history of pneumonia 6 months ago.

Hospitalization

A. Dx: _____

Physician's services

B. Dx: _____

C. E/M: _____

Combined Facility/Professional Billing/Outpatient Setting:
CASES 11.56–11.70

Assign ICD-9-CM diagnoses and CPT/HCPCS codes for the following outpatient cases. Cases 11.56 through 11.60 are outpatient clinic cases. Assign the ICD-9-CM diagnoses and CPT/HCPCS codes that apply to both the physician and the facility for these cases.

Cases 11.61 through 11.70 are emergency department cases. Assign the ICD-9-CM diagnosis (including E codes as appropriate for the facility side) for both the physician(s) and the hospital. Assign the E/M code for the ED physician based on current CPT coding guidelines. The hospital E/M codes are provided for you, as these are specific to each facility. *Do not code for other hospital services provided in the ED, such as radiology procedures.*

Case 11.56

A patient with asthma has increased shortness of breath and undergoes a diagnostic bronchoscopy.

A. Dx: _____

B. Proc.: _____

Case 11.57

Patient has been experiencing gastroesophageal reflux. The physician does an endoscopic diagnostic evaluation of the patient's esophagus and stomach. The scope does not go beyond the cardia of the stomach.

A. Dx: _____

B. Proc.: _____

Case 11.58

A 12-year-old boy with chronic adenotonsilitis for the past 16 months is seen today at the ASC. He is scheduled for T&A under general anesthesia. The physician used a laser to excise both the tonsils and adenoids and to control bleeding.

A.   Dx: _____

B.   Proc.: _____

Case 11.59

The lacrimal sac of the left eye has an abscess that must be drained in order for the eye to drain properly. The surgeon makes a small incision directly into the lacrimal sac, and the pressure caused by the abscess is relieved as the area drains. The incision is sutured closed.

A.   Dx: _____

B.   Proc.: _____

Case 11.60

Years of chronic maxillary sinusitis had created a severe blockage of the maxillary sinus cavity on the both sides, discovered on CT exam. A sinus endoscopy was performed to remove tissue from the maxillary sinuses.

A.   Dx: _____

B.   Proc.: _____

Case 11.61

A female patient burned her left upper leg when she spilled boiling water accidentally at home. She sustained a 2nd degree burn that was treated with burn dressings. An expanded problem-focused history and physical examination was completed by the ED physician. Decision making was low. *Remember that the hospital ED E/M codes are provided in Cases 11.61 through 11.70, because they are hospital-specific. These codes are not necessarily the same as the physician's E/M code you assign.*

Hospital Codes

A.   Dx: _____

B.   E/M: 99283-25

ED Physician Codes

C.   Dx: _____

D.   E/M: _____

Case 11.62

The patient presented to the ER after the police found him on the front lawn at the college. He was diagnosed with alcohol intoxication. The ED physician documented an expanded problem-focused history, detailed examination, and medical decision of low complexity.

Hospital Codes

A.   Dx: _____

B.   E/M: 99283

ED Physician Codes

C.   Dx: _____

D.   E/M: _____

Case 11.63

The patient is a 3-year-old boy who got something in his eye while he was playing at home. Examination revealed a foreign body in the superficial conjunctiva of the right eye. The ED physician removed the foreign body without incision. A problem-focused history and exam was documented along with decision making that was straightforward.

Hospital Codes

A.   Dx: _____

B.   E/M: 99281-25

ED Physician Codes

C.   Dx: _____

D.   E/M: _____

Case 11.64

The patient was a passenger in a car that collided with another vehicle at a stop sign. She presented with neck pain and single view of the cervical spine x-ray was negative for fracture. The ED physician documented an expanded problem-focused history and physical, and decision making was low for this patient with a cervical sprain.

Hospital Codes

A.   Dx: _____

B.   E/M: 99283-25

ED Physician Codes

C.   Dx: _____

D.   E/M: _____

Case 11.65

The patient crushed his finger when a brick fell accidentally while he was at work on a construction site. X-ray of the hand (2 views) revealed a closed nondisplaced distal phalanx fracture of the left ring finger. The ED physician documented an expanded problem-focused history and physical, and decision making that was low, and she placed a finger splint (static).

Hospital Codes

A.   Dx: _____

B.   E/M: 99282-25

ED Physician Codes

C.   Dx: _____

D.   E/M: _____

Case 11.66

The patient presented in threatened labor at 34 weeks. Limited fetal ultrasound of her uterus was normal. The ED physician documented false labor and the patient returned home. ED physician documented a detailed history and examination with moderate medical decision making.

Hospital Codes

A.   Dx: _____

B.   E/M: 99284

ED Physician Codes

C.   Dx: _____

D.   E/M: _____

Case 11.67

Patient presented with a bloody nose that would not stop bleeding. She has known hypertension and blood pressure was elevated. The ED physician completed an anterior nasal packing on the left. Documentation by the ED physician included a detailed history, an expanded problem-focused exam, and moderate decision making.

Hospital Codes

A.   Dx: _____

B.   E/M: 99283-25

ED Physician Codes

C.   Dx: _____

D.   E/M: _____

Case 11.68

Patient presented with hemoptysis. He has known COPD and he is a smoker. Further evaluation by AP and lateral view chest x-ray was negative. He was very ill and required admission to the hospital. The ED physician documented a detailed examination, a detailed physical, and decision making of moderate complexity, as well as the diagnosis of hemoptysis, rule out pneumonia.

Hospital Codes: None–patient was admitted

ED Physician Codes

A. Dx: _____

B. E/M: _____

Case 11.69

The patient presented to the ED with headaches. CT of the brain without contrast was negative. Her headaches were due to migraines as documented by the ED physician. An intramuscular injection of 15 mg Toradol was administered prior to leaving the ED. Documentation included a detailed history and physical with moderate decision making.

Hospital Codes

A. Dx: _____

B. E/M: 99284-25

ED Physician Codes

C. Dx: _____

D. E/M: _____

Case 11.70

The patient is an 89-year-old who presented with abdominal pain, nausea and vomiting. He had not eaten much in the past two days. The physician documented the diagnoses of viral gastroenteritis with dehydration. Patient was treated with intravenous infusion of 1000 cc of normal saline over 100 minutes. The ED physician documented an expanded problem-focused history, a detailed examination, and moderate decision making.

Hospital Codes

A. Dx: _____

B. E/M: 99284-25

ED Physician Codes

C. Dx: _____

D. E/M: _____

A

abnormal finding Out of normal range; often refers to a finding based on a laboratory or radiology test.

abuse Action that improperly uses another person's resources.

acute Illness or condition with severe symptoms and short duration; can also refer to a sudden exacerbation of a chronic condition.

addenda Updates to the ICD-9-CM diagnostic coding system.

add-on code CPT code preceded by + that is always performed along with another primary procedure and that is reported with the primary code.

administration Means or method by which a drug or chemical is introduced into the body.

admitting physician Physician who orders the patient to be admitted to the hospital.

advance beneficiary notice (ABN) Medicare form used to inform a patient that a service, item, or supply is not likely to be reimbursed by the Medicare program.

AHA Coding Clinic® for ICD-9-CM Quarterly publication of the American Hospital Association (AHA) that offers coding advice, guidelines, and practical information and that gives correct code assignments for new diseases and technologies.

AHIMA *See American Health Information Management Association.*

Alphabetic Index ICD-9-CM section that contains an index of the disease descriptions in the Tabular List, an index of drugs and chemicals that cause poisoning in table format, and an index of external causes of injury, such as accidents; officially Volume 2, but often appears first in the ICD-9-CM book.

Alphabetic Index to Diseases and Injuries A main section of the ICD-9-CM Alphabetic Index that contains main terms used to classify diseases.

Alphabetic Index to External Causes of Disease and Injury A section of the ICD-9-CM Alphabetic Index that includes terms that identify causes and circumstances of injuries, poisonings, and adverse effects.

Alphabetic Index and Tabular List of Procedures (Volume 3) The HIPAA-mandated inpatient procedure code set.

ambulatory Able to be treated as an outpatient; not bedridden.

Ambulatory Payment Classifications (APC) Prospective payment system used by Medicare for reimbursement of hospital outpatient services.

ambulatory surgery Services provided on an outpatient basis.

American Academy of Professional Coders (AAPC) National association that fosters the establishment and maintenance of professional, ethical, educational, and certification standards for medical coding.

American Health Information Management Association (AHIMA) National association of health information management professionals that promotes valid, accessible, yet confidential health information.

American Hospital Association (AHA) National organization that represents all types of hospitals, health care networks, and their patients and communities; advocates for members in national health policy development, legislative and regulatory debates, and judicial matters.

American Medical Association (AMA) Member organization for physicians that aims to promote the art and science of medicine, improve public health, and promote ethical, educational, and clinical standards for the medical profession; maintains the CPT code set.

American Society of Anesthesiologists Professional organization of anesthesiologists that publishes the annual *Relative Value Guide.*

analgesia Absence of pain by use of a medication or agent without loss of consciousness.

analgesic Medication or agent that reduces pain or inhibits the ability to feel pain without loss of consciousness.

analyte A chemical or substance being measured or analyzed.

ancillary services Services provided by a laboratory, radiology facility, pharmacy, pathology facility, physical therapy facility, or speech therapy facility.

anesthesia The loss of the ability to feel pain caused by the administration of a drug or other medical intervention; partial or complete loss of sensation with or without loss of consciousness.

anesthesia modifiers HCPCS Level II modifiers that identify the provider of anesthesia services.

anesthesiologist Physician who specializes in providing anesthesia and pain management services.

anesthesiology Practice of medicine dealing with providing anesthesia and maintaining respiratory and cardiac functions and pain relief during surgical procedures.

anesthetist Critical care nurse with additional training in anesthesiology; also known as CRNA (certified registered nurse anesthetist).

anteroposterior From front to back.

assay To test drug purity or the drug's ability to be absorbed by the body.

attending physician Physician responsible for patient care during hospitalization.

authorization (1) Document signed by a patient to permit release of particular medical information under stated specific conditions. (2) A health plan's system of approving payment of benefits for services that satisfy the plan's requirements for coverage.

automated Performed using a machine or computer (such as an automated lab test).

B

biofeedback Treatment modality in which people are trained to improve their current state of health by recognizing signals from their own bodies.

braces ICD-9-CM punctuation mark used to enclose a series of terms, each of which is modified by the statement to the right of the brace. The terms to both the left and the right of the brace must be present in order to assign the code.

brachytherapy Internal radiation therapy that involves inserting a radioactive substance into the patient via tubes, wires, seeds, needles, or other small containers.

brackets ICD-9-CM punctuation mark used to enclose synonyms or explanatory notes.

bundle Use of a single procedure code to cover a group of related procedures.

bundled code A single procedure code that covers a group of related procedures.

C

capitation Payment method in which a prepayment covers the provider's services to a plan member for a specified period of time.

cardiac catheterization Procedure that involves passing a catheter into the heart through a vein or artery to withdraw samples of blood, measure pressures in the heart's chambers or great vessels, and inject contrast media.

carryover line Line indented six character spaces from the term above to denote a continuation of the line in the ICD-9-CM indexes.

category (1) In ICD-9-CM, a three-digit code used to represent a disease or injury or a two-digit code used to represent a procedure. (2) Methodology used by CPT to classify the sections of E/M services.

Category I codes Procedure codes found in the main body of CPT (Evaluation and Management, Anesthesia, Surgery, Pathology and Laboratory, Radiology, and Medicine).

Category II codes Optional or supplemental CPT codes that track performance measures for a medical goal such as reducing tobacco use.

Category III codes Temporary CPT codes for emerging technology, services, and procedures that are used instead of unlisted codes when available.

catheterization Introduction of a catheter into a vein, artery, or vessel. Catheters are thin tubes that allow drainage or injection of fluids or access by surgical instruments.

causal condition The medical illness that brought on the documented condition.

CCI column 1/column 2 code pair edit Medicare code edit under which CPT codes in column 2 will not be paid if reported for the same patient on the same day of service by the same provider as the column 1 code.

CCI modifier indicator Number that shows whether the use of a modifier can bypass a CCI edit.

CCI mutually exclusive code (MEC) edit CCI edit for codes for services that could not have reasonably been done during a single patient encounter, so both will not be paid by Medicare. Only the lower-paid code is reimbursed.

Centers for Disease Control (CDC) Federal agency in the Department of Health and Human Services (HHS) that administers national programs for the prevention and control of communicable and vector-borne diseases and for implementing programs for dealing with environmental health problems.

Centers for Medicare and Medicaid Services (CMS) (formerly HCFA) Federal agency in the Department of Health and Human Services (HHS) that runs Medicare, Medicaid, clinical laboratories (under the CLIA program), and other government health programs. CMS promotes health care services and delivery for its beneficiaries and maintains payment processes that pay claims for covered medically necessary services only, at correct payment amounts, and in a timely manner.

certificate of medical necessity (CMN) Signed certificate from a physician to a supplier of medical equipment that contains information about medical necessity.

certification Process of earning a credential through a combination of education and experience followed by successful performance on a national certification exam. Certified individuals must maintain their credentials by meeting annual continuing education requirements.

chapter A section of the ICD-9-CM Tabular List that covers diseases and injuries to a specific body system.

chapter-specific guidelines Section 1C of the *ICD-9-CM Official Guidelines for Coding and Reporting,* which provides detailed instructions for coding conditions and situations that are specific to certain ICD-9-CM chapters.

charge capture Administrative procedures that ensure that billable services are recorded and reported for payment.

charge description master (CDM) or charge master In a facility, a computerized list of all billable services, procedures, devices, medications, and supplies that can be provided to inpatients and outpatients.

chief complaint (CC) Patient's description of the symptoms or other reasons for seeking medical care.

chronic Of long duration (referring to an illness or condition).

CLIA-waived test Simple laboratory test often performed in a physician office that does not require CLIA certification to conduct; the provider must comply with the test manufacturers' exact instructions.

Clinical Laboratory Improvement Amendments (CLIA) 1988 federal law establishing standards for laboratory testing performed in hospital-based facilities, physician office laboratories, and other locations; administered by CMS.

closed procedure Surgery that does not involve making an incision and surgically opening the site of an injury or area in need of repair or treatment.

CMS-1500 (08/05) Medicare-mandated paper billing form for physician services.

CMS-1491 Claim form used to submit ambulance charges to Medicare.

CMS HCPCS Workgroup Federal government committee that maintains the Level II HCPCS code set.

code first notes ICD-9-CM instructional notations directing the coder to list particular disease codes before other codes.

code first underlying disease ICD-9-CM instructional notation directing the coder to code both the cause and the manifestation of the disease, coding the manifestation second.

code range Numerical code sequence list with a beginning and end point; the coder must evaluate each code in the sequence before selecting the most appropriate one.

code set Alphabetic and/or numeric representations for data. Medical code sets are systems of medical terms that are required for HIPAA transactions. Administrative (nonmedical) code sets, such as taxonomy codes and ZIP codes, are also used in HIPAA transactions.

coding Process of assigning codes to diagnoses and procedures or services.

coexisting condition Additional illness that either has an effect on the patient's primary illness or is also treated during the encounter.

colon ICD-9-CM punctuation mark placed after an incomplete term that needs one or more of the modifiers that follow in order to be assigned.

combination code Single ICD-9-CM code that classifies both the etiology and the manifestation of an illness or injury.

comorbidity Admitted patient's coexisting condition that affects the length of the hospital stay or the course of treatment.

comorbidity/complication (CC) A condition in addition to the basic diagnosis that is likely to cause a longer hospitalization period.

comparative or contrasting condition Usually two separate conditions that may or may not be related to one another.

complete blood count (CBC) The most common blood test, which includes white blood cell (WBC) count, red blood cell (RBC) count, hemoglobin, hematocrit, and platelet count.

complete lab test The entire procedure for a lab test, including ordering the procedure or test, obtaining the sample or specimen, handling the specimen, performing the procedure or test, and analyzing and interpreting the results.

complete procedure Procedure in which one physician provides the supervision and interpretation and also performs the actual procedure.

compliance Actions that satisfy official guidelines and requirements.

compliance plan Written plan created by a health care provider or health care plan for the following: the appointment of a compliance officer and committee; a code of conduct for physicians' business arrangements and employees' compliance; training plans; properly prepared and updated coding tools such as job reference aids, encounter forms, and documentation templates; rules for prompt identification and refunding of overpayments; and ongoing monitoring and auditing of claim preparation.

complication Condition a patient develops after hospital admission that affects the recovery and discharge period.

computer assisted coding (CAC) Use of a product that examines documents electronically and suggests codes for the medical coder to validate.

computerized axial tomography scan (CT or CAT scan) Type of radiographic imaging that can produce cross-sectional views and three-dimensional images of soft tissues such as the internal organs as well as other parts of the body.

conscious sedation (CS) Sedative and/or analgesic injected to relieve patient anxiety and control pain during a diagnostic or therapeutic procedure while not putting the patient to sleep.

consultation Service performed by a physician to advise a requesting physician about a patient's condition and care; the consultant does not assume responsibility for the patient's care and must send a written report back to the requestor.

consulting physician Physician who provides a consultation.

continuous positive airway pressure (CPAP) Use of air pressure to push the tongue forward and open the throat to prevent sleep apnea.

contraindication Something (such as a symptom or condition) that makes a particular treatment or procedure inadvisable.

contrast material (media) In imaging, a substance that helps provide a clearer image. It can be administered, or introduced, with an injection, rectally, or orally.

contributory components The last four E/M components: counseling, coordination of care, nature of the presenting problem, and time.

convention Typographic techniques or standard practices that provide visual guidelines for understanding printed material, specifically, all punctuation, symbols, abbreviations, instructions and cross-references applicable to ICD-9-CM coding.

cooperating parties Committee of representatives from NCHS, CMS, AHIMA, and AHA that maintains the ICD-9-CM coding system.

coordination of care The component of a physician's work that involves coordinating a patient's care with other providers or agencies.

Correct Coding Initiative (CCI) Medicare's official listing of each CPT code and what services are bundled or considered an inherent part of another service.

counseling Physician's discussion with a patient and/or family about diagnostic results, risks and benefits of management options, instructions for management, importance of compliance, and patient and family education.

covered entity (CE) Under HIPAA, a health plan, clearinghouse, or provider that transmits any health information in electronic form in connection with a HIPAA transaction; does not specifically include workers' compensation programs, property and casualty programs, or disability insurance programs.

CPT modifier Characters that may be appended to a CPT code to show that the base code is in some way different from the code descriptor.

critical care Medical care provided to a patient who is critically ill or critically injured. Both the illness or injury and the care must meet the definition of critical in order for services to be reported as critical care services.

cross-references Directions in printed material that tell a coder where to find additional information.

crosswalk A comparison connecting two sets of items, such as a list of deleted codes and the current correct codes that replace them.

Current Dental Terminology (CDT) HIPAA-mandated code set for procedures performed in a dental office.

Current Procedural Terminology (CPT) HIPAA-mandated procedural code set developed and maintained by the American Medical Association.

D

decubitus Lying down (refers to sores that result from long periods of lying down).

definitive diagnosis The actual medical condition rather than its signs or symptoms.

de-identified health information Medical data from which individual identifiers have been removed.

descriptor Narrative part of a CPT code that identifies the procedure or service.

diagnosis code Number assigned to a diagnosis in ICD-9-CM.

diagnosis-related group (DRG) Medicare payment category for inpatients.

diagnostic procedure Procedure performed to confirm a physician's working diagnosis or to assist in determining a course of treatment, but not specifically to treat the problem.

direct care In-person, face-to-face care.

discharge summary a progress note of a patient's condition upon discharge including disposition or arrangements (such as returning home, died, or moving to another facility).

disposition The place or circumstance of patient discharge.

DME Medicare Administrative Contractors (DME MACs) DME suppliers that have contracts with Medicare. Each DME MAC covers a specific geographical region of the country and is responsible for processing durable medical equipment and prosthetic and orthotic supplies claims.

documentation Systematic, logical, and consistent recording of a patient's health status—history, examinations, tests, results of treatments, and observations—in chronological order in a patient medical record.

dosimetry Process of determining the amount of radiation needed during treatment.

durable medical equipment (DME) Equipment that is primarily and customarily used to serve a medical purpose, can withstand repeated use, and is appropriate for use in the home.

durable medical equipment, prosthetic and orthotic supplies (DMEPOS) DMEPOS dealers provide patients with durable medical equipment and supplies.

Durable Medical Equipment Regional Carriers (DMERCs) Medicare contractors that process claims for durable medical equipment, prosthetics, orthotics, and supplies.

E

echocardiography Ultrasound procedure used to examine the cardiac chambers and valves, the great vessels, and the pericardium.

E code Alphanumeric ICD-9-CM code for an external cause of injury or poisoning.

edits Computer processes that review submitted information against certain criteria.

837I HIPAA-mandated electronic format for claims for institutional (facility) services.

837P HIPAA-mandated electronic format for claims for professional services.

electrocardiogram (ECG or EKG) Test that records the electrical activity of the heart.

electronic health record or electronic medical record (EHR or EMR) Collection of health information that is immediately electronically accessible by authorized users.

E/M components Seven factors—history, examination, medical decision making, counseling, coordination of care, nature of the presenting problem, and time—used in the selection of the level of service.

encoder Computer software that assists coders in assigning medical codes.

encounter Visit of a patient and a medical professional.

encounter form Form that contains a provider's most frequent or major services. Also called a superbill, the services are checked off after a patient's encounter, and the form is used as a receipt and in billing.

endoscope Viewing instrument made up of hundreds of tiny light-transmitting glass fibers bundled tightly together with a camera on the end that is inserted into a joint, a natural orifice, or an artificially created puncture site to guide surgery without large incisions.

enteral Via the intestine (such as in the administration of substances).

eponym Name or phrase formed from or based on a person's name; usually describes a condition or procedure associated with that person.

established patient Patient who has received a professional service from the physician or another physician of the same specialty in the same group within three years.

ethics Standards of conduct based on moral principles.

etiology Cause or origin of a disease.

evaluation and management (E/M) The part of a physician's work that includes assessing the nature of a patient's condition and devising a plan to treat it.

examination Face-to-face inspection and investigation by a physician for the purpose of diagnosis and management.

excludes ICD-9-CM coding convention that lists terms that are excluded or are to be coded elsewhere.

F

face sheet Cover sheet of a facility's medical record that contains patient identification data.

face-to-face time Direct time a physician spends with a patient obtaining history, examining the patient, and discussing plans.

facility Health care institution.

facility modifier CPT modifier used in coding hospital outpatient services and procedures.

family history Medical events in a patient's family.

Federal Register Official publication for federal government rules, proposed rules, and notices.

fee-for-service Method of charging in which a provider's payment is based on each service performed.

fee schedule List of charges for services performed.

first-listed diagnosis ICD-9-CM code reported first, which represents the reason for the outpatient visit.

fluoroscopy Imaging technique that uses a continuous low-level X-ray beam to view the body in motion.

Food and Drug Administration (FDA) Federal agency that protects against public health hazards by ensuring the safety and in most cases the quality and effectiveness of products and services.

fraud Intentional deceptive act to obtain a benefit.

freestanding facility Hospital-owned medical center that provides outpatient services.

frontal Facing forward.

G

general anesthesia Anesthesia that renders the patient unconscious, pain-free, and pharmacologically paralyzed for the entire surgical procedure. Constant attendance of anesthesia personnel and monitoring are required.

global period Specific time period assigned by a payer to a CPT code that groups payment for any services provided to a patient relative to the surgical procedure performed. Time frames range from ten to ninety days surrounding a procedure.

global surgery days Global period surrounding surgery during which a single fee is paid for all related services furnished by the surgeon before, during, and after the procedure.

grouper Software used to assign DRGs based on inpatients' diagnoses and procedures during hospitalization.

H

HCFA *See Centers for Medicare and Medicaid Services.*

HCPCS Level I CPT codes used to report physician services.

HCPCS Level II Coding system for identifying medical services and supplies for government payers.

HCPCS modifiers Modifiers required on claims for government payers such as Medicare.

health care claim Electronic transaction or a paper document filed with a health plan to receive benefits.

Healthcare Common Procedure Coding System (HCPCS) Two-level coding system comprising CPT procedure codes and the HCPCS supply code set.

health information management (HIM) Hospital department that organizes and maintains patient medical records; also profession devoted to managing, analyzing, and utilizing data vital for patient care and making the data accessible to health care providers.

Health Insurance Portability and Accountability Act (HIPAA) of 1996 Federal act that sets forth guidelines for standardizing the electronic data interchange of administrative and financial transactions, exposing fraud and abuse in government programs, and protecting the security and privacy of health information.

health plan Under HIPAA, an individual or group plan that either provides or pays for the cost of medical care; group health plan, health insurance issuer, health maintenance organization, Medicare, Medicaid, TRICARE, and other government and nongovernment plan.

hemodialysis Dialysis in which blood is circulated through an artificial kidney machine to be cleaned.

HIPAA Electronic Health Care Transactions and Code Sets (TCS) HIPAA rule governing the electronic exchange of health information.

HIPAA Privacy Rule Law that regulates the use and disclosure of patients' protected health information (PHI).

HIPAA Security Rule Law that requires covered entities to establish administrative, physical, and technical safeguards to protect the confidentiality, integrity, and availability of health information.

history Subjective information about illness and symptoms provided by a patient to a physician.

history codes ICD-9-CM V codes that represent past conditions or status affecting medical care.

history of present illness Documentation of a patient's response to a physician's questions about the patient's chief complaint.

hospital-based facility Health care outpatient facility owned by a hospital.

hospital-based outpatient services Services provided by a hospital in which the patient is not formally admitted (such as in an emergency room, an ambulatory surgery center, or for outpatient testing).

Hospital Outpatient Prospective Payment System (HOPPS) *See Outpatient Prospective Payment System.*

hybrid record Medical record that is made up of both electronic and paper documents.

I

ICD-9-CM *See International Classification of Diseases, Ninth Revision, Clinical Modification.*

ICD-9-CM Alphabetic Index to Disease and Injuries (Volume 2) Official title of Volume 2 of ICD-9-CM.

ICD-9-CM Alphabetic Index and Tabular List of Procedures (Volume 3) Official title of Volume 3 of ICD-9-CM.

ICD-9-CM Coordination and Maintenance Committee Federal group that considers and adopts changes to the ICD-9-CM code set.

ICD-9-CM Official Guidelines for Coding and Reporting Written by NCHS and CMS and approved by the cooperating parties, it provides rules for selecting and sequencing diagnosis codes in both the inpatient and the outpatient environments.

ICD-9-CM Tabular List of Disease and Injuries (Volume 1) Official title of Volume 1 of ICD-9-CM.

ICD-10-CM International Classification of Diseases, Tenth Revision, Clinical Modification.

ill-defined condition Medical condition that is vague and is often described by a sign or symptom.

immunotherapy Process by which an allergic patient can become desensitized to antigens that trigger allergic responses.

impending Medical condition that is considered as threatened at the time of discharge.

incidental procedure Related procedure that is performed with a more complex primary procedure at an operative session and that would not usually be reported alone.

includes ICD-9-CM coding convention that further defines or gives examples of terms that are included in a code or code section.

informed consent Process by which a patient authorizes medical treatment after discussion with a physician about the nature, indications, benefits, and risks of a recommended treatment.

inhalant (INH) Substance introduced or administered into the body by inhaling it through the nose or mouth.

injection (INJ) Introduction or administration of a substance into the body via a needle.

inpatient Person admitted to a medical facility for services that require an overnight stay.

Inpatient Prospective Payment System (IPPS) Medicare payment system for hospitals and other inpatient facilities.

integral In diagnosis coding, a symptom that is part of the process of an underlying disease.

International Classification of Diseases Adapted for Indexing of Hospital Records and Operation Classification (ICDA) Diagnosis classification system used before ICD-9-CM.

International Classification of Diseases, Ninth Revision, Clinical Modification

(ICD-9-CM) HIPAA-mandated standardized code set for diseases and injuries developed by the World Health Organization and modified for use in the United States.

interventional radiology Radiology subspecialty that uses CT, ultrasound, and fluoroscopy to guide procedures such as percutaneous stent placement, biopsy, and catheterization.

intra-arterial or intra-arterially (IA) Administered directly into an artery.

intramuscular (IM) Administered directly into the muscle.

intrathecal (IT) Administered directly into the spinal canal.

intravenous (IV) Administered directly into a vein.

J

The Joint Commission Formerly called the Joint Commission on Accreditation of Healthcare Organizations (JCAHO), an organization that reviews hospitals, other organizations and programs for accreditation".

K

key components The essential parts of an E/M service, including history, examination, and medical decision making.

L

late effect Condition that remains after an acute illness or injury has completed its course.

lateral At the side (the view of a body part being examined).

level of service (LOS) One of four types of E/M services provided by a physician: problem-focused (PF), expanded problem-focused (EPF), detailed (DET), or comprehensive (COMP).

Level I Current Procedural Terminology (CPT), one of the two main parts of the HCPCS code set.

Level II Coding system that covers products, supplies, and services not included in the CPT codes; one of the two main parts of the HCPCS code set.

LCD *See local coverage determination.*

local anesthesia Anesthesia administered by injection, topical anesthesia, or spray to a very specific body area.

local coverage determination (LCD) Notice sent to providers with detailed and updated information about the coding and medical necessity of a specific Medicare service.

lozenge ICD-9-CM symbol denoting a code unique to ICD-9-CM and not part of ICD-9.

M

magnetic resonance imaging (MRI) Type of imaging that uses radio frequency waves and a strong magnetic field rather than X-rays to provide detailed pictures of internal organs and tissues.

main term Word in boldface type that denotes a disease, injury, or condition in the ICD-9-CM Alphabetic Index.

major CC (MCC) Secondary diagnosis classified by the IPPS as severe when assigning the DRG.

mammography Low-dose X-ray system for the examination of breasts.

mandatory multiple coding Single condition that must be represented by two or more codes.

manifestation Characteristic sign or symptom of a disease.

manual Without the use of machines (such as performing a laboratory test and analyzing the specimen without the use of a machine).

medical coder Medical office staff member with specialized training who handles the diagnostic and procedural coding of medical records.

medical coding Process of assigning diagnosis and procedure codes to patients' records in medical documentation.

medical decision making (MDM) Complex process that a physician uses to establish a diagnosis and determine how to treat or manage the condition.

medical insurance Financial plan that covers the cost of hospital and medical care.

medically unlikely edits (MUEs) CMS unit-of-service edits that check for clerical or software-based coding or billing errors, such as anatomically related mistakes.

medical necessity Payment criterion that requires medical treatments to be appropriate and to be provided in accordance with generally accepted standards of medical practice. To be medically necessary, the reported procedure or service must match the diagnosis, be provided at the appropriate level, not be elective, not be experimental, and not be performed for the convenience of the patient or the patient's family.

medical observation Medical services for hospital outpatients that provide close monitoring before potential admission.

medical standards of care State-specified performance measures for the delivery of health care by medical professionals.

Medicare Carrier Manual (MCM) Manual on coverage of and payment for services reported with HCPCS codes.

Medicare-Severity DRG (MS-DRG) Medicare Inpatient Prospective Payment System revision that takes into account whether certain conditions were present on admission.

minimum necessary standard Principle that individually identifiable health information should be disclosed only to the extent needed to support the purpose of the disclosure.

modality Method, technique, or protocol used to treat or diagnose a disease or injury.

modifier Character that is appended to a code to report special circumstances involved with a procedure or service.

monitored anesthesia care (MAC) Heavy IV sedation administered by a CRNA or MD that is deeper than conscious IV sedation.

morbidity Rate of incidence of disease.

mortality Death rate.

N

National Center for Health Statistics (NCHS) Division of the Centers for Disease Control that tracks health care statistics and participates as a member of the cooperating parties.

national coverage determination (NCD) Policy stating whether and under what circumstances a service is covered by the Medicare program.

negligence Failure to perform duties according to the state-required standard of care.

Neoplasm Table Table in the ICD-9-CM Alphabetic Index that points to codes for neoplasms, referring to anatomical location and behavior.

new patient Patient who has not received a professional service from the physician or another physician of the same specialty in the same group within a three-year period.

1995 Documentation Guidelines Code selection guidelines developed by the AMA and the Health Care Financing Administration (HCFA, now CMS) to make E/M codes more consistent.

1997 Documentation Guidelines Refinement of 1995 Documentation Guidelines for single-specialty and multisystem exams.

nonoutpatient Inpatient.

nonscheduled admission admission to a hospital without prior arrangements (as from the ED).

not elsewhere classified (NEC) ICD-9-CM abbreviation indicating the code to be used when an illness or condition cannot be placed in any other category.

notes Explanations located throughout all volumes of ICD-9-CM to define terms or to provide coding instructions.

Notice of Exclusions from Medicare Benefits (NEMB) CMS form—given by a participating provider to a Medicare patient before providing a noncovered service—that provides written notification that Medicare will not pay and estimates the charge for which the patient will be responsible.

not otherwise specified (NOS) ICD-9-CM abbreviation indicating the code to be used when no information is available for assigning a more specific code; unspecified.

nuclear medicine Branch of medicine that uses radioactive elements for either diagnostic imaging or radiopharmacological treatment.

O

oblique Slanted (view of object being X-rayed).

observation Monitoring in a hospital to see if the patient will need to be admitted or will require further treatment.

observation unit Hospital unit set up to treat patients on an outpatient basis. Typically, patients stay in this special unit for monitoring for eight to forty-eight hours.

Office for Civil Rights (OCR) Federal agency that enforces the HIPAA Privacy Act.

Office of the Inspector General (OIG) Federal agency that investigates and prosecutes fraud against government health care programs such as Medicare.

omit code Instruction in the ICD-9-CM Alphabetic Index to Procedures instructing the coder to not report an incision performed for completion of additional surgery.

open procedure Procedure that involves making an incision and surgically opening the body at the site of the injury or ailment.

OPPS APC status indicators Letters assigned to each CPT/HCPCS code identifying the payment rules established by the

Centers for Medicare and Medicaid Services (CMS) for that code.

other (OTH) routes Suppository or catheter injections aside from routine methods of administration.

outpatient (OP) Patient who receives health care in a medical setting without admission.

outpatient code editor (OCE) Medicare computer program that checks claims from the outpatient departments of hospitals and other facilities.

outpatient procedure Services for patients who are not formally admitted, which are usually provided in a specialty unit (such as a cardiac catheterization lab or physical therapy).

Outpatient Prospective Payment System (OPPS) System used by Medicare to pay providers for services to patients who are not admitted.

P

panel Group of lab tests commonly performed together.

parenteral Administered into the body other than through the digestive tract.

parentheses ICD-9-CM punctuation mark used to enclose supplemental words or nonessential modifiers. The absence or presence of terms in parentheses does not affect code assignment.

past history Patient's personal medical history.

patient's reason for visit Patient's stated purpose for an encounter, which is used to provide the equivalent of a principal diagnosis in the outpatient setting.

payer Health plan or program.

payment-for-performance (P4P) Health plan financial incentives program to encourage providers to follow recommended care management protocols.

peritoneal dialysis Dialysis that uses a filtration process in which fluid is placed into the peritoneal cavity through a catheter and is cycled or drained several times a day, cleaning the blood inside the body rather than in a machine.

permanent codes Type of HCPCS codes maintained by the CMS HCPCS Workgroup that are available for use and change only if a majority of Workgroup members agree.

physical status modifier Code used in the Anesthesia Section of CPT with procedure codes to indicate the patient's health status.

place of service (POS) code HIPAA administrative code that indicates where medical services were provided.

POA exempt from reporting Conditions that do not require a POA (present on admission) indicator.

port Site where the treatment beam will enter the skin and focus on a malignant area.

positron emission tomography (PET) Type of imaging that produces high-energy three-dimensional computer-reconstructed images of the metabolic function of an organ such as thyroid, liver, spleen, bone, cardiovascular, or kidney.

posteroanterior From back to front.

postoperative observation Special services that provide close monitoring of surgical patients in a designated unit.

postoperative period Period after surgery during which visits relating to the surgery are reimbursed (generally ten days for minor procedures and ninety days for major surgery).

presenting problem Reason for the patient's encounter with a physician, such as an injury or illness.

present on admission (POA) Indicator required by Medicare that identifies whether a coded condition was present at the time of hospital admission.

preventive medicine Medical services such as annual physicals that aim to prevent disease and/or detect problems early.

primary procedure The most comprehensive, complex, and resource-intensive procedure, which according to the ICD-9-CM *Official Guidelines* is listed first, before any other procedures.

principal diagnosis Condition established after study to be chiefly responsible for occasioning the admission of the patient to the hospital for care.

problem-oriented Relating to an encounter in which the patient has a condition, symptom, or diagnosis that will be evaluated or treated during the visit.

procedure code Code that identifies medical treatment or diagnostic services.

professional (1) Person trained (and often certified or licensed) to practice medicine or work in other areas of health care. (2) Appropriate to the standards of a profession.

professional component (PC) The part of a charge that represents the physician's time and skill in performing the procedure.

professional service Face-to-face service (used for E/M coding).

protected health information (PHI) Individually identifiable health information that is transmitted or maintained by electronic media.

provider Person or entity that supplies medical or health services and bills for or is paid for the services in the normal course of business. A provider may be a professional member of the health care team, such as a physician, or a facility, such as a hospital or skilled nursing home.

Q

qualifying circumstance Anesthesia services provided under particularly difficult circumstances such as extraordinary condition of the patient, notable operative conditions, and/or unusual risk factors.

query Written communication with a physician asking for clarification of documentation to support code assignment.

R

radiation oncology Subspecialty of radiology that utilizes high-energy ionizing radiation to treat malignant neoplasms and certain nonmalignant conditions.

radiology Subspecialty of medicine that concentrates on medical imaging to prevent, diagnose, and treat diseases and injuries.

radiology report Written report signed by the interpreting physician that accompanies all diagnostic or therapeutic radiological services.

radiotherapy Treatment of disease by radiation and/or X-ray.

real-time Immediate imaging results.

red blood cell (RBC) count Blood test for the number of red blood cells.

referral Transfer of a patient's care from one physician to another for either a specific diagnosis or for total care.

referring physician Physician who refers the patient to another physician for treatment.

regional anesthesia Numbing of a region or part of the body without inducing unconsciousness.

Relative Value Guide Annual publication of the American Society of Anesthesiologists that lists anesthesia guidelines, modifiers, and common procedures performed by anesthesiologists and elements used in calculating anesthesia fees.

release of information (ROI) Transmission of a patient's information.

residual condition Condition that remains after the acute phase of an illness or injury has terminated.

resource-based relative value system (RBRVS) System of Medicare reimbursement that sets physicians' fees for providing care to Medicare patients based on the physician's work, overhead, and the cost of malpractice insurance.

revenue cycle Process of providing services, billing, collecting payments, and using the funds for the cost of operations.

review of systems Physician's review of the major functions of the body's systems in the examination of a patient.

roll-up rule Payment concept that directs how to code an office visit that turns into hospital observation for a patient. The office care is coded together with the observation care, thereby being "rolled-up" into one set of codes.

S

S&I *See supervision and interpretation.*

scheduled admission admission to a hospital of a patient for whom prior arrangements were made.

screening procedure Procedure performed to detect a disease or condition in the absence of signs and symptoms.

secondary diagnosis Diagnosis that is reported in addition to a principal diagnosis; must meet the UHDDS guidelines.

secondary diagnosis code Code that is listed after the principal diagnosis; also called "additional diagnosis code" or "other diagnosis code."

secondary procedure Procedure that is less extensive or resource-intensive and is listed in addition to the primary procedure.

section guidelines Notes and coding instructions that appear at the beginning of each of the six sections of Category I codes in CPT.

section mark In ICD-9-CM, a punctuation mark located to the left of the code to signify a footnote.

semicolon In ICD-9-CM, punctuation used to identify and divide the common portion and the unique portion of the code.

separate procedure Status of some CPT codes indicating that the procedure can be billed only if it was performed alone, for a specific purpose, and independent of any other related service provided; the procedure is usually part of another procedure and not separately reported.

sequence Put in order; the order in which multiple diagnoses or procedure codes are listed on health care claims.

sequenced Ordering the codes reported.

sign Objective indication that can be evaluated by the physician, such as weight loss.

significant procedure Incision, excision, repair, manipulation, amputation, endoscopy, destruction, suturing, or introductions.

single proton emission computerized tomography (SPECT) Type of diagnostic imaging that provides three-dimensional computer-reconstructed images of an organ.

social history Patient's age, employment, marital status, and other factors relating to social environment as documented during the physician's examination.

special report Documentation that meets the payer's requirement to describe the nature, extent, need for the procedure, time involved, effort, and equipment necessary.

specificity Use of additional ICD-9-CM digits to provide more detail.

specimen Tissue submitted for individual examination and pathologic diagnosis.

spirometry Pulmonary function test that measures volume of air in the lungs by measuring how much air is expelled from the lung and how quickly.

standby Category of physician service meaning at the ready, referring to a physician who is asked by another physician to wait in case special services are needed, such as an obstetrician asking a pediatrician to stand by in the case of a difficult delivery.

Statistical Analysis Durable Medical Equipment Regional Carriers (SADMERC) CMS contractors who provide assistance in determining which HCPCS codes describe DMEPOS items for Medicare billing purposes.

subcategory In ICD-9-CM, a four-digit code.

subclassification In ICD-9-CM, a five-digit code.

subcutaneous (SC) Beneath the skin.

subterm Term indented under a main term in the ICD-9-CM Alphabetic Index that modifies the disease, condition, or procedure.

supervision and interpretation (S&I) Physician's work in supervising a technician who is performing a procedure and in preparing a report based on the findings.

supplemental classification system Group of codes used to classify events or circumstances; they identify factors influencing health status and contact with health services (V codes) or external causes of injury and poisoning (E codes).

surgery modifier Modifier that can be appended to a surgical procedure code only, not to an E/M code; includes HCPCS Level II anatomic modifiers.

surgical package Services routinely carried out in conjunction with a surgical procedure, including one pre-op office visit after the decision for surgery is made, infiltration of anesthesia, the actual surgical procedure, writing orders, and typical postoperative follow-up care.

symptom Subjective statement by the patient that cannot be confirmed during an examination, such as pain.

T

Table of Drugs (and Chemicals) Reference listing of drugs and chemicals in the ICD-9-CM Alphabetic Index.

Tabular List Section of ICD-9-CM in which diagnosis codes are presented in numerical order; officially called Volume 1.

technical component (TC) The part of the charge associated with a procedure code that reflects the technician's work and the equipment and supplies used in performing it; in contrast to the *professional component*.

temporary codes HCPCS codes that can be added, changed, or deleted on a quarterly basis. Once established and approved, temporary codes are usually implemented within ninety days.

therapeutic procedure Surgical treatment or correction of a confirmed disease, condition, or injury.

therapeutic services Restorative procedures to repair or cure a disease or condition.

threatened Likely to occur.

time Length of time a physician spends with a patient; one of the contributory E/M components.

time (tm) units Intervals of anesthesia time, ranging from ten to twenty minutes, used to calculate anesthesia reimbursement.

transitional pass-through payments Temporary payments (in addition to the APC payment) made for certain medical devices, drugs, and biologicals provided exclusively to Medicare patients.

treatment, payment, and health care operations (TPO) Under HIPAA, patients' protected health information may be shared without authorization for the purposes of treatment, payment, and operations.

treatment plan The documented steps of patient care and treatment.

U

UB-04 (CMS-1450) Paper billing form completed for hospital services.

UHDDS *See Uniform Hospital Discharge Data Set.*

ultrasound Imaging technique that uses ultra-high-frequency sound waves for diagnostic scanning.

unbundle To take apart and report codes that are included in a bundled code.

unbundling Breaking apart an "all-inclusive" or "comprehensive package" into its component parts or less-extensive individual services.

uncertain diagnosis Conditions documented as possible, probable, suspected, or rule out.

unclassified HCPCS code Code assigned to services or items without a specific Level II HCPCS code or CPT code until a new code can be implemented.

Uniform Hospital Discharge Data Set (UHDDS) Uniform set of data definitions applied to inpatient health care settings; the minimum data set collected on each inpatient.

unit/floortime Care provided to the patient in a facility setting (such as a hospital or nursing home), including bedside care and services, reviewing the patient's medical record, writing orders, and reviewing films or test results.

unlisted code CPT code located in each section and subsection that ends in 9 and is used when a code does not completely describe the service provided.

unscheduled outpatient visit Visit in which the facility is not expecting the patient, such as an emergency room encounter.

unspecified Incompletely described condition that must be coded with an unspecified ICD code.

upcoding Use of a procedure code that provides a higher payment than the code for the service actually provided.

usual fee Charge for a physician's particular services that is billed to most patients most of the time under typical conditions.

use additional code In ICD-9-CM, an instruction to assign an additional code providing more information, if known.

V

various routes/variously, into joint, cavity tissue, or topical (VAR) Indication that various routes are available and used for a drug, such as intra-articularly or into cavities, or topical application.

V code Alphanumeric code in ICD-9-CM that identifies factors that influence health status and encounters that are not due to illness or injury.

visit Seeing a health care provider or obtaining health care services in person.

W

white blood cell (WBC) count Blood test that counts the number of white blood cells.

World Health Organization (WHO) United Nations agency concerned with global health issues; publishes revisions of the International Classification of Diseases.

Abbreviations/Acronyms

AAMA American Association of Medical Assistants

AAPC American Academy of Professional Coders

ab antibody

ABN advanced beneficiary notice

a.c. before meals

adm admitted

ag antigen

AHA American Hospital Association

AHDI Association for Healthcare Documentation Integrity

AHIMA American Health Information Management Association

AHQR Agency for Health Care Research and Quality

AI alphabetic index (ICD-9-CM)

AKA above-knee amputation

AMA American Medical Association

AMI acute myocardial infarction

AMT American Medical Technologists

Anes anesthesia

ANSI American National Standards Institute

AOA American Osteopathic Association

AP anterior-posterior

APC ambulatory patient classification

APR DRG All Patient Refined Diagnosis Related Group System

APRN advanced practice registered nurse

A/R accounts receivable

ASA American Society of Anesthesiologists

ASC ambulatory surgical center

ASU ambulatory surgical unit

BCBS Blue Cross and Blue Shield

b.i.d. twice a day

bilat bilateral

bld blood

BLK Lung black lung

BMI body mass index

BP blood pressure

BPH benign prostatic hypertrophy

BUN blood urea nitrogen

BVU basic value unit

bx biopsy

ca cancer

cabg coronary artery bypass graft

CAC computer-assisted coding

CAH critical access hospital

CBC complete blood count

CC (1) physicians' records: chief complaint, (2) hospital documentation: comorbidities and complications

cc cubic centimeter

CCA Certified Coding Associate

CCI Correct Coding Initiative (National; Medicare)

CCS Certified Coding Specialist

CCS-P Certified Coding Specialist: Physician-based

CCYY year, indicates entry of four digits for the century (CC) and year (YY)

CDC Centers for Disease Control

CDM charge description master

CDT Current Dental Terminology

CE covered entity

CHAMPUS Civilian Health and Medical Program of the Uniformed Services, now TRICARE

CHAMPVA Civilian Health and Medical Program of the Department of Veterans Affairs

CHF congestive heart failure

CLIA Clinical Laboratory Improvement Amendment

cm centimeter

CMA Certified Medical Assistant

CMI case mix index

CMN certificate of medical necessity

CMS Centers for Medicare and Medicaid Services

CNS central nervous system

COB coordination of benefits

COBRA Consolidated Omnibus Budget Reconciliation Act of 1985

COMP comprehensive (E/M)

COP conditions of participation

COPD chronic obstructive pulmonary disease

CPAP continuous positive airway pressure

CPC Certified Professional Coder

CPC-H Certified Professional Coder: -Hospital Outpatient Facility

CPE complete physical exam

CPT Current Procedural Terminology

CRCS Civil Service Retirement System

CRNA Certified Registered Nurse Anesthetist

C&S culture and sensitivity

CS conscious sedation

CT computerized axial tomography/computerized tomography

c/v cervical or vaginal

CV cardiovascular

D&C dilation and curettage

DD day, indicates entry of two digits for the day

DEERS Defense Enrollment Eligibility Reporting System

DET detailed (E/M)

DME durable medical equipment

DME MAC durable medical equipment Medicare administrative contractor

DMEPOS durable medical equipment, prosthetic and orthotic supplies

DMERC durable medical equipment regional carrier

DOB date of birth

DOS date of service

dose dosage

DPT diphtheria, pertussis, and tetanus

DRG Diagnosis-Related Group

DRS designated record set

dtap diphtheria, tetanus, acellular pertussis

dx diagnosis

ED emergency department

EDI electronic data interchange

EEG electroencephalogram

EENT eyes, ears, nose, and throat

EFT electronic funds transfer

eia enzyme immunoassay

EIN Employee Identification Number

EKG/ECG electrocardiogram

EMC electronic media claim

E/M code Evaluation and Management code

EMG emergency

EMR/EHR electronic medical (health) record

EMTALA Emergency Medical Treatment and Labor Act of 1986, PL 99-272

ENMT ears, nose, mouth, and throat

ENT ears, nose, and throat

EOB explanation of benefits

EOC episode of care

EOM extraocular muscles

EP established patient

EPSDT Early and Periodic Screening, Diagnosis, and Treatment

ER emergency room

ERISA Employee Retirement Income Security Act of 1974

EPF expanded problem-focused (E/M)

est established

ET tube endotracheal tube

ETOH alcohol

ext external

F female

fac facility

fb foreign body

FDA Food and Drug Administration

FECA Federal Employee Compensation Act

FEHBP Federal Employees Health Benefits Program

FERS Federal Employees Retirement System

FH family history

FI fiscal intermediary

FICA Federal Insurance Contribution Act

FMAP Federal Medicaid Assistance Percentage

FNA fine needle aspiration

FOBT Fecal Occult Blood Test

FQHC federally qualified health center

F/U follow-up

FUO fever, unknown origin

Fx fracture

g, or gm gram

GA general anesthesia

GI gastrointestinal

GPCI geographic practice cost index

gr grain

GTIN Global Trade Item Number

GU genitourinary

GYN gynecologic, gynecologist

h hour

HBA health benefits adviser

HCFA Health Care Financing Administration, currently CMS

HCPCS Healthcare Common Procedure Coding System

HEDIS Health Employer Data and Information Set

HEENT head, eyes, ears, nose, and throat

Hep A/B hepatitis A and B vaccines

HGB hemoglobin

HIM health information management

HINN hospital-issued notice of noncoverage

HHA home health agency

HHS Department of Health and Human Services

HiB hemophilus influenza type B vaccine

HIM health information management

HIPAA Health Insurance Portability and Accountability Act

HMO health maintenance organization

hosp, hsp hospital

H&P history and physical

HPI history of present illness

HS hour of sleep

HTN hypertension

hx history

IA intra-arterial/intra-arterially

ICDA International Classification of Diseases Adapted for Indexing of Hospital Records and Operation Classification

ICD-9-CM International Classification of Diseases, Ninth Revision, Clinical Modification

ICD-10-PCS International Classification of Disease, Tenth Edition, Procedure Coding System

ICU intensive care unit

I&D incision and drainage

ID # identification number

ID, I.D identification

IDTF Independent Diagnostic Testing Facility

IM intramuscular

INFO information

INH inhalant solution

INJ injection

int internal

interv interventional

IOM Institute of Medicine

ip interphalangeal

IP inpatient

IPA individual practice association

IPF inpatient psychiatric facility

IPPS Inpatient Prospective Payment System

ipv inactivated poliovirus vaccine

IRF inpatient rehabilitation facility

IT intrathecal

IV intravenous

JC Joint Commission

kg kilogram

L liter

LCD local coverage determination

LLQ left lower quadrant

LMP last menstrual period

LOS level of service

LPN licensed practical nurse

LUQ left upper quadrant

LVAH laparoscopic vaginal hysterectomy

M male

m meter

MA medical assistant

MAC (1) Medicare Administrative Contractor; (2) monitored anesthesia care

MCC Major complication or comorbidity

mcg microgram

MCM Medicare Carriers Manual

MCO managed care organization

mcp metacarpalphalangeal

MD medical doctor

MDC major diagnostic category

MDH Medicare-dependent, small rural hospital

MDM medical decision making

MEC mutually exclusive code

MedPAC Medicare Payment Advisory Commission

MedPAR Medicare Provider Analysis and Review File

mEq milliequivalent

MFS Medicare Fee Schedule

mg milligram

MGMA Medical Group Management Association

min minute

mL milliliter

mm millimeter

MM month, indicates entry of two digits for the month

MMA Medicare Modernization Act

MMR measles, mumps, and rubella

MRA magnetic resonance angiography

MRI magnetic resonance imaging

MRN Medicare Remittance Notice

MS musculoskeletal

MSA Medicare Savings Account

MS-DRG Medicare-Severity Diagnosis-Related Group

MSN Medicare Summary Notice

MTF Military Treatment Facility

MTS Medicare Transaction System

MUE medically unlikely edits

n.p.o. nothing per os (by mouth)

NB nerve block

NCCI National Correct Coding Initiative

NCD national coverage determination

NCHS National Center for Health Statistics

NCVHS National Committee on Vital and Health Statistics

NCQA National Committee for Quality Assurance

NDC National Drug Codes

NEC not elsewhere classified

NEMB notice of exclusion from Medicare benefits

neuro neurologic, neurological

NIST National Institute for Standards and Technology

NKDA no known drug allergies

NO number

nonPAR nonparticipating

NOS not otherwise specified

NP (1) new patient, (2) nurse-practitioner

NPI National Provider Identifier

NPP Notice of Privacy Practices

NUCC National Uniform Claim Committee

OB obstetrics

OCE outpatient code editor

OCR Office for Civil Rights

OIG Office of the Inspector General

OMB Office of Management and Budget

op operative

OP outpatient

OPPS Outpatient Prospective Payment System

opt optional

OR operating room

OSHA Occupational Safety and Health Administration

OTH other routes (of administration)

OV office visit

OWCP Office of Workers' Compensation Programs

OZ Product product number, Health Care Uniform Code Council

P&A percussion and auscultation

PA physician's assistant

PACU postanesthesia care unit

pat patient

p.c. after meals

PC professional component

PCM Primary Care Manager (TRICARE)

PCP primary care physician/provider

PE physical exam

PECOS Provider Enrollment Chain and Ownership System

ped pediatric

PET positron emission tomography

PF problem-focused (E/M)

P4P pay-for-performance

PH # phone number

PHI protected health information

PIN provider identifier number

PM pain management

PMH past medical history

PMPM per member per month

p.o. per os (by mouth)

po postoperative

POA present on admission

POS place of service

PPD purified protein derivative of tuberculin test

PPO preferred provider organization

PPS prospective payment system

PQRI physician quality reporting initiative

premal premalignant

prev preventive

p.r.n. as desired or as needed

proc procedure

PSA prostate- specific antigen

PSO provider-sponsored organization

psych psychiatric

psytx psychotherapy

pt patient

pt physical therapy

q. every

q.d. every day

q.h. every hour

q.i.d. four times a day

q.o.d. every other day

QIO quality improvement organization

q.2h. every two hours

QUAL. qualifier

quant quantitative

RA remittance advice

RBC red blood cell

RBRVS Resource-Based Relative Value Scale (Medicare)

REF reference

Resp respiratory

RHIA Registered Health Information Manager

RHIT Registered Health Information Technologist

RLQ right lower quadrant

RMA Registered Medical Assistant

RN registered nurse

R/O rule out

ROI (1) release of information; (2) return on investment

ROS review of systems

RTC return to clinic

RUG Resource Utilization Group

RUQ right upper quadrant

RVS relative value scale

RVU relative value unit

Rx prescription

SC subcutaneous

SCHIP State Children's Health Insurance Program

SADMERC Statistical Analysis Durable Medical Equipment Regional Carrier

SDA same-day appointment

SDI state disability insurance

sed sedimentation

SH social history

S&I supervision and interpretation

SNF skilled nursing facility

SOAP Subjective/Objective/Assessment/Plan

SOB shortness of breath

SOF signature on file

S/P status post

SPECT single proton emission computerized tomography

SSDI Social Security Disability Insurance

SSI Supplemental Security Income

SSN Social Security number

stat, STAT immediately

STD sexually transmitted diseases

TAH total abdominal hysterectomy

T&A tonsillectomy and adenoidectomy

TANF Temporary Assistance for Needy Families

TC technical component

TCS (HIPAA Electronic) Transaction and Code Sets

temp temperature

t.i.d. three times a day

TL tabular list (ICD-9-CM)

TM tympanic membrane

TM time

TPA third-party claims administrator

TPO treatment, payment, and operations

TPR temperature, pulse, and respirations

UA urinalysis

UC urine culture

UCR usual, customary, and reasonable

UHDDS Uniform Hospital Discharge Data Set

unilat unilateral

UPC Universal Product Code

UPIN Unique Physician Identification Number

URI upper respiratory infection

USIN Unique Supplier Identification Number

UTI urinary tract infection

vac, vacc vaccine

VAR various

VD venereal disease

VIS vaccine information sheet

VP Vendor Product Number

VS vital signs

wbc white blood cells

WBC white blood cell count

WHO World Health Organization

wt weight

yo year old

YY year, indicates entry of two digits for the year; may also be noted as CCYY, which allows for entry of four digits for the century (CC) and year (YY)

Appendix A Place of Service Codes

Codes designated as F are facility codes; those with NF are nonfacility physician practice codes. The rate calculations for nonfacility locations take into account the higher overhead expenses such as the cost of clinical staff, supplies, and equipment, collectively called practice expense, generally borne by providers in these settings. The facility rates paid to providers usually are lower because the hospital/facility is reimbursed separately for overhead costs associated with patient care.

Code	Definition	Use
01	pharmacy	NF
03	school	NF
04	homeless shelter	NF
05	Indian Health Service freestanding facility	
06	Indian Health Service provider-based facility	
07	Tribal 638 freestanding facility	
08	Tribal 638 provider-based facility	
09	prison/correctional facility	NF
11	office	NF
12	home	NF
13	assisted living facility	NF
14	group home	NF
15	mobile unit	NF
20	urgent care facility	NF
21	inpatient hospital	F
22	outpatient hospital	F
23	emergency room, hospital	F
24	ambulatory surgical center	F, or NF for payable procedures not on ASC list
25	birthing center	NF
26	military treatment facility	F
31	skilled nursing facility	F
32	nursing facility	NF
33	custodial care facility	NF
34	hospice	F
41	ambulance, land	F
42	ambulance, air or water	F
49	independent clinic	NF
50	federally qualified health center	NF
51	inpatient psychiatric facility	F
52	psychiatric facility, partial hospitalization	F

(Continued)

Code	Definition	Use
53	community mental health center	F
54	intermediate care facility/mentally retarded	NF
55	residential substance abuse treatment facility	NF
56	psychiatric residential treatment center	F
57	nonresidential substance abuse treatment facility	NF
60	mass immunization center	NF
61	comprehensive inpatient rehabilitation facility	F
62	comprehensive outpatient rehabilitation facility	NF
65	end-stage renal disease treatment facility	NF
71	state or local public health clinic	NF
72	rural health clinic	NF
81	independent laboratory	NF
99	other place of service	NF

Appendix B Professional Resources

Government Sites and Resources

CCI

The Medicare Correct Coding Initiative automated edits are online at
cms.hhs.gov/NationalCorrectCodInitEd/

CMS

Coverage of the Centers for Medicare and Medicaid Services: Medicare,
Medicaid, SCHIP, HIPAA, CLIA topics
www.cms.hhs.gov
Medicare Learning Network: cms.hhs.gov/mlngeninfo
Online Medicare manuals: cms.hhs.gov/manuals/IOM
Medicare Physician Fee Schedule: cms.hhs.gov/FeeScheduleGenInfo
Conditions of Participation: cms.hhs.gov/CFCsandCOPs

HCPCS

General information on HCPCS
www.cms.hhs.gov/MedHCPCSGenInfo
Annual alphanumeric Healthcare Common Procedure Coding System file
www.cms.hhs.gov/HCPCSReleaseCodeSets
SADMERC
www.palmettogba.com

HIPAA

Home page
www.cms.hhs.gov/hipaageninfo
Questions and Answers on HIPAA Privacy Policies
answers.hhs.gov
HIPAA Privacy Rule
"Standards for Privacy of Individually Identifiable Health Information; Final
Rule." 45 CFR Parts 160 and 164. *Federal Register 65,* no. 250 (2000).
www.hhs.gov/ocr/hipaa/finalreg.html

ICD

NCHS (National Center for Health Statistics) posts the ICD-9-CM addenda
and guidelines
www.cdc.gov/nchs/datawh/ftpserv/ftpicd9/ftpicd9.htm#guidelines

WHO The International Statistical Classification of Diseases and Related Health
Problems, tenth revision. is posted on the World Health Organization site
www.who.int/whosis/icd10/

ICD-9-CM addenda
www.cms.hhs.gov/ICD9ProviderDiagnosticCodes
ICD-9-CM Official Guidelines for Coding and Reporting
www.cdc.gov/nchs/datawh/ftpserv/ftpicd9/ftpicd9.htm

NUBC

The National Uniform Billing Committee develops and maintains a standardized data set for use by institutional providers to transmit claim and encounter information. This group is in charge of the 837I and the CMS-1450 (UB 04)
claim formats.
www.nubc.org

NUCC

The National Uniform Claim Committee develops and maintains a standardized data set for use by the non-institutional health care community to transmit claim and encounter information. This group is in charge of the 837P and the CMS-1500 claim formats.
www.nucc.org

OCR

The Office of Civil Rights of the HHS enforces the HIPAA Privacy Rule; Privacy Fact Sheets are online at
www.hhs.gov/ocr/hipaa

OIG

The Office of Inspector General of the HHA home page links to fraud and abuse, advisory opinions, exclusion list, and other topics
www.oig.hhs.gov
Model compliance programs are found at
oig.hhs.gov/fraud/complianceguidance.html

TRICARE AND CHAMPVA

General TRICARE information
www.tricare.osd.mil
CHAMPVA Overview
www.military.com/benefits/veterans-health-care/champva-overview

WPC

Washington Publishing Company is the link for HIPAA Transaction and Code Sets implementation guides. It also assists several organizations in the maintenance and distribution of HIPAA-related code lists that are external to the X12 family of standards:

- Provider Taxonomy Codes
- Claim Adjustment Reason Codes
- Claim Status Codes
- Claim Status Category Codes
- Health Care Services Decision Reason Codes
- Insurance Business Process Application Error Codes
- Remittance Remark Codes

www.wpc-edi.com

Electronic Medical Records

AHIMA Coverage of Related Topics Located under HIM resources under the Practice Brief tab on the AHIMA Home Page
www.ahima.org

Maintaining a Legally Sound Health Record
The Legal Process and Electronic Health Records
Implementing Electronic Signatures
HIM Practice Transformation/EHR's Impact on HIM Functions
Core Data Sets for the Physician Practice Electronic Health Record

Computer-based Patient Record Institute (CPRI)
www.cpri.org

Medical Record Institute
www.medrecinst.com

Associations

AAFP American Academy of Family Physicians
www.aafp.org

AAHAM American Association of Healthcare Administrative Management
www.aaham.org

AAMA American Association of Medical Assistants
www.aama-ntl.org

AHDI Association for Healthcare Documentation Integrity
www.aamt.org

AAPC American Academy of Professional Coders
www.aapc.com

ACA International (formerly American Collectors Association)
www.acainternational.org

AHIP America's Health Plans
Links to Member Health Plans
ww.ahip.org

ACHE American College of Healthcare Executives
www.ache.org

AHIMA American Health Information Management Association
www.ahima.org

AMB Association of Medical Billers
www.ambanet.net/AMBA.htm

AHLA American Health Lawyers Association
www.healthlawyers.org

AHA American Hospital Association
www.aha.org

AMA American Medical Association
www.ama-assn.org

AMT American Medical Technologists
www.amt1.com

ANA American Nursing Association
www.ana.org

HBMA Healthcare Billing and Management Association
www.hbma.com

HFMA Healthcare Financial Management Association
www.hfma.org

MGMA Medical Group Management Association
www.mgma.org

PAHCOM Professional Association of Health Care Office Management
www.pahcom.com

Selected Professional Coding Resources

Note that many commercial vendors of the annual coding books offer package prices for the year's CPT, ICD-9-CM, and HCPCS references. Professional organizations may also offer discounts.

American Academy of Professional Coders (AAPC)
309 West 700 South
Salt Lake City, UT 84101
800 626 CODE
www.aapc.com
Certification courses/examinations and coding-related publications

AHA Coding Clinic for ICD-9-CM
AHA Order Services
PO Box 92683
Chicago, IL 60675-2683
800 242 2626
www.ahaonlinestore.com
Official Coding Guidelines for ICD-9-CM

American Association of Health Information Management (AHIMA)
233 North Michigan Avenue, Suite 2150
Chicago, IL 60601-5800
312 233 1100
www.ahima.org
Certification courses/examinations and coding-related publications

AMA Press
PO Box 930884
Atlanta, GA 31193-0884
800 621 8335
www.amapress.com
Annual Editions of CPT, ICD, and HCPCS
www.ama-assn.org/go/CPT
CPT Assistant and CPT Clinical Examples

The Coding Institute
2272 Airport Road South
Naples, FL 34112
800-508-2582
www.codinginstitute.com
Coding resources in medical specialties; seminars

Coding Strategies, Inc.
5401 Dallas Hwy, Suite 606
Powder Springs, GA 30132
877 6 CODING
www.codingstrategies.com
Medical coding education and specialty publications

Conomikes Reports, Inc.
12233 W. Olympic Blvd., Suite 116Los Angeles, California 90064
800 421 6512
www.conomikes.com
Newsletters and handbooks

HCPro
200 Hoods Lane
Marblehead, MA 01945
800 650 6787
www.hcpro.com
Training materials and E-newsletters

Ingenix, Inc.
St. Anthony Publishing/Medicode
2525 Lake Park Blvd.
Salt Lake City, UT 84120
800 INGENIX
www.ingenix.com
Annual editions of ICD-9-CM, CPT, and HCPCS books; newsletters, and electronic reference manuals

MMHSI/Coders Central
800 253 4945
Online resource for coding reference books
www.coderscentral.com

The Medical Management Institute/a Contexo Media Company
P.O. Box 25128
Salt Lake City, Utah 84125-0128
800 334 5724
Annual editions of ICD-9-CM, CPT, and HCPCS books; seminars
CodeItRightOnline®

NCHS
National Center for Health Statistics
3311 Toledo Road
Hyattsville, MD
301 458 4000
ICD-9-CM code set, addenda, and coding guidelines available for downloading
www.cdc.gov/nchs/datawh/ftpserv/ftpicd9/ftpicd9.htm#guidelines

Practice Management Information Corp. (PMIC)
4727 Wilshire Boulevard
Los Angeles, CA 90010
800 MEDSHOP
http://pmiconline.stores.yahoo.net
Annual Editions of CPT, ICD-9-CM, and HCPCS Code Books; publications on prac-
tice management and coding reimbursement.

www.icd9coding.com
Online Web site for ICD and DRG codes

UCG/DecisionHealth
11300 Rockville Pike, Suite 1100
Rockville, MD 20852
301 287-2700
www.decisionhealth.com
Newsletters, especially ICD-9/CPT Coding Pro and Specialty Coders' Pink Sheets;
publications

United States Government Printing Office:
Federal Register
www.access.gpo.gov

Photo Credits

Page ix: © Comstock/PictureQuest; p. 1: © BrandX/Getty; p. 12: © BrandX Pictures/Punchstock; p. 13: Courtesy CDC/Dr. Sherif Zaki; p. 49: © EP046 PhotoDisc/Getty; p. 60: © Vol. 29; PhotoDisc/Getty; p. 66: Courtesy CDC; p. 67: © Corbis RF; p. 84: © Corbis RF; p. 85: © Vol. 29 PhotoDisc/Getty; p. 108: © Vol. 40 PhotoDisc/Getty; p. 109 (left): © IL045 RF/Getty; p. 109 (right): © BrandX/Getty; p. 114: © Stockbyte/Punchstock; p. 120: © Vol. 54 PhotoDisc/Getty; p. 121: © Dynamic Graphics/Jupiter Images; p. 142: © Vol. 59 PhotoDisc/Getty; p. 150: © Vol. 29 PhotoDisc/Getty; p. 151: Courtesy CDC/Dr. Steven Kraus; p. 184: © Vol. 59 PhotoDisc/Getty; p. 186: Courtesy CDC/Dr. Thomas F. Sellers, Emory University; p. 187: Courtesy CDC/Susan Linsley; p. 203: © Stockbyte/Punchstock; p. 447: © BrandX/Getty.